REPERTORY MADE EASY

VOLUME 1

HOMEOPATHIC REPERTORY

Dr. ARUN KUMAR LALL

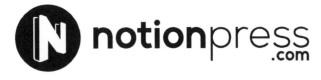

notionpress
.com

INDIA • SINGAPORE • MALAYSIA

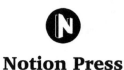

Notion Press

Old No. 38, New No. 6
McNichols Road, Chetpet
Chennai - 600 031

First Published by Notion Press 2018
Copyright © Arun Kumar Lall 2018
All Rights Reserved.

ISBN 978-1-64249-945-2

LIST OF HOMEOPATHIC MEDICINES

List of Homeopathic Medicines	Abbreviation	List of Homeopathic Medicines	Abbreviation
Abelmoschus	Abel.	Agrostemma Githago	Agro.
Abies Canadensis	Abies-c.	Ailanthus	Ail.
Abies Nigra	Abies-n.	Alcohol	Alco.
Abroma Augusta	Abr-a.	Aletris Farinosa	Alet.
Abroma Radix	Abr-r	Alfalfa	Alf.
Abrotanum	Abrot.	Allium Cepa	All-c.
Absinthium	Absin.	Allium Sativum	All-s.
Acalypha Indica	Acal.	Alloxan	Allx.
Acenasia	Acen.	Alnus Rubra	Aln.
Aceticum Acidum	Acet-ac.	Aloe Socotrina	Aloe.
Achyranthes Aspera	Ach.	Alstonia Constricta	Alst.
Aconitum Cammarum	Acon-c.	Alstonia Scholaris	Alst-s.
Aconitum Ferox	Acon-f.	Althaea Officinalis	Alth.
Aconitum Lycotonum	Acon-l.	Alumen	Alumn.
Aconitum Nappellus	Acon.	Alumina Silicata	Alum-s.
Aconitum Neomont	Acon-n.	Alumina	Alum.
Aconitum Radix	Acon-r.	Aluminium Muriaticum	Alum-mu.
Actaea Racemos	Act--r.	Aluminum Metallicum	Alum-m.
Actaea Spicata	Act-sp.	Aluminum Silicata	Alum-sil.
Adonis Vernalis	Ado.	Amalki	Amal.
Adrenalinum	Adren.	Ambra Grisea	Ambr.
Adrenocorticotrophin	Adreno.	Ambrosia Artemisiae Folia	Ambro.
Aegle Folia	Aeg-f.	Ammon.tart.	Ammon.t.
Aegle Marmelos	Aeg-m.	Ammoniacum Gummi	Ammc.
Aesculus Compose	AEsc-c	Ammonium Aceticum	Am-a.
Aesculus Glabra	AEsc-g.	Ammonium Benzoicum	Am-be.
Aesecules Hippocastanum	AEsc.	Ammonium Bromatum	Am-br.
Aethiops Antimonialis	Aethi-a.	Ammonium Carbonicum	Am-c.
Aethiops Merc.	Aethi.	Ammonium Causticum	Am.caust.
Aethusa Cynapium	AEth.	Ammonium Iodatum	Am-i.
Agaricus Emeticus	Agar-em.	Ammonium Muriaticum	Am-m.
Agaricus Muscarius	Agar.	Ammonium Phosphoricum	Am-ph.
Agaricus Phalloides	Agar-ph.	Ammonium Picricum	Am-pi.
Agave Americana	Agav-a.	Ampelopsis Quin.	Amp.
Agave Tequilana	Agav-t.	Amphisboena	Amph.
Agnilgia	Agni.	Amygdalae Amarae Aqua	Amyg.
Agnus Castus	Agn.	Amygdalus Persica	Amyg-p.
Agraphis Nutans	Agra.	Amyl Nitrite	Aml-n.
Agrimonia Eupatoria	Agri.	Amyl Nitrosum	Aml-nit.

List of Homeopathic Medicines	Abbreviation	List of Homeopathic Medicines	Abbreviation
Anacardium Occidentale	Anac-oc.	Argentum Cyanidum	Arg-c.
Anacardium Orientale	Anac.	Argentum Iodatum	Arg-i.
Anagallis Arvensis	Anag.	Argentum Metallicum	Arg-m.
Anantherum Muricatum	Anan.	Argentum Muriaticum	Arg-mur.
Anas Barbariae Hepatis	Anas.	Argentum Nitricum	Arg-n.
Andersonia / Amoora Rohitika	Ander.	Argentum Phos.	Arg-p.
Angelica Archangelica	Angel-Arc.	Aristolochia Clematitis	Aristo-c.
Angelica Atropurpurea	Angel-at.	Aristolochia Milhomens	Aristo-m.
Angophora	Ango.	Aristolochia Serpentaria	Aristo-s
Angustura Vera	Ang.	Arjun/Terminalia Arjuna	Arj.
Anhalonium	Anha.	Armoracea Sativa	Armo.
Anilinum	Anil.	Arnica Montana Radix	Arn-r.
Anisum Stellatum	Anis.	Arnica Montana	Arn.
Anthemis Nobilis	Anth.	Arsenicum Album	Ars.
Anthracinum	Anthr.	Arsenicum Bromatum	Ars-b.
Anthrokokali	Anthro.	Arsenicum Hydrogenisatum	Ars-h.
Anthroxanthum Odoratum	Anthrx.	Arsenicum Iodatum	Ars-i.
Antifebrinum	Antifeb.	Arsenicum Metallicum	Ars-m.
Antimonium Arsenicosum	Ant-a.	Arsenicum Nitricum	Ars-n.
Antimonium Chloridum	Ant-chl.	Arsenicum Sulphuratum Flavum	Ars-s-f.
Antimonium Crudum	Ant-c.	Arsenicum Sulphuratum Rubrum	Ars-s-r.
Antimonium Iodatum	Ant-i.	Artemisia Vulgaris	Art-v.
Antimonium Muriaticum.	Ant-m.	Arum Dracontium	Arum-d.
Antimonium Oxydatum	Ant-ox.	Arum Dracunculus	Arum-dr.
Antimonium Sulph. Auratum	Ant-s.	Arum Italicum	Arum-i.
Antimonium Tartaricum	Ant.t.	Arum Maculatum	Arum-m.
Antipyrinum	Antip.	Arum Triphyllum	Arum-t.
Aphis Chenopodii glauci	Aphis.	Arundo Donax	Arund-d.
Apis Mellifica	Apis.	Arundo Mauritanica	Arund.
Apis Venenum Purum	Apis-v.	Asafoetida	Asaf.
Apium Graveolens	Ap-g.	Asai	Asai.
Apocynum Anderosemifolium	Apoc-a.	Asarum Canadense	Asarum.
Apocynum Cannabinum	Apoc.	Asarum Europaeum	Asar.
Apomorphium	Apom.	Asclepias Cornuti (Syriaca)	Asc-c.
Aqua Marina	Aqua-m.	Asclepias Inc.	Asc-i.
Aqua/Ptychosis	Aqua.	Asclepias Pseudosarsa	Asc-p.
Aquilegia Can.	Aquil.	Asclepias Syriaca	Asc-s.
Aquilegia Vulgaris	Aquil-v.	Asclepias Tuberosa	Asc-t.
Aralia Quinquefolia	Aral-q.	Asimina Triloba	Asim.
Aralia Racemosa	Aral.	Asoka Jonosia	Asoka.
Aranea Diadema	Aran.	Asparagus Officinalis	Aspar.
Aranea Scinencia	Aran-s.	Asperula Od.	Asp.
Aranearum Tela	Aranea.	Aspidosperma	Aspido.
Arbutinum	Arbu.	Astacus Fluviatilis	Astac.
Arbutus Andrachne	Arbut.	Asterias Rubens	Aster.
Arctium Lappa	Arc-l.	Astrangalus Menziesii	Astra.
Areca Catechu	Are.	Athamanta	Atha.

List of Homeopathic Medicines	Abbreviation
Aswagandha	Aswa.
Atista Indica/Glycosmis Pentaphylla	Ati-i.
Atista Radix	Ati-r.
Atropia Sulphurica	Atro-s.
Atropinium	Atro.
Aurantium	Auran.
Aurum Arsenicum	Aur-a.
Aurum Bromatum	Aur-b.
Aurum Iodatum	Aur-i.
Aurum Kalinatum	Aur-k
Aurum Metallicum	Aur.
Aurum Muriaticum Natronatum	Aur-m-n.
Aurum Muriaticum	Aur-m.
Aurum Natro	Aur-n.
Aurum Sulphuratum	Aur-s.
Avena Sativa	Avena.
Aviere	Aviera
Azadirachta Indica	Azad-i.
Bacillinum	Bacc.
Bacillinum Testinum	Bacc-t.
Bacopa Monnieri	Bacopa.
Badiaga	Bad.
Balsamum Peruvianum	Bals.
Baptisia Conf.Aset	Bapt-c-a.
Baptisia Tinctoria	Bapt.
Barosma	Bars.
Bartfelder (acid spring)	Bart.
Baryta Acetica	Bar-ac.
Baryta Carbonica	Bar-c.
Baryta Iodata	Bar-i
Baryta Muriatica	Bar-m.
Baryta Sulphurica	Bar-s.
Belladona	Bell.
Belladonna Radix	Bell-r.
Bellis Perennis	Bell-p.
Benzinum	Benz.
Benzinum Dinitricum	Benz-d.
Benzoic Acid.	Benz-a.
Benzoic Nitricum	Benz-n.
Berberis Aquifolium	Berb-a.
Berberis Vulgaris	Berb-v.
Beryllium Metallicum	Bery.
Beta Vulgaris	Berb.
Betonica	Bet.
Betula	Betul.
Bioplasma	Bio.
Bismuthum Oxidatum	Bism.

List of Homeopathic Medicines	Abbreviation
Bizmuthum Metallicum	Biz-m.
Bizmuthum Subnitricum	Biz-s.
Blatta Americana	Blat.
Blatta Orientalis	Blatta.
Blumea Odorata	Blum.
Boerahavia Diffusa	Boer.
Boldo	Bold.
Boletus Larcis / Polyporius Officinalis	Bol.
Boletus Luridus	Bol-l.
Boletus Satanas	Bol-s.
Bombyx Processionea	Bom.
Borago Officianalis	Bora.
Borax	Bor.
Boricum Acidum	Bor-ac.
Bothrops Lanceolatus	Both.
Bovista	Bov.
Brachyglottis Repens	Brach.
Brahmi	Bra.
Brassica Napus	Brass.
Bromium	Brom.
Brucea Antidysenterica	Bruc.
Brucinum	Bruci.
Bryonia	Bry.
Bryophyllum Calycinum	Bryoph.
Bufo Rana	Bufo.
Bufo Sahytiensis	Buf-s.
Buthus Australis	Buth.
Butyricum Acidum	Buty.
Buxus Sempervirens	Bux.
Cactus Grandiflorus	Cact.
Cadmium Bromatum	Cadm-b.
Cadmium Iodatum	Cadm-i.
Cadmium Metallicum	Cadm-m.
Cadmium Phosphate	Cadm-p.
Cadmium Sulphuratum	Cadm.
Cadmium Sulphuricum	Cadm-s
Caesalpinia Bonducela/Quininia Indica/Nata	Caes.
Caffeinum	Caff.
Cahinca	Cahin.
Cainca	Cain.
Cajuputum	Caj.
Caladium Sequinum	Calad.
Calcarea Acetica	Calc-ac.
Calcarea Arsenica	Calc-ar.
Calcarea Bromata	Calc-b.
Calcarea Carbonica	Calc.
Calcarea Chlorinata	Calc-ch.

List of Homeopathic Medicines	Abbreviation	List of Homeopathic Medicines	Abbreviation
Calcarea Caustica	Calc-caust.	Castanea Vesca	Cast-v.
Calcarea Fluorata	Calc-f.	Castor Equi	Cast-eq.
Calcarea Hypophosphorosa	Calc-h	Castoreum	Cast.
Calcarea Iodata	Calc-i.	Castoreum Nepeta	Cast-n.
Calcarea Lactica	Calc-l.	Catalpa Big.	Cat.
Calcarea Lactica Naronate	Calc-l-n.	Caulophyllum Thalictroides	Caul.
Calcarea Muriatica	Calc-m.	Causticum	Caust.
Calc.Ovi Testae	Calc-o.	Ceanothus Americanus	Cean.
Calcarea Oxalica	Calc.ox.	Cedron	Cedr.
Calcarea Phosphorica	Calc-p.	Cenchris Contortrix	Cench.
Calcarea Picrata	Calc-pic.	Cenic Acid	Cenic-ac.
Calcarea Renalis	Calc-r.	Centaurea Tagana	Cent.
Calcarea Silicata	Calc-sil.	Cephalandra Indica	Ceph.
Calcarea Sulphurica	Calc-s.	Cephalanthus Occidentalis	Cephl-o.
Calendula Officinalis	Calend.	Ceresus Virginiana	Cere-v.
Calliandra Houstoni	Calli.	Cereus Bonplandii	Cere-b.
Calotropis Gigantea	Calo.	Cereus Serpentaria	Cer-s.
Calotropis Lactum	Calo-l.	Cerium Oxalicum	Cerium-ox.
Caltha Palustris	Calt.	Cervus	Cervus.
Camphora Bromate	Camph-b.	Cetraria Islandica	Cet.
Camphora Monobromata	Camph-m	Chamomilla	Cham.
Camphora Officinalis	Camph.	Chaparo Amargosa	Chap.
Canchalagua	Canch.	Cheiranthus Cheiri	Cheir.
Candida Albicans	Candid.	Chelidonium Majus	Chel.
Cannabis Indica	Cann-i.	Chelone Glabra	Chelon-g.
Cannabis Sativa	Cann-s.	Chenopodium Anthelminticum	Chen-a.
Cantharis	Canth.	Chenopodium Glauci Aphis	Chen.
Capsicum	Caps.	Chenopodium Vulvaria	Chen-v
Carbo Animalis	Carb-an.	Chimaphila Maculata	Chim-m
Carbo Vegetabilis	Carb-v.	Chimaphila Umbellata	Chim.
Carbolic Acid.	Carb-ac.	China Boliviana	Chin-b.
Carboneum Chloratum	Carb-ch.	China Officinalis	Chin.
Carboneum Hydrogenisatum	Carb-h.	Chininum Arsenicosum	Chin-a.
Carboneum Oxygenisatum	Carbo-o.	Chininum Brom.	Chin-b.
Carboneum Sulphuratum	Carb-s.	Chininum Muriaticum	Chin-m.
Carcinocin	Car.	Chininum Purum	Chin-p.
Cardiospermum	Cardio.	Chininum Salicylicum	Chin-salcy.
Carduus Benedictus	Card-b.	Chinnium Sulphuricum	Chin-s.
Carduus Marianus	Card-m.	Chionanthus Latifolia	Chion-l.
Carica Papaya	Caric.	Chionanthus Virginica	Chion.
Carlsbad	Carl.	Chirata	Chir.
Carum Carvi	Caru.	Chlerod	Chlero.
Carya Alba	Carya.	Chloralum	Chlol.
Cascara Amarga	Casc-a.	Chlorinum	Chlori.
Cascara Sagrada	Casc-s.	Chloroform	Chlf.
Cascarilla	Casc.	Chlorpromazinum(Thorazine)	Chlorpro.
Cassia Sophora	Cass.	Chlorum	Chlor.

List of Homeopathic Medicines	Abbreviation	List of Homeopathic Medicines	Abbreviation
Cholestrinum	Chol.	Colocynthinum	Colcy.
Chondrus Crisp	Chond.	Colocynthis	Colo.
Chromicum Acidum	Chr-ac.	Colostrum	Colos.
Chromicum Oxydatum	Chr-ox.	Comocladia Dentata	Com.
Chromium Kali Sulphuricun	Chr-k-s.	Conchiolinum	Conch.
Chromium Sulf.	Chr-s.	Condurango	Condu.
Chrysanthemum Leuc.	Chrysa.	Conium Bromatum	Con-b.
Chrysarobin	Chrys.	Conium Maculatum	Con.
Chrysophanicum Acidum	Chryso.	Convalaria Majalis	Conv.
Cichorium Intybus	Cicho.	Convolvulus Arvensis	Conv-a.
Cicuta Mac.	Cic-m.	Convolvulus Duartinus	Conv-d.
Cicuta Virosa	Cic.	Copaiva Officinalis	Cop.
Cimex	Cimx.	Coqueluchinum	Coq.
Cimicifuga Racemosa	Cimic.	Corallium Rubrum	Cot-r.
Cina	Cina.	Coriaria Ruscifolia	Cori-r.
Cinchona (China) Officinalis	China.	Cornus Alternifolia	Corn.-a
Cinchona Boliviana	Cinch-b.	Cornus Circinata	Corn.
Cinchonium Sulphuricum	Cinch.	Cornus Florida	Corn-f.
Cineraria Maritima	Ciner.	Cornus Seriea	Corn-s.
Cinnabaris	Cinnb.	Cortisone Acetate	Cort-a.
Cinnamonum	Cinnm.	Cortisone Aceticum	Cort-ac.
Cistus Canadensis	Cist.	Corydalis Can.	Coryd.
Citricum Acidum	Cit-ac.	Coto Bark	Coto.
Citrus Decumana	Cit-d.	Cotyledon Umbilicus	Cot.
Citrus Limonum	Cit-l.	Cratagus Oxyacantha	Crat.
Citrus Vulgaris	Cit-v.	Cresolum	Cres.
Clematis Erecta	Clem.	Crocus Sativa	Croc.
Clematis Vit. Folia	Clem-v-i.	Crotalus Cascavella	Crot-c.
Clerodendron Infortunatum	Clero.	Crotalus Horridus	Crot-h.
Cobaltum Nitricum	Cob-n.	Croton Chloral	Crot-ch.
Cobaltum	Cob.	Croton Tiglinum	Crot-t.
Coca	Coca.	Cubeba	Cub.
Cocaine	Cocaine.	Cucurbita Citrulus	Cucur-c
Cocainum Muriaticum	Cocain.	Cucurbita Pepo -Semen	Cucur.
Coccinella Septempunctata	Cocc-s	Culex Moscae	Culx.
Cocculus Indicus	Cocc.	Cundurango	Cund.
Coccus Cacti	Coc-c.	Cuphea	Cuph.
Cochlearia Armoracia	Coch.	Cupressus Australia	Cupres-a.
Cochlearia Officinalis	Coch.	Cupressus Lawsoniana	Cupres.
Codeinum	Cod.	Cuprum Aceticum	Cupr-ac.
Coffea Cruda	Coff.	Cuprum Arsenicosum	Cupr-ar.
Coffea Mocha	Coff-m.	Cuprum Cyanatum	Cupr-c.
Coffea Tosta	Coff-t.	Cuprum Metallicum	Cupr.
Coffeinum	Coffein.	Cuprum Nitricum	Cupr-n.
Colchicum Autumnale	Colch.	Cuprum Oxydatum Nigrum	Cupr-o-n.
Coleus Aromaticus	Coleus.	Cuprum Sulphuricum	Cupr-s.
Collinsonia Canadensis	Coll.	Curare	Cur.

List of Homeopathic Medicines	Abbreviation	List of Homeopathic Medicines	Abbreviation
Cyclamen Europaeum	Cycl.	Eryngium Aquaticum	Ery-a.
Cydonia Vulgaris	Cydon	Eryngium Maritimum	Ery-m.
Cyndon Dactylon	Cyndon.	Erythrinus	Eyth.
Cypripedium Pubescens	Cypr.	Escholtzia Californica	Escho.
Cytisus Scoparius	Cyst.	Esculetine	Escu.
Damiana	Dam.	Eserinum	Eser.
Daphne Indica	Daph.	Etherum	Ether.
Derris Pinnata	Der.	Ethylicum	Ethy.
Datura Arborea	Dat.	Ethylum Nitricum	Ethy-n.
Datura Ferox	Dat.	Eucalyptus Globulus	Eucal.
Datura Metel	Dat.	Eugenia Jambos	Eug.
Derris Pinnata	Derr.	Euonymus Atropurpureus	Euon.
Desmodium Gangeticum	Desm.	Euonymus Europaeus	Euon.
Dictamnus Albus	Dicta.	Eupatorinum Aromaticum	Eup-aro.
Digitalinum	Digit.	Eupatorium Ayapana	Eup-A.
Digitalis Purpurea	Dig.	Eupatorium Perfoliatum	Eup-per.
Digitoxinum	Digito	Eupatorium Purpureum	Eup-pur.
Dioscorea Villosa	Dios.	Euphorbia Amygdale	Eupho-a.
Diosma Lincaris	Dio.	Euphorbia Coro	Eupho-c.
Diphtherinum	Diph.	Euphorbia Cypa	Eupho-cy.
Dirca Palustris	Dirc.	Euphorbia Heter	Eupho-h.
Dolichos Pruriens	Dol.	Euphorbia Hyper	Eupho-hy.
Doryphora	Dor.	Euphorbia Ipecac	Eupho-i.
Drosera Rotundifolia	Dros.	Euphorbia Lat.	Eupho-l.
Duboisinum	Dub.	Euphorbia Pep	Eupho-Pe.
Dulcamara	Dulc.	Euphorbia Pilulifera	Eupho-p.
Echinacea Angustifolia	Echi.	Euphorbium Officinarum	Euphorb.
Echinacea Purpurea	Echi-p.	Euphorbium	Euph.
Elaeis Guineensis	Elaeis.	Euphrasia Officinalis	Euphr.
Elaps Corallinus	Elaps.	Eupionum	Eupi.
Elaterium	Elat.	Fabiana Imbricata	Fab.
Electricitas	Elec.	Fagopyrum	Fago.
Embelia Ribes	Emb.	Fagus Sylvatica	Fag.
Emetinum	Emet.	Fel Tauri	Fel.
Eosinum Natrum	Eos.	Ferrum Aceticum	Ferr-ac.
Ephedra Vulgaris	Eph.	Ferrum Arsenicicum	Ferr-ar.
Epigea Repens	Epig.	Ferrum Arsenicosum	Ferr-ars.
Epilobium Palustre	Epil.	Ferrum Bromatum	Ferr-b.
Epiphegus Virginiana	Epiph.	Ferrum Carbonicum	Ferr-c.
Epiphysterinum	Epiphy.	Ferrum Citricum	Ferr-cit.
Equisetum Arvense	Equis-a.	Ferrum Iodatum	Ferr-i.
Equisetum Hyemale	Equis.	Ferrum Magneticum	Ferr-ma.
Erechthites Hieracifolia	Erechthites.	Ferrum Metallicum	Ferr.
Ergotinum	Ergo.	Ferrum Muriaticum	Ferr-m.
Erigeron Canadense	Erig.	Ferrum Pernit	Ferr-pe.
Eriodictyon Californicum	Eriod-c.	Ferrum Phosphoricum	Ferr-p.
Erodium	Erod.	Ferrum Picricum	Ferr-pic.

List of Homeopathic Medicines	Abbreviation	List of Homeopathic Medicines	Abbreviation
Ferrum Pyrophos	Ferr-py.	Glycerinum	Glycerine.
Ferrum Sulphuricum	Ferr.s.	Glycyrrhiza	Glycy.
Ferrum Tartaricum	Ferr-t.	Gnaphalium Leontopodium	Gnaph-l.
Ferula Glau	Ferula.	Gnaphalium Polycephalum	Gnaph-p.
Ficus Indica	Ficus-i.	Gnaphalium	Gnaph.
Ficus Religiosa	Ficus-r.	Gossypium Herbaceum	Goss.
Filix Mas	Fil.	Granatum Punica	Gran.
Fluoricum acidum	Fl-ac.	Graphites	Graph.
Foeniculum Vulgare	Foen.	Gratiola Officinalis	Grat.
Folliculinum	Foll.	Grindelia Robusta	Grin.
Formalinum	Formal.	Guaco	Gua.
Formic Acid	Form-ac.	Guaiacum	Guaj.
Formica Rufa	Form.	Guano Australis	Guano.
Fragaria Vesca	Frag-v.	Guarana	Guar.
Franciscae Uniflora	Fran.	Guarea Trichilioides	Guare-t.
Franzenbad	Frenz.	Guarea	Guare
Fraxinus Americana	Frax-a.	Guatveria Gaumeri	Guat.
Fraxinus Excelsior	Frax-e.	Gummi Gutii	Gum.
Fucus Vesiculosus	Fuc.	Gun Powder	Gun.
Fuschsine	Fusch.	Gymnema Sylvestre	Gymne.
Fuligo Ligno	Ful.	Gymnocladus	Gymn.
Fumaria Off.	Fum.	Gynocardia	Gyno.Hedera.
Gadus Morrhua	Gad.	Haematoxylon	Hem.
Galanthus nivalis	Galan.	Hall	Hall
Galega Officinalis	Galeg.	Hamamelis Virginica	Ham.
Galium Aparine	Gall	Hecla Lava	Hecla.
Gallicum Acidum	Gall-ac.	Hedeoma Pulegioides	Hedeom.
Galphimia glauca	Galph.	Hedera Helix	Hedera.
Galvanismus	Gal.	Hedysarum	Hedy.
Gambogia	Gamb.	Helianthus Annuus	Heli.
Gastein	Gas.	Heliotropium Peruvianum	Helio.
Gaultheria	Gau.	Helleborus Foetidus	Hell-f.
Gelsimium Sempervirens	Gels.	Helleborus Niger	Hell.
Genista Tinctoria	Genist.	Helleborus Orien	Hell-o.
Gentiana Cruciata	Cent-c.	Helleborus Viridis	Hell-b.
Gentiana Lutea	Gent-l.	Helix Tosta	Helix.
Gentiana Quinq	Gent-q.	Heloderma	Helo.
Geranium Maculatum	Ger.	Helonias Dioica	Helon.
Geranium Robertianum	Ger-r.	Hemidesmus Indica	Hem.
Gettisburg Water	Get.	Hepar Sulphuris Calcareum	Hep.
Geum Rivale	Geum-r.	Hepar Sulphuris Kalinum	Hep-k.
Geum Urbanum	Geum.	Hepatica Triloba	Hepat.
Gingko Biloba	Ging.	Heracleum	Hera.
Ginseng	Gins.	Hippomanes	Hipp.
Glanderine	Gland.	Hippozaenium	Hippoz.
Glechoma Hederacea	Glech.	Hippuric Acid	Hipp-ac.
Glonoin	Glon.	Histaminum	Hista.

List of Homeopathic Medicines	Abbreviation	List of Homeopathic Medicines	Abbreviation
Hoang-Nan	Hoang.	Jaborandi (Pilocarpus)	Jab.
Holarrhena Antidysentrica	Holarr.	Jacaranda Caroba	Jac-c.
Homarus	Hom.	Jacaranda Gualandai	Jac.
Homeria	Home.	Jalapa	Jal.
Humulus Lupulus	Hum.	Jasminum	Jas.
Hura Braziliensis	Hura.	Jatropha Curcas	Jatr.
Hura Crepitans	Hura-c.	Jatropha Urens	Jatr-u.
Hydrangea Arborescens	Hydrang.	Jequirity	Jeq.
Hydrastininum Mur	Hydra-m.	Jonesia Asoca	Jon.
Hydrastinum Mur	Hydra-mu.	Juglans Cinerea	Jug-c.
Hydrastin Sulph	Hydra-s.	Juglans Regia	Jug-r.
Hydrastis Canadensis	Hydr.	Juncus Effusus	Junc.
Hydrocotyle Asiatica	Hydrc.	Juniperus Communis	Juni-c.
Hydrocyanicum Acidum	Hydr-ac.	Juniperus Virginiana	Juni.
Hydrofluoricum Acidum	Hydrof.	Justicia Adhatoda	Just-a.
Hydrophila Spinosa	Hydroph.	Justicia Rubrum	Just-r.
Hydrophyllum Virg.	Hydro-v.	Kali Aceticum	Kali-a.
Hymosa	Hymosa.	Kali Arsenicosum	Kali-ar.
Hyoscaminum	Hyosc.	Kali Bichromicum	Kali-bi.
Hyoscyamus Niger	Hyos.	Kali Bromatum	Kali-br.
Hypericum Perforatum	Hyper.	Kali Carbonicum	Kali-c.
Hypothalamus	Hypo.	Kali Chloricum	Kali-chl.
Iberis Amara	Iber.	Kali Chlorosum	Kali-ch.
Ichthyolum	Ichthy.	Kali Cit	Kali-ci.
Ictodes Foetida	Ictod.	Kali Cyanatum	Kali-cy.
Ignatia Amara	Ign.	Kali Ferrocyanicum	Kali-fer.
Ilex Aquifolium	ill.	Kali Iodatum	Kali-i.
Illicium Anisatum	Illic.	Kali Manganicum	Kali-ma.
Imperatoria Ostruthium	Imp.	Kali Muriaticum	Kali-m.
Indigo	Indg.	Kali Nitricum	Kali-n.
Indium Metallicum	Ind.	Kali Oxalicum	Kali-ox.
Indolum	Indo.	Kali Permanganicum	Kali-per.
Influenzinum	Inf.	Kali Phosphoricum	Kali-p.
Ingluvin	Ing.	Kali Picricum	Kali-s.
Insulin	Ins.	Kali Silicatum	Kali-pic.
Inula Helenium	Inul.	Kali Sulphuricum	Kali-s.
Iodium	Iod.	Kali Tar	Kali-Tar.
Iodoformum	Iodof.	Kali Telluricum	Kali-t.
Ipecacuanha	Ip.	Kalmegh /Andrographis Paniculata	Kalmegh
Ipomia Purpurea	Ipom.	Kalmia Latifolia	Kalm.
Iridium	Iridium.	Kamala	Kamal.
Iris Florentina	Ir-fl.	Kaolin	Kaol.
Iris Foetidissima	Ir-foe.	Karaka	Kar.
Iris Germanica	Ir-g.	Kerosolenum	Kero.
Iris Tenax	Ir-t.	Kino	Kino.
Iris Versicolor	Iris.	Kissingen	Kiss.
Itu	Itu	Kobaltum	Kob.

List of Homeopathic Medicines	Abbreviation	List of Homeopathic Medicines	Abbreviation
Kousso	Kous.	Lithium Muriaticum	Lith-m.
Kreosotum	Kreos.	Lobelia Cardinalis	Lob-c.
Laburnum Anagyroides	Lab.	Lobelia Erinus	Lob-e.
Lac Caninum	Lac-c.	Lobelia Inflata	Lob.
Lac Defloratum	Lac-d.	Lobelia Purp	Lob-p.
Lac Delphinum	Lac-del.	Lobelia Syphilitica	Lob-s.
Lac Equinum	Lac-e.	Lolium Temulentum	Lol.
Lac Felinum	Lac-f.	Lonicera Xylost.	Lon.
Lac Vaccinum	Lac-v.	Lophophytum Leandri	Loph.
Lacerta Agilis	Lacer.	Luffa Amara / Fuetida	Luffa.
Lachesis	Lach.	Luffa Bindal	Luffa-b.
Lacerta	Lac.	Luffa Operculata	Luffa-o.
Lachnanthes Tinctoria	Lachn.	Luna	Luna.
Lactic Acid.	Lac-ac.	Lupulus	Lup.
Lactis Vas	Lactis.	Lycopersicum	Lycpr.
Lactuca Virosa	Lact-v.	Lycopodium Clavatum	Lyc.
Lamium Album	Lam.	Lycopus Virginicus	Lycps.
Lapathum	Lap.	Lysidinum	Lysi.
Lapis Albus	Lap-a.	Lyssin (Hydrophobinum)	Lyss.
Lappa Arctium	Lappa-a.	Macrotinum	Mac.
Lappa Major	Lappa-m.	Maercurius Sulphuratus Ruber (Cinnabaris)	Mae-s-r.
Lapsana	Lapsa	Mag Oxydata	Mag-o.
Lathyrus Sativus	Lath.	Magnesia Carbonica	Mag-c.
Latrodectus Ka	Lat-k.	Magnesia Muriatica	Mag-m.
Latrodectus Mactans	Lat-m.	Magnesia Phosphorica	Mag-p.
Laurocerasus	Laur.	Magnesia Sulphurica	Mag-s.
Lecithin	Lec.	Magnesium Met.	Mag-met.
Ledum Palustre	Led.	Magnetis Poli. Ambo.	Mag-p-a.
Lemna Minor	Lem-m.	Magnetis Polus Arcticus	Mag-arct.
Leonurus Cardiaca	Leon.	Magnetis Polus Australis	Mag-aust.
Lepidium Bonariense	Lepi.	Magnolia Grandiflora	Mag-G
Leptandra Virginica	Lept.	Magnolia Grandiflora	Mag.
Lespedeza Capitata	Lesp.	Makardhwaja	Makar.
Leucas Aspera	Leu.	Malandrinum	Maland.
Levico	Levico.	Malaria Officinalis	Malar.
Levisticum officinale	Lev.	Mancinella (Hippomanes)	Manc.
Liatris Spicata	Lia.	Mandragora Officinarium	Mandra.
Lilium Tigrinum	Lil-t.	Manganum	Mang.
Limulus	Lim.	Manganum Aceticum	Mang-a.
Linaria Vulgaris	Lin-v.	Manganum Carbonicum	Mang-c.
Linum Cathar	Linu-c.	Manganum Metallicum	Mang-met.
Linum Usitat	Lin-u.	Manganum Muriaticum	Mang-m.
Lippia Mexi	Lip.	Manganum Oxydatum Nigrum	mang-o-n.
Lithium Benz	Lith-b.	Manganum Sulfuricum	Mang-s.
Lithium Bromatum	Lith-br.	Mangifera Indica	Mangi.
Lithium Carbonicum	Lith.	Mangnese Dioxide	Magnese.
Lithium Lact	Lith-l.	Marrubium Vulgare	Med-v.

List of Homeopathic Medicines	Abbreviation	List of Homeopathic Medicines	Abbreviation
Marum Varum Teuc	Mar.	Musa	Mus.
Matthiola Gr	Mat.	Mutha	Mutha.
Medorrhinum	Med.	Mygale Lasiodora	Mygal
Medusa	Medusa.	Myosotis	Myos.
Melastoma	Mel.	Myrica Cerifera	Myric.
Melilotus Alba	Meli.	Myristica Sebifera	Myris.
Melilotus Officinalis	Meli-o.	Myrrha	Myrrha.
Melissa Off.	Mellisa.	Myrtus Communis	Myrt-c.
Melitagrinum	Melitag.	Nabulus	Nab.
Menispermum	Menis	Naja Tripudia	Naja.
Mentha Piperita	Ment.	Naphthalin	Naph.
Mentha Pulegium	Mentha	Narcissus Pseudo-Narcissus	Narc.
Mentha Vir.	Mentha-p.	Narcotinum	Narcot.
Mentholum	Mentho.	Nasturtium Aquaticum	Nast.
Menyanthes	Meny.	Natrum Aceticum	Nat-ac.
Mephitis	Meph.	Natrum Arsenicatum	Nat-a.
Mercurialis	Meri.	Natrum Bromatum	Nat-b.
Mercurious Sulphutatus Ruber	Merc.s-r.	Natrum Carbonicum	Nat-c.
Mercurius Aceticus	Merc-ac.	Natrum Chloratum	Nat-ch.
Mercurius Auratus	Merc-a.	Natrum Cocodicum	Nat-co.
Mercurius Bromatus	Merc-b.	Natrum Fluoratum	Nat-f.
Mercurius Corrosivus	Merc-c.	Natrum Hypochlorosum	Nat-h.
Mercurius Cyanatus	Merc-cy.	Natrum Iodatum	Nat-i.
Mercurius Dulcis	Merc-d.	Natrum Lacticum	Nat-l.
Mercurius Iodatus Flavus	Merc-i-f.	Natrum Muriaticum	Nat-m.
Mercurius Iodatus Ruber	Merc-i-r.	Natrum Muriaticum Bit	Nat-m.b.
Mercurius Nitrosus	Merc-n.	Natrum Nitricum	Nat-n.
Mercurius Praecipitatus Albus	Merc-p-a.	Natrum Nitrosum	Nat-nitro.
Mercurius Praecipitatus Ruber	Merc-p-r.	Natrum Phosphoricum	Nat-p.
Mercurius Solubilis	Merc-s.	Natrum Salicylicum	Nat-salic.
Mercurius Sulphuricus	Merc-sul.	Natrum Selenicum	Nat-sel.
Mercurius Vivus	Merc.	Natrum Silicofluoricum	Nat-sili.
Methylene Blue	Meth.	Natrum Sulphuricum	Nat-s.
Mezereum	Mez.	Natrum Sulphurosum	Nat-Sulph.
Millefolium	Mill.	Nectrianinum	Nect.
Mimosa Humilis	Mim.	Negundo	Negu.
Mitchella Repens	Mit.	Nepeta Cataria	Nepe.
Momordi Charantia	Mom.	Niacin	Niacin.
Momordica Balsamina	Mom-b.	Niccolum	Nicc.
Morbilinum	Mor.	Niccolum Metallicum	Nicc-m.
Morgan (Bach)	Morgan.	Niccolum Sulph	Nicc-s.
Morphinum	Morph.	Nicotinum	Nico.
Moschus	Mosch.	Nitri Spiritus Dulcis	Nit-s-d.
Mucuna Urens	Muc.	Nitricum Acidum	Nit-ac.
Mullen Oil	Mullen.	Nitro Muriatic Acid	Nit-m-ac.
Murex	Murx.	Nitrogenium Oxygenatum	Nitro-o.
Muriaticum Acidum	Mur-ac.	Nuphar Luteum	Nuph.

List of Homeopathic Medicines	Abbreviation	List of Homeopathic Medicines	Abbreviation
Nux Juglans	Nux-j.	Parietaria Officinalis	Pari.
Nux Moschata	Nux-m.	Paris Quadrifolia	Par.
Nux Vomica	Nux-v.	Paronichia Illecebrum	Paro.
Nyctanthes Abor Tristis	Nycta.	Parotidinum	Parot.
Nymphaea Odorata	Nym.	Parthenium	Parth.
Ocimum Basil	Oci-b.	Pas Avena	Pas.
Ocimum Canum	Oci.	Passiflora Compound	Pass.
Ocimum Caryophyllatum	Oci-c.	Passiflora Incarnata	Pass-i.
Ocimum Gratis	Oci-g.	Pastinaca Sativa	Past.
Ocimum Sanctum	Oci-s.	Paullinia Pinnata	Paull.
Oenanthe Crocata	OEna.	Paullinia Sorbilis	Paull-s.
Oenotherra Biennis	Oeno.	Pecten	Pec.
Oldenlandia Herbacea	Olden.	Pediculus Capitis	Ped.
Oleander	Olnd.	Pelargonium Reni	Pelar.
Oleum Animale	Ol-an.	Penthorum	Pen.
Oleum Jecoris Aselli.	Ol-j	Pepsi	Pep.
Oleum Morrhue	Ol-m.	Persea Americana	Persea.
Oleum Ricini	Ol-r.	Persica	Per.
Oleum Santali	Ol.s.	Pertussinum	Pert.
Olibanum	Olib.	Pestinum	Pest.
Oniscus	Onis.	Petiveria	Peti.
Ononis Spinosa	Onis-s.	Petroleum	Petr.
Onosmodium	Onos.	Petroselinum	Petros.
Oophorinum	Oop.	Phallus Impudicus	Phal.
Operculina	Oper.	Phaseolus Nanus	Phase.
Opium	Op.	Phellandrium	Phel.
Opuntia Vulgaris	Opunita.	Phenacetinum	Phena.
Orchitinum	Orch.	Phloridzinum	Phlo.
Oreodaphne Californica	Oreo.	Phosphoricum Acidum	Ph-ac.
Origanum Majorana	Orig.	Phosphorus	Phos.
Ornithogalum Umbellatum	Ornitho.	Phosphorus Hydrogen	Phos-h.
Osmium	Osm.	Phosphorus Muria	Phos-m.
Ostrya	Ost.	Physalia	Physal.
Ova Tosta	Ova.	Physalis Alkekengi	Phy.
Ovi Gallinae Pellicula	Ovi.	Physostigma	Phys.
Ovinine	Ov.	Phytolacca Decandra	Phyt.
Oxalicum Acidum	Ox-ac.	Pichi	Pichi.
Oxalis Acetosa	Ox-a.	Picricum Acidum	Pic-ac.
Oxydendrum Arboreum	Oxy.	Picrotoxinum	Picro.
Oxytropis Lamberti	Oxyl.	Pilocarpinum Muriaticum	Pilo-m.
Ozone (Oxygenium)	Ozone.	Pilocarpinum Nitricum	Pilo-n.
Paeonia Officinalis	Paeon.	Pilocarpinum	Pilo.
Palladium	Pall.	Pimpinella Saxifraga	Pimp.
Pancreatinum	Pan.	Pinus Lambertiana	Pin-l.
Papaverinum	Papa.	Pinus Silvestris	Pin-s.
Paraffinum	Para.	Piper Methysticum	Pip-m.
Pareira Brava	Pareir.	Piper Nigrum	Pip-n.

List of Homeopathic Medicines	Abbreviation	List of Homeopathic Medicines	Abbreviation
Piperazinum	Piper.	Quebracho	Quebra.
Piscida Erythrina	Pis.	Quercus Glandus Spiritus	Qeuer.
Pituitarum-posterior	Pitu.	Quercus Robur	Guer-r.
Pix Liquida	Pix.	Quillia Saponaria	Quilla.
Placebo	Placebo.	Radium Bromatum	Rad-b.
Plantago Major	Plan.	Radium	Rad.
Platanus	Plata.	Ranunculus Acris	Ran-a.
Platanus Occi	Plat-o.	Ranunculus Bulbosus	Ran-b.
Platinum Metallicum	Plat.	Ranunculus Fincaria	Ran-f.
Platinum Muriaticum	Plat-m.	Ranunculus Flam	Ran-fl.
Platinum Natro	Pllat-n	Ranunculus Glac	Ran-g.
Plectranthus	Plect.	Ranunculus Repens	Ran-r.
Plumbago Littoralis	Plumbg.	Ranunculus Sceleratus	Ran-s.
Plumbum Aceticum	Plb-ac.	Raphanus Sat	Raph.
Plumbum Carbonicum	Plb-c.	Ratanhia	Rat.
Plumbum Chrom	Plb-ch.	Rauwolfia Serpentina	Rau.
Plumbum Iodatum	Plb-i.	Rhamnus Californica	Rham.
Plumbum Metallicum	Plb.	Rhamnus Cathartica	Rham-c.
Plutonium Nitricum	Plb-n.	Rhamnus Frangula	Rham-f.
Pneumococcin	Pneumo.	Rhamnus Purshiana	Rham-p.
Pneumus Boldo	Pneum-b.	Rheum	Rheum.
Podophyllum Peltatum	Podo.	Rhodium Oxyd. Nit	Rho-o-n.
Polygonum Hydropiperoides	Polyg.	Rhododendron	Rhod.
Polygonum Punc.	Polyg-t.	Rhus Aromatica	Rhus-a.
Polyporus Officianlalis	Poly	Rhus Diversaloba	Rhus-d.
Polyporus Pinicola	Poly-p.	Rhus Glabra	Rhus-g.
Populus Candicans	Pop-c.	Rhus Radicans	Rhus-r.
Populus Tremuloides	Pop.	Rhus Tox	Rhus-t.
Pothos Foetidus	Poth.	Rhus Venenata	Rhus-v.
Primula Obc.	Prim.	Rhusaromatica	Rhusaro.
Primula Veris	Prim-V.	Ricinus Communis	Ricinus.
Primula Virg	Prim-Vi.	RNA	Rana.
Primulaveris	Primu.	Robinia Pseudacacia	Rob.
Prunus Padus	Primus.	Rosa Canina	Rosa.
Prunus Spinosa	Prun.	Rosa Damascena	Rosa-d.
Prunus Virginiana	Prun-v.	Rosmarinus Officinalis	Rosma.
Psorinum	Psor.	Rubia Tinctorum	Rubia.
Ptelea Trifoliata	Ptel.	Rubinia	Rubin.
Pulex Irritans	Pulx.	Rumex Acetosa	Rumex-a.
Pulmoa Vulpis	Pulm.	Rumex Crispus	Rumex.
Pulsatilla Nigricans	Puls.	Rumex Obtusifolius	Rumex-o.
Pulsatilla Nuttaliana	Puls-n.	Rassula	Russ.
Pyarara	Pya.	Ruta Graveolens	Ruta.
Pyrethrum Parthenium	Pyreth.	Sabadilla	Sabad.
Pyrogenium	Pyrog.	Sabal Serrulata	Sabal.
Pyrus Americana	Pyrus.	Sabina	Sabin.
Quassia Amara	Quass.	Saccharinum	Sacc.

List of Homeopathic Medicines	Abbreviation	List of Homeopathic Medicines	Abbreviation
Saccharum Album	Sac.	Serpentaria	Serp.
Saccharum Lactis	Sac-l.	Septicaeminum	Sept.
Saccharum Officiniale	Sac-o.	Serum Anguillae	Serum.
Salamander	Salam.	Silica Marina	Silica.
Salicinum	Salic.	Silicea	Sil.
Salicylicum Acidum	Sal-ac.	Silphium Laciniatum	Silphi.
Salix Alb	Sal-n.	Simaruba	Sima.
Salix Mol	Sal-m	Sinapis Alba	Sin-a.
Salix Nigra	Salix.	Sinapis Nigra	Sin-n.
Salix Purpurea	Salix-p.	Sium	Sium.
Salol	Salol.	Skatolum	Skat.
Salvia Officinalis	Salix-o.	Skookum Chuck	Skook.
Sambucus Can	Samb-c.	Slag	Slag.
Sambucus Nigra	Samb.	Sol	Sol.
Sanguinaria Canadensis	Sang.	Solaninum	Solani.
Sanguinaria Nitrica	Sang-n.	Solaninum Ars	Solani-a.
Sanguinarinum	San.	Solanum Car.	Sol-c.
Sanguinarinum Tar	San-t.	Solanum Mammosum	Sol-m.
Sanguisuga	Sangu.	Solanum Nigrum	Sol-n.
Sanicula Aqua	Sanic.	Solanum Oleraceum	Sol-o.
Santalum	Santo	Solanum Pseu	Sol-p.
Santoninum	Sant.	Solanum Tuberosum Aegrotans	Sol-t-ae.
Saponaria Off.	Sapo.	Solanum Tuberosum	Sol-t.
Saponinum	Sapn.	Solanum Xanthocarpum	Sol-x.
Sarcolacticum Acidum	Sarco.	Solidago Virg. aur.	Sol-v.
Sarcolatic Acid	Sarco-ac.	Spigelia Anthelmia	Spig.
Sarracenia Purpurea	Sarr.	Spigelia Marilandica	Spig-m.
Sarsaparilla	Sars.	Sphingurus	Sphing.
Sassafras	Sass.	Spiraea Ulmaria	Spi.
Scammonium	Scam.	Spiranthes	Spira.
Scarlatinum	Scarl.	Spiritus Glandium Quercus	Spirit-g-q.
Schinus Molle	Schin.	Spongia Tosta	Spong.
Scilla Maritima	Scill.	Squilla Hispanica	Squil.
Scirrhinum	Scirr.	Stachys Betonica	Stach.
Scolopendra	Sciol.	Stannum Iodatum	Stann-i.
Scorpid	Scor.	Stannum Metallicum	Stann.
Scrophularia Nodosa	Scorp.	Staphysagria	Staph.
Scutellaria Lateriflora	Scut.	Stellaria Media	Stel.
Secale Cornutum	Sec.	Sterculia Acuminata	Ster.
Sedum Acre	Sed.	Sticta Pulmonaria	Stict.
Selenium	Sel.	Stigmata Maydis	Stig.
Sempervivum Tectorum	Sem.	Stillingia Sylvatica	Still.
Senecio Aureus	Senec.	Stramonium	Stram.
Senecio Jacobaea	Senec-j.	Strontium	Stront.
Senega	Seneg.	Strontium Bromatum	Stront-b.
Senna	Senn.	Strontium Carbonicum	Stron-c.
Sepia	Sep.	Strontium Nitricum	Stront-n.

List of Homeopathic Medicines	Abbreviation	List of Homeopathic Medicines	Abbreviation
Strophanthus Hispidus	Strph.	Thea Sinensis	Thea.
Strychinum	Stryc.	Theobrominum	Theo.
Strychinum Ars	Stryc-a.	Theridion	Ther.
Strychinum Nit.	Stryc-n.	Thiosinaminum	Thio.
Strychnia Phosphoricum	Strych-p.	Thuja Lobbi	Thuja-l.
Strychninum Arsenicum	Stry-a.	Thuja Occidentalis	Thuja.
Strychninum Nitricum	Stry-n.	Thymolum	Thymol.
Strychninum Sulphuricum	Stry-s.	Thymus Serpyllum	Thymus.
Strychninum Valerium	Stry-v.	Thyroidinum	Thy.
Succinum Acidum	Succi.	Thyro-Iodinum	Thyro.
Succus Amogara	Succus.	Tilia Europoea	Til.
Sulfanilamidum	Sulfa.	Tinospora Cordifolia	Tino.
Sulfonal	Sulfo.	Titanium Metallicum	Tita.
Sulfurosum Acidum	Sulfu.	Tongo Odorata	Tong.
Sulphur	Sulph.	Torula Cerevisiae	Tor.
Sulphur Hydro	Sulph-h.	Toxicophis	Tox.
Sulphur Iodatum	Sul-i.	Trachinus	Trach.
Sulphur Tereb	Sul-t.	Tradescantia	Trade.
Sulphuricum Acidum	Sul-ac.	Tribulus Terrestris	Trib.
Sumbul	Sumb.	Trichophyton Rubrum	Tricho.
Symphoricarpus Rasemosus	Sym-r.	Trichsanthes Dioica	Trich.
Symphytum Officinale	Symph.	Trifolium Pretense	Trif-p.
Syphilinum	Syph.	Trifolium Repens	Trif-r.
Syzygium Jambolinum	Syz.	Trillium Pendulum	Tril.
Tabacum	Tab.	Trimethylaminum	Trime.
Tamus Comm.	Tamus.	Triosteum Perfoliatum	Trio.
Tanacetum Vulgare	Tanac.	Triticum Repens	Trit.
Tanghinna	Tang.	Trombidium Muscae Domesticae	Trom.
Tannicum Acidum	Tanni.	Tropaeolum Maj.	Tropa.
Tanninum	Tann.	Tuberculinum	Tub.
Tanthelin	Tanth.	Turnera Aphrodis	Turn.
Taraxacum	Tarax.	Tussilago Farfara	Tuss.
Tarentula Cubensis	Tarent-c.	Tussilago Fragrans	Tus-f.
Tarentula Hispanica	Tarent.	Tussilago Petasites	Tus-p.
Tartaricum Acid.	Tart-ac.	Typhofebrinum	Typho.
Taxus Baccata	Tax.	Ulmus Fulv.	Ulmus.
Tellurium	Tell.	Upas Tiente	Upa.
Teplitz	Tep.	Uranium Nitricum	Uran.
Teradymite	Tera.	Urea	Urea.
Terebinthina	Ter.	Uricum Acidum	Uri.
Terminalia Chebula	Termi.	Urinum	Urin.
Teucrium Marum Verum	Teucr.	Urtica Dioica	Urt-d
Teucrium Scoro	Teucr-s.	Urtica Urens	Urt-u.
Thalaspi Bursa Pastoris	Thlaspi.	Usala Barb	Usala.
Thallium	Thal.	Usnea Barbata	Usnea.
Thaspium Aureum	Thasp.	Usnea Barbata	Usnea-b.
Thavetia	Thav.	Ustilago Maydis	Ust.

List of Homeopathic Medicines	Abbreviation	List of Homeopathic Medicines	Abbreviation
Uva Ursi	Uva.	Viscum Album	Visc.
Vaccininum	Vac.	Voeslum	Voes.
Vaccinium Myrtillus	Vacci.	Wiesbaden	Wies.
Valeriana	Vacler..	Wildbad	Wild.
Vanadium Metallicum	Vanad.	Withania Som	With.
Variolinum	Vario.	Wyethia Helenioides	Wye.
Venus Mercenaria	Venus.	Xanthoxylum Fraxineum	Xan.
Veratrinum	Veratr.	Xerophyllum Asphodeloides	Xero.
Veratrum Album	Verat.	X-ray	X-ray.
Veratrum Nig	Verat-n.	Yerba Santa	Yerba.
Veratrum Viride	Verat-v.	Yohimbinum	Yohomb.
Verbascum Thapsus	Verb.	Yucca	Yuc.
Verbena Officinalis	Verb.	Zea	Zea.
Verbena Hastata	Verb-h.	Zincum Aceticum	Zinc-ac.
Veronia Anthelmintica	Vero.	Zincum Brom	Zinc-b.
Vesicaria Communis	Vesi-c.	Zincum Carb	Zinc-carb.
Vesicaria	Vesi.	Zincum Cyanatum	Zinc-c.
Vespa Crabro	Vesp.	Zincum Iodatum	Zinc-i.
Viburnum Opulus	Vib.	Zincum Metallicum	Zinc.
Viburnum Prunifolium	Vib-p.	Zincum Muriaticum	Zinc-m.
Viburnum Tinus	Vib-t.	Zincum Oxydatum	Zinc-ox.
Vichy	Vichy.	Zincum Phosphoratum	Zinc-p.
Vinca Minor	Vinc.	Zincum Picricum	Zinc-pic.
Vincetoxicum	Vince.	Zincum Sulphuricum	Zinc-s.
Viola Odorata	Viol-o.	Zincum Valerianicum	Zinc-v.
Viola Tricolor	Viol-t.	Zingiber	Zing.
Vipera	Vip.	Zizia Aurea	Ziz.

PREFACE

This book has been published in fond memory of my father Dr. Basant Lall and mother Mrs. Ram Keshi Devi who inspired me to give something new to the Homeopath doctors practicing in different parts of this universe.

It is a great honour for me for being the youngest son of Dr. Basant Lall who was a renowned homeopathic practioner. He shared enormous experiences of his life time.

My heart felt blessing to my sons Mr. Prashun L.Raj, MBA in Logistic from IIL Chennai and working in Dubai as an executive and Pranav L. Raj, B.Tech from NIFT Chennai working as Marketing Manager in Dubai for their timely coming forward and helping me in compiling my experiences and lastly to my wife Dr. Sheela Kanchan without whom this Homeopathic repertory would have never seen the light of the day.

I am hopeful that this repertory based on my practice and research will prove a boon to the society across the globe. It is very easy to search with desciptive index facility. I had been a great admirer of Dr. J.T. Kent. Symptoms and remedies described in this repertory is based on my practice and research of Dr. J.T. Kent.

Homeopathy as a system of medicine has got several advantages over every other system due to its following qualities:

1. These are prepared and standardised according to the methods prescribed in the American Pharmacopeia by reputed firms over a century's standing in USA.

2. They are most suitable for domestic and professional practice as they are easily available for use in the form of globules.

3. They are most cheaper and effective than any medicine in any other system of medicine. They are the most suitable for a developing country like India and other developing countries as well. It is possible to extend necessary medical help to the poor people even in the remotest part of any country.

4. As the doses administered are very small there is no danger of over dosing.

5. There are absolutely no bad effect left in the patient as a result of excessive medication.

6. Homeopathic system of case taking coupled with physical examination of the patient gives a true picture of the remedy.

7. They are highly efficient in their action which in extreme cases work as wonderful change in the condition of the patient at a critical stage.

8. They are both preventive in the initial stage and also curative in later stage. Most diseases can be aborted by proper application in their initial stages before they develop into a complicated one.

9. Gradually peoples across the globe are showing their great interest and adopting homeopathic treatment even in most lingering and fatal cases.

– Dr. Arun Kumar Lall

A

Body part/Disease	Symptom	Medicines
Abdomen	abscess in walls of abdomen	Hep., rhus-t., sil., sulph.
Abdomen	Aching in back ameliorated from lying on abdomen	Nit-ac.
Abdomen	Aching in lumbar region can lie only on abdomen	Nit-ac.
Abdomen	ameliorated from lying on abdomen	Acet-ac., aloe., am-c., ambr., ars., bar-c., **Bell.**, bry., calc., chel., cina., coloc., crot-t., elaps., lach., mag-c., nit-ac., phos., phyt., plb., rhus-t., sel., sep., stann.
Abdomen	aneurism in abdomen	Bar-m., sec.
Abdomen	asthmatic with stitching in abdomen to back	Calc.
Abdomen	band around abdomen	Crot-c.
Abdomen	blindness, with abdominal pain	Crot-t., plb.
Abdomen	blotches (An irregularly shaped Reddish patch on the skin) on abdomen	Crot-t., merc., nat-c.
Abdomen	breathing difficult alternating with pain in hypochondria	Zinc.
Abdomen	bubbling (a gurgling sound made by a boiling or effervescent liquid) in abdomen while lying on back	Sul-ac.
Abdomen	bubbling in abdomen	Hell., Lyc., nat-m., ph-ac., puls., stann., sul-ac., tarax.
Abdomen	bubbling in inguinal region	Berb., lyc.
Abdomen	burning after itching in lumbar region extending to abdomen and thighs	Nat-m.
Abdomen	burning pain in abdomen after eating	Hydr-ac.
Abdomen	burning pain in abdomen after ice cream	Ars.
Abdomen	burning pain in abdomen after stool	Cupr-ar., jug-c., kali-bi., nat-a., sabad.
Abdomen	burning pain in abdomen ameliorated on lying	Podo.
Abdomen	burning pain in abdomen before stool	Aloe.
Abdomen	burning pain in abdomen during stool	Eug., sul-ac.
Abdomen	burning pain in abdomen while eating	Phos.
Abdomen	burning pain in lumbar region extending across abdomen	Bar-c.
Abdomen	chill beginning in and extending from abdomen	**Apis.**, bell., calad., calc., camph., cann-s., coloc., cur., **Ign.**, merc., par., teucr., verat.
Abdomen	chill developing slowly in morning on rising from bed with cold developing slowly on abdomen	Meny.
Abdomen	chill in and extending from abdomen to fingers and toes	Calad.
Abdomen	chill in evening with burning in abdomen	Nat-c., phos.
Abdomen	chill in evening with colic	Led.
Abdomen	coldness in back extending to abdomen	Crot-t., phos., sec., spig.

Body part/Disease	Symptom	Medicines
Abdomen	coldness in hands with cutting and tearing in abdomen	Ars.
Abdomen	coldness in lumbar extending to abdomen after urinating	Sulph.
Abdomen	coldness in thigh at night during colic	Calc.
Abdomen	coldness with pain in abdomen	Ars.
Abdomen	constriction in chest alternating with pain in abdomen	Calc.
Abdomen	convulsion begin in the abdomen	Aran., bufo.
Abdomen	convulsion during colic	Plb.
Abdomen	convulsion epileptic from solar plexus (a point on the upper abdomen just below where the ribs separate)	Art-v., bell., bufo., calc., caust., **Cic.**, cupr., indg., **Nux-v.**, sil., **Sulph.**
Abdomen	convulsion epileptic with aura (warning sensation before epileptic episode) abdomen to head	Indg.
Abdomen	cough ameliorated from warming abdomen	Sil.
Abdomen	cracks on surface of abdomen	Sil.
Abdomen	cramp in lower limbs with colic	Coloc.
Abdomen	cramp in sole preceding colic	Plb.
Abdomen	cramping (painful muscle contraction) pain in abdomen after breakfast	Agar., eupi., grat., ham., kali-bi., nux-m., stront., Zinc.
Abdomen	cramping pain in abdomen after fruit	Calc-p., chin., coloc., puls.
Abdomen	cramping pain in abdomen after ice cream	Ars., calc-p., ip., puls.
Abdomen	cramping pain in abdomen after menses	Am-c., cocc., kreos., merl., puls.
Abdomen	cramping pain in abdomen after milk	Cupr., lac-d., mag-s., raph.
Abdomen	cramping pain in abdomen after sour food	Asaf.
Abdomen	cramping pain in abdomen after taking cold	All-c., alumn., Asaf., dulc.
Abdomen	cramping pain in abdomen ameliorated by warm milk	Crot-t., op.
Abdomen	cramping pain in abdomen ameliorated from hot milk	Crot-t.
Abdomen	cramping pain in abdomen ameliorated from kneading abdomen	Nat-s.
Abdomen	cramping pain in abdomen ameliorated from passing flatus	Acon., am-c., cimx., coloc., con., echi., graph., hydr., lyc., mag-c., merc-c., nat-a., nat-m., nux-m., ol-an., psor., rumx., sil., spong., squil., sulph.
Abdomen	cramping pain in abdomen ameliorated while lying	Cupr., ferr.
Abdomen	cramping pain in abdomen ameliorated while lying on the abdomen	Am-c., chion., coloc., dor.
Abdomen	cramping pain in abdomen before menses	Aloe., alum., am-c., bar-c., bell., brom., calc-p., carb-v., caust., cham., chin., cinnb., cocc., coloc., croc., cupr., cycl., hyper., ign., Kali-c., lach., mag-c., mag-p., manc., nux-v., ph-ac., plat., puls., sep., spong.
Abdomen	cramping pain in abdomen before menses from hip to hip	Thuj.
Abdomen	cramping pain in abdomen during constipation	Merc., op., plb., podo.
Abdomen	cramping pain in abdomen during fever	Caps., carb-v., elat., rhus-t., rob.
Abdomen	cramping pain in abdomen from fasting	Dulc.

Body part/Disease	Symptom	Medicines
Abdomen	cramping pain in abdomen from lying on back	Phys.
Abdomen	cramping pain in abdomen from melons	Zing.
Abdomen	crusts (a dry hardened outer layer of blood, pus, or other bodily secretion that forms over a cut or sore) on abdomen	Anac., arn., kali-c.
Abdomen	cutting pain from left to right abdomen	Ip.
Abdomen	cutting pain from right to left abdomen	Lyc.
Abdomen	cutting pain in abdomen after warm milk	Ang.
Abdomen	cutting pain in abdomen ameliorated from passing flatus	Anac., ars-i., bapt., bov., bry., calc-p., Con., eupi., gamb., hydr., laur., plb., psor., sel., sulph., viol-t.
Abdomen	cutting pain in abdomen extending to anus	Coloc.
Abdomen	cutting pain in abdomen extending to thigh	Coloc., ter.
Abdomen	cutting pain in abdomen from fasting	Dulc.
Abdomen	cutting pain in abdomen like electric shock darting through the anus	Coloc.
Abdomen	desquamation on abdomen	Merc., vesp.
Abdomen	discoloration of abdomen with redness	Anac., plb., rhus-t.
Abdomen	discoloration on abdomen in spots	Vip.
Abdomen	discoloration, blackness on abdomen	Vip.
Abdomen	discoloration, blotches (An irregularly shaped Reddish patch on the skin) on abdomen	Aloe., crot-t.
Abdomen	discoloration, blue spots on abdomen	Ars., mosch.
Abdomen	discoloration, brown spots on abdomen	Ars., carb-v., cob., hydr-ac., kali-c., lach., Lyc., nit-ac., phos., sabad., Sep., thuj.
Abdomen	discoloration, greenish spots on abdomen	Rob.
Abdomen	discoloration, inflamed spots on abdomen	Ars., bell., canth., kali-c., lach., led., lyc., nat-m., Phos., sabad., sep.
Abdomen	distension ameliorated by eructation (to expel stomach gases through the mouth)	Carb-v., sep., thuj.
Abdomen	distension of abdomen (to expand, swell, or inflate as if by pressure from within) after beer	Nat-m.
Abdomen	distension of abdomen after breakfast	Agar., chin-a., nat-m.
Abdomen	distension of abdomen after dinner	Alum., anac., calc., carb-an., Carb-v., euphr., grat., lyc., mag-c., mag-m., nat-m., nicc., nux-m., phos., sep., sulph., thuj., til.
Abdomen	distension of abdomen after drinking	Ambr., ars., carb-v., Chin., hep., nux-v., petr.
Abdomen	distension of abdomen after menses	Cham., kreos., lil-t., rat.
Abdomen	distension of abdomen after milk	Con.
Abdomen	distension of abdomen ameliorated by passing flatus (Intestinal gas, composed partly of swallowed air and partly of gas produced by bacterial fermentation of intestinal contents. It consists mainly of hydrogen, carbon dioxide, and methane in varying proportionsGas produced in the digestive system usually expelled from the body through the anus)	All-c., am-m., ant-t., bov., bry., carb-v., kali-i., Lyc., mag-c., mang., nat-c., nat-m., ph-ac., sulph.

Body part/Disease	Symptom	Medicines
Abdomen	distension of abdomen ameliorated from stool	Alum., am-m., asaf., calc-p., corn., hyper., nat-m.
Abdomen	distension of abdomen before dinner	All-c.
Abdomen	distension of abdomen before menses	Am-m., arn., berb., carb-an., carb-v., chin., cycl., hep., kreos., lach., lyc., mang., puls., zinc.
Abdomen	distension of abdomen before urination	Chin-s.
Abdomen	distension of abdomen during constipation	Bry., ery-a., graph., hyos., iod., lach., mag-m., nit-ac., phos., ter.
Abdomen	distension of abdomen during menses	Aloe., alum., berb., brom., carb-an., chin., Cocc., coff., croc., cycl., graph., ham., hep., ign., kali-c., kali-p., kreos., lac-c., lachn., lyc., mag-c., nat-c., nicc., nit-ac., nux-v., rat., Sulph., zinc.
Abdomen	distension of abdomen fasting while	Dulc.
Abdomen	distension of abdomen in children	Bar-c., Calc., Caust., cina., cupr., sil., staph., Sulph.
Abdomen	distension of abdomen in morning	Aloe., ars., asaf., cham., chin-a., chin., grat., nat-s., nit-ac., nux-v., ol-an., rhod., sulph.
Abdomen	distension of abdomen, after milk	Con.
Abdomen	distension of abdomen, after rising	Coc-c.
Abdomen	distension of abdomen, ameliorated by lying on abdomen	Con.
Abdomen	distension of abdomen, ameliorated from motion	Cedr.
Abdomen	distension of abdomen, ameliorated from stool	Corn.
Abdomen	distension of abdomen, ameliorated from walking	Calad., cedr.
Abdomen	distension of abdomen, before menses	Zinc.
Abdomen	distension of abdomen, from oysters	Bry., lyc.
Abdomen	distension of abdomen, painful	Acon., alum., ant-t., Ars., bar-c., bell., Bry., calad., canth., Caust., cham., hell., hyos., kali-i., Lach., merc-c., Merc., nat-c., nat-m., nux-v., Rhus-t., sulph., verat.
Abdomen	distension of abdomen, painful before stool	Ars., corn., fl-ac., phyt.
Abdomen	distesion of abdomen, after contradiction	Nux-m.
Abdomen	distesion of abdomen, after dinner	Ant-c., dig., kalm., zinc.
Abdomen	distesion of abdomen, after drinking	Manc., tab.
Abdomen	distesion of abdomen, after pickled fish	Calad.
Abdomen	distesion of abdomen, ameliorated after eating	Cedr., rat.
Abdomen	distesion of abdomen, ameliorated after eructations	Arg-n., Carb-v., mag-c., nat-s.
Abdomen	distesion of abdomen, ameliorated after passing flatus	Rat.
Abdomen	distesion of abdomen, before dinner	Rat.
Abdomen	distesion of abdomen, during convulsion	Cic.
Abdomen	distesion of abdomen, in night, on waking	Asaf.
Abdomen	distesion of abdomen, in afternoon	Nat-m., petr., sulph.
Abdomen	distesion of abdomen, in evening	Dios., eupi., kali-bi., osm.
Abdomen	distesion of abdomen, in forenoon	Myric.
Abdomen	distesion of abdomen, in morning	Nux-v., phos.
Abdomen	distesion of abdomen, not ameliorated after eructations	Chin., echi., lyc.

Body part/Disease	Symptom	Medicines
Abdomen	distesion of abdomen, while eating	Con.
Abdomen	dropsy (a buildup of excess serous fluid between tissue cells) due to ascites (an accumulation of fluid serous fluid in the peritoneal cavity, causing abdominal swelling) with chronic diarrhoea	Apoc., oena.
Abdomen	dropsy due to ascites (accumulation of fluid serous fluid in the peritoneal cavity, causing abdominal swelling) with induration (hardness in body tissue) of liver	Aur., lact.
Abdomen	dysuria with suppressed menses and drawing pain in abdomen	Puls.
Abdomen	emaciation (become thin) of the muscles of abdomen	Plb.
Abdomen	emptyness of abdomen, after breakfast	Am-m., coca., colch., dig., lyc., puls.
Abdomen	emptyness of abdomen, after dinner	Lyc., ptel., thea., zinc.
Abdomen	emptyness of abdomen, after nursing	Carb-an., olnd.
Abdomen	emptyness of abdomen, after siesta (afternoon rest)	Ang.
Abdomen	emptyness of abdomen, after stool	Aloe., ambr., dios., fl-ac., Petr, ph-ac., puls., sep., sulph.
Abdomen	emptyness of abdomen, after vomitting	Ther.
Abdomen	emptyness of abdomen, aggravated from inspiration	Calad.
Abdomen	emptyness of abdomen, ameliorated from eructations	Sep.
Abdomen	emptyness of abdomen, before sleep	Dig.
Abdomen	emptyness of abdomen, during fever	Zinc.
Abdomen	emptyness of abdomen, during headache	Cocc., nat-m., phos., ptel., sang., Sep.
Abdomen	emptyness of abdomen, during menses	Kali-p., spong., tab.
Abdomen	emptyness of abdomen, when thinking of food	Sep.
Abdomen	emptyness of abdomen, with aversion to food	Bar-c., carb-s., carb-v., chin., cocc., coff., dulc., grat., hell., hydr, nat-m., nux-v., rhus-t., sil., stann., sulph., verb.
Abdomen	emptyness of abdomen, with diarrhoea	Fl-ac., lyc., petr., stram., sulph.
Abdomen	emptyness of abdomen, without hunger	Act-sp., agar., alum., am-m., ars., bar-c., berb., bry., chin-s., chin., cocc., dulc., hell., kali-n., Lach., mur-ac., nat-m., nicc., olnd., op., phos., psor., rhus-t., sil., sul-ac., sulph., tax.
Abdomen	enlarged abdomen of children	Bar-c., Calc., cupr., mag-m., psor., sanic., sars., Sil., sulph.
Abdomen	enlarged abdomen of children with marasmus (a gradual wasting away of the body, generally associated with severe malnutrition or inadequate absorption of food and occurring mainly in young children)	Calc., sanic., sars.
Abdomen	enlarged abdomen of fat children	Am-m., calc.
Abdomen	erection strong with pain in abdomen	Zinc.
Abdomen	eruptions on abdomen	Agar., anac., apis., ars., bar-m., bry., calc., graph., kali-ar., kali-bi., kali-c., merc-c., merc., nat-c., nat-m., phos., rhus-t., sulph.

Body part/Disease	Symptom	Medicines
Abdomen	eruptions on abdomen, itching	Agar., calc., merc., rhus-t., sulph.
Abdomen	eruptions on abdomen,moist	Merc.
Abdomen	eruption, pustular (a small round raised area of inflamed skin filled with pus) on abdomen	Crot-c., crot-t., kali-bi., merc., puls., squil.
Abdomen	erysipelas on abdomen	Graph.
Abdomen	excoriated perineum (region of the abdomen surrounding the urogenital and anal openings)	Calc., carb-v., caust., Graph., hep., Lyc., merc., petr., sep., sulph., thuj.
Abdomen	excoriation (to remove skin off) over inguinal (area between thigh and abdomen) region	Ars., arum-t., bov., graph.
Abdomen	excoriation over inguinal region during menses	Bov.
Abdomen	faintness from pain in abdomen	Cocc., plb.
Abdomen	fatty abdomen	Am-m., calc., Chel.
Abdomen	feeling of tightnes in abdomen during stool	Sulph.
Abdomen	feeling of tightnes in abdomen aggravated while rising	Zinc.
Abdomen	feeling of tightnes in abdomen ameliorated by passing flatus	Sil.
Abdomen	feeling of tightnes in abdomen as by string	Caust., Chel.
Abdomen	feeling of tightnes in abdomen at night	Phos., sulph.
Abdomen	feeling of tightnes in abdomen during cough	Lach.
Abdomen	feeling of tightnes in abdomen during fasting	Carb-an.
Abdomen	feeling of tightnes in abdomen during menses	Cact., cocc., croc., sulph.
Abdomen	feeling of tightnes in abdomen in morning	Calc.
Abdomen	feeling of tightnes in abdomen relaxed after stool	Mag-m., phos., sep., sulph.
Abdomen	feeling of tightnes in abdomen while lying	Zinc.
Abdomen	feeling of tightnes in hypochondria	Acon., arg-n., Cact., calc., chel., con., Crot-c., dig., dros., kreos., Lyc., nux-v., puls., sep., staph., sulph., tarent.
Abdomen	feeling of tightnes in hypochondria (the area of the upper abdomen on each side of the epigastrium below the lower ribs) extending to umbilicus	Mag-c.
Abdomen	feeling of tightnes in hypogastrium	Bar-c., bell., chel., clem., coloc., euon., hydr., sars., thuj., verb.
Abdomen	feeling of tightnes in hypogastrium (the part of the front of the abdomen that lies below the navel) in evening	Sars.
Abdomen	feeling of tightnes in hypogastrium in forenoon	Sars.
Abdomen	feeling of tightnes in inguinal region extending around pelvis (any basin or cup-shaped anatomical cavity, e.g. the region of the kidney into which urine is discharged before its passage into the ureter)	Cact.
Abdomen	feeling of tightnes in inguinal ameliorated by stretching	Bov.
Abdomen	feeling of tightnes in inguinal region	Bov., cact., gamb., kali-n., mag-c., rat.

Body part/Disease	Symptom	Medicines
Abdomen	feeling relaxed in abdomen, ameliorated by lying on back	Cast-v.
Abdomen	fermentation in abdomen (the breakdown of carbohydrates by microorganisms) causing rumbling	Agar., ambr., aran., brom., bry., calc., carb-an., carb-v., Chin., coff., croc., gran., hell., hep., Lyc., mag-m., merl., mur-ac., nat-m., nat-s., phos., plb., rhus-t., sars., seneg., stram., sulph.
Abdomen	fermentation in abdomen (the breakdown of carbohydrates by microorganisms) causing rumbling (deep rolling sound) after fruit	Chin.
Abdomen	fermentation in abdomen (the breakdown of carbohydrates by microorganisms) causing rumbling during menses	Lachn., Lyc., phos.
Abdomen	flexed thigh, upon abdomen	Arg-n., ars., carb-v., cham., cina., cupr., hydr-ac., hyos., merc-c., mur-ac., ox-ac., plb., verat., zinc.
Abdomen	formication in thigh extending to abdomen	Ars.
Abdomen	formication over abdomen	Aloe., ars., calad., calc., camph., carb-v., caust., colch., coloc., crot-t., cycl., dulc., mag-m., paeon., pall., pic-ac., Plat., stann., zinc.
Abdomen	fullness in hypogastrium region	Aesc., bar-c., bell., carb-v., sulph.
Abdomen	hardness of abdomen after eating	Con., phos.
Abdomen	hardness of abdomen in children	Calc., sil.
Abdomen	hardness of abdomen in umbilicus region	Bry., plb., rhus-t.
Abdomen	head heated from pain in abdomen	Grat.
Abdomen	headache alternating with pain in abdomen	Aesc., ars., cina., gels., iris., plb., rhus-r.
Abdomen	hernia inguinal in right side of abdomen in children	Aur., lyc.
Abdomen	hernia inguinal in left side of abdomen in children	Nux-v.
Abdomen	herpes (a viral infection causing small painful blisters and inflammation) on abdomen	Sep.
Abdomen	impeded, obstructed breath from constriction in abdomen	Anan.
Abdomen	inflammation of serous membranes (a thin moist transparent membrane that lines the body cavities and surrounds the internal organs, e.g. the peritoneum that lines the abdomen)	**Acon.**, am-c., **Apis.**, apoc., arg-m., ars-i., **Ars.**, asaf., aur-m., aur., bell., **Bry.**, calc-p., **Calc.**, carb-v., colch., ferr., fl-ac., **Hell.**, indg., iod., kali-c., lach., led., **Lyc.**, mag-m., merc., nat-m., ph-ac., phos., plat., psor., puls., samb., seneg., **Sil.**, squil., stram., sulph., ter., zinc.
Abdomen	intussusception (a condition of the bowel in which this happens, creating swelling that leads to obstruction)	Acon., arn., Ars., bell., bry., colch., coloc., cupr., kali-bi., kreos., lach., lob., lyc., merc., nux-v., Op., phos., Plb., rhus-t., samb., sulph., tab., tarent., thuj., Verat.
Abdomen	itching in hypochondrium (upper region of the abdomen just below the lowest ribs on either side of the epigastrium)	Agar., tab.
Abdomen	itching in hypochondrium at night	Agar.
Abdomen	itching in Hypogastrium (The part of the front of the abdomen that lies below the navel) ameliorated by scratching	Ph-ac.
Abdomen	itching in Hypogastrium (The part of the front of the abdomen that lies below the navel)	Agar., anac., carb-ac., elaps., indg., kali-c., merc., nat-c., nat-m., ph-ac., rhus-t., rhus-v., zinc.

Body part/Disease	Symptom	Medicines
Abdomen	itching in inguinal (lower abdominal wall) region	Agar., agn., ammc., cycl., form., laur., lyc., mag-c., mag-m., merc., rhus-t., rumx., spig., spong., ter.
Abdomen	itching in inguinal region ameliorated by scratching	Laur., mag-c., mag-s.
Abdomen	itching in inguinal region extending to knee	Ars-m.
Abdomen	itching in inguinal region in bed	Sep., verat-v.
Abdomen	itching in inguinal region in evening	Pall., sep.
Abdomen	itching in inguinal region not ameliorated by scratching	Mag-m.
Abdomen	itching in left inguinal region	Cycl., pall., spig.
Abdomen	itching in umbilicus region	Aloe., aur-m., carb-v., cist., ign., kali-c., phos., puls., sulph.
Abdomen	itching of abdomen ameliorated by scratching	Arn., ferr-ma., mez., sars.
Abdomen	itching of abdomen at night	Agar., crot-t., nux-v., phos., Sulph., thuj.
Abdomen	itching of abdomen at night on going to bed	Thuj.
Abdomen	itching of abdomen undressing while	Cact., nux-v.
Abdomen	movements in abdomen before stool	Mang.
Abdomen	movements in abdomen disturbs sleep	Con.
Abdomen	movements in abdomen painful	Arn., op., puls., Sil.
Abdomen	movements up and down of something in abdomen	Lyc.
Abdomen	nausea after operation of abdomen	Bism., staph.
Abdomen	numbness in hips extending to abdomen while standing	Sulph.
Abdomen	numbness in upper arm with colic	Aran.
Abdomen	ovaries painful extending to abdomen	Con., ham., lil-t.
Abdomen	pain behind sternum (chitinous ventral plate covering the abdomen)	Agar., arg-n., cact., chel., cimx., eup-per., Ind., kali-bi., lob., phos., rumx., Sang., seneg., sil., syph., ter.
Abdomen	pain between scapula extending to sternum (abdominal covering)	Kali-bi., lac-c.
Abdomen	pain in abdomen after beer	Carb-s., nux-v.
Abdomen	pain in abdomen after bread	Acon., ant-c., bar-c., Bry., Caust., coff., kali-c., merc., phos., puls., rhus-t., ruta., sars., staph., sul-ac., zinc., zing.
Abdomen	pain in abdomen after breakfast	Agar., all-c., aloe., anac., ars., calc-s., carb-s., caust., crot-h., cycl., kali-bi., myric., nat-c., puls., sulph.
Abdomen	pain in abdomen after cereal grains	Merc-c.
Abdomen	pain in abdomen after coffee	Cham., cocc., dig., ign., nux-v.
Abdomen	pain in abdomen after cold drinks	Acon., aloe., am-br., ant-c., arg-n., Ars., bry., calad., calc-ar., calc-p., calc., carb-s., caust., ferr-ar., ferr., graph., iris., kali-ar., kali-c., lyc., manc., nat-c., nit-ac., nux-v., ol-an., rhod., Rhus-t., sil., sul-ac., tarent., tep.
Abdomen	pain in abdomen after cold food	Carb-v., caust., kreos., lyc., mang., sul-ac.
Abdomen	pain in abdomen after dinner	Acon., agar., alum., am-c., arg-n., ars., Calc-p., cast-eq., chin., clem., cob., coc-c., coloc., crot-h., dig., elaps., hyper., laur., mag-c., mez., myric., nat-c., nux-m., petr., phos., rhod., sep., sulph., trom., verat.

Body part/Disease	Symptom	Medicines
Abdomen	pain in abdomen after disappointment	Carb-v.
Abdomen	pain in abdomen after drinking	Acon., aloe., apis., Apoc., arn., bell., canth., chel., chin., coloc., daph., ferr., iris., kali-c., kali-s., lac-c., lact-ac., manc., merc-c., nat-c., nat-m., nit-ac., nux-v., ol-an., plb., rhod., rhus-t., sec., sil., sul-ac., sulph.
Abdomen	pain in abdomen after eating	Con., grat., nux-m., Nux-v., tarent.
Abdomen	pain in abdomen after fat food	Ars., caust., Puls.
Abdomen	pain in abdomen after flatulent food	Carb-v.
Abdomen	pain in abdomen after fruit	Bor., Calc-p., chin., Coloc., lyc., mag-m., merc-c., puls., Verat.
Abdomen	pain in abdomen after ice cream	Arg-n., Ars., calc-p., ip., puls., sep.
Abdomen	pain in abdomen after meat	Calc., ferr., kali-bi., ptel.
Abdomen	pain in abdomen after menses	Bell., bor., kali-c., lach., sulph.
Abdomen	pain in abdomen after milk	Alum., Ang., Ang., ars., bry., bufo., carb-v., con., ferr., hyper., lac-d., mag-c., Mag-m., mag-s., nat-c., petr., samb.,sul-ac., sulph.
Abdomen	pain in abdomen after pears	Bor.
Abdomen	pain in abdomen after plums	Rheum.
Abdomen	pain in abdomen after potatoes	Alum., coloc.
Abdomen	pain in abdomen after potatoes	Alum., coloc., mag-s., merc-c.
Abdomen	pain in abdomen after rich food	Ars., ip., ptel., Puls.
Abdomen	pain in abdomen after shell fish	Brom.
Abdomen	pain in abdomen after soup	Ars., indg.
Abdomen	pain in abdomen after stool	Calc-s., calc., con., ferr., puls., sulph.
Abdomen	pain in abdomen after sugar	Alum., bry., calc., chin., coff., ferr., gels., kali-n., Ox-ac., puls., zinc.
Abdomen	pain in abdomen after taking cheese	Ptel.
Abdomen	pain in abdomen after vomitting	Ant-t., lach.
Abdomen	pain in abdomen after wine	Bry., Lyc.
Abdomen	pain in abdomen aggravated by eructations	Cham., cocc., phos.
Abdomen	pain in abdomen aggravated from hot drinks	Brom., graph., kali-c.
Abdomen	pain in abdomen aggravated from lying on abdomen	Ambr.
Abdomen	pain in abdomen aggravated from warm food	Brom., chin., fl-ac., ign., Phos., Puls.
Abdomen	pain in abdomen aggravated from yawning	Ars.
Abdomen	pain in abdomen aggravated on passing flatus	Aur., canth., fl-ac., nat-a., squil.
Abdomen	pain in abdomen amelioated from lying	Am-c., bry., canth., cupr., dios., gran., merc., nux-v., phys.
Abdomen	pain in abdomen amelioated from lying on abdomen	Aloe., am-c., ars-h., Bell., bry., chin-a., chion., coloc., Ind., phos., plb., rhus-t., stann.
Abdomen	pain in abdomen amelioated from lying on back	Coloc., kalm., mez., onos.
Abdomen	pain in abdomen amelioated from lying on left side	Pall., sec.
Abdomen	pain in abdomen amelioated from lying on right side	Nux-v., phos., phys.

Body part/Disease	Symptom	Medicines
Abdomen	pain in abdomen amelioated from lying on side	Nat-s.
Abdomen	pain in abdomen ameliorated after dinner	Chel., graph., mang.
Abdomen	pain in abdomen ameliorated when flow becomes free	when : Bell., kali-c., kali-p., lach., lap-a., mosch., sep., sulph.
Abdomen	pain in abdomen ameliorated after bread	Nat-c.
Abdomen	pain in abdomen ameliorated after cold food	Phos.
Abdomen	pain in abdomen ameliorated after eating	Aur-m., bov., chel., iod., mang., mez., nat-c., plan., psor.
Abdomen	pain in abdomen ameliorated after eating	Aesc., agar., anac., aur., brom., cham., chel., chin-a., cina., dios., fago., gamb., Graph., hep., ign., iod., iris., kali-bi., kalm., lach., lith., mag-m., mang., med., mez., nat-c., nat-s., nicc., ox-ac., petr., phos., raph., verat.
Abdomen	pain in abdomen ameliorated after food	Mag-c., ph-ac.
Abdomen	pain in abdomen ameliorated after ice cream	Phos.
Abdomen	pain in abdomen ameliorated after milk	Chel., crot-t., op.
Abdomen	pain in abdomen ameliorated after stool	Chel.
Abdomen	pain in abdomen ameliorated after urination	Carb-an.
Abdomen	pain in abdomen ameliorated after warm drinks	Acon., chel., mag-p., spong.
Abdomen	pain in abdomen ameliorated by drawing up the limbs	Bry., chel.
Abdomen	pain in abdomen ameliorated by knee-elbow position	Con.
Abdomen	pain in abdomen ameliorated by passing flatus	Agar., chel., dig., hep., lact., tarent.
Abdomen	pain in abdomen ameliorated from bending backward	Bell., bism., caust., kali-c.
Abdomen	pain in abdomen ameliorated from bending double	Alumn., carb-v., cham., chel., colch., Coloc., lach., lyc., nux-v., psor., ptel., verat-v.
Abdomen	pain in abdomen ameliorated from heat	Ars., bry., caust., chel., lyc., mag-p., nux-v., sil.
Abdomen	pain in abdomen ameliorated from legs drawn up	Ars., bry., caust., chel., lyc., mag-p., nux-v., sil.
Abdomen	pain in abdomen ameliorated from lying on abdomen	Elaps.
Abdomen	pain in abdomen ameliorated from lying on back	Calc., laur.
Abdomen	pain in abdomen ameliorated from pressure	Alumn., coloc., dios., mag-p., mang., plb., stann.
Abdomen	pain in abdomen ameliorated from rubbing	Lyc.
Abdomen	pain in abdomen ameliorated from sitting bent over	Bry., coloc., ox-ac., staph., sulph.
Abdomen	pain in abdomen ameliorated from sitting erect	Dios.
Abdomen	pain in abdomen ameliorated from stretching	Dios., nat-c.
Abdomen	pain in abdomen ameliorated from warm application	Chel., Mag-p., nux-m., nux-v., sil.
Abdomen	pain in abdomen ameliorated from warm drinks	Alum., ars., bry., graph., mang., nux-m., Nux-v., ph-ac., rhus-t., spong., sulph., verat.
Abdomen	pain in abdomen ameliorated from warm milk	Chel., graph.
Abdomen	pain in abdomen ameliorated from warmth of bed	Carb-v., graph., lyc., Nux-v.
Abdomen	pain in abdomen ameliorated from yawning	Lyc., nat-m.
Abdomen	pain in abdomen ameliorated on bending backward	Bell., dios., lac-c., nux-v., onos.

Body part/Disease	Symptom	Medicines
Abdomen	pain in abdomen ameliorated on motion	Aur-m., bov., cycl., kali-n., petr., phos., ptel., rhus-t., sulph.
Abdomen	pain in abdomen ameliorated when over heated	Alumn., arg-n., calc-s., caust., Phos., puls., tep.
Abdomen	pain in abdomen ameliorated while lying	Am-c., bell., caust., chin., graph., kali-i., lach., lyc., sil., stann.
Abdomen	pain in abdomen appears and disappears gradually	stannum
Abdomen	pain in abdomen appears gradually and disappears suddenly	Arg-m.
Abdomen	pain in abdomen as if squeezed (To press something hard in the hand in order to reduce its size or alter its shape) between two stones	Coloc.
Abdomen	pain in abdomen at beginning of menses	Calc., caust., graph., kali-c., lap-a., lyc., mag-c.
Abdomen	pain in abdomen before breakfast	Arg-n., bufo., iris., Nat-s.
Abdomen	pain in abdomen before dinner	Graph., lyc., nat-m., phos.
Abdomen	pain in abdomen before menses	Aur-s., bell., bor., cupr., lach., mag-c., nux-m., puls., sep., sulph., tarent.
Abdomen	pain in abdomen before passing flatus	Calc-p., Chin., nit-ac.
Abdomen	pain in abdomen before stool	Alum., ars., coloc., nat-c., rhus-t.
Abdomen	pain in abdomen comes gradually and goes gradually	Plat., stann.
Abdomen	pain in abdomen comes quickly and goes quickly	Bell., vib.
Abdomen	pain in abdomen during deep inspiration	Card-m.
Abdomen	pain in abdomen during dinner	Corn., thuj.
Abdomen	pain in abdomen during hunger	Hura., Merc., petr., psor., stram.
Abdomen	pain in abdomen during inspiration	Aesc., agar., am-m., anac., brom., bry., calc., carb-s., caust., nux-v., rhus-t., rumx., sulph., thuj.
Abdomen	pain in abdomen during labour pain	Sep.
Abdomen	pain in abdomen during menses	Am-c., ars., bor., caps., carb-s., caul., caust., cham., cocc., cupr., graph., kali-c., kali-i., kali-p., lac-c., nux-m., nux-v., phos., puls., sars., Sulph., thuj., zinc.
Abdomen	pain in abdomen during nausea	Glon.
Abdomen	pain in abdomen during night after acids	Ant-c., kreos., sulph.
Abdomen	pain in abdomen during night alternating with pain in limbs	Kali-bi.
Abdomen	pain in abdomen during night ameliorated in open air	Naja.
Abdomen	pain in abdomen during pregnancy	Con., dios., ip.
Abdomen	pain in abdomen during stool	Bell., con., dios., kali-c., lyc., mag-m., puls., ran-b., rhod., sars.
Abdomen	pain in abdomen during urination	Ip., laur.
Abdomen	pain in abdomen extendimg into chest	Aloe., alum., dulc., grat., hyos., kali-c., lach., mag-c., merl., nat-m., par., phos., plb., raph.
Abdomen	pain in abdomen extendimg into groins	Plb.
Abdomen	pain in abdomen extendimg to back	Absin., aloe., bell., bor., chel., con., cycl., ferr., hep., ign., indg., mag-m., nat-m., ph-ac., phos., puls., sulph., ter.

Body part/Disease	Symptom	Medicines
Abdomen	pain in abdomen extendimg to back between shoulders	Bell.
Abdomen	pain in abdomen extendimg to bladder and testes	Kali-c.
Abdomen	pain in abdomen extendimg to heart	Lach., sol-n., stry.
Abdomen	pain in abdomen extendimg to hypochondria (area of the upper abdomen on each side of the epigastrium below the lower ribs)	Aesc., phos., verat.
Abdomen	pain in abdomen extendimg to left scapula	Arg-n.
Abdomen	pain in abdomen extendimg to left shoulder	Sol-n.
Abdomen	pain in abdomen extendimg to limbs	Plb.
Abdomen	pain in abdomen extendimg to navel	Brom.
Abdomen	pain in abdomen extendimg to oesophagus (passage down which food moves between the throat and the stomach)	Aeth., brom.
Abdomen	pain in abdomen extendimg to sternum	Nat-m., rheum.
Abdomen	pain in abdomen extendimg to throat	Aloe., alum., con., cupr-ac., grat., mag-m., nat-m.
Abdomen	pain in abdomen extending spine	Iod., lyc., sil.
Abdomen	pain in abdomen extending testicles (the male or sperm-producing gland testis usually with its surrounding membranes)	Dig., plb., Puls., sec., sil., teucr.
Abdomen	pain in abdomen extending thigh	Aloe., bar-c., cham., coloc., con., kali-i., nat-m., nux-v., sep., stram., ter., ust.
Abdomen	pain in abdomen extending throat	Caust., kali-bi., kreos., merc.
Abdomen	pain in abdomen extending to front of left shoulder	Agar.
Abdomen	pain in abdomen extending to genitals	Alumn., calc., crot-t., dig., lyc., plb., Puls., rhus-t., sep., tep., teucr., verat.
Abdomen	pain in abdomen extending to head	Ars., mang.
Abdomen	pain in abdomen extending to hip	Kali-c., lyc.
Abdomen	pain in abdomen extending to inguinal (area between thighs and abdomen) region	Arg-n., bar-c., kali-i., tarent., thuj.
Abdomen	pain in abdomen extending to left side of abdomen	Colch.
Abdomen	pain in abdomen extending to leg	Carb-v., ter., thuj.
Abdomen	pain in abdomen extending to loins (the area on each side of the backbone between the ribs and hips)	Kali-bi., kali-i.
Abdomen	pain in abdomen extending to lower limbs	Bar-c., Carb-v., kali-i., plb., sang., sep.
Abdomen	pain in abdomen extending to mammae (a woman's breast)	Ferr-m.
Abdomen	pain in abdomen extending to penis	Alumn., puls.
Abdomen	pain in abdomen extending to pubic (lower front of hipbone) region	Coloc., sep.
Abdomen	pain in abdomen extending to rectum (the lower part of the large intestine, between the colon and the anal canal)	Aloe., brom., eupi., mag-m., nat-m., nux-v., sang.
Abdomen	pain in abdomen extending to right mammae	Coloc.

Body part/Disease	Symptom	Medicines
Abdomen	pain in abdomen extending to scrotum (pouch containing testicles)	Verat.
Abdomen	pain in abdomen extending to shoulder	Lach.
Abdomen	pain in abdomen extending vagina	Ars., berb., calc-p., kreos., nit-ac.
Abdomen	pain in abdomen from clothing	Am-c., calc., kali-bi., lyc., nat-m., sep.
Abdomen	pain in abdomen from constipation	Ars., bell., con., cupr., kali-c., merc., op., plb., sil., sul-ac., thuj.
Abdomen	pain in abdomen from coughing	Am-c., apoc., arn., ars., arund., bell., Bry., cadm., calc., camph., chin-a., chin., chlor., cor-r., dros., hell., hyos., ip., kali-bi., lach., lob., Lyc., mang., nit-ac., nux-v., phos., puls., rhus-t., rumx., ruta., sabad., sep., sil., squil., Stann.
Abdomen	pain in abdomen from fright	Carb-v., ign.
Abdomen	pain in abdomen from haemorrhoids (painful varicose veins in the canal of the anus)	Aesc., carb-v., coloc., lach., nux-v., puls., sulph., valer.
Abdomen	pain in abdomen from inspiring deep	Arg-n., asar., bry., carb-an., caust., cor-r., dros., ign., kali-n., nat-m., op., phyt., puls., zinc.
Abdomen	pain in abdomen from lifting	Arn., bry., calc.
Abdomen	pain in abdomen from raising arm high	Arg-n.
Abdomen	pain in abdomen from sitting erect	Gels.
Abdomen	pain in abdomen from suppressed eructations	Bar-c., con.
Abdomen	pain in abdomen from taking cold	All-c., alum., carb-v., Cham., Chin., coloc., Dulc., hep., lyc., merc., nat-c., nit-ac., nux-v., Verat.
Abdomen	pain in abdomen from turning on bed	Alum., bapt.
Abdomen	pain in abdomen in damp weather	Kali-c., mang.
Abdomen	pain in abdomen in drunkards	Calc., carb-v., lach., nux-v., sul-ac., sulph.
Abdomen	pain in abdomen instead of menses	Lach.
Abdomen	pain in abdomen on bending backward	Anac., thuj.
Abdomen	pain in abdomen on bending double	Kalm., lyc.
Abdomen	pain in abdomen on breathing	Anac., ars., caps., coc-c., lyc., mang., puls.
Abdomen	pain in abdomen on breathing deep	Caust.
Abdomen	pain in abdomen on every attempt to eat	Calc-p.
Abdomen	pain in abdomen on expiration (relating to the process of breathing out)	Brom., dig.
Abdomen	pain in abdomen on fasting	Dulc., gran., hell.
Abdomen	pain in abdomen on sneezing (forcefully, and involuntarily expel air through the nose and mouth because of irritation of the nasal passages)	Bell., canth., cham., eupi., Ind., pall.
Abdomen	pain in abdomen on waking	Agar., caust., cycl., lach., lyc., nat-m., nicc., nit-ac., phyt., staph.
Abdomen	pain in abdomen radiating (parts spreading out from a common)	Dios., ip., Mag-p., plb.
Abdomen	pain in abdomen when over heated	Acon., kali-c., nat-c.
Abdomen	pain in abdomen while eating	Acon., ant-t., arn., ars., bry., calc-p., cic., coff., con., corn., crot-c., led., mang., merc., op., phos., plb., puls., sep., thuj., verat.

Body part/Disease	Symptom	Medicines
Abdomen	pain in abdomen while exercising	Ang., bry., cann-s., caust., cupr.
Abdomen	pain in abdomen while fasting	Bar-c., calc., caust., cocc., fago., Graph., hura., ign., lach., lob., nit-ac., petr., psor., rhod., seneg., sep.
Abdomen	pain in abdomen while lying	Apis., bar-c., bell., coloc., dios., phos., puls., spig.
Abdomen	pain in abdomen while sitting	Acon., ambr., ars., asaf., caust., elaps., hep., nat-c., nat-s., phos., puls., sulph.
Abdomen	pain in abdomen while straining (make extreme effort) for stool	Acon., aloe., bell., bry., podo.
Abdomen	pain in abdomen with fainting	Bism., nux-v., ran-s.
Abdomen	pain in abdomen, periodical	Arg-n., calc., cupr., graph., hyos., ign., iod., lyc.
Abdomen	pain in abdomen, radiating	Dios., kali-c., plb.
Abdomen	pain in abdomen, sudden	Cic., cupr., elaps.
Abdomen	pain in abdomen, violent ameliorated from walking	Nit-ac.
Abdomen	pain in abdomen, violent ameliorated while walking	All-c., bor., bov., dios., elaps., lyc., nat-c., op., stann.
Abdomen	pain in back ameliorated from lying on abdomen	Acet-ac., chel., mag-c., nit-ac., sel.
Abdomen	pain in back extending to abdomen	Cham.
Abdomen	pain in bladder ameliorated from lying on abdomen	Chel.
Abdomen	pain in cervical region extending to epigastrium (upper mid-abdomen)	Crot-c.
Abdomen	pain in chest alternating with pain in abdomen	Aesc., ran-b.
Abdomen	pain in chest ameliorated while lying on abdomen	Bry.
Abdomen	pain in coccyx ameliorated from pressure on abdomen	Merc.
Abdomen	pain in eye alternates with pain in abdomen	Euphr.
Abdomen	pain in heart extending to sternum	Spig.
Abdomen	pain in ilium extending around abdomen	Berb.
Abdomen	pain in ilium extending to abdomen	Berb., bry., cham., kreos., lach.
Abdomen	pain in ilium extending to the epigastric region at night	Lyc.
Abdomen	pain in joints alternating with colic	Plb.
Abdomen	pain in kidney ameliorated while lying on abdomen	Chel.
Abdomen	pain in kidney extending over abdomen	Hydr-ac.,Berb., canth., kali-bi., nux-v.
Abdomen	pain in kidney extending over epigastrium (upper mid-abdomen)	Hydr-ac.
Abdomen	pain in kidneys ameliorated from lying on abdomen	Chel.
Abdomen	pain in kidneys extending over abdomen	Hydr-ac.
Abdomen	pain in kidneys extending to epigastrium	Hydr-ac.
Abdomen	pain in larynx extending to abdomen	Crot-c.
Abdomen	pain in lumbar region ameliorated while lying on abdomen	Chel., nit-ac., sel.
Abdomen	pain in lumbar region over to the hypochondrium in morning on waking	Kali-n.
Abdomen	pain in lumbar region to the perineum (the region of the abdomen surrounding the urogenital and anal openings)	Canth.

Body part/Disease	Symptom	Medicines
Abdomen	pain in region of diaphragm	Echi., nux-m.
Abdomen	pain in region of diaphragm in forenoon	Nux-m.
Abdomen	pain in spine extending to epigastrium (the upper middle part of the abdomen)	Nicc., rat., thuj.
Abdomen	pain in testes extending to abdomen	Iod.
Abdomen	pain in uvula extending to abdomen (the part of the body that contains the stomach, intestines, and other organs.It is situated between the pelvis and the thorax)	Iod.
Abdomen	pain, burning in larynx extending to abdomen	Ambr.
Abdomen	palpitation of heart with colic (a sudden attack of abdominal pain, often caused by spasm, inflammation, or obstruction)	Plb.
Abdomen	paralysis of diaphragm (A curved muscular membrane that separates the abdomen from the area around the lungs)	Bell., cact., cimic., cupr., mez., mosch., rhus-t., sil.
Abdomen	paralysis of lower limb with colic	Plb.
Abdomen	paralysis of lower limb with pain in abdomen like lightening	Thal.
Abdomen	perspiration during colic	Mez., nux-v., plan., plb., sulph.
Abdomen	perspiration in lower limbs during menstrual colic	Ant-t.
Abdomen	perspiration in sternum	Graph.
Abdomen	pimples on abdomen	Ambr., calad., chel., graph., kali-bi., lach., merc., nat-m., nit-ac., sil., thuj., til.
Abdomen	readily take cold (viral infection of nose and throat), large heads and abdomens, open fontanelles and sutures, and crooked legs	Calc.
Abdomen	retention of urine from colic	Arn., coloc., Plb., thuj.
Abdomen	rumbling in abdomen before stool	Ars., asc-t., brom., cact., carb-s., card-m., colch., dulc., ferr-i., form., gnaph., grat., hell., indg., iris., jatr., kali-ar., kali-c., kali-s., Mag-c., mag-m., merc., mur-ac., nat-m., nat-s., nux-v., olnd., ox-ac., phos., rat., rhod., sabad., spig., spong., stront., sulph., tax.
Abdomen	rumbling in abdomen during diarrhoea	Crot-t., glon., hyos., iris., kali-c.
Abdomen	sensation as if abdomen full of water	Kali-c., mill., ol-an., phel.
Abdomen	sensation as if something alive in abdomen	Chel., coloc., Croc., tarent.
Abdomen	sensation of ball in abdomen	Bell., coc-c., lach., senec.
Abdomen	sensation of bubbling in abdomen	Caust., lyss.
Abdomen	sensation of burning ball in abdomen	Bell.
Abdomen	sensation of burning ball rising up from abdomen into throat	Lach., senec.
Abdomen	sensation of emptynes behind sternum	Zinc.
Abdomen	sensation of lump (tumor) in abdomen	Ant-t., bry., nux-m., plb., rhus-t., sulph., thuj.
Abdomen	sensation of lump in abdomen after cold drinks	Acet-ac., ars.
Abdomen	sensation of lump in abdomen after eating	Abies-n., ars., med., nat-m., nux-v., ph-ac., puls., rumx.

Body part/Disease	Symptom	Medicines
Abdomen	sensation of lump in abdomen ameliorated after eructation	Bar-c.
Abdomen	sensation of lump in abdomen while lying on back	Sulph.
Abdomen	sensation of lump in middle of sternum	Chin., puls.
Abdomen	sensation of lump under sternum	Lec.
Abdomen	sensation of movement in abdomen	Arn., chel., cocc., colch., coloc., Croc., kali-n., laur., lyss., nat-m., nicc., olnd., phos., sul-ac., tarent.
Abdomen	sleepiness during pain in abdomen	Ant-t.
Abdomen	sleeplessness from pulsation of body & abdomen	Sil.
Abdomen	sleeps on abdomen	Acet-ac., ars., bell., bry., calc-p., calc., cina., cocc., coloc., crot-t., ign., lac-c., podo., puls., stann., stram.
Abdomen	sleeps on abdomen with one arm under the head	Cocc.
Abdomen	sleeps with arm on abdomen	Cocc., **Puls.**
Abdomen	stitching pain in chest extending to hypochondrium	Berb.
Abdomen	stitching pain in chest extending to sternum	Laur.
Abdomen	stretching during colic	Haem.
Abdomen	sweating during night with pain in abdomen	Crot-t.
Abdomen	trembling after colic	Plb.
Abdomen	twisting in abdomen aggravated by eating	Grat.
Abdomen	twisting in abdomen extending to abdomen	Arg-n.
Abdomen	twisting in abdomen sudden	Chin.
Abdomen	ulcer in sternum	Calc-p.
Abdomen	ulcer in abdomen	Arg-n., ars., calc-ar., calc., caust., cur., Hydr., Kali-bi., kali-c., kreos., Lyc., merc-c., mez., nat-p., nit-ac., nux-v., Phos., sil., sul-ac., syph., uran.
Abdomen	ulcer in abdomen	Arg-n., Ars., bar-m., calc., Carb-v., chin., coloc., cupr., hep., kali-bi., lach., lyc., merc., Nit-ac., phos., plb., sil., sulph., Ter.
Abdomen	ulcer in abdomen spreading	Ars.
Abdomen	urging for during colic	Coloc., Ind., Nux-v.
Abdomen	urging to urinate in bladder on touching abdomen	Acon.
Abdomen	urticaria in abdomen	Bry., kali-i.
Abdomen	varicose vein on abdomen	Berb., sep.
Abdomen	veins (a blood vessel that carries blood to the heart and around the body) of abdomen distended	Berb., sep.
Abdomen	vesicles on abdomen	Clem., mag-c., ph-ac., sep., vip.
Abdomen	vomiting bile with colic	Chin., coloc., iod., nux-v.
Abdomen	warts on sternum	Nit-ac.
Abortion	abortion (an involuntary ending of a pregnancy through the discharge of the fetus from the womb at too early a stage in its development for it to survive) after injuries	Arn., rhus-t.
Abortion	abortion from exertion	Erig., helon., mill., nit-ac., rhus-t.
Abortion	abortion from fright	Acon., gels., ign., op.

Body part/Disease	Symptom	Medicines
Abortion	abortion in early months	Apis.
Abortion	abortion in fifth to seventh month	Sep.
Abortion	abortion in last month	Op.
Abortion	abortion in second month	Apis., kali-c.
Abortion	abortion in third month	Apis., cimic., croc., eup-pur., merc., sabin., sec., thuj., ust.
Abortion	convulsion after miscarriage	Ruta.
Abortion	convulsion of upper limbs after miscarriage	Ruta.
Abortion	cough following difficult labour or abortion, with backache and sweat	Kali-c.
Abortion	delirium after miscarriage	Ruta.
Abortion	tendency to abortion	Alet., apis., arg-n., asar., aur., bapt., bufo., calc., carb-v., caul., cimic., ferr., helon., hyos., kali-c., kreos., lyc., nux-m., Plb., puls., sabin., sep., sil., sulph., vib., zinc.
Abscess	abcscess (Pus filled cavity) in external throat	Cham., Hep., kali-c., kali-i., lach., lyc., Merc., nit-ac., phos., psor., sep., Sil., sul-ac., sulph.
Abscess	abscess in lumbar (relating to or situated in the loins or the small of the back) region	Calc-p.
Abscess	abscess at root of nails	Puls.
Abscess	abscess behind ear	Eup-per., rhus-t., tub.
Abscess	abscess below ear	Nat-h.
Abscess	abscess in ankle joint (joint that connects the leg bones with the highest bone in the foot)	Ang., guai., ol-j., sil.
Abscess	abscess in axilla (Arm pit)	Am-c., apis., ars., bell., bufo., cadm., calc-s., calc., cedr., coloc., crot-h., Hep., kali-bi., kali-c., lac-c., merc-i-r., Merc., nat-m., nat-s., Nit-ac., petr., ph-ac., prun-s., Rhus-t., sep., Sil., sulph., thuj.
Abscess	abscess in back of hand	Plb.
Abscess	abscess in calf (the fleshy part at the back of the leg below the knee)	Chin.
Abscess	abscess in cervical (relating to neck or cervix of the womb) region	Lach., lyc., petr., ph-ac., psor., sec., sil., tarent-c.
Abscess	abscess in left lung (either of the paired spongy respiratory organs, situated inside the rib cage, that transfer oxygen into the blood and remove carbon dioxide from it)	Calc.
Abscess	contraction of muscles & tendons of hamstrings after abscess	Lach.
Abscess	old cicatrices (cause a wound to heal and form a scar) due to abscess in cervical region	Sil.
Abuse of Drug	abuse of quinine	Am-c., ant-t., apis., **Arn.**, ars., asaf., bell., bry., **Calc.**, caps., **Carb-v.**, cham., cina., cupr., cycl., dig., ferr-ar., **Ferr.**, gels., hell., **Ip.**, lach., merc., **Nat-m.**, nux-v., ph-ac., phos., plb., **Puls.**, samb., sep., stann., sul-ac., sulph., verat.
Abuse of Drug	abuse of sulphur	Ars., calc., chin., merc., **Puls.**, sep.
Abuse of Drug	after abuse of iron	Ars., puls., sulph., zinc.

Body part/Disease	Symptom	Medicines
Abuse of drug	arsenic poisoning	Camph., chin., ferr., graph., iod., ip., merc., nux-v., samb., verat.
Abuse of Drug	chronic effects of lead poisoning	Alum., alumn., ars., bell., **Caust.**, chin., nux-v., op., plat., sul-ac., sulph.
Abuse of Drug	headache after abuse of drugs	Nux-v.
Abuse of Drug	hearing impaired (lessened) after abuse of quinine	Calc..
Abuse of Drug	warts after abuse of mercury	Aur., nit-ac., staph.
Acne	acne (a disease of the oil-secreting glands of the skin that often affects adolescents, producing eruptions on the face, neck, and shoulders that can leave pitted scars) in coccyx	Carb-v.
Acne	acne in cervical region	Amph., jug-r.
Acne	acne in small bone at base of spine	Carb-v.
Acne	acne on chest	Bar-c.
Acne	acne on face aggravated on becoming heated	Caust.
Acne	acne on face	Ant-c., ars-i., ars., Aur., bar-c., bell., calc-s., Calc-sil., calc., Carb-an., Carb-s., Carb-v., Caust., chel., con., cop., crot-h., eug., Hep., iod., Kali-br., kreos., lach., led., med., nat-m., nit-ac., Nux-v., ph-ac., psor., puls., sabin., sanic., sel., Sep., Sil., sul-i., sulph., thuj., tub., uran.
Adhesion	inflammation , after with adhesions (joining of normally unconnected body parts by bands of fibrous tissue) of iris	Calc., clem., merc-c., nit-ac., sil., spig., staph., sulph., ter.
Agggravation	Aching in back aggravated from coffee	Cham.
Agggravation	Aching in lumbar region aggravated from pressure	Canth., graph.
Agggravation	Aching in lumbar region aggravated from stepping	Acon., carb-ac., spong.
Agggravation	Aching in lumbar region aggravated from straightening up	Carb-ac., kali-bi.
Agggravation	Aching in spine aggravated from respiration	Calc.
Agggravation	acne on face aggravated on becoming heated	Caust.
Agggravation	affected parts aggravated on motion	Acon., **Aesc.**, agar., am-c., anac., ant-t., **Arn.**, ars., asaf., asar., bar-c., bell., **Bry.**, camph., cann-s., caps., caust., **Cham.**, chel., chin., cic., cimic., clem., cocc., coff., **Colch.**, coloc., com., con., croc., cupr., dig., ferr-ar., form., gels., glon., guai., hep., ign., iod., kali-c., kalm., lach., **Led.**, mag-c., mang., meny., merc., mez., nat-c., nat-m., nux-m., nux-v., olnd., petr., phos., phyt., plan., plat., puls., ran-b., rheum., rhod., **Rhus-t.**, rumx., ruta., sabad., sabin., samb., sang., sars., sel., sep., sil., **Spig.**, stann., staph., sulph., thuj., zinc.
Agggravation	aggaravated from entering a cold place	**Ars.**, calc-p., carb-v., caust., con., dulc., ferr-ar., ferr., graph., hep., **Kali-ar.**, kali-c., kali-p., mosch., nux-m., nux-v., petr., phos., psor., puls., **Ran-b.**, rhus-t., sabad., **Sep.**, sil., spong., stront., tub., verb.
Agggravation	aggravated after afternoon sleep	Anac., bry., chin., lach., phos., puls., spong., **Staph.**, sulph.

Body part/Disease	Symptom	Medicines
Agggravation	aggravated after breakfast	Agar., am-m., ambr., anac., ars., bell., bor., bry., calc., carb-an., carb-s., carb-v., caust., **Cham.**, chin., con., cycl., eupho., form., graph., hell., ign., kali-c., kali-n., laur., lyc., mag-c., mang., nat-c., nat-m., nit-ac., nux-m., **Nux-v.**, par., petr., ph-ac., **Phos.**, plb., puls., rhod., rhus-t., sars., sep., sil., stront., sulph., thuj., valer., verat., **Zinc.**
Agggravation	aggravated after long sleep	Ambr., anac., arn., ars., asaf., bell., bor., bry., calc., camph., carb-v., caust., cham., cocc., con., dig., euphr., ferr., graph., hep., hyos., ign., kali-c., kreos., **Lach.**, lyc., mag-c., nux-v., ph-ac., puls., rhus-t., spig., stram., **Sulph.**, verat.
Agggravation	aggravated after lying	Acon., agar., agn., alum., am-c., am-m., **Ambr.**, ant-c., ant-t., arg-m., arn., **Ars.**, asaf., asar., **Aur.**, bar-c., bell., bism., bor., bov., bry., calad., calc., canth., caps., carb-an., carb-v., caust., cham., chel., chin., clem., cocc., coff., colch., coloc., con., croc., cupr., cycl., dros., **Dulc.**, eupho., euphr., ferr., graph., guai., hell., hep., hyos., ign., ip., kali-c., kali-n., lach., laur., led., **Lyc.**, mag-c., mag-m., mang., meny., merc., mez., mosch., mur-ac., nat-a., nat-c., nit-ac., nux-m., nux-v., olnd., op., par., petr., ph-ac., phos., **Plat.**, plb., **Puls.**, ran-b., ran-s., rhod., **Rhus-t.**, ruta., sabad., sabin., **Samb.**, sars., sel., seneg., sep., sil., spig., stann., staph., **Stront.**, sul-ac., sulph., tarax., teucr., thuj., valer., verat., verb., viol-o., viol-t., zinc.
Agggravation	aggravated after motion	**Agar.**, am-c., anac., arn., **Ars.**, aspar., calad., camph., **Cann-s.**, carb-v., caust., cocc., coff., croc., dros., hyos., iod., kali-c., laur., merc., nit-ac., nux-v., olnd., phos., plb., **Puls.**, **Rhus-t.**, ruta., sabin., sep., spig., **Spong.**, **Stann.**, staph., stram., sul-ac., **Valer.**, zinc.
Agggravation	aggravated after peaches (a sweet round juicy fruit with yellow flesh, a single stone, and a soft downy orange-yellow skin)	Psor.
Agggravation	aggravated after perspiration	Ars., bell., bry., calc., carb-v., **Chin.**, con., ign., iod., kali-c., lyc., merc., nat-c., nat-m., nux-v., petr., **Ph-ac.**, phos., puls., sel., **Sep.**, sil., spig., squil., staph., sulph.
Agggravation	aggravated after riding on a horse back	Graph., kali-n., nat-c., nat-m., nit-ac., plat., **Sil.**
Agggravation	aggravated after sleep	Acon., aesc., am-m., ambr., anac., apis., arn., ars., asaf., bell., bor., bov., bry., cadm., calc., camph., carb-s., carb-v., caust., cham., chel., chin., cina., cocc., coff., con., **Crot-c.**, dig., euphr., ferr-ar., ferr., graph., hep., hyos., ign., kali-ar., kali-c., kali-p., kreos., lac-c., **Lach.**, lyc., mag-c., mur-ac., naja., nat-a., nux-m., nux-v., olnd., op., paeon., ph-ac., phos., phyt., puls., rheum., rhus-t., sabad., samb., **Sel.**, sep., spig., **Spong.**, stann., staph., **Stram.**, **Sulph.**, thuj., verat.
Agggravation	aggravated after undressing	Am-m., **Ars.**, calc., cocc., **Dros.**, hep., mag-c., mez., mur-ac., nat-s., **Nux-v.**, olnd., plat., puls., **Rhus-t.**, sep., sil., spong., stann.
Agggravation	aggravated after undressing in open air	Phos.

Body part/Disease	Symptom	Medicines
Agggravation	aggravated at beginning of motion	Agar., ant-t., asar., cact., calc., **Caps.**, carb-v., caust., chin., cina., cocc., **Con.**, cupr., dros., **Eupho.**, **Ferr.**, fl-ac., graph., kali-p., lach., led., **Lyc.**, mag-c., nit-ac., petr., ph-ac., phos., plat., plb., psor., **Puls.**, rhod., **Rhus-t.**, ruta., sabad., sabin., samb., sars., sil., ther., thuj., valer., verat., zinc.
Agggravation	aggravated at beginning of sleep	Agar., agn., am-m., aral., arg-m., arg-n., arn., **Ars.**, aur., bapt., bar-c., **Bell.**, bor., **Bry.**, calad., calc., caps., carb-an., carb-v., caust., cench., chin., cocc., coff., con., **Crot-h.**, dulc., graph., grin., guai., hep., ign., ip., kali-ar., **Kali-c.**, kreos., lac-c., **Lach.**, laur., lyc., mag-c., mag-m., merc., mur-ac., nat-c., nat-m., nux-v., op., ph-ac., phos., **Puls.**, ran-b., rhus-t., sabin., sars., sel., **Sep.**, sil., spong., staph., stront., sulph., tarax., teucr., thuj., valer., verat.
Agggravation	aggravated at night	Mag-m., merc-i-f., rhus-t., vinc.
Agggravation	aggravated before sleep	Acon., agar., agn., alum., am-c., am-m., ambr., anac., ant-c., arn., **Ars.**, asar., aur., bar-c., bell., bism., bor., **Bry.**, calad., **Calc.**, camph., canth., caps., carb-an., **Carb-v.**, caust., cham., chel., chin., clem., cocc., coff., coloc., con., cycl., dig., dulc., eupho., euphr., graph., guai., hep., ign., ip., kali-c., kali-n., kreos., lach., laur., led., lyc., mag-c., mag-m., mang., **Merc.**, mez., mosch., mur-ac., nat-a., nat-c., nat-m., nit-ac., nux-m., nux-v., par., petr., ph-ac., **Phos.**, plat., plb., **Puls.**, ran-b., rheum., rhod., **Rhus-t.**, sabad., sabin., samb., sars., sel., seneg., **Sep.**, sil., spig., spong., stann., staph., stront., sul-ac., **Sulph.**, tarax., thuj., verat., verb., viol-t., zinc.
Agggravation	aggravated by exposure to cold, damp, rainy weather, of sudden changes in hot weather	Dul.
Agggravation	aggravated by tobacco	Acon., agar., alum., ambr., ant-c., arg-m., arg-n., **Ars.**, bell., bry., calad., calc., camph., carb-an., carb-s., chel., chin., cic., clem., coc-c., coca., cocc., coloc., con., cycl., dig., euphr., ferr., gels., hell., hep., hydr., **Ign.**, iod., ip., lach., lact-ac., lyc., mag-c., meny., nat-m., **Nux-v.**, osm., par., petr., phos., **Plan.**, **Puls.**, ran-b., rhus-t., ruta., sabad., sabin., sars., sel., sep., sil., **Spig.**, **Spong.**, **Staph.**, sul-ac., sulph., tarax., thuj., verat.
Agggravation	aggravated by tobacco chewing	**Ars.**, carb-v., lyc., nux-v., plan., verat.
Agggravation	aggravated by uncovering	Alum., berb., Hep., kali-ar., Kali-c., merc., nat-m., nat-s., Nux-v., phos., Rhus-t., rumx., Sil., spong., Squil., thuj., Zinc.
Agggravation	aggravated from ascending	Acet-ac., acon., aloe., alum., am-c., anac., ant-c., arg-m., arg-n., arn., **Ars.**, asar., aur., bar-c., bar-m., bell., bor., **Bry.**, cadm., calc-p., **Calc.**, cann-i., cann-s., canth., carb-s., carb-v., caust., chin., **Coca.**, coff., conv., cupr., dig., dios., dros., eupho., gels., glon., graph., hell., hep., hyos., ign., kali-ar., kali-c., kali-i., kali-n., kali-p., kalm., kreos., lach., led., lyc., mag-c., mag-m., meny., merc., mosch., mur-ac., nat-a., nat-c., nat-m., nat-p., nit-ac., nux-m., nux-v., ox-ac., par., petr., ph-ac., phos., plat., plb., ran-b., rhus-t., ruta., sabad., seneg., sep., sil., spig., **Spong.**, squil., stann., staph., sul-ac., sulph., tab., tarax., thuj., verb., zinc.

Body part/Disease	Symptom	Medicines
Agggravation	aggravated from ascending high	Acon., bry., calc., coca., conv., olnd., spig., sulph.
Agggravation	aggravated from bad meat	**Ars.**, carb-v., chin., crot-h., lach., puls., pyrog.
Agggravation	aggravated from bathing	Aesc., aeth., **Am-c.**, am-m., **Ant-c.**, ant-t., aran., ars-i., bar-c., bell., bor., bov., bry., **Calc-s.**, **Calc.**, canth., carb-s., carb-v., caust., cham., **Clem.**, con., dulc., graph., kali-c., kali-n., kali-s., lac-d., laur., lyc., mag-c., mag-p., mang., merc-c., merc., mez., mur-ac., nat-c., nat-m., nit-ac., nux-m., nux-v., petr., phos., puls., **Rhus-t.**, rumx., sars., **Sep.**, sil., spig., stann., staph., stront., sul-ac., **Sulph.**, zinc.
Agggravation	aggravated from beans and peas	Ars., **Bry.**, calc., carb-v., chin., cupr., hell., kali-c., **Lyc.**, nat-m., petr., puls., sep., sil., verat.
Agggravation	aggravated from becoming cold	Acon., aesc., *agar., alumn.,* am-c., ant-c., arg-n., *arn.,* ars-i., **Ars.**, asar., **Aur.**, *bad.,* **Bar-c.**, bar-m., bell., bor., bov., *bry., calc-p., calc., camph.,* canth., *caps., carb-an., carb-s., carb-v., caust.,* cham., chin-a., chin., cic., *cimic.,* clem., *cocc.,* con., *dig., dulc.,* elaps., ferr-ar., ferr-p., *ferr., graph.,* hell., **Hep.**, *hyos., hyper.,* ign., **Kali-ar.**, **Kali-bi.**, **Kali-c.**, kali-p., kali-s., *kreos.,* lach., **Lyc.**, *mag-c.,* mag-m., *mag-p.,* mang., *med.,* meny., merc-i-r., merc., mez., **Mosch.**, mur-ac., *nat-a.,* nat-c., nat-m., *nat-p.,* nicc., nit-ac., nux-m., **Nux-v.**, *petr.,* **Ph-ac.**, *phos., psor.,* **Pyrog.**, **Ran-b.**, rhod., **Rhus-t.**, *rumx.,* ruta., **Sabad.**, samb., sars., **Sep.**, **Sil.**, spig., spong., squil., staph., stram., *stront.,* **Sul-ac.**,
Agggravation	aggravated from becoming warm in open air	Acon., agn., alum., ambr., ant-c., aur-m., aur., bar-c., bell., bor., bov., **Bry.**, calad., calc., cann-s., carb-v., caust., cham., chin., cina., cocc., coff., colch., coloc., croc., dros., dulc., eupho., glon., graph., ign., **Iod.**, ip., kali-c., lach., led., **Lyc.**, mang., merc., mez., nat-c., nat-m., nat-s., nit-ac., olnd., op., petr., ph-ac., phos., plat., **Puls.**, sabad., sabin., sec., sel., seneg., sep., sil., spig., spong., staph., sulph., teucr., thuj., verat.
Agggravation	aggravated from beer	Acon., aloe., ars., asaf., bell., bry., cadm., carb-s., chel., chin., chlol., coc-c., coloc., crot-t., eupho., ferr., ign., kali-br., led., lyc., mez., mur-ac., nux-v., puls., rhus-t., sep., sil., stann., staph., stram., sulph., teucr., verat.
Agggravation	aggravated from black bread (dark rye bread particularly popular in Germany)	Bry., ign., kali-c., lyc., nat-m., nit-ac., nux-v., ph-ac., phos., puls., sulph.
Agggravation	aggravated from bread	Ant-c., bar-c., **Bry.**, carb-an., caust., chin., clem., coff., crot-h., crot-t., kali-c., merc., nat-m., nit-ac., nux-v., olnd., ph-ac., phos., **Puls.**, ran-s., rhus-t., ruta., sars., sec., sep., staph., sul-ac., sulph., teucr., zinc., zing.
Agggravation	aggravated from buck wheat (cereal foods)	Ip., **Puls.**, verat.
Agggravation	aggravated from butter	Acon., ant-c., ant-t., ars., asaf., bell., carb-an., **Carb-v.**, caust., chin., colch., cycl., dros., eupho., ferr-ar., ferr., hell., hep., ip., mag-m., meny., nat-a., nat-c., nat-m., nat-p., nit-ac., nux-v., phos., ptel., **Puls.**, sep., spong., sulph., tarax., thuj.

Body part/Disease	Symptom	Medicines
Agggravation	aggravated from butter & bread	Carb-an., caust., chin., crot-t., cycl., meny., nat-m., nit-ac., nux-v., phos., **Puls.**, sep., sulph.
Agggravation	aggravated from cabbage	Ars., **Bry.**, calc., carb-v., chin., cupr., hell., kali-c., **Lyc.**, mag-c., nat-m., nat-s., **Petr.**, puls., sep., sil., verat.
Agggravation	aggravated from carrot	Calc., lyc.
Agggravation	aggravated from carrying on the back	Alum.
Agggravation	aggravated from carrying on the head	Calc.
Agggravation	aggravated from change from cold to warm	**Bry.**, carb-v., chel., ferr., gels., **Kali-s.**, lach., lyc., nat-m., nat-s., **Psor.**, puls., **Sulph.**, **Tub.**
Agggravation	aggravated from change of position	Acon., bry., **Caps.**, carb-v., caust., chel., con., **Eupho.**, **Ferr.**, lach., lyc., petr., ph-ac., phos., plat., plb., **Puls.**, ran-b., rhod., rhus-t., sabad., samb., sil., thuj.
Agggravation	aggravated from change of temperature	Acon., alum., **Ars.**, carb-v., caust., graph., lyc., mag-c., nux-v., phos., puls., **Ran-b.**, ran-s., rhus-t., sabin., spong., sulph., verat., **Verb.**
Agggravation	aggravated from change of weather	Abrot., alumn., am-c., ant-c., ant-t., apis., ars., bell., benz-ac., bor., brom., bry., calc-p., calc., carb-s., caust., chel., colch., dig., **Dulc.**, eupho., gels., graph., hep., hyper., kali-bi., kali-c., lach., mang., meli., merc., mez., nat-c., nit-ac., **Nux-m.**, nux-v., petr., ph-ac., **Phos.**, **Psor.**, puls., **Ran-b.**, rheum., **Rhod.**, **Rhus-t.**, rumx., sep., **Sil.**, stront., sulph., **Tub.**, verat.
Agggravation	aggravated from coffee	Aeth., all-c., ars., arum-t., aster., bell., bov., bry., cact., calc-p., calc., **Canth.**, caps., carb-v., **Caust.**, **Cham.**, cist., cocc., colch., cycl., fl-ac., form., glon., grat., hep., **Ign.**, ip., kali-bi., kali-n., lyc., mag-c., mang., merc., nat-m., nat-s., nit-ac., **Nux-v.**, ox-ac., ph-ac., plat., puls., rhus-t., sep., stram., sul-ac., sulph., thuj., vinc.
Agggravation	aggravated from cold bathing	**Ant-c.**, bar-c., bell., caps., carb-s., caust., colch., elaps., form., kreos., lac-d., **Mag-p.**, mur-ac., nit-ac., phos., **Rhus-t.**, sars., sep., **Tub.**
Agggravation	aggravated from cold drinks	Agar., alum., anac., ant-c., apis., apoc., arg-n., ars., bell., bor., calc-p., calc., **Canth.**, carb-an., carb-v., chel., clem., cocc., coloc., croc., dig., dulc., ferr-ar., **Ferr.**, graph., grat., hyos., ign., kali-ar., kali-c., kali-i., kali-p., lyc., mag-p., mang., merc., mur-ac., nat-a., nat-c., nat-p., nux-m., nux-v., ph-ac., puls., rhod., **Rhus-t.**, sars., sil., spig., stram., sul-ac., sulph., tarent., teucr., thuj., verat.
Agggravation	aggravated from cold drinks in hot weather	Bry., kali-c., nat-c.
Agggravation	aggravated from cold drinks when heated	Kali-ar., kali-c., nat-c., samb.
Agggravation	aggravated from cold food	Acet-ac., agar., alum., ant-c., arg-n., **Ars.**, bar-c., bov., brom., bry., calad., calc-f., calc-p., calc., canth., carb-s., carb-v., caust., cham., chel., cocc., coloc., con., dig., **Dulc.**, graph., hell., hep., ign., kali-ar., kali-c., kali-i., kali-n., kreos., **Lach.**, **Lyc.**, mag-c., mag-m., mang., merc., mur-ac., nat-a., nat-c., nat-m., nat-p., nat-s., nit-ac., nux-m., **Nux-v.**, par., ph-ac., plb., puls., rhod., **Rhus-t.**, rumx., sabad., sep., **Sil.**, spig., sulph., thuj., verat.

Body part/Disease	Symptom	Medicines
Agggravation	Aggravated from Consolation	Arn., ars., bell., cact., calc-p., calc., cham., chin., hell., Ign., kali-c., lil-t., lyc., merc., Nat-m., nit-ac., nux-v., plat., Sep., Sil., staph., tarent., thuj.
Agggravation	Aggravated from conversation	Acon., alum., am-c., Ambr., aur., calc., cann-s., canth., chin., cocc., coff., dios., ferr., fl-ac., graph., Ign., iod., kali-c., mag-m., mang., mez., Nat-m., nat-p., nux-m., nux-v., ph-ac., plat., puls., rhus-t., sars., sep., sil., spig., sulph., thuj.
Agggravation	aggravated from copper fumes	Camph., ip., lyc., merc., nux-v., op., puls.
Agggravation	aggravated from corn (the grain of a tall annual cereal plant that produces densely packed ears of grains attached to a central core) meal	Calc-ar.
Agggravation	aggravated from descending	Acon., alum., am-m., arg-m., bar-c., bell., **Bor.**, bry., canth., coff., con., ferr., lyc., meny., nit-ac., plb., rhod., rhus-t., ruta., sabin., stann., sulph., verat., verb.
Agggravation	aggravated from dry food	Agar., calc., chin., ip., lyc., nat-c., nit-ac., nux-v., petr., ph-ac., puls., sars., sil., sulph.
Agggravation	aggravated from egg	Chin-a., colch., ferr-m., ferr.
Agggravation	aggravated from farinaceous (containing starch) food	Caust., lyc., nat-c., **Nat-m.**, **Nat-s.**, nux-v., sulph.
Agggravation	aggravated from fast walking	Alum., apis., arg-m., arn., ars-i., **Ars.**, aur-m., aur., **Bell.**, **Bry.**, cact., calc-s., calc., cann-s., caust., chel., chin., cina., cocc., coff., **Con.**, croc., cupr., dros., ferr-ar., ferr., hep., hyos., ign., iod., ip., kali-ar., kali-c., kali-p., laur., led., lyc., merc., mez., nat-a., nat-c., nat-m., nit-ac., nux-m., nux-v., olnd., **Phos.**, plb., **Puls.**, rheum., rhod., rhus-t., ruta., sabin., seneg., sep., **Sil.**, spig., spong., squil., staph., sul-ac., **Sulph.**, verat., zinc.
Agggravation	aggravated from fat food	Acon., ant-c., ant-t., ars., asaf., bell., bry., carb-an., carb-s., **Carb-v.**, caust., chin., colch., **Cycl.**, dros., eupho., ferr-ar., ferr-m., **Ferr.**, hell., hep., ip., kali-ar., kali-c., kali-chl., kali-n., mag-c., mag-m., meny., merc-c., merc., nat-a., nat-c., nat-m., nat-p., nit-ac., nux-v., phos., ptel., **Puls.**, rob., ruta., sep., sil., spong., staph., sulph., **Tarax.**, thuj., verat.
Agggravation	aggravated from fish	Calad., carb-an., chin-a., kali-c., plb.
Agggravation	aggravated from fish shell	Carb-v., lyc., urt-u.
Agggravation	aggravated from flatulent food	Ars., **Bry.**, calc., carb-v., chin., cupr., hell., kali-c., **Lyc.**, nat-m., **Petr.**, puls., sep., sil., verat.
Agggravation	aggravated from fresh meat	Caust.
Agggravation	aggravated from frozen (extremely cold) food	Arg-n., ars., bry., calc-p., carb-v., dulc., ip., **Puls.**, rumx.
Agggravation	aggravated from fruit	Acon., aloe., ant-c., ant-t., **Ars.**, bor., **Bry.**, calc-p., calc., carb-v., chin-a., **Chin.**, cist., **Coloc.**, crot-t., cub., ferr., ign., ip., iris., kreos., lach., lith., lyc., mag-c., mag-m., mur-ac., nat-a., nat-c., nat-p., **Nat-s.**, olnd., ph-ac., phos., podo., psor., **Puls.**, rheum., rhod., ruta., sel., sep., sul-ac., tarax., trom., **Verat.**
Agggravation	aggravated from gently stroking (a gentle caressing)	Teucr.
Agggravation	aggravated from green vegetables	Alum., ars., bry., cupr., hell., lyc., nat-c., **Nat-s.**, verat.

Body part/Disease	Symptom	Medicines
Agggravation	aggravated from heavy food	Bry., calc., caust., cupr., **Iod.**, lyc., nat-c., puls., sulph.
Agggravation	aggravated from honey	Nat-c.
Agggravation	aggravated from hot food	Arum-t., bry., caps., carb-v., coff., ferr., graph., nat-s., phyt., puls., sep.
Agggravation	aggravated from lemonade (drink made from lemons)	Phyt., sel.
Agggravation	aggravated from letting limbs hang down	Alum., am-c., berb., **Calc.**, carb-v., caust., cina., dig., hep., ign., lyc., nat-m., nux-v., ox-ac., par., ph-ac., phos., phyt., plat., plb., puls., ran-s., ruta., sabin., stann., sul-ac., sulph., thuj., valer., vip.
Agggravation	aggravated from loss of sleep	Ambr., bry., caust., chin., cimic., **Cocc.**, colch., cupr., ip., lac-d., laur., nat-m., nit-ac., **Nux-v.**, olnd., op., ph-ac., puls., ruta., sabin., sel., sep., sulph., zinc.
Agggravation	aggravated from lying on back	Acet-ac., acon., aloe., alum., am-c., am-m., arg-m., arn., ars., aur-m., bar-c., bell., bor., bry., bufo., calc., canth., caust., cham., chin., cina., clem., coloc., cupr., dulc., eup-per., eupho., hyper., iod., kali-c., lach., merc., nat-c., nat-m., nat-s., **Nux-v.**, op., par., **Phos.**, plat., ran-b., rhus-t., sep., sil., spig., spong., stront., sulph., thuj.
Agggravation	aggravated from lying on left side	Acon., ail., anac., ant-t., arg-n., arn., bar-c., bell., bry., cact., canth., carb-an., chin., colch., con., eup-per., ip., kali-ar., kali-c., kalm., kreos., lyc., mag-m., merc., naja., nat-c., nat-m., nat-p., nat-s., op., par., petr., **Phos.**, plat., **Puls.**, rhus-t., seneg., sep., sil., sulph., tab., thuj.
Agggravation	aggravated from lying on painful side	Acon., agar., am-c., am-m., ambr., anac., ant-c., arg-m., arn., ars-i., ars., bapt., **Bar-c.**, bell., bry., **Calad.**, calc-f., calc., cann-s., caps., carb-an., carb-v., caust., chin., cina., clem., croc., cupr., dios., dros., graph., guai., **Hep.**, hyos., ign., **Iod.**, kali-c., kali-i., kali-n., led., lyc., mag-c., mang., merc., mez., mosch., mur-ac., nat-m., nit-ac., **Nux-m.**, nux-v., olnd., par., petr., ph-ac., phos., plat., puls., ran-b., ran-s., rheum., rhod., rhus-t., rumx., **Ruta.**, sabad., sabin., samb., sars., sel., sep., **Sil.**, spong., staph., stram., tarax., teucr., thuj., valer., verat., verb.
Agggravation	aggravated from lying on painless side	Ambr., arg-m., arn., bell., **Bry.**, calc., cann-s., carb-v., caust., **Cham.**, chel., **Coloc.**, cupr., hyper., ign., kali-c., lyc., merc-i-r., naja., nat-c., nux-v., phos., plan., **Puls.**, rhus-t., sep., stann., sul-ac., viol-o., viol-t.
Agggravation	aggravated from lying on right side	Acon., alum., am-c., am-m., anac., benz-ac., bor., bry., bufo., carb-an., cina., clem., con., ip., kali-c., kali-i., kreos., lyc., mag-m., **Merc.**, mur-ac., nux-v., phos., prun-s., psor., ran-b., seneg., spong., sul-ac., sulph., thuj.
Agggravation	aggravated from lying on side	**Acon.**, am-c., am-m., **Anac.**, arg-n., arn., aur., bar-c., bell., bor., **Bry.**, calad., **Calc.**, canth., **Carb-an.**, caust., chin., cina., clem., colch., con., ferr., ign., ip., **Kali-c.**, kreos., lach., **Lyc.**, merc-c., merc., mosch., nat-m., nat-s., nux-v., par., ph-ac., phos., plat., puls., ran-b., **Rhus-t.**, sabad., seneg., sep., sil., spig., spong., **Stann.**, sulph., thuj., verat., viol-t.

Body part/Disease	Symptom	Medicines
Agggravation	aggravated from meat	Carb-an., caust., colch., cupr., ferr., kali-bi., lyss., mag-c., mag-m., merc., ptel., puls., ruta., sil., staph., sulph., ter.
Agggravation	aggravated from milk	**Aeth.**, alum., ambr., ant-c., ant-t., arg-m., brom., bry., **Calc-s., Calc.,** carb-an., carb-s., carb-v., cham., chel., **Chin.,** cic., **Con.,** crot-t., cupr., ham., hell., ign., iris., kali-ar., kali-c., kali-i., kali-p., **Lac-d.,** lach., lyc., mag-c., **Mag-m.,** nat-a., nat-c., nat-m., nat-p., nat-s., **Nit-ac.,** nux-m., nux-v., ol-j., phos., psor., puls., rhus-t., sabin., samb., **Sep.,** sil., spong., stram., sul-ac., **Sulph.,** valer., zinc.
Agggravation	aggravated from mutton	Lyss., ov.
Agggravation	aggravated from narcotics (something that soothes, induces sleep, relieves pain or stress, or causes a sensation of mental numbness)	Acon., agar., ars., aur., **Bell.,** bry., calc., canth., carb-v., caust., **Cham.,** chin., **Coff.,** colch., croc., cupr., dig., dulc., eupho., ferr., graph., hep., hyos., ign., ip., **Lach.,** lyc., merc., mosch., nat-c., nat-m., nit-ac., nux-m., **Nux-v.,** op., ph-ac., phos., plat., plb., puls., rhus-t., seneg., sep., staph., sulph., valer., verat., zinc.
Agggravation	aggravated from odor of coffee	Sul-ac.
Agggravation	aggravated from odor of cooking meat	Ars., colch.
Agggravation	aggravated from odor of egg	Colch.
Agggravation	aggravated from old cheese	Ars., bry., coloc., ph-ac., ptel., rhus-t.
Agggravation	aggravated from onion	**Lyc.,** nux-v., puls., thuj.
Agggravation	aggravated from oysters (shellfish with a rough irregularly shaped shell in two parts)	Aloe., brom., bry., lyc., podo., sul-ac.
Agggravation	aggravated from pancakes (thin fried cake)	Bry., ip., kali-c., **Puls.,** verat.
Agggravation	aggravated from pastry (sweet baked food made from pastry)	Ant-c., arg-n., ars., carb-v., ip., kali-chl., lyc., phos., **Puls.**
Agggravation	aggravated from pears (a sweet juicy fruit with a usually green skin, firm white flesh, and roughly teardrop shape, eaten fresh or canned)	Bor., bry., verat.
Agggravation	aggravated from pepper (condiments such as chili sauce or cayenne pepper made from the more strongly pungent peppers)	Ars., cina., nat-c., sep., sil.
Agggravation	aggravated from pork (pig) meat	Acon., ant-c., ant-t., ars., asaf., bell., **Carb-v.,** caust., colch., **Cycl.,** ham., ip., nat-a., nat-c., nat-m., **Puls., Sep.,** tarax., thuj.
Agggravation	aggravated from potatoes	Alum., am-m., calc., coloc., mag-s., merc-c., nat-s., sep., verat.
Agggravation	aggravated from pressure on painless side	Ambr., arn., bell., **Bry.,** calc., cann-s., carb-an., carb-v., caust., cham., coloc., **Ign.,** kali-c., lyc., nux-v., **Puls.,** rhus-t., sep., stann., viol-o., viol-t.
Agggravation	aggravated from raw potatoes	Ars., bry., chin., lyc., puls., **Ruta.,** verat.
Agggravation	aggravated from rich potatoes	Ant-c., arg-n., bry., carb-an., **Carb-v.,** cycl., dros., ferr., ip., kali-chl., nat-m., nat-s., nit-ac., phos., **Puls.,** sep., staph., tarax., thuj.
Agggravation	aggravated from riding down hill on a horse back	**Bor.,** psor.

Body part/Disease	Symptom	Medicines
Agggravation	aggravated from riding in a wagon, or on the cars	Arg-m., arg-n., arn., ars., aur., bor., bry., calc., carb-v., **Cocc.**, colch., con., croc., ferr., hep., hyos., ign., iod., kali-c., lach., lyc., lyss., mag-c., meph., nat-m., nux-m., op., **Petr.**, phos., plat., psor., puls., rhus-t., rumx., sel., **Sep.**, sil., staph., sulph., ther., thuj., valer.
Agggravation	aggravated from riding on horse back	Ars., bell., bry., graph., lil-t., mag-m., meph., nat-c., **Sep.**, sil., spig., sul-ac., valer.
Agggravation	aggravated from rubbing	Am-m., **Anac.**, arn., ars., bism., bor., calad., calc., cann-s., canth., caps., carb-an., caust., cham., chel., coff., **Con.**, cupr., dros., guai., kreos., led., mag-c., mang., merc., mez., mur-ac., nat-c., par., ph-ac., **Puls.**, seneg., **Sep.**, sil., spig., spong., squil., stann., staph., stram., **Stront.**, **Sulph.**
Agggravation	aggravated from running	Alum., arg-m., arn., ars-i., **Ars.**, aur., bell., bor., **Bry.**, calc., cann-s., caust., chel., chin., cina., cocc., coff., con., croc., cupr., dros., ferr., hep., hyos., ign., iod., ip., kali-c., laur., led., lyc., merc., mez., nat-c., nat-m., nit-ac., nux-m., nux-v., olnd., phos., plb., **Puls.**, rheum., rhod., rhus-t., ruta., sabin., seneg., sep., sil., spig., spong., squil., staph., sul-ac., **Sulph.**, verat., zinc.
Agggravation	aggravated from salad	Ars., bry., calc., carb-v., lach., lyc.
Agggravation	aggravated from salt	Alum., ars., calc., carb-v., dros., lyc., mag-m., nux-v., **Phos.**, sel.
Agggravation	aggravated from sauerkraut (pickled cabbage salad)	Ars., **Bry.**, calc., carb-v., chin., cupr., hell., lyc., nat-m., **Petr.**, phos., puls., sep., verat.
Agggravation	aggravated from sea bath	Ars., mag-m., rhus-t., sep.
Agggravation	aggravated from sexual excitement	Bufo., **Lil-t.**, sars.
Agggravation	aggravated from slight touch	Ars., **Bell.**, **Chin.**, coff., colch., ign., **Lach.**, mag-m., **Merc.**, mez., **Nux-v.**, ph-ac., phos., stann.
Agggravation	aggravated from smoke	Calc., caust., euphr., nat-m., nux-v., olnd., sep., **Spig.**, sulph.
Agggravation	aggravated from smoked (to cure or treat food such as meat, fish, or cheese with wood smoke) food	Calc., sil.
Agggravation	aggravated from snow air	Calc-p., calc., caust., cic., **Con.**, lyc., mag-m., merc., nat-c., nux-v., ph-ac., phos., puls., rhod., rhus-t., **Sep.**, sil., sulph., urt-u.
Agggravation	aggravated from sour	**Ant-c.**, ant-t., arg-n., ars., bell., bor., brom., calad., caust., chin., cub., dros., ferr-ar., ferr-p., ferr., kreos., lach., merc-c., nat-c., nat-m., nat-p., nux-v., ph-ac., phos., ran-b., sel., sep., staph., sulph.
Agggravation	aggravated from sour fruit	Ant-c., ip., ph-ac., psor.
Agggravation	aggravated from sour odors	Dros.
Agggravation	aggravated from sour wine	**Ant-c.**, ant-t., ars., ferr., sep., sulph.
Agggravation	aggravated from spices	Phos.
Agggravation	aggravated from spoiled fish	Ars., carb-v., chin., puls.
Agggravation	aggravated from spoiled sausage	**Ars.**, **Bell.**, bry., ph-ac., rhus-t.
Agggravation	aggravated from strawberries	Ant-c., ox-ac., sep.
Agggravation	aggravated from suppression of sexual desire	**Apis.**, berb., calc., **Camph.**, carb-o., **Con.**, hell., lil-t., ph-ac., pic-ac., plat., **Puls.**

Body part/Disease	Symptom	Medicines
Aggravation	aggravated from sweets	Acon., am-c., ant-c., **Arg-n.**, calc., cham., fl-ac., graph., **Ign.**, merc., nat-c., ox-ac., phos., sel., spig., sulph., thuj., zinc.
Aggravation	aggravated from talk of others	Agar., alum., am-c., Ars., aur., cact., chin., cocc., colch., con., elaps., ferr-ar., ferr., hell., Hyos., kali-c., kalm., mag-m., mang., nat-a., nat-c., nat-s., nit-ac., Nux-v., rhus-t., sep., sil., stram., teucr., verat., zinc.
Aggravation	aggravated from tea	Aesc., chin., coff., dios., ferr., lach., rumx., **Sel.**, thuj., verat.
Aggravation	aggravated from touching anything	Acon., am-c., am-m., arg-m., arn., bell., bor., bry., calc., cann-s., carb-v., caust., **Cham.**, chin., dros., kali-c., kali-n., led., lyc., merc., nat-c., phos., plat., puls., sec., sil., spig., verat.
Aggravation	aggravated from touching cold things	Calc., **Hep.**, lac-d., merc., nat-m., pyrog., **Rhus-t.**, **Sil.**, thuj., zinc.
Aggravation	aggravated from touching warm things	Sulph.
Aggravation	aggravated from turnip	Bry., calc-ar., lyc., puls.
Aggravation	aggravated from uncleanliness	**Caps.**, chin., psor., puls., sulph.
Aggravation	aggravated from uncovering	Acon-f., acon., agar., am-c., ant-c., arg-m., arg-n., arn., **Ars.**, asar., atro., aur., bell., benz-ac., bor., bry., camph., canth., caps., carb-an., cham., chin., cic., clem., cocc., coff., colch., con., dios., dulc., graph., hell., **Hep.**, hyos., ign., **Kali-ar.**, kali-bi., **Kali-c.**, kali-i., kreos., lach., **Lyc.**, lycps., mag-c., mag-m., **Mag-p.**, meny., merc., mur-ac., nat-c., nat-m., **Nux-m.**, **Nux-v.**, ph-ac., phos., puls., rheum., **Rhod.**, **Rhus-t.**, rumx., sabad., **Samb.**, sep., **Sil.**, **Squil.**, staph., stram., **Stront.**, thuj., **Zinc.**
Aggravation	aggravated from uncovering of single part	Bry., **Hep.**, nat-m., **Rhus-t.**, **Sil.**, squil., stront., thuj.
Aggravation	aggravated from veal (meat from calf)	Ars., calc., caust., chin., **Ip.**, **Kali-n.**, nux-v., sep., sulph., verat., zinc.
Aggravation	aggravated from vinegar (a sour-tasting liquid that is used to flavor and preserve foods. It is a dilute acetic acid made by fermenting beer, wine, or cider)	Aloe., **Ant-c.**, ars., bell., bor., calad., caust., dros., ferr-ar., ferr., kreos., lach., nat-a., nat-c., nat-m., nat-p., nux-v., ph-ac., phos., ran-b., sep., staph., sulph.
Aggravation	aggravated from vomiting	Acon., ant-t., arn., **Ars.**, asar., bell., bry., calc., caps., cham., chin., cina., cocc., colch., coloc., con., **Cupr.**, dig., dros., ferr., graph., hyos., iod., **Ip.**, lach., lyc., mez., mosch., nat-m., nux-v., op., phos., plb., **Puls.**, ran-s., ruta., sabin., sars., sec., sep., sil., stann., **Sulph.**, verat.
Aggravation	aggravated from walking in wind	Acon., agar., ars., asar., aur., **Bell.**, calc., carb-v., cham., chin., con., euphr., graph., lach., lyc., mur-ac., nat-c., nux-m., **Nux-v.**, phos., plat., puls., rhus-t., **Sep.**, spig., stann., thuj.
Aggravation	aggravated from warm	Acon., agar., agn., all-c., **Alum.**, ambr., ant-c., ant-t., **Apis.**, arg-n., arn., **Ars-i.**, aur-m., aur., bar-c., bell., bism., bor., bry., calad., camph., cann-s., canth., carb-s., carb-v., caust., cham., cina., coc-c., cocc., colch., coloc., croc., dig., dros., dulc., eupho., euphr., ferr-i., gels., glon., graph., guai., hell., ign., Ind., **Iod.**, ip., kali-br., kali-s., lac-c., lach., laur., **Led.**, lyc., merc., mez., mur-ac., nat-c., nat-m., nat-s., op., ph-ac., phos., plat., **Puls.**, sabad., sabin., **Sec.**, sel., seneg., spig., spong., staph., sulph., tab., teucr., thuj., verat., zinc.

Body part/Disease	Symptom	Medicines
Agggravation	aggravated from warm air	Agn., aloe., ambr., ant-c., ant-t., arg-n., ars-i., aur-m., aur., bry., calad., calc-s., calc., cann-s., carb-v., cham., cina., cocc., colch., croc., dros., eupho., fl-ac., **Glon.**, ign., Ind., **Iod.**, ip., kali-bi., **Kali-s.**, **Lach.**, led., lyc., **Merc.**, mez., nat-m., nat-s., nux-m., nux-v., op., phos., pic-ac., plat., podo., **Puls.**, sabin., sars., **Sec.**, sel., seneg., sulph., teucr., thuj., xan.
Agggravation	aggravated from warm food	Acon., agn., all-c., alum., am-c., ambr., anac., ant-t., asar., bar-c., bell., bism., bor., **Bry.**, calc., canth., carb-s., carb-v., caust., cham., clem., coc-c., cupr., dros., eupho., ferr., gran., hell., kali-c., **Lach.**, laur., mag-c., mag-m., merc., mez., nat-m., nit-ac., nux-m., nux-v., par., ph-ac., **Phos.**, **Puls.**, rhod., rhus-t., sars., sep., sil., spig., squil., stann., sul-ac., sulph., thuj., verat., zinc.
Agggravation	aggravated from warm milk	Ambr.
Agggravation	aggravated from warm stove	Ant-c., apis., arg-n., bry., bufo., cocc., con., eupho., **Glon.**, iod., kali-i., laur., mag-m., merc., nat-m., op., puls., **Sec.**
Agggravation	aggravated from Weeping	Ant-t., arn., bell., bor., canth., cham., croc., cupr., hep., lach., nit-ac., stann., teucr., verat.
Agggravation	aggravated from wrapping	Acon., **Apis.**, arg-m., arg-n., ars-i., aur-m., aur., bor., bry., calc-s., calc., camph., carb-s., carb-v., cham., chin., coc-c., coff., ferr-i., ferr., fl-ac., glon., ign., **Iod.**, **Kali-s.**, lac-c., lach., **Led.**, **Lyc.**, merc., mosch., mur-ac., nit-ac., nux-v., op., phos., plat., **Puls.**, rhus-t., **Sec.**, seneg., sep., spig., staph., **Sulph.**, tab., thuj., verat.
Agggravation	aggravated in autumn	Ant-t., aur., bapt., bar-m., bry., calc., chin., cic., colch., graph., hep., kali-bi., **Lach.**, merc., nux-v., **Rhus-t.**, stram., verat.
Agggravation	aggravated in cold dry weather	**Acon.**, ars., **Asar.**, bell., bor., bry., carb-an., carb-v., **Caust.**, cham., crot-h., **Hep.**, ip., **Kali-c.**, laur., mag-c., mez., mur-ac., **Nux-v.**, rhod., sabad., sep., sil., spig., spong., staph., sulph., zinc.
Agggravation	aggravated in cold wet weather	Agar., all-s., **Am-c.**, ant-c., apis., aran., arg-m., arg-n., ars-i., **Ars.**, asc-t., aster., aur-m-n., aur., **Bad.**, bar-c., bell., bor., bov., bry., **Calc-p.**, calc-s., **Calc.**, canth., carb-an., carb-s., carb-v., cham., chin., clem., **Colch.**, con., cupr., **Dulc.**, ferr., fl-ac., form., gels., graph., hep., hyper., iod., ip., kali-bi., kali-c., kali-i., kali-n., kali-p., lach., lath., laur., lyc., mag-c., mang., **Med.**, merc-i-f., merc., mez., mur-ac., nat-a., nat-c., **Nat-s.**, nit-ac., **Nux-m.**, nux-v., paeon., petr., phos., phyt., puls., **Pyrog.**, ran-b., **Rhod.**, **Rhus-t.**, ruta., sars., seneg., sep., **Sil.**, spig., stann., staph., stront., sul-ac., sulph., tarent., thuj., **Tub.**, verat., zinc.
Agggravation	aggravated in dry weather	Alum., ars., **Asar.**, bry., carb-an., carb-v., **Caust.**, **Hep.**, kali-c., **Nux-v.**, phos., sabad., sep., sil., spong., staph., sulph., zinc.
Agggravation	aggravated in evening after eating	Indg.
Agggravation	aggravated in evening after lying down	Ars., ign., led., phos., stront., sulph., thuj.

Body part/Disease	Symptom	Medicines
Agggravation	aggravated in evening from twilight (half-light)	Am-m., ars., calc., caust., dig., nat-m., phos., plb., **Puls.**, rhus-t., staph., sul-ac., valer.
Agggravation	aggravated in evening in open air	Am-c., carb-an., carb-v., merc., nit-ac., sulph.
Agggravation	aggravated in foggy weather	Bry., cham., chin., **Hyper.**, mang., mosch., nux-m., plb., rhod., **Rhus-t.**, sep., sil., sulph., verat.
Agggravation	aggravated in moonlight	Ant-c., hell., thuj.
Agggravation	aggravated in room full of people	Ambr., ant-c., arg-n., ars., bar-c., carb-an., con., hell., lyc., mag-c., nat-c., nat-m., petr., phos., plb., puls., sabin., sep., stann., stram., sulph.
Agggravation	aggravated in warm bed	Aeth., agn., alum., ambr., ant-c., ant-t., **Apis.**, arg-n., arn., ars-i., asaf., aur-m., aur., bar-c., bov., bry., calad., calc-s., calc., camph., cann-s., carb-v., cedr., **Cham.**, chin., cina., clem., coc-c., cocc., colch., croc., daph., **Dros.**, dulc., eupho., fl-ac., glon., goss., graph., hell., hyos., ign., iod., ip., kali-chl., kali-s., lac-c., lach., **Led.**, lyc., mag-c., **Merc.**, mez., mur-ac., nat-c., nat-m., nit-ac., **Op.**, ph-ac., phos., phyt., plat., psor., **Puls.**, sabad., **Sabin.**, sars., **Sec.**, sel., seneg., spig., spong., staph., stram., **Sulph.**, teucr., thuj., verat.
Agggravation	aggravated in warm evening	Lyc., sulph.
Agggravation	aggravated in warm room	Acon., agn., alum., ambr., ant-c., ant-t., **Apis.**, arg-n., arn., ars-i., asaf., aur-m., aur., bar-c., bell., bor., brom., bry., bufo., calad., calc-p., **Calc-s.**, calc., cann-s., carb-ac., **Carb-s.**, carb-v., caust., cina., coc-c., cocc., colch., **Croc.**, dros., dulc., fl-ac., glon., **Graph.**, hell., hyos., ign., Ind., **Iod.**, ip., kali-c., **Kali-i.**, **Kali-s.**, laur., led., lil-t., **Lyc.**, mag-m., merc-i-f., merc., mez., mosch., mur-ac., nat-a., nat-c., nat-m., nat-s., nit-ac., op., oxyt., ph-ac., phos., pic-ac., plat., ptel., **Puls.**, ran-b., **Sabin.**, sanic., **Sec.**, sel., **Seneg.**, spig., spong., staph., **Sulph.**, tab., thuj., til., tub., verat.
Agggravation	aggravated in warm room	Clem., mag-m.
Agggravation	aggravated in wet weather	**Carb-v.**, gels., iod., kali-bi., **Lach.**, **Nat-s.**, sil.
Agggravation	aggravated on beginning of walking	Acon., *agar.*, am-c., ambr., anac., ant-c., ant-t., arn., ars., asar., aur., bar-c., bell., bov., *bry.*, *cact.*, *calc.*, cann-s., canth., **Caps.**, carb-an., *carb-v.*, *caust.*, cham., chin., cic., cina., cocc., **Con.**, croc., cupr., cycl., dig., dros., **Eupho.**, **Ferr.**, graph., kali-c., kali-n., lach., laur., led., **Lyc.**, mag-c., mang., merc., mur-ac., nat-c., nat-m., nit-ac., nux-v., olnd., petr., ph-ac., *phos.*, plat., plb., **Puls.**, ran-b., rhod., **Rhus-t.**, *ruta.*, *sabad.*, sabin., *samb.*, *sars.*, sep., *sil.*, spig., staph., stram., stront., sulph., *thuj.*, valer., verat., *zinc.*
Agggravation	aggravated on feather bed	Asaf., cocc., coloc., led., lyc., **Mang.**, merc., psor., sulph.
Agggravation	aggravated on first sitting down	Agn., alum., **Am-m.**, ant-t., arg-m., aur., bar-c., bov., bry., caust., chel., chin., coff., croc., cycl., graph., hell., ip., iris., kali-c., lyc., mag-c., mang., merc., murx., nit-ac., ph-ac., phos., puls., ruta., sabin., samb., sars., **Spig.**, spong., squil., thuj., valer., verat., viol-t.

Body part/Disease	Symptom	Medicines
Agggravation	Aggravated on high places	Arg-n., aur., gels., puls., staph., sulph.
Agggravation	aggravated on rising	**Acon.**, alum., am-m., anac., ant-t., arg-m., arn., ars., asar., bar-c., bar-m., **Bell.**, bov., **Bry.**, cact., calad., cann-i., cann-s., caps., carb-an., caust., cham., chel., chin., cic., **Cocc.**, colch., coloc., con., croc., **Dig.**, dros., ferr., hell., hep., ign., kali-c., lach., laur., **Lyc.**, mag-m., mang., meny., merc., mur-ac., nat-c., nat-m., nit-ac., **Nux-v., Op.**, osm., ph-ac., phos., plat., plb., puls., ran-b., **Rhus-t.**, rumx., sabad., sang., sars., seneg., sep., **Sil.**, spong., squil., stann., staph., stram., sul-ac., **Sulph.**, tarax., verat-v., verat., viol-t., zinc.
Agggravation	Aggravatied from Darkness	Acon., aeth., ars., bapt., berb., calc., camph., carb-an., carb-v., caust., cupr., graph., lyc., nat-m., phos., plat., puls., rhus-t., sanic., Stram., valer.
Agggravation	anal haemorrhoids aggravated at night	Aesc., aloe., alum., am-c., ant-c., ars., carb-an., carb-v., coll., euphr., ferr., graph., merc., phys., puls., rhus-t., Sulph.
Agggravation	anal haemorrhoids aggravated during wiping after stool	Aesc., Graph., Mur-ac., Paeon., puls., sulph.
Agggravation	anal haemorrhoids aggravated from milk	Sep.
Agggravation	anal haemorrhoids aggravated from touch	Abrot., Bell., berb., calc., carb-an., carb-s., Caust., graph., hep., kali-c., lil-t., lyc., merc., Mur-ac., nit-ac., nux-v., phos., Rat., sep., sil., sul-ac., Sulph., syph., Thuj.
Agggravation	anal haemorrhoids aggravated in bed	Graph., rumx.
Agggravation	anal haemorrhoids aggravated in morning	Aloe., Dios., mur-ac., sabin., sulph., sumb., thuj.
Agggravation	blotches of face aggravated at night	Mag-m.
Agggravation	blotches of face aggravated by washing	Am-c., phyt.
Agggravation	blotches of face aggravated from warmth of bed	Mag-m.
Agggravation	boring pain in lumbar aggravated from bending back	Plat.
Agggravation	burning in ears aggravated by rubbing	Alum.
Agggravation	burning pain in ankle aggravated from rubbing	Sulph.
Agggravation	burning pain in back in morning after coition aggravated by rest ameliorated by motion	Mag-m.
Agggravation	burning pain in cervical region aggravated from moving head	Nat-s., plb.
Agggravation	burning pain in foot aggravated from touch	Bor.
Agggravation	burning pain in forearm aggravated from pressure	Bell.
Agggravation	burning pain in hand aggravated from washing in cold water	Caps.
Agggravation	burning pain in leg aggravated from stretching	Berb.
Agggravation	burning pain in leg aggravated from touch	Bov., con.
Agggravation	burning pain in nose aggravated during menses	Carb-an.
Agggravation	burning pain in thigh aggravated from touch	Phos.
Agggravation	burning pain in toes aggravated in warm bed	Nux-v.
Agggravation	burning pain in upper limbs aggravated from covering	Rhus-v.

Body part/Disease	Symptom	Medicines
Agggravation	burning pain in upper limbs aggravated from touch	Crot-t.
Agggravation	burning pain in upper limbs aggravated from uncovering	Crot-t.
Agggravation	burning pain in wrist aggravated from rubbing	Berb.
Agggravation	chest symptoms aggravated from clothing	Ail., aur-m., benz-ac., bov., calc., Caust., chel., con., kali-bi., Lach., lact., lycps., merc., tarent., zinc.
Agggravation	chill aggravated during drinking	Alum., ant-t., arn., **Ars.**, **Asar.**, bry., cadm., **Calc.**, cann-s., **Caps.**, chel., chin-a., **Chin.**, cimx., cocc., con., croc., elaps., **Eup-per.**, hep., kali-ar., lob., lyc., mez., nat-m., nit-ac., **Nux-v.**, puls., rhus-t., sep., sil., sulph., tarax., tarent., thuj., **Verat.**
Agggravation	chill aggravated from rising from bed	Bar-c., bism., bor., **Calc.**, canth., cham., ferr-i., mag-c., **Merc.**, mez., **Nux-v.**, phos., rhus-t., sil.
Agggravation	chill aggravated from swallowing	Merc-c.
Agggravation	chill aggravated from touch	**Acon.**, ang., apis., bell., cham., **Chin.**, colch., hep., hyos., lyc., **Nux-v.**, phos., puls., sep., spig., staph., sulph.
Agggravation	chill aggravated from warm drinks	Alum., cham.
Agggravation	chill aggravated from warm things	Alum., bell., bry., **Puls.**
Agggravation	chill aggravated in warm room	Acon., **Apis.**, arg-n., bry., cinnb., **Ip.**, merc., nat-m., puls., **Sec.**, sep., staph.
Agggravation	chill aggravated when thinking of it	Chin-a.
Agggravation	chilliness in evening aggravated from warm stove	Merc.
Agggravation	choking (stop breathing through blockage of throat) of throat aggravated by clothing	Agar., ambr., apis., bell., cact., chel., elaps., kali-bi., kali-c., Lach., sep.
Agggravation	chorea aggravated from wine	Zinc.
Agggravation	chorea aggravated in afternoon	Zinc.
Agggravation	chorea aggravated in clear weather	Acon., asar., bry., caust., hep., nux-v., plb., sabad., spong.
Agggravation	chorea aggravated in cloudy weather	Am-c., bry., calc., cham., chin., dulc., mang., merc., nux-m., plb., puls., rhod., **Rhus-t.**, sep., sulph., verat.
Agggravation	coldness in back aggravated from warmth	Apis.
Agggravation	coldness in lumbar region aggravated from draft of cold air	Tarent.
Agggravation	coldness in lumbar region aggravated from motion	Podo.
Agggravation	coldness in lumbar region aggravated from walking	Camph.
Agggravation	complaints of face aggravated by shaving	Carb-an.
Agggravation	compression of thigh aggravated on motion	Sabad.
Agggravation	Constriction in brain aggravated from bending forward	Asaf.
Agggravation	Constriction in brain aggravated from sitting	Fl-ac.
Agggravation	Constriction in brain aggravated from standing	Mag-c.
Agggravation	Constriction in brain aggravated from stooping	Berb., coloc., dig., med., thuj.
Agggravation	Constriction in brain aggravated in open air	Mang., merc., nat-m., valer.
Agggravation	Constriction in brain aggravated in wet weather	Sulph.

Body part/Disease	Symptom	Medicines
Agggravation	constriction in chest aggravated after supper	Mez.
Agggravation	constriction in chest aggravated from covering of bed	Ferr.
Agggravation	constriction in chest aggravated from motion	Agar., ang., ars., ferr., led., lyc., nux-v., spong., verat.
Agggravation	constriction in chest aggravated from touch	Arn., cupr.
Agggravation	constriction in chest aggravated lying on left	Myric.
Agggravation	constriction in chest aggravated lying on right	Lycps.
Agggravation	constriction in chest aggravated lying quiet	Caps.
Agggravation	constriction in heart aggravated from eating	Alum.
Agggravation	constriction in larynx aggravated on singing	Agar.
Agggravation	constriction in lower part of chest aggravated from lying on right side	Lycps.
Agggravation	constriction in stomach aggravated when inspirating deep	Bry.
Agggravation	convulsion (uncontrollable shaking) aggravated by coffee	Stram.
Agggravation	coryza aggravated in cold	Calc-p., coff., dulc., graph., hyos., kali-ar., mang., Merc., Ph-ac.
Agggravation	coryza aggravated in warm yet dreads cold	Apis., merc.
Agggravation	cough aggravated by crying	Ant-t., Arn., ars., bell., cham., cina., dros., ferr., guare., hep., lyc., phos., samb., sil., sulph., verat.
Agggravation	cough aggravated from acids	Ant-c., brom., con., lach., mez., nat-m., nux-v., sep., sil., sulph.
Agggravation	cough aggravated from all kinds of smoke	Euphr., ment.
Agggravation	cough aggravated from bathing	Ant-c., ars., calc-f., calc-s., calc., caust., dulc., lach., nit-ac., nux-m., psor., Rhus-t., sep., stram., sul-ac., sulph., verat., zinc.
Agggravation	cough aggravated from becoming warm in bed	Ant-t., brom., Caust., cham., dros., led., merc., naja., nat-m., nux-m., nux-v., Puls., verat.
Agggravation	cough aggravated from bending head forward	Caust., dig.
Agggravation	cough aggravated from brandy	Ferr.
Agggravation	cough aggravated from bread	Kali-c.
Agggravation	cough aggravated from close air	Brom., nat-a.
Agggravation	cough aggravated from coffee	Caps., caust., cham., cocc., ign., nux-v., sul-ac.
Agggravation	cough aggravated from consolation	Ars.
Agggravation	cough aggravated from eating hastily	Sil.
Agggravation	cough aggravated from eating high seasoned food	Sulph.
Agggravation	cough aggravated from elongated (to make something longer) uvula (a small fleshy "V"-shaped extension of the soft palate that hangs above the tongue at the entrance to the throat) in morning	Brom.
Agggravation	cough aggravated from elongated uvula	Alum., bapt., brom., hyos., merc-i-r., nat-m.
Agggravation	cough aggravated from entering in warm room from cold air or vice versa (the position being reversed)	Acon., all-c., carb-v., lach., nat-c., nux-v., Phos., rumx., sep., verat-v.

Body part/Disease	Symptom	Medicines
Agggravation	cough aggravated from fog (condensed water vapor in the air at or near ground level)	Sep.
Agggravation	cough aggravated from fruit	Arg-m., mag-m.
Agggravation	cough aggravated from happy surprise	Acon., merc.
Agggravation	cough aggravated from hot tea	Spong.
Agggravation	cough aggravated from lying and ameliorated from sitting	Hyos., laur., Puls., rhus-t., sang., Sep.
Agggravation	cough aggravated from milk	Ambr., ant-c., ant-t., brom., kali-c., spong., sul-ac., zinc.
Agggravation	cough aggravated from motion	Arn., ars-i., ars., bar-c., bell., brom., bry., bufo., calc., carb-o., carb-v., chin-a., chin., cina., coc-c., cur., dros., eup-per., ferr-ar., Ferr., form., iod., ip., kali-ar., kali-bi., kali-c., kali-n., kreos., lach., laur., led., lob., lyc., merc., mez., mosch., mur-ac., nat-m., nat-s., nit-ac., nux-v., osm., phos., plan., psor., pyrog., seneg., sep., sil., spong., squil., stann., staph., sul-ac., zinc.
Agggravation	cough aggravated from motion of arms	Ars., calc., ferr., kali-c., led., lyc., Nat-m., nux-v.
Agggravation	cough aggravated from motion of chest	Anac., bar-c., Chin., cocc., dros., lach., mang., merc., mur-ac., nat-m., Nux-v., phos., sil., Stann.
Agggravation	cough aggravated from mucous in upper chest	Anac., bar-c., Chin., cocc., dros., lach., mang., merc., mur-ac., nat-m., Nux-v., phos., sil., Stann.
Agggravation	cough aggravated from music	Ambr., calc., cham., kali-c., kreos., ph-ac.
Agggravation	cough aggravated from other person approaching or passing	Carb-v.
Agggravation	cough aggravated from other person coming into room	Phos.
Agggravation	cough aggravated from potatoes	Alum.
Agggravation	cough aggravated from raising the arms	Bry., ferr., lyc., ol-j.
Agggravation	cough aggravated from reading aloud	Ambr., cina., dros., mang., meph., nit-ac., nux-v., par., Phos., stann., tub., verb.
Agggravation	cough aggravated from reading aloud in evening	Phos.
Agggravation	cough aggravated from rinsing (flush mouth with water)	Coc-c.
Agggravation	cough aggravated from running	Cina., iod., merc., seneg., sil., stann., sul-ac.
Agggravation	cough aggravated from sensation from sulphur fumes or vapour	Am-c., aml-n., Ars., asaf., brom., bry., calc., carb-v., chin., cina., Ign., ip., kali-chl., lach., Lyc., mosch., par., Puls.
Agggravation	cough aggravated from singing	Alum., arg-m., arg-n., dros., hyos., mang., meph., phos., rhus-t., rumx., sil., spong., stann., stram.
Agggravation	cough aggravated from sitting bent	Rhus-t., spig., stann.
Agggravation	cough aggravated from standing	Acon., aloe., euphr., ign., mag-s., nat-m., nat-s., sep., stann., sulph., zinc.
Agggravation	cough aggravated from sugar	Zinc.
Agggravation	cough aggravated from sun	Ant-t., coca.
Agggravation	cough aggravated from swallowing	Aesc., Brom., cupr., eug., kali-ma., lyc., lyss., nat-m., op., phos., puls., sul-ac.
Agggravation	cough aggravated from tight clothing	Stann.

Body part/Disease	Symptom	Medicines
Agggravation	cough aggravated from turning left to right side in bed	Kreos.
Agggravation	cough aggravated from uncovering feet or head	Sil.
Agggravation	cough aggravated from uncovering hands	Bar-c., Hep., Rhus-t., sil.
Agggravation	cough aggravated in dark room	Bry.
Agggravation	cough aggravated where many persons are present	Ambr.
Agggravation	cough croupy aggravated after midnight	Ars.
Agggravation	cough short aggravated from inspiration	Nat-a.
Agggravation	cough short aggravated in open air	Ang., seneg., spig.
Agggravation	cough short aggravated on smoking	Thuj.
Agggravation	cough with copious greenish salty expectorations aggravated in morning	Stann.
Agggravation	cramp aggravated from cold air	Bufo.
Agggravation	cramp aggravated from pressure	Zinc.
Agggravation	cramp in forearm aggravated from motion	Kali-i., plb.
Agggravation	cramp in hand aggravated from extending	Plb.
Agggravation	cramp in sole in bed aggravated from putting foot out of bed	Chel.
Agggravation	cramps in chest aggravated from motion	Ferr., sulph.
Agggravation	croup aggravated after sleep	Lach., spong.
Agggravation	croup aggravated on lying	Hep.
Agggravation	delirium aggravated from heat	Stram.
Agggravation	Desire to be alone while Aggravated	Ambr., Ars., bov., brom., cadm., calc., camph., con., dros., elaps., kali-c., lyc., mez., pall., Phos., rat., sil., stram., tab., zinc.
Agggravation	discharge from nose aggravated from stooping	Am-c.
Agggravation	discoloration of skin with spots aggravated from warmth	Fl-ac.
Agggravation	dry cough aggravated from heat of room	Coc-c., nat-a.
Agggravation	dry cough at night aggravated from inspiration	Nat-a.
Agggravation	dry cough at night aggravated from lying	Con., hyos., kali-br., laur., ol-j., phyt., puls., Sulph., zinc.
Agggravation	dry cough at night aggravated from lying on right side	Carb-an.
Agggravation	dry cough at night aggravated from motion	Bell., seneg.
Agggravation	dry cough in evening aggravated from inspiring	Dig.
Agggravation	dysuria painful, aggravated from effort to urinate	Plb.
Agggravation	dysuria painful, aggravated from thinking of it	Hell., nux-v.
Agggravation	emptyness of abdomen, aggravated from inspiration	Calad.
Agggravation	eruption in forearm aggravated from scratching	Mang., mez.
Agggravation	eruption, vesicles in upper limbs aggravated from washing in cold water	Clem.
Agggravation	eruptions burning aggravated from touch	Cann-s., canth., merc.

Body part/Disease	Symptom	Medicines
Agggravation	eruptions herpetic aggravated by cold water	Clem., dulc., sulph.
Agggravation	eruptions itching aggravated from fire	Mez.
Agggravation	eruptions itching aggravated from touch	Mez.
Agggravation	eruptions itching aggravated from warmth	Alum., bov., caust., clem., led., lyc., **Merc.**, mez., nat-a., psor., puls., sulph.
Agggravation	eruptions itching aggravated from warmth of bed	Aeth., alum., anac., ant-c., caust., clem., cocc., kali-a., kreos., mag-m., merc., mur-ac., **Psor.**, puls., rhus-t., sars., staph., **Sulph.**, til., verat.
Agggravation	eruptions itching aggravated from washing	Mez., sulph.
Agggravation	eruptions itching aggravated in cold water	Clem.
Agggravation	eruptions itching aggravated in warm room	Sep.
Agggravation	eruptions on face aggravated at night	Ars., mag-m.
Agggravation	eruptions on face aggravated at night in warm room	Mag-m.
Agggravation	eruptions on face aggravated by cold air	Ars., dulc.
Agggravation	eruptions on face aggravated from warmth	Euphr., mez., psor., sulph., teucr. amel. : Ars.
Agggravation	eruptions on face aggravated from washing	Nux-v., sulph.
Agggravation	eruption, pustules aggravated from bathing	Dulc.
Agggravation	erysipelas aggravated after scratching	Am-c., ant-c., arn., ars., bell., bor., bry., calc., canth., carb-an., carb-v., graph., hep., hyos., lach., lyc., mag-c., **Merc.**, nat-a., nat-c., nit-ac., petr., phos., puls., ran-b., **Rhus-t.**, samb., sil., spong., sulph., thuj.
Agggravation	excessive flow of blood in brain aggravated toward evening with terrible pain , would press the head against wall , fears going mad	Stram.
Agggravation	Expanded (Out stretched) sensation aggravated from shaking head	Carb-ac.
Agggravation	expectoration aggravated from air	Chin-s., cob., merc., nux-v., plan., sacc., sep.
Agggravation	feeling of tightness in abdomen aggravated while rising	Zinc.
Agggravation	felon with caries of bone and deep seated pain aggravated from warmth of bed	Sep.
Agggravation	fever aggravated from drinking	Bar-c., calc., cham., cocc.
Agggravation	fever aggravated from drinking beer	Bell., ferr., rhus-t., sulph.
Agggravation	fever aggravated from drinking coffee	Canth., cham., rhus-t.
Agggravation	fever aggravated from drinking cold water with shivering	Bell., calen., **Caps.**, eup-per., nux-v.
Agggravation	fever aggravated from drinking water	*Calc., canth., ign., rhus-t., sep.*
Agggravation	fever aggravated from drinking wine	Ars., carb-v., fl-ac., gins., iod., nat-m., nux-v., sil.
Agggravation	fever aggravated from standing	Arg-m., con., mang., puls., rhus-t.
Agggravation	fever aggravated from warm covering	Acon., **Apis.**, calc., cham., coff., ferr., **Ign.**, led., lyc., mur-ac., nux-v., op., petr., **Puls.**, rhus-t., staph., sulph., verat.
Agggravation	fever aggravated from warm drinks	Sumb.
Agggravation	fever aggravated from warmth	**Apis.**, bry., ign., op., **Puls.**, staph.

Body part/Disease	Symptom	Medicines
Agggravation	fever aggravated from washing	Am-c., rhus-t., sep., sulph.
Agggravation	fever aggravated in warm room	Am-m., ang., **Apis.**, bry., ip., lyc., mag-m., nat-m., nicc., plan., **Puls.**, sul-ac., sulph., zinc.
Agggravation	fever aggravated on motion	Agar., alum., am-m., ant-c., ant-t., ars., bell., bry., camph., canth., chin-s., **Chin.**, con., cur., nux-v., sep., stann., stram., sul-ac.
Agggravation	fever aggravated while sitting	Phos., sep.
Agggravation	formication aggravated from heat of bed	Rhod.
Agggravation	formication aggravated from scratching	Dulc.
Agggravation	formication in sole of foot aggravated from rest	Sep.
Agggravation	hacking cough aggravated from heat	Hyper.
Agggravation	hacking cough aggravated in cold air	All-c., hyper.
Agggravation	headache aggravated from blowing nose	Ambr., aster., Aur., bell., calc., chel., ferr., Hep., mur-ac., nit-ac., Puls., Sulph.
Agggravation	headache aggravated from clothing about the neck	Arg-n., bell., crot-c., glon., lach., sep.
Agggravation	headache aggravated from hot drinks	Arum-t., Phos., Puls., sulph.
Agggravation	headache aggravated from warm food	Arum-t., mez., phos., puls., sulph.
Agggravation	headache aggravated in darkness	Aloe., carb-an., carb-v., lac-c., onos., sil.
Agggravation	headache aggravated while lying in dark room	Onos.
Agggravation	headache on left side of head and face extending to neck aggravated by lying on left side	Ars., calad., kali-bi.
Agggravation	heaviness in back aggravated from rising	Ant-t.
Agggravation	heaviness in hand aggravated from warmth of bed	Goss.
Agggravation	heaviness in kidneys aggravated by sitting	Carl.
Agggravation	heaviness in leg aggravated from exertion	**Gels.**, pic-ac.
Agggravation	heaviness in lumbar region aggravated from motion	Phos., pic-ac.
Agggravation	heaviness in lumbar region aggravated from turning in bed	Corn.
Agggravation	heaviness in region of kidneys aggravated by motion	Cimic.
Agggravation	heaviness of Head aggravated from looking steadily	Mur-ac.
Agggravation	heaviness of Head aggravated from thinking on	Hell.
Agggravation	heaviness of Head aggravated on smoking	Ferr-i., gels.
Agggravation	hysteriacal, aggravated in morning	Tarent.
Agggravation	inflamation of joints aggravated from heat	Guai., led.
Agggravation	inflammation of lungs aggravated by lying on right side	Kali-c.
Agggravation	Inflammation of eye aggravated from becoming wet	Calc., dulc., rhus-t.
Agggravation	Inflammation of eye aggravated from cold	Ars., sil.
Agggravation	Inflammation of eye aggravated from dry cold wind	Acon.
Agggravation	Inflammation of eye aggravated from warmth of bed	Merc.
Agggravation	Inflammation of eye aggravated from washing	Sulph.

Body part/Disease	Symptom	Medicines
Agggravation	inflammation of iris with bursting pain in eyeball, temple and side of face	Staph.
Agggravation	inflammation of larynx aggravated in evening	Cedr., kali-bi., rhus-t.
Agggravation	internal chill aggravated by external heat	Ip.
Agggravation	irritability Aggravated after consolation	Bell., cact., calc-p., calc., chin., hell., Ign., kali-c., lil-t., lyc., merc., Nat-m., nit-ac., nux-v., plat., Sep., Sil., staph.
Agggravation	itching in eye aggravated from rubbing	Mag-c.
Agggravation	itching about anus aggravated by rubbing	Alum., petr.
Agggravation	itching in ankle aggravated from scratching	Led.
Agggravation	itching in ankle aggravated from warmth	**Led.**, rhus-v.
Agggravation	itching in axilla aggravated from perspiration	Jug-r.
Agggravation	itching in back of foot aggravated from scratching	Berb., bism., led.
Agggravation	itching in back of hand aggravated from scratching	Ph-ac.
Agggravation	itching in back of hand aggravated from warmth	Sulph.
Agggravation	itching in buttock aggravated from scratching	Petr.
Agggravation	itching in chest biting aggravated by cold	Nicc.
Agggravation	itching in chest biting aggravated from scratching	Con.
Agggravation	itching in coccyx aggravated from warmth of bed	Petr.
Agggravation	itching in elbow aggravated in evening	Sulph.
Agggravation	itching in external throat aggravated by swallowing	Aur., con.
Agggravation	itching in female genitalia aggravated by scrartching	Am-c., onos.
Agggravation	itching in female genitalia aggravated on contact of urine	Merc.
Agggravation	itching in fingers aggravated from scratching	Ars., arum-t.
Agggravation	itching in fingers aggravated in warm room	Nux-v.
Agggravation	itching in foot aggravated from rubbing	Corn.
Agggravation	itching in foot aggravated from scratching	Bism., corn., led.
Agggravation	itching in foot aggravated from warming up	Rhus-v.
Agggravation	itching in forearm in evening aggravated in bed	Sars.
Agggravation	itching in hand aggravated from scratching	Ars., ham., ph-ac., **Sulph.**
Agggravation	itching in hip in morning aggravated from becoming cool	Dios.
Agggravation	itching in leg aggravated from rubbing	Corn.
Agggravation	itching in leg aggravated from touch	Nat-m.
Agggravation	itching in leg aggravated from undressing	Agar., cact., cupr-ar., dios., rumx.
Agggravation	itching in lower limbs aggravated from rubbing	Corn.
Agggravation	itching in lower limbs aggravated from scratching	Alum., bism., corn., led.
Agggravation	itching in lower limbs aggravated from touch	Nat-m.
Agggravation	itching in lower limbs aggravated from warm bed	Agar., alum., led., sulph.
Agggravation	itching in lower limbs aggravated from warmth	Rhus-v.
Agggravation	itching in male genitalia aggravated from rubbing	Con.
Agggravation	itching in male genitalia aggravated from rubbing	Staph.

Body part/Disease	Symptom	Medicines
Agggravation	itching in male genitalia aggravated from scratching	Rhus-v.
Agggravation	itching in male genitalia aggravated when warm	Rhus-v.
Agggravation	itching in region of bladder with urge to urinate aggravated at night	Sep.
Agggravation	itching in shoulder aggravated from scratching	Stront.
Agggravation	itching in teeth aggravated after super	Kali-c.
Agggravation	itching in teeth aggravated in open air	Anac.
Agggravation	itching in thigh aggravated from scratching	Ars.
Agggravation	itching in toes aggravated from heat	Rhus-v.
Agggravation	itching in toes aggravated from scratching	Alum., arg-m., zinc.
Agggravation	itching in toes in evening aggravated after scratching	Alum.
Agggravation	itching in upper arm aggravated from scratching	Stront.
Agggravation	itching in upper limbs aggravated from lying down	Calad.
Agggravation	itching in upper limbs aggravated from motion	Crot-t.
Agggravation	itching in upper limbs aggravated from rubbing	Crot-t., nat-m., rhus-v.
Agggravation	itching in upper limbs aggravated from scratching	Ars., ham., ph-ac., rhus-v., stront., **Sulph.**
Agggravation	itching in upper limbs aggravated from touch	Crot-t., psor.
Agggravation	itching in upper limbs aggravated from warmth	Sulph.
Agggravation	itching in upper limbs aggravated in warm room	Nux-v.
Agggravation	itching in wrist aggravated from scratching	**Sulph.**
Agggravation	itching of occiput aggravated by scratching	Staph.
Agggravation	itching of occiput aggravated in warm room	Fago., sulph.
Agggravation	itching of Scalp aggravated by scratching	Calc., lyc., Phos., sil.
Agggravation	itching of Scalp aggravated from warmth of bed	Bov., calc., carb-v., lyc., mez., sil., staph., sulph.
Agggravation	itching on face aggravated at night	Mez., sulph., viol-t.
Agggravation	itching on face aggravated by warmth	Ant-c., euphr., mez., psor., sulph., teucr.
Agggravation	jar (shake) aggravated from stepping	Acon., alum., am-c., ambr., anac., ant-c., arg-m., arg-n., **Arn.**, ars., asar., bar-c., **Bell.**, bor., **Bry.**, cact., calad., calc., camph., canth., carb-s., caust., cham., chel., chin., **Cic.**, cocc., coff., **Con.**, dros., dulc., euphr., ferr-ar., ferr., glon., graph., ham., hell., hep., ign., kali-c., kali-i., kali-n., **Lach.**, led., lil-t., lyc., mag-c., mag-m., meny., merc., nat-a., nat-c., nat-m., nat-p., **Nit-ac.**, nux-m., nux-v., onos., par., petr., ph-ac., phos., plat., plb., puls., rhod., **Rhus-t.**, ruta., sabad., sabin., sanic., seneg., sep., **Sil.**, spig., spong., stann., staph., sulph., **Ther.**, thuj., verb., viol-t.
Agggravation	lameness aggravated in cold wet weather	**Rhus-t.**
Agggravation	leg hot aggravated from sitting	Berb.
Agggravation	leucorrhoea aggravated from walking	Aesc., alum., anan., aur., Bov., calc., carb-an., graph., kreos., lac-c., mag-m., nat-m., phos., sars., sep., stront., sulph., tub.
Agggravation	loose cough aggravated from exercise & warm room	Brom.
Agggravation	menses, copious, aggravated by lying	Kreos.

Body part/Disease	Symptom	Medicines
Agggravation	menses, copious, aggravated from cold air	Am-c.
Agggravation	menses, copious, aggravated from sitting	Mag-m.
Agggravation	menses, copious, aggravated from standing	Am-c., Cocc., mag-c.
Agggravation	menses, copious, aggravated from walking	Am-c., Cocc., croc., erig., lil-t., mag-c., nat-s., pall., puls., sabin., ust., zinc.
Agggravation	metrorrhagia aggravated at night	Mag-m.
Agggravation	metrorrhagia aggravated by lying on back	Cham.
Agggravation	metrorrhagia aggravated from motion	Arg-n., bell., bry., cact., calc., coff., croc., Erig., helon., Ip., psor., sabin., sec., sulph., tril., ust.
Agggravation	nausea aggravated from motion of eyes	Con., graph., jab., puls., sep.
Agggravation	nausea aggravated from thinking of tea	Arg-m., calc., dros., graph., lach., mosch., sars., sep.
Agggravation	numbness aggravated from warmth	Sec.
Agggravation	numbness in elbow aggravated on motion	All-c.
Agggravation	numbness in forearm aggravated from raising arm	Puls., sep.
Agggravation	numbness in leg aggravated in cold water	Apis.
Agggravation	numbness in upper arm aggravated from motion	Plb., ruta.
Agggravation	orgasm of blood aggravated on motion or speaking	Iod., nat-c.
Agggravation	ovaries painful aggravated from breathing	Bry., lac-c.
Agggravation	ovaries painful aggravated from motion	Ars., Bell., Bry., cench., lac-c., pall., ther.
Agggravation	pain aggravated from jar while walking	Aloe., alumn., anac., Bell., hell., kali-s., mang-m., sep.
Agggravation	pain aggravated in prostate gland on riding	Staph.
Agggravation	pain aggravated in prostate gland on shaking	Bell.
Agggravation	pain aggravated in prostate gland on walking	All-c., brom., cycl., staph.
Agggravation	pain between scapula (shoulder blade) aggravated from wine	Ph-ac.
Agggravation	pain between scapula aggravated from beer	Phos.
Agggravation	pain between scapula aggravated from lying on left side	Ph-ac.
Agggravation	pain in abdomen aggravated by eructations	Cham., cocc., phos.
Agggravation	pain in abdomen aggravated from hot drinks	Brom., graph., kali-c.
Agggravation	pain in abdomen aggravated from lying on abdomen	Ambr.
Agggravation	pain in abdomen aggravated from warm food	Brom., chin., fl-ac., ign., Phos., Puls.
Agggravation	pain in abdomen aggravated from yawning	Ars.
Agggravation	pain in abdomen aggravated on passing flatus	Aur., canth., fl-ac., nat-a., squil.
Agggravation	pain in ankle aggravated from warmth	Guai., lac-c., **Led., Puls.**
Agggravation	pain in anus aggravated from warm bathing	Brom.
Agggravation	pain in apex of left lung aggravated from inspiration	Cimic.
Agggravation	pain in arm aggravated from touch	Agn., arg-m., chin., sabin., staph.
Agggravation	pain in arm aggravated from turning in bed	Sang.
Agggravation	pain in back aggravated bending backward	Arg-m., bar-c., calc-p., calc., chel., cimic., con., dios., kali-c., lam., mang., plat., puls., sel., stann.

Body part/Disease	Symptom	Medicines
Agggravation	pain in back aggravated bending forward	Pic-ac.
Agggravation	pain in back aggravated during thunderstorm	Agar., rhod.
Agggravation	pain in back aggravated from coffee	Cham.
Agggravation	pain in back aggravated from jarrying (to have an irritating, unsettling, or unpleasantly disturbing effect on somebody or something)	Acon., Bell., carb-ac., carb-an., Graph., podo., seneg., sep., Sil., sulph., ther., thuj.
Agggravation	pain in back aggravated from laughing	Cann-i., phos., plb., tell.
Agggravation	pain in back aggravated from leaning back against chair	Agar., ther.
Agggravation	pain in back aggravated from lying on left side	Ph-ac.
Agggravation	pain in back aggravated from lying on side	Cina., ign., nat-s., puls., staph.
Agggravation	pain in back aggravated from noise of running water	Lyss.
Agggravation	pain in back aggravated from pulling	Dios.
Agggravation	pain in back aggravated from warmth of bed	Lil-t., sulph.
Agggravation	pain in back aggravated in warm room	Gels., kali-s.
Agggravation	pain in back of foot aggravated from stepping	Nux-m.
Agggravation	pain in bladder aggravated from drinking	Canth.
Agggravation	pain in bladder aggravated from standing	Puls.
Agggravation	pain in bladder with burning aggravated by standing	Eup-pur.
Agggravation	pain in bone aggravated from touch	Staph.
Agggravation	pain in cervical region aggravated in room	Psor.
Agggravation	pain in chest aggravated by arms near chest	Psor.
Agggravation	pain in chest aggravated from bending right	Rhod.
Agggravation	pain in chest aggravated from bending sideways	Acon.
Agggravation	pain in chest aggravated from blowing nose	Chel.
Agggravation	pain in chest aggravated from lying on painful side	Bell., nux-v., ran-b., rumx.
Agggravation	pain in chest aggravated from motion	Abrot., arn., bad., bapt., Bell., Bry., Calc., caps., carb-s., card-m., chel., chin., cimic., equis., gamb., graph., hep., hyos., kali-c., kali-p., kalm., lact-ac., laur., lyc., manc., meny., merc., naja., nat-m., nit-ac., nux-v., phos., psor., ran-b., sabad., sars., sec., Spig., squil., stront., sulph., viol-t.
Agggravation	pain in chest aggravated from pressure	Ant-c., meny., merc-i-f., nat-p., ran-b., seneg., sul-ac., tarax.
Agggravation	pain in chest aggravated from singing	Am-c.
Agggravation	pain in chest aggravated in warm room	Mag-s., nat-m., sil.
Agggravation	pain in dorsal region aggravated on stepping hard	Seneg.
Agggravation	pain in dorsal region in right scapula aggravated from bending forward	Lob.
Agggravation	pain in elbow aggravated from warmth	Guai.
Agggravation	pain in elbow aggravated on motion	Agn., **Bry.**, carb-s., guai., kali-bi., led., plb., sulph., ust.
Agggravation	pain in extremities aggravated after sleep	Agar., lach., merc-c., op.
Agggravation	pain in extremities aggravated from cold water	Ant-c., ars., phos., rhus-t., tarent.

Body part/Disease	Symptom	Medicines
Agggravation	pain in extremities aggravated from drinking	**Crot-c.**
Agggravation	pain in extremities aggravated from thinking about the pain	Ox-ac.
Agggravation	pain in extremities aggravated from thunderstorm	**Med.**, nat-c., **Rhod.**
Agggravation	pain in extremities aggravated from touch during thunderstorm	**Chel.**, chin., cocc., vip.
Agggravation	pain in extremities aggravated from warmth	Ant-t., apis., bry., guai., iod., kali-i., ptel., puls., **Sec.**, sep., stel., sulph., thuj.
Agggravation	pain in extremities aggravated from warmth of bed	Apis., lac-c., led., **Merc.**, phyt., stel., sulph., verat.
Agggravation	pain in eye aggravated by closing	Bell., canth., carb-v., cimic., clem., con., fago., lact-ac., sil., staph., sumb.
Agggravation	pain in eye aggravated from dim light	Am-m., apis., sars., stram.
Agggravation	pain in eye aggravated from pressure	Brom., dros., ham., plan., sars.
Agggravation	pain in eye aggravated from rest	Coloc., dros., dulc., merc-i-f., mur-ac., thuj.
Agggravation	pain in eye aggravated from sun light	Aml-n., calc., clem., hep., kali-p., mang., nat-a., nat-m., sulph.
Agggravation	pain in eye aggravated from thinking of the pain	Lach., spig.
Agggravation	pain in eye aggravated from warmth	Arn., chel., merc., mez., nat-m., puls.
Agggravation	pain in eye aggravated from wet weather	Calc., dulc., merc., rhus-t., spig.
Agggravation	pain in face in left zygoma aggravated by rest	Mag-c.
Agggravation	pain in face in left zygoma aggravated at night	Mag-c., mez., plat., sil.
Agggravation	pain in fingers aggravated from cold	Stram.
Agggravation	pain in flexor muscles aggravated from motion	Nux-v.
Agggravation	pain in foot aggravated from touch	Acon., bor., bry., chin., ferr-ma.
Agggravation	pain in foot aggravated from warmth	Guai.
Agggravation	pain in forearm aggravated from touch	Cupr., sabin., staph.
Agggravation	pain in hand aggravated from running	Agar.
Agggravation	pain in heart aggravated on moving	Cact., kali-i., lil-t., phyt.
Agggravation	pain in heart aggravated by ascending	Crot-h.
Agggravation	pain in heart aggravated by bending forward	Lil-t., Lith.
Agggravation	pain in heart aggravated from lying	Agar., aur., lil-t., puls., rumx., Spong.
Agggravation	pain in heart aggravated from lying on left side	Cact., colch., crot-h., dig., dios., iber., kali-ar., lach., naja., nat-m., Spig., tell.
Agggravation	pain in heart aggravated from respiration	Crot-h., rumx.
Agggravation	pain in joints aggravated from warmth of bed	Calc., lac-c., **Led.**, plb., sabin., sulph.
Agggravation	pain in joints aggravated from warmth	Caust., cedr., guai., lac-c., **Led., Puls.**
Agggravation	pain in kidney aggravated from motion	Aesc., arg-n., berb., cahin., coc-c., colch., dor., gels., ham., kali-bi., nux-v.
Agggravation	pain in kidney aggravated from sneezing	Aeth., ars., bell.
Agggravation	pain in kidneys aggravated from motion	Aesc., arg-n., berb., cahin., coc-c., colch., dor., gels., ham., kali-bi., nux-v.
Agggravation	pain in kidneys aggravated from sneezing	Aeth., ars., bell.

Body part/Disease	Symptom	Medicines
Agggravation	pain in kidneys aggravated from straightening out legs	Colch.
Agggravation	pain in knee aggravated from flexing limb	Phys.
Agggravation	pain in knee aggravated from pressure	Ol-j., ran-b.
Agggravation	pain in knee aggravated from stretching	Ant-c., calc-p., med.
Agggravation	pain in knee aggravated from warmth	Guai., **Led.**
Agggravation	pain in larynx aggravated on respiration	Bell., carb-v., hep., kali-n.
Agggravation	pain in left lung aggravated in evening	Sulph.
Agggravation	pain in left shoulder aggravated from lying on painless side	Nat-m.
Agggravation	pain in leg aggravated in cold air	Ars., kalm., rhus-t., tub.
Agggravation	pain in lower limb aggravated after sleep	**Lach.**, led.
Agggravation	pain in lower limb aggravated from motion	Acon., alum., apis., berb., **Bry.**, calc-p., carb-s., cocc., guai., kali-p., kreos., lac-c., led., mang., merc., nat-s., nux-v., phos., phyt., plb., puls., ran-b., sulph.
Agggravation	pain in lower limb aggravated from pressure	Coloc., dros., kali-bi., kali-c., kali-i., lyc., Phos., phyt., plb.
Agggravation	pain in lower limb aggravated from sitting	**Am-m.**, berb., bry., coloc., dios., ferr., indg., iris., kali-bi., kali-i., lach., **Lyc.**, lyss., meny., merc., ruta., sep., staph., valer.
Agggravation	pain in lower limb aggravated from standing	Aesc., agar., bar-c., ferr., kali-bi., kali-i., nux-v., sulph., valer.
Agggravation	pain in lower limb aggravated from stepping	Asar., bar-c., gnaph., nux-m.
Agggravation	pain in lower limb aggravated from stooping	Agar., card-m., dros., nat-s., tell.
Agggravation	pain in lower limb aggravated from stretching the leg	Arn., berb., caps., cham., guai., valer.
Agggravation	pain in lower limb aggravated from touch	Bell., berb., caps., **Chin-s.**, cocc., coloc., ferr., gels., guai., kali-c., **Lach.**, led., mag-p., mez., sulph., verat.
Agggravation	pain in lower limb aggravated from turning in bed	Nat-s.
Agggravation	pain in lower limb aggravated from walking	Bar-c., berb., chin-s., coff., coloc., ign., lach., led., nat-a., nat-s., psor., sulph., zinc.
Agggravation	pain in lower limb aggravated from warmth	Guai., **Led.**, verat., zinc.
Agggravation	pain in lower limb aggravated in warm room	**Puls.**
Agggravation	pain in lumbar region aggravated after urinating	Syph.
Agggravation	pain in lumbar region aggravated from drawing up limbs	Arg-m.
Agggravation	pain in lumbar region aggravated from lying on left side	Agar., Sulph.
Agggravation	pain in lumbar region aggravated from pulling	Dios.
Agggravation	pain in lumbar region aggravated from sitting bent	Chin-s., kali-i., lac-c., phos.
Agggravation	pain in mammae aggravated from pressure	Plb.
Agggravation	pain in nail of toes aggravated from motion	Aster., chin., sabin.
Agggravation	pain in nail of toes aggravated on touch	Chin., mang., sabin.
Agggravation	pain in nose aggravated from lying down	Bor.

Body part/Disease	Symptom	Medicines
Agggravation	pain in nose aggravated from pressure	Chin., con., cupr-ar., led.
Agggravation	pain in penis aggravated from motion	Berb.
Agggravation	pain in prostate gland aggravated from jar	Bell.
Agggravation	pain in prostate gland aggravated from riding	Staph.
Agggravation	pain in region of heart aggravated from motion	Bapt., bry., sep., stront.
Agggravation	pain in region of heart aggravated on becoming straight	Acon.
Agggravation	pain in right scapula aggravated from bending forward	Lob.
Agggravation	pain in sacral region aggravated from lying on right side	Agar.
Agggravation	pain in sacral region aggravated from touch	Colch.
Agggravation	pain in sacral region aggravated while extending right thigh by pressing at stool or cough	Tell.
Agggravation	pain in shoulder aggravated from lying quite on painful side	Lach., nat-m., nux-v., ph-ac., rhod., thuj.
Agggravation	pain in shoulder aggravated from pulling arm	Chel.
Agggravation	pain in shoulder aggravated from putting the arm behind him	**Ferr.**, rhus-t., **Sanic.**
Agggravation	pain in shoulder aggravated from raising the arm	Alum., bar-c., bry., calc., card-m., chel., cocc., dros., ferr., hep., ign., iris., kali-bi., kali-n., kreos., lac-c., led., lyc., mag-c., mag-m., nat-c., nat-m., nit-ac., petr., phos., phyt., prun-s., puls., rhus-t., **Sang.**, sanic., sep., sul-ac., sulph., syph., thuj., zinc.
Agggravation	pain in soles of foot aggravated from touch	Crot-t., puls.
Agggravation	pain in spermatic cord aggravated from motion	Ox-ac.
Agggravation	pain in spine aggravated by jarring	Acon., Bell., Graph., podo., sulph., ther., thuj.
Agggravation	pain in spine aggravated from noise	Ars.
Agggravation	pain in spleen aggravated from inspiration	Cob., mez.
Agggravation	pain in spleen aggravated from pressure of clothing	Calad., fl-ac., kali-bi., nat-m., puls.
Agggravation	pain in sternum aggravated from stretching	Staph.
Agggravation	pain in sternum aggravated from pressure	Manc., ph-ac.
Agggravation	pain in teeth aggravated from breathing deep	Nux-v.
Agggravation	pain in teeth aggravated from brushing teeth	Bry., carb-v., Lach., lyc., staph.
Agggravation	pain in teeth aggravated from coughing	Bry., lyc., sep.
Agggravation	pain in teeth aggravated from lying on painful side	Ars., guare., ign., nux-v., puls.
Agggravation	pain in teeth aggravated from lying on painless side	Bry., cham., ign., puls.
Agggravation	pain in teeth aggravated from motion	Bry., chel., chin., clem., daph., hyper., merc., mez., nux-v., sabin., spig., staph.
Agggravation	pain in teeth aggravated from sneezing	Thuj.
Agggravation	pain in teeth aggravated from sucking teeth	Bell., bov., carb-v., cast., kali-c., mang., nux-m., nux-v., sil., zinc.
Agggravation	pain in teeth aggravated from swallowing	Alum., chin-s., phos., staph.

Body part/Disease	Symptom	Medicines
Agggravation	pain in teeth aggravated from warmth of bed	Ant-c., bell., bry., Cham., chel., clem., graph., jug-r., led., mag-c., Merc., ph-ac., phos., Puls., rhod., sabin., sulph.
Agggravation	pain in teeth aggravated from water held in mouth	Camph.
Agggravation	pain in teeth aggravated from wine	Acon., anan., camph., ign., nux-v.
Agggravation	pain in teeth aggravated from working in damp places	Ars., Calc., dulc., Rhus-t.
Agggravation	pain in testes (either of the paired male reproductive glands, roundish in shape, that produce sperm and male sex hormones, and hang in a small sac scrotum) aggravated from wine	Thuj.
Agggravation	pain in testes aggravated from pressure of clothing	Arg-m.
Agggravation	pain in testes aggravated from standing	Rhod.
Agggravation	pain in thigh aggravated from ascending stairs	Bar-c., kali-c., sep.
Agggravation	pain in thigh aggravated from change of weather	Berb.
Agggravation	pain in throat aggravated after drinking	Canth.
Agggravation	pain in throat aggravated on expectoration	Bell.
Agggravation	pain in throat aggravated on hawking	Bell., canth., cob., Lach., thuj.
Agggravation	pain in upper limb aggravated from pressure	Berb., merc-i-f., rhus-v., sil., spig.
Agggravation	pain in upper limb aggravated from warmth	Ant-t., apis., bry., calc., caust., cham., dulc., guai., lact-ac., **Led.**, nux-v., **Puls.**, sabad., stel., stront., sulph., thuj., zinc.
Agggravation	pain in uterus aggravated from jar	Bell., lach., lil-t.
Agggravation	pain in uterus aggravated from motion	Bell., Bry., cimic., Cocc., con., lil-t.
Agggravation	pain in wrist aggravated from twisting	Merc-i-f.
Agggravation	pain in wrist aggravated from warmth	Guai., puls.
Agggravation	pain of ear aggravated from warmth of bed	Merc-i-f., Merc., nux-v., phos., puls.
Agggravation	pain of face aggravated by bathing	Am-c., coff.
Agggravation	pain of face aggravated by blowing nose	Merc.
Agggravation	pain of face aggravated by change of weather	Rhod.
Agggravation	pain of face aggravated by chewing	Acon., agar., Ars., bell., carb-s., colch., dulc., kali-ar., kali-c., kali-p., mag-c., Mag-p., merc., phos., rhod., Rhus-t., ruta., sulph., verb.
Agggravation	pain of face aggravated by cold application	Aesc., bell., con., ferr., hep., mag-c., Mag-p., phos., rhod., Rhus-t., sanic., Sil., stann.
Agggravation	pain of face aggravated during stool	Spig.
Agggravation	pain of face aggravated from dry cold wind	Acon., caust., Hep., lac-c., Mag-p., rhod.
Agggravation	pain of face aggravated from motion	Acon., Bell., Bry., cact., calc-p., calc., chin-a., chin., colch., coloc., ferr-p., gels., lac-c., mez., Nux-v., phos., rhod., sep., Spig., squil., staph., verb.
Agggravation	pain of face aggravated from odors	Sep.
Agggravation	pain of face aggravated from pressure	Bell., caps., cina., coloc., cupr., dros., gels., mag-c., merc-i-f., nux-v., verb.
Agggravation	pain of face aggravated from rising from bed	Chin., olnd., rhus-t., spig.
Agggravation	pain of face aggravated from swallowing	Kali-n., phos., staph.
Agggravation	pain of face aggravated from talking	Bry., chel., euphr., mez., phos., puls., rhod., spig., squil., verb.

Body part/Disease	Symptom	Medicines
Agggravation	pain of face aggravated from touch	Arn., aur., Bell., bry., caps., chel., chin-s., chin., cina., cocc., Coff., coloc., cor-r., cupr., dig., dros., Hep., Lach., lyc., mag-c., mag-p., nat-m., nux-v., par., ph-ac., phos., puls., sep., spig., spong., staph., verb., zinc.
Agggravation	pain of face aggravated from walking	Agar., mag-c., sulph.
Agggravation	pain of face aggravated from warm drinks	Cham.
Agggravation	pain of face aggravated from warm food	Mez., puls., sep.
Agggravation	pain of face aggravated from warmth	Clem., glon., merc., mez., plat., puls., verat.
Agggravation	pain of face aggravated from wine	Bell., cact.
Agggravation	pain of face aggravated from yawning	Arn., ign., op., rhus-t., sabad., staph.
Agggravation	pain of face aggravated in bed	Carb-v., mag-c., mag-p., puls., sil., spong., verb., viol-t.
Agggravation	pain of face aggravated in damp weather	Calc-p., calc., chin-s., dulc., merc., nat-s., sep., sil., spig., verat.
Agggravation	pain of face aggravated in open air	Alum., ars., bell., calc., carb-an., chin-a., chin., cocc., guai., hep., kali-ar., kali-c., kali-p., kreos., laur., mag-c., mag-p., merc-c., merc., phos., plat., puls., rhus-t., sars., sep., sil., spig., spong., Sulph., thuj., valer.
Agggravation	pain of face aggravated while lying on affected side	Acon., arn., chin., clem., puls., spig., syph.
Agggravation	pain under left scapula aggravated from expiration	Sep.
Agggravation	pain under left scapula aggravated from pressure	Chin.
Agggravation	pain, cutting in bladder aggravated from rest	Ter.
Agggravation	pain, cutting in bladder aggravated from walking	Mang., thuj.
Agggravation	pain, drawing aggravated by walking	Calc., coca.
Agggravation	pain, drawing aggravated in bad weather	Rhod.
Agggravation	painful varices of lower limbs aggravated by warmth	**Fl-ac., Sulph.**
Agggravation	palpitation of heart aggravated from bathing	Am-c.
Agggravation	palpitation of heart aggravated from motion of arms	Acon., am-m., bor., bry., camph., chel., dig., ferr., led., naja., puls., rhus-t., seneg., spig., spong., Sulph., thuj.
Agggravation	palpitation of heart aggravated from warm bath	Iod., lach.
Agggravation	palpitation of heart aggravated while lying on right side	Alumn., arg-n., bad., kali-n., lil-t., plat., spong.
Agggravation	paralysis aggravated from rising	Phos.
Agggravation	persistent cough at midnight aggravated from lying on back and ameliorated from lying on side	Nux-v.
Agggravation	perspiration aggravated from cold wind	Cur.
Agggravation	perspiration in chest aggravated from cold	Agar., camph., canth., cocc., hep., lyc., merc., petr., sep., stann.
Agggravation	pimples of face aggravated at night	Mag-m.
Agggravation	pimples on face aggravated by cold air	Ars.
Agggravation	pimples on face itching aggravated before menses	Mag-m.
Agggravation	pimples on face itching aggravated during menses	Dulc., eug., graph.
Agggravation	pulsation aggravated from excitement	Ferr., kreos.
Agggravation	pulsation aggravated from exertion	Ferr., iod.

Body part/Disease	Symptom	Medicines
Agggravation	pulsation aggravated from motion	Ant-t., graph., iod.
Agggravation	pulsation aggravated from music	Kreos.
Agggravation	pulsation in cervical region aggravated from motion	Ferr.
Agggravation	pulsation in cervical region aggravated from writing	Manc.
Agggravation	pulsation in head aggravated from closing eyes	Sep.
Agggravation	pulsation in head aggravated from motion	Acon., anac., apis., ars., bell., bry., calc-p., caust., chin., cimic., cocc., colch., dirc., eupi., ferr-p., ferr., gels., glon., grat., iod., kali-bi., lach., lyc., nat-m., nit-ac., nux-m., sep., stram., sulph.
Agggravation	pulsation in head aggravated from warm food	Sulph.
Agggravation	pulsation on back aggravated from coughing	Nit-ac.
Agggravation	Pulsation sensation aggravated in open air	Carb-an., cocc., eup-pur., iris. amel. : Kali-bi., kali-i., mang., nicc., phos., pic-ac.
Agggravation	pulse aggravated on motion	Ant-t., arn., bry., dig., fl-ac., gels., graph., iod., lycps., **Nat-m.**, nux-v., petr., phos., sep., staph., stram
Agggravation	quick breath aggravated from lying	Cact., calc.
Agggravation	quick breath aggravated from lying on back	Agar., kali-c.
Agggravation	rash on face aggravated from warmth	Euphr., teucr.
Agggravation	rash red on chest aggravated by warmth	Stram.
Agggravation	restlessness aggravated by drinking	Crot-c.
Agggravation	restlessness aggravated from covering	Aster.
Agggravation	restlessness aggravated from warm bed	Ars-i., Aster., ferr., iod., kali-s., lach., nat-m., puls.
Agggravation	rheumatic pain in joints aggravated from touch	Cocc., mang.
Agggravation	rheumatic pain in shoulder aggravated from external warmth	Guai.
Agggravation	rheumatic pain in shoulder aggravated from wine	Ph-ac.
Agggravation	scales aggravated in winter	Sil.
Agggravation	sciatic pain in lower limb aggravated from cold	Ars., asar., caust., coloc., mag-p., pall., phos., ran-b., **Rhus-t.**, sil.
Agggravation	sciatic pain in lower limb aggravated from cold application	Ars., bry., mag-p., nux-v., phos., **Rhus-t.**, ruta.
Agggravation	sciatic pain in lower limb aggravated from continued motion	Coloc.
Agggravation	sciatic pain in lower limb aggravated from coughing	Caps., caust., sep., tell.
Agggravation	sciatic pain in lower limb aggravated from heat	Led., verat., zinc.
Agggravation	sciatic pain in lower limb aggravated from laughing	Tell.
Agggravation	sciatic pain in lower limb aggravated from motion	Acon., **Bry.**, calc., chel., cocc., coff., coloc., dios., eup-pur., gels., gnaph., guai., iris., kali-c., lac-c., lach., led., mag-p., merc., mez., nux-m., nux-v., pall., phos., phyt., plb., puls., ran-b., sep., staph., syph.
Agggravation	Sciatica aggravated on sitting, relief on lying	Ammon Mur. Q
Agggravation	skin, crawling aggravated from perspiration	**Mang.**, merc., rhod.

Body part/Disease	Symptom	Medicines
Agggravation	skin, itching aggravated by undressing	Am-m., anac., ars., asim., cact., cocc., dros., gamb., hyper., kali-ar., kali-br., mag-c., mez., mur-ac., nat-s., nux-v., olnd., pall., ph-ac., rhod., **Rumx.**, sil., stann., staph., tub.
Agggravation	skin, itching aggravated from scratching	Agar., alum., am-m., **Anac.**, anag., arg-m., arn., **Ars.**, bar-c., bism., bov., calad., calc., cann-s., canth., **Caps.**, carb-an., carb-v., caust., cham., chel., cinnb., coff., con., cupr., dol., dros., guai., ip., kreos., lachn., led., mag-c., mang., merc., mez., mur-ac., nat-a., nat-c., par., ph-ac., phos., phyt., **Puls.**, **Rhus-t.**, rhus-v., seneg., sep., sil., spig., spong., squil., stann., staph., stram., stront., **Sulph.**, til.
Agggravation	skin, itching aggravated from wool	Hep., phos., psor., puls., sulph.
Agggravation	slow expiration in evening aggravated while lying quite	Con., ferr.
Agggravation	stiffness in back aggravated from standing erect	Bry.
Agggravation	stiffness in joints aggravated from heat	Lac-c.
Agggravation	stitching pain in chest extending to back aggravated from lying on left side	Kali-c.
Agggravation	stitching pain in prostate gland aggravated from walking	Kali-bi.
Agggravation	stitching pain in trachea aggravated by swallowing	Ign.
Agggravation	stitching pain in urethra aggravated from sudden sitting	Plan.
Agggravation	stitching sensation in chest aggravated from bending sideways	Acon.
Agggravation	stitching sensation in chest aggravated from sneezing	Acon., bor., bry., chel., Dros., Merc., rhus-t.
Agggravation	swelling in first toe aggravated in evening in bed	Am-c.
Agggravation	symptoms aggravated by wetting feet	Cham., merc., nat-c., nat-m., phos., puls., rhus-t., sep., **Sil.**, xan.
Agggravation	symptoms aggravated in presence of strangers	Ambr., bar-c., bry., bufo., con., lyc., petr., sep., stram., thuj.
Agggravation	symptoms aggravated while sweating	Acon., ant-t., arn., **Ars.**, calc., **Caust.**, **Cham.**, chin-a., chin., cimx., croc., eup-per., ferr-ar., ferr., **Form.**, ign., ip., lyc., **Merc.**, nat-a., nat-c., nux-v., **Op.**, phos., psor., puls., **Rhus-t.**, **Sep.**, spong., **Stram.**, **Sulph.**, **Verat.**
Agggravation	tension in lumbar region aggravated from stretching	Agar.
Agggravation	tension in lumbar region aggravated from touch	Agar.
Agggravation	tension in muscles of back aggravated from lying on other side	Sep.
Agggravation	tension in muscles of back extending to chest aggravated from stooping	Chel.
Agggravation	tension in sacrum aggravated from ascending	Carb-s.
Agggravation	thigh hot aggravated after sitting	Graph.
Agggravation	thirst aggravated after beer	Bry.
Agggravation	tingling in foot aggravated from heat	Lachn.

Body part/Disease	Symptom	Medicines
Agggravation	tingling in hand aggravated on motion	Bapt.
Agggravation	tingling in lower limbs aggravated in warm room	Com.
Agggravation	trembling aggravated from company	Ambr., lyc.
Agggravation	trembling in hand aggravated from mental worry	Plb.
Agggravation	twisting in abdomen aggravated by eating	Grat.
Agggravation	twitching aggravated from touch	Stry.
Agggravation	twitching in hand aggravated from exertion	Merc.
Agggravation	twitching in lower limbs aggravated from warmth of bed	Rhus-t., verat.
Agggravation	ulcer in skin aggravated from warmth	Cham., dros., eupho., fl-ac., hydr., led., lyc., merc., sabin., sec.
Agggravation	ulcer in skin aggravated from washing	Hydr.
Agggravation	ulcer in leg aggravated from warmth	Carb-v., hydr., merc., mez.
Agggravation	ulcer in lower limbs aggravated from warmth	Carb-v., sabin.
Agggravation	ulcer in throat aggravated by cold	Anan.
Agggravation	urticaria aggravated from drinking cold water	Bell.
Agggravation	urticaria vesicular aggravated from washing	Canth., **Clem.**, dulc., hydr., mez., phos., psor., sars., **Sulph.**, urt-u.
Agggravation	urticaria vesicular aggravated from washing in cold water	**Clem.**, dulc., sulph.
Agggravation	uterine (relating to, in, or affecting the womb or uterus) symptoms aggravated from lying	Ambr.
Agggravation	vertigo aggravated after sleep	Ambr., ant-t., apis., ars., atro., calc., carb-v., chin., cimic., dulc., graph., hep., kali-c., kali-i., Lach., lact., med., merc., nat-m., Nux-v., op., sep., spong., stann., stict., stram., stront., tarent., ther., thuj., zinc.
Agggravation	vertigo aggravated from deep breath	Cact.
Agggravation	vertigo aggravated from rest	Acon., bell., calc., cycl., lach., manc., nat-c., puls., rhus-t., sil.
Agggravation	vertigo aggravated while lying on left side	Alumn., iod., phos., sil.
Agggravation	vertigo aggravated while lying on right side	Mur-ac.
Agggravation	vertigo aggravated while lying on side	Stram.
Agggravation	vision, dimness aggravated by sunlight	Asar., both., cic., merc.
Agggravation	vision, dimness (inadequate light) aggravated by fire light	Merc., nat-s.
Agggravation	vision, dimness aggravated by rubbing	Caust.
Agggravation	vision, foggy aggravated from sunlight	Am-m., tarent.
Agggravation	vomiting aggravated from wine	Ant-c.
Agggravation	vomiting blood aggravated on lying	Stann.
Agggravation	warts aggravated from cold washing	Dulc.
Agggravation	weakness aggravated from lying	Agar., alum., bar-c., bry., carb-v., carl., coca., cycl., gels., nat-c., nat-m., nit-ac., nux-v., petr., phys., pip-m., puls., spig., zinc-m.
Agggravation	weakness aggravated in a warm weather	**Ant-c.**, iod., nat-a., nat-m., nat-p., sel., sulph.

Body part/Disease	Symptom	Medicines
Agggravation	weakness aggravated in open air	Am-c., am-m., ambr., bry., calc., chin., clem., coff., coloc., con., ferr., grat., kali-c., mag-c., merc., mur-ac., nux-v., plat., sang., spig., verat.
Agggravation	weakness in back aggravated from eating	Nat-m.
Agggravation	weakness in chest aggravated from reading	Sulph.
Agggravation	weakness in chest aggravated from sitting long	Dig., ph-ac.
Agggravation	weakness in chest aggravated from wine	Bor.
Agggravation	weakness in hip aggravated on rising from seat	Sep.
Agggravation	weakness in leg aggravated after eating	Hyos.
Agggravation	weakness in lumbar (lower back) region aggravated from eating	Nat-m.
Agggravation	weakness in upper arm aggravated from bending of limb	Phyt.
Agggravation	weakness in wrist aggravated on motion	Dig.
Agggravation	Weeping aggravated from consolation	Bell., cact., calc-p., calc., chin., hell., ign., kali-c., lil-t., lyc., merc., Nat-m., nit-ac., nux-v., plat., Sep., Sil., staph., sulph., tarent., thuj.
Agggravation	whistling breath aggravated on ascending	Sulph.
Aggravations	anxiety aggravated from excitement	Phos.
Albumin	albuminous discharge from urethra	Canth., nit-ac., petros.
Albumin	bloody, ink-like, albuminous urine from kidney	Colch.
Albumin	discharge from urethra albuminous	Canth., nit-ac., petros.
Albumin	inflammation of kidneys with bloody ink like albuminous urine	Colch.
Albumin	swelling in lower limbs in albuminaria	Apis., ars., calc-ar., ferr., lach., sars., ter.
Albumin	ulcer with albuminous discharge	Calc., puls.
Albumin	urine albuminous (the presence of albumin in urine, usually an indication of kidney disease) after diphtheria	Apis., ars., carb-ac., hell., hep., kali-chl., lach., lyc., merc-c., merc-cy., phyt.
Albumin	urine albuminous after scarlet fever	Apis., ars., asc-t., aur-m., bell., bry., canth., carb-ac., coch., colch., con., cop., crot-h., dig., dulc., glon., hell., helon., hep., kali-c., kali-chl., kali-s., lach., Lyc., merc-c., Nat-s., phos., phyt., rhus-t., sec., senec., stram., ter., uran.
Albumin	urine albuminous causing amaurosis (partial or complete vision impairment, especially when there is no obvious damage to the eye)	Apis., ars., cann-i., colch., gels., hep., kalm., merc-c., ph-ac., phos., plb.
Albumin	urine albuminous chronic	Atro., cedr., glon., helon., petr., plb.
Albumin	urine albuminous consecutive to heart disease	Apis., ars-i., ars., aur., Calc-ar., coc-c., colch., crot-h., cupr., dig., glon., kali-bi., kali-p., kalm., lach., lyc., lycps., petr., ph-ac., ter., uran.
Albumin	urine albuminous during and after delivery	Merc-c., ph-ac., pyrog.
Albumin	urine albuminous during insanity	Phyt.
Albumin	urine albuminous during menses	Helon.
Albumin	urine albuminous from exposure to cold and dampness	Calc., colch., dulc., kali-c., merc-c., nux-v., rhus-t., sep.

Body part/Disease	Symptom	Medicines
Albumin	urine albuminous in syphilitics	Aur-i., aur-m-n., Aur-m., aur., kali-bi., kali-i., merc-c., nit-ac., sars.
Albumin	urine albuminous indication of kidney from abuse of alcohol	Ars., aur., bell., berb., calc-ar., Carb-v., chin., crot-t., cupr., ferr., lach., led., merc., nat-c., nux-v., sulph.
Albumin	vomiting albuminous	Ars., ip., jatr., merc-c., plb., verat.
Alkaline	urine alkaline (having the properties of an alkali)	Am-c., am-caust., Bapt., benz-ac., canth., Carb-ac., chin-s., chlor., cina., ferr., fl-ac., hyos., kali-bi., kali-c., kreos., morph., nat-m., plb., stram., uran., xan.
Amelioration	Aching in back ameliorated from lying on back	Equis., nat-m.
Amelioration	Aching in back ameliorated from bending backward	Aeth.
Amelioration	Aching in back ameliorated from leaning against something	Eupi., zing.
Amelioration	Aching in back ameliorated from lying on abdomen	Nit-ac.
Amelioration	Aching in back ameliorated from pressure	Kali-c., nat-m., sep.
Amelioration	Aching in back ameliorated from urinating	Lyc.
Amelioration	Aching in back ameliorated from washing	Vesp.
Amelioration	Aching in back ameliorated on motion	Graph.
Amelioration	Aching in back in evening ameliorated after exertion	Ruta.
Amelioration	Aching in cervical region ameliorated after supper	Sep.
Amelioration	Aching in cervical region ameliorated from bending head back	Cycl., lac-c.
Amelioration	Aching in cervical region extending to head and shoulders	Dios.
Amelioration	aching in kidney ameliorated during urination	Lyc., tarent.
Amelioration	Aching in lumbar region ameliorated after flatus	Coc-c.
Amelioration	Aching in lumbar region ameliorated after hard stool	Ox-ac.
Amelioration	Aching in lumbar region ameliorated after urinating	Lyc.
Amelioration	Aching in lumbar region ameliorated from bending backward	Fl-ac., puls., sabad., sabin.
Amelioration	Aching in lumbar region ameliorated from leaning against something	Zing.
Amelioration	Aching in lumbar region ameliorated from leaning on the side	Raph.
Amelioration	Aching in lumbar region ameliorated from pressure	Carb-ac., fl-ac.
Amelioration	Aching in lumbar region ameliorated from straightening up	Nat-m.
Amelioration	Aching in lumbar region ameliorated from walking	Ant-c., arg-n., cob., kali-p., kreos., phos., ruta., staph., tab.
Amelioration	Aching in lumbar region ameliorated from walking bent	Sulph.
Amelioration	Aching in lumbar region ameliorated from warm applications	Calc-f., caust., rhus-t.
Amelioration	Aching in lumbar region ameliorated on motion	Alum., calc-caust., calc-f., kali-n., kreos., nux-v., rhod., staph., stront.

Body part/Disease	Symptom	Medicines
Amelioration	Aching in lumbar region ameliorated on rising up	Cob., ferr., ptel., ruta., sulph.
Amelioration	Aching in lumbar region ameliorated when stooping	Chel., puls., sang.
Amelioration	Aching in lumbar region ameliorated while lying	Cob.
Amelioration	Aching in lumbar region ameliorated while sitting	Mag-c., meny.
Amelioration	Aching in lumbar region ameliorsated from standing	Arg-n.
Amelioration	Aching in lumbar region in morning ameliorated after rising	Nat-s.
Amelioration	Aching in sacrum region ameliorated from pressure	Colch., sep.
Amelioration	affected parts ameliorated on motion	Abrot., acon., agar., agn., am-m., arn., ars-i., ars., asaf., asar., aur., calc., **Caps.**, cham., chin., cina., con., croc., **Dulc.**, eupho., **Ferr.**, kali-bi., kali-c., lyc., mag-c., mag-m., meny., mosch., mur-ac., nat-c., ph-ac., **Puls.**, rhod., **Rhus-t.**, sabad., samb., sep., squil., stann., stront., **Sulph.**, tarax., thuj., valer., verb., viol-t.
Amelioration	ameliorated after becoming cold	Acon., agar., alum., alumn., am-c., ant-t., arg-n., arn., **Ars.**, aur., **Bar-c.**, **Bell.**, bor., **Bry.**, **Calc-p.**, calc-s., **Calc.**, camph., carb-s., carb-v., **Cham.**, **Chin.**, cocc., coff., coloc., con., croc., cupr., cycl., dig., dros., **Dulc.**, ferr., **Graph.**, **Hep.**, **Hyos.**, hyper., ign., ip., kali-bi., kali-c., kali-p., kalm., led., lyc., mag-c., mang., med., **Merc.**, nat-c., nat-m., nat-p., nit-ac., nux-m., **Nux-v.**, op., petr., ph-ac., **Phos.**, plat., psor., **Puls.**, **Pyrog.**, **Ran-b.**, **Rhus-t.**, ruta., sabin., samb., sars., sel., **Sep.**, **Sil.**, **Spig.**, stann., staph., stront., **Sul-ac.**, sulph., tarent., thuj., valer., verat.
Amelioration	ameliorated after breakfast	Calc., croc., ferr., iod., nat-m., staph., valer.
Amelioration	ameliorated after perspiration	Acon., aesc., am-m., ambr., ant-t., ars., bar-c., bell., bov., bry., calad., canth., **Cham.**, chel., clem., cocc., coloc., **Gels.**, graph., hell., hep., hyos., ip., kali-n., led., lyc., mag-m., **Nat-m.**, nit-ac., nux-v., olnd., op., **Psor.**, puls., rhod., **Rhus-t.**, sabad., sabin., samb., sel., spong., stram., stront., sul-ac., sulph., tarax., thuj., valer., verat.
Amelioration	ameliorated after sleep	Acon., agar., am-m., ambr., apis., ars., bry., calad., calc., cham., chin., cocc., colch., con., ferr., hell., ign., ip., kreos., lach., merc., nat-c., nux-v., oxyt., **Ph-ac.**, **Phos.**, puls., ruta., sabin., samb., sang., sel., sep., spig., thuj.
Amelioration	ameliorated at 4.00 p.m. till going to bed	Alum.
Amelioration	ameliorated at open seashore	Med.
Amelioration	ameliorated by tobacco	Aran., bor., carb-ac., coloc., hep., merc., nat-c., sep., spig.
Amelioration	ameliorated during sleep	Am-m., calad., hell., phos., samb.
Amelioration	ameliorated from cold drinks in hot weather	Acon-f., all-c., aloe., ambr., anac., ant-t., apis., ars., asar., **Bism.**, bor., **Bry.**, calc., **Caust.**, cham., clem., coc-c., coff., cupr., kali-c., laur., onos., **Phos.**, puls., **Sep.**, sumb., thuj., verat., zinc.
Amelioration	ameliorated from bacon (pig meat)	Ran-b., ran-s.
Amelioration	ameliorated from bathing	Acon., agar., alum., am-m., ant-t., apis., ars., **Asar.**, aur., bor., bry., cann-i., caust., cham., chel., euphr., fl-ac., form., kali-chl., lac-c., laur., **Led.**, mag-c., mez., mur-ac., nux-v., phyt., pic-ac., psor., **Puls.**, rhod., sabad., sep., spig., staph., zinc.

Body part/Disease	Symptom	Medicines
Amelioration	ameliorated from bathing face	Asar., calc-s., mez., sabad.
Amelioration	ameliorated from becoming cold	Acon., agn., alum., ambr., ant-c., ant-t., arg-n., arn., aur., bar-c., bell., bov., bry., calad., cann-s., carb-v., cham., clem., cocc., coff., colch., coloc., croc., dros., dulc., eupho., glon., hell., **Iod.**, ip., lac-c., lach., led., **Lyc.**, mang., merc., mez., mur-ac., nat-c., nat-m., nit-ac., olnd., op., petr., ph-ac., phos., plat., **Puls.**, sabad., sabin., sars., sec., sel., seneg., spig., spong., staph., sulph., teucr., thuj., verat.
Amelioration	ameliorated from change of position	Agar., ars., cham., **Ign.**, meli., nat-s., ph-ac., puls., **Rhus-t.**, teucr., valer., zinc.
Amelioration	Ameliorated from closing eyes	Kali-c., zinc.
Amelioration	ameliorated from coffee	Acon., agar., arg-m., ars., cann-i., canth., **Cham.**, coloc., eucal., euphr., hyos., lach., op., phos.
Amelioration	ameliorated from cold bathing	Arg-n., arn., asar., aur-m., bism., calc-s., fl-ac., Ind., iod., meph., nat-m.
Amelioration	Ameliorated from Consolation	Puls.
Amelioration	ameliorated from fast walking	Arg-n., canth., carb-ac., ign., nat-m., petr., **Sep.**, sil., stann., sul-ac., **Tub.**
Amelioration	ameliorated from fruit	Lach.
Amelioration	ameliorated from hemorrhage	Bov., sars., sel.
Amelioration	ameliorated from laying hand on part	Bell., calc., canth., croc., dros., mang., meny., mur-ac., nat-c., olnd., par., phos., rhus-t., sabad., sep., spig., sulph., thuj.
Amelioration	ameliorated from letting arms hang down	Acon., anac., bar-c., bor., bry., caps., chin., **Con.**, cupr., ferr., graph., lac-d., lach., led., lyc., phos., plb., ran-b., rhus-t., sulph., thuj.
Amelioration	ameliorated from letting limbs hang down	Acon., am-m., anac., ant-c., arg-m., arg-n., arn., asar., bar-c., bell., bor., bry., camph., caps., caust., chin., cic., cina., cocc., coff., colch., coloc., **Con.**, cupr., dros., eupho., ferr., graph., hep., ign., iris., kali-c., kreos., lach., led., lyc., mag-c., mag-m., merc., mez., nat-c., nat-m., nit-ac., nux-v., olnd., petr., phos., plb., puls., ran-b., rhus-t., ruta., sil., stann., sul-ac., sulph., teucr., thuj., verat., verb.
Amelioration	ameliorated from lying	Acon., agar., agn., alum., am-c., **Am-m.**, ambr., anac., ant-c., ant-t., arg-m., arn., ars., **Asar.**, bar-c., **Bell.**, bor., **Bry.**, calad., calc-p., **Calc.**, camph., cann-s., canth., caps., carb-ac., carb-an., carb-s., carb-v., caust., chel., chin., cic., cimic., cina., clem., cocc., coff., colch., coloc., con., conv., croc., cupr., dig., dios., dros., dulc., eupho., **Ferr.**, glon., graph., guai., hell., hep., hyos., ign., iod., ip., kali-c., kali-n., kalm., kreos., lach., laur., led., lyc., mag-c., mag-m., **Mang.**, merc., mez., mur-ac., nat-c., **Nat-m.**, nit-ac., nux-m., **Nux-v.**, olnd., op., par., petr., ph-ac., phos., **Pic-ac.**, plb., psor., ran-b., rheum., rhus-t., ruta., sabad., sabin., sars., sec., sel., seneg., sep., spig., spong., **Squil.**, sulph.
Amelioration	ameliorated from lying on abdomen	Acet-ac., aloe., am-c., ambr., ars., bar-c., **Bell.**, bry., calc., chel., cina., coloc., crot-t., elaps., lach., mag-c., nit-ac., phos., phyt., plb., rhus-t., sel., sep., stann.

Body part/Disease	Symptom	Medicines
Amelioration	ameliorated from lying on back	Acon., aeth., am-c., **Am-m.**, anac., apis., arn., bar-c., bell., bor., **Bry.**, cact., calad., **Calc.**, canth., carb-an., caust., chin., cimic., cina., clem., colch., con., conv., ferr., grat., hell., ign., ip., kali-c., kalm., kreos., lach., lyc., **Merc-c.**, merc., mosch., nat-c., nat-m., nat-s., nux-v., ox-ac., par., phos., plat., **Puls.**, ran-b., **Rhus-t.**, sabad., sang., senec., seneg., sep., sil., spig., spong., stann., sulph., thuj., verat., viol-t.
Amelioration	ameliorated from lying on bed	Acon., agar., am-m., ambr., anac., ant-c., ant-t., arg-m., arn., ars., asar., aur., bar-c., bell., bov., **Bry.**, calad., calc., camph., cann-s., canth., caps., carb-an., carb-v., caust., cham., chel., chin., **Cic.**, cina., clem., coc-c., **Cocc.**, coff., colch., coloc., con., croc., cupr., dig., dulc., ferr., graph., guai., hell., **Hep.**, hyos., ign., iod., ip., kali-c., kali-n., kreos., lach., laur., led., lyc., mag-c., merc., mez., mur-ac., nat-c., nat-m., nit-ac., nux-m., **Nux-v.**, olnd., par., petr., ph-ac., phos., puls., ran-b., rheum., rhod., rhus-t., sabad., sabin., samb., sars., sec., sel., sep., sil., spig., spong., **Squil.**, **Stann.**, staph., stram., stront., sul-ac., sulph., tarax., thuj., valer., verat., verb., viol-t.
Amelioration	ameliorated from lying on painful side	Ambr., arn., bell., **Bry.**, calc., cann-s., carb-v., caust., cham., coloc., ign., kali-c., lyc., nux-v., puls., rhus-t., sep., stram., sulph., viol-o., viol-t.
Amelioration	ameliorated from lying on side	Acon., alum., am-c., am-m., arn., ars., bar-c., bell., bor., bry., calc-p., canth., caust., cham., chin., cina., clem., **Cocc.**, colch., cupr., dulc., eupho., ign., iod., kali-c., lach., nat-m., **Nux-v.**, par., phos., plat., ran-b., rhus-t., sep., spig., spong., stront., sulph., thuj.
Amelioration	ameliorated from magnetism (force of magnetic field)	Acon., bar-c., bell., calc-p., calc., chin., con., **Cupr.**, graph., ign., iod., nat-c., nux-v., **Phos.**, sabin., sep., sil., sulph., teucr., viol-o.
Amelioration	ameliorated from milk	Apis., ars., iod., mez., ruta., verat.
Amelioration	ameliorated from over indulgence in eating	Ars., iod., phos.
Amelioration	ameliorated from perspiration	Ars., bov., **Bry.**, calad., calc., **Cupr.**, lyc., nat-c., rhus-t.
Amelioration	ameliorated from physical exertion	Canth., ign., nat-m., plb., **Rhus-t.**, **Sep.**, sil., stann., tril.
Amelioration	ameliorated from pressure	Abies-c., acon., agar., agn., alum., am-c., am-m., ambr., anac., ant-c., apis., arg-m., arg-n., arn., ars., asaf., aur., bell., bism., bor., bov., **Bry.**, cact., calc-f., calc., camph., canth., carb-ac., carb-s., caust., chel., **Chin.**, cina., cinnb., clem., **Coloc.**, **Con.**, croc., crot-t., dig., dios., **Dros.**, dulc., form., glon., graph., guai., hell., ign., ip., kali-bi., kali-c., kali-i., kali-p., kreos., lach., laur., led., **Lil-t.**, mag-c., **Mag-m.**, **Mag-p.**, mang., **Meny.**, merc., mez., mosch., mur-ac., **Nat-c.**, nat-m., nat-p., nat-s., nit-ac., nux-m., nux-v., olnd., par., ph-ac., phos., **Plb.**, **Puls.**, rhus-t., ruta., sabad., sabin., sang., sep., **Sil.**, spig., stann., sul-ac., sulph., thuj., tril., verat., verb., zinc.
Amelioration	ameliorated from riding in a wagon, or on the cars	Ars., brom., kali-n., **Nit-ac.**, phos.
Amelioration	ameliorated from riding in cold wind	Arg-n.
Amelioration	ameliorated from riding on horse back	Brom., calc., lyc.

Body part/Disease	Symptom	Medicines
Amelioration	ameliorated from rubbing	Acon., agar., agn., alum., am-c., am-m., ambr., anac., ant-c., ant-t., arn., ars., asaf., bell., bor., bov., bry., **Calc.**, camph., cann-s., **Canth.**, caps., **Carb-ac.**, carb-an., caust., cedr., chel., chin., cic., cina., colch., cycl., dios., dros., guai., ham., hep., ign., kali-c., kali-n., kreos., laur., lil-t., mag-c., mag-m., mang., meny., merc., mosch., mur-ac., **Nat-c.**, nit-ac., nux-v., ol-an., olnd., osm., pall., ph-ac., **Phos.**, plat., **Plb.**, ran-b., rhus-t., ruta., sabad., sabin., samb., sars., sec., sel., seneg., spig., spong., stann., staph., sul-ac., sulph., tarax., thuj., valer., viol-t., zinc.
Amelioration	ameliorated from running	Caust., ign., nat-m., **Sep.**, sil., stann.
Amelioration	ameliorated from sitting	Asar., nat-m.
Amelioration	ameliorated from slow walking	Agar., **Aur-m.**, **Aur.**, cact., calc-s., ferr-ar., **Ferr.**, iris., kali-p., **Puls.**, sep., tarent.
Amelioration	ameliorated from standing	Agar., agn., am-c., anac., ant-t., arn., **Ars.**, asar., bar-c., **Bell.**, bor., bry., calad., calc., camph., cann-s., canth., carb-an., carb-v., chel., chin., cic., cina., cocc., coff., colch., croc., cupr., dig., dios., eupho., graph., guai., hell., hep., ign., iod., ip., kreos., led., mang., meny., merc., mez., mur-ac., naja., nat-m., nux-m., nux-v., par., petr., phos., plb., ran-b., rheum., ruta., sars., sec., sel., spig., spong., squil., stann., staph., stram., sul-ac., tarax., tarent., thuj.
Amelioration	ameliorated from suppression of sexual desire	Calad.
Amelioration	ameliorated from tea	Carb-ac., dig., ferr.
Amelioration	ameliorated from thinking	Camph., cic., hell., mag-c., pall., prun-s.
Amelioration	ameliorated from touch	Agar., alum., am-c., am-m., anac., ant-c., arn., *ars.*, bell., *bism., bry.*, **Calc.**, canth., caust., chel., chin., *coloc., con.*, **Cycl.**, dros., eupho., euphr., lyc., *mang., meny.*, **Mur-ac.**, nat-c., nat-m., olnd., petr., ph-ac., *phos.*, plb., sep., spong., sulph., tarax., **Thuj.**, viol-t.
Amelioration	ameliorated from vinegar	Asar., bry., ign., meny., op., puls., stram.
Amelioration	ameliorated from vomiting	Acon., agar., ars., carb-s., coc-c., colch., dig., hyos., nux-v., op., puls., sang., sec.
Amelioration	ameliorated from warm drinks	Alum., arg-n., **Ars.**, bry., carb-s., cedr., chel., graph., guare., lyc., mang., nux-m., **Nux-v.**, pyrus., **Rhus-t.**, spong., sulph., verat.
Amelioration	ameliorated from warm milk	Chel.
Amelioration	ameliorated from warm stove	Acon., agar., am-c., **Ars.**, aur., bar-c., bell., bor., camph., canth., caps., caust., cic., cocc., con., conv., dulc., hell., **Hep.**, hyos., **Ign.**, kali-c., mag-c., **Mag-p.**, mang., mosch., nux-m., **Nux-v.**, petr., ran-b., rhod., **Rhus-t.**, sabad., **Sil.**, stront., sulph.
Amelioration	ameliorated from wine	Acon., agar., ars., bell., brom., bry., canth., carb-ac., chel., cocc., con., gels., glon., graph., lach., mez., nux-v., op., osm., phos., sel., sul-ac., sulph., thea.
Amelioration	ameliorated in afternoon	Cinnb.
Amelioration	ameliorated in constipation	Calc., merc., psor.
Amelioration	ameliorated in evening	Alum., arg-m., arn., asaf., **Aur.**, chel., lyc., med., sep.

Body part/Disease	Symptom	Medicines
Amelioration	ameliorated in evening after eating	Sep.
Amelioration	ameliorated in evening after lying down	Kali-n.
Amelioration	ameliorated in evening in twilight	Alum., bry., phos.
Amelioration	ameliorated in forenoon	Alum., **Lyc.**
Amelioration	ameliorated in open air	Acon.
Amelioration	ameliorated in open air	Acon., agar., aloe., **Alum.**, am-m., ambr., anac., ant-c., arg-m., **Arg-n.**, arn., asaf., asar., aur., bapt., bar-c., bell., bism., bor., bov., brom., bry., calc-s., calc., caps., carb-ac., carb-s., carb-v., caust., cic., cina., con., dulc., **Fl-ac.**, gamb., graph., hyos., ign., kali-c., **Kali-i.**, kali-n., **Kali-s.**, laur., lil-t., **Lyc.**, mag-c., mag-m., mang., meny., merc-i-r., merc., mez., mosch., mur-ac., naja., nat-a., nat-c., nat-m., nit-ac., op., ox-ac., par., petr., ph-ac., phos., plat., plb., **Puls.**, rhod., **Rhus-t.**, sabin., sang., sars., sel., seneg., sep., spig., stann., staph., stront., sul-ac., sulph., tarax., teucr., thuj., verat., verb., viol-t., zinc.
Amelioration	ameliorated in warm bed	Agar., am-c., arn., **Ars.**, aur., bar-c., bell., **Bry.**, calc-p., camph., canth., caust., cic., cocc., coloc., con., dulc., graph., **Hep.**, hyos., kali-bi., **Kali-c.**, kali-i., kali-p., lach., **Lyc.**, mag-p., mosch., nit-ac., **Nux-m.**, **Nux-v.**, petr., ph-ac., phos., **Rhus-t.**, rumx., sabad., sep., **Sil.**, spong., squil., stann., staph., stram., stront., sulph., tarent., **Tub.**
Amelioration	ameliorated on bending backward	Thuj.
Amelioration	ameliorated on continued motion	Agar., am-m., ambr., bry., cact., **Caps.**, carb-v., caust., chin., cina., com., **Con.**, cycl., dros., **Eupho.**, **Ferr.**, gels., Ind., iris., kali-c., lyc., plat., plb., ptel., **Puls.**, rhod., **Rhus-t.**, ruta., sabad., sabin., **Samb.**, sep., sil., tarax., thuj., valer., verat.
Amelioration	ameliorated on falling asleep	Merc.
Amelioration	ameliorated on first sitting down	Acon., ambr., anac., ant-c., ant-t., arn., ars., asar., aur., bar-c., bell., bov., bry., calc., cann-s., canth., **Caps.**, carb-an., carb-v., caust., cham., chin., cic., cocc., **Con.**, croc., dig., dros., eupho., ferr., graph., kali-c., kali-n., lach., laur., led., lyc., mang., merc., mur-ac., nat-c., nat-m., nit-ac., nux-v., olnd., petr., ph-ac., phos., plat., puls., ran-b., rhod., rhus-t., ruta., sabad., sep., sil., spig., staph., stram., stront., sulph., thuj., verat.
Amelioration	ameliorated on rising	Acon., alum., **Am-c.**, am-m., *ant-t.*, **Ars.**, asaf., aur., bar-c., bell., *bor.*, bov., bry., **Calc.**, cann-s., canth., carb-v., caust., *cham.*, chel., chin., cic., coloc., con., *cupr.*, *dig.*, ferr., hell., hep., *hyos.*, *ign.*, *kali-c.*, laur., *lyc.*, mag-c., mang., merc., mosch., naja., nat-c., nat-m., nux-m., nux-v., olnd., petr., phos., puls., rhus-t., sabin., **Samb.**, **Sep.**, *sil.*, spig., squil., stann., sul-ac., sulph., teucr.
Amelioration	ameliorated on waking	Am-m., ambr., ars., bry., calad., calc., cham., chin., cocc., colch., hell., ign., ip., kreos., lach., nat-c., nux-v., onos., ph-ac., **Phos.**, puls., ruta., sabin., samb., sel., **Sep.**, spig., thuj.

Body part/Disease	Symptom	Medicines
Amelioration	Ameliorated when alone	Ambr., bar-c., bov., carb-an., con., cycl., ferr-p., ferr., hell., lyc., mag-s., nat-c., nat-m., petr., phos., plb., Sep., stann., staph., stram., sulph.
Amelioration	ameliorated when half asleep	Sel.
Amelioration	ameliorated while eating	Aloe., alum., am-m., ambr., **Anac.**, arn., aur., bell., cadm., calc-p., cann-i., caps., carb-an., carb-v., cham., chel., chin., cocc., croc., dig., dros., ferr., graph., **Ign.**, iod., **Lach.**, laur., led., lyc., mag-c., mang., merc., mez., nat-c., nit-ac., nux-v., par., ph-ac., phos., puls., rheum., rhod., rhus-t., sabad., sabin., sep., sil., spig., spong., squil., stann., staph., sul-ac., sulph., tarax., **Zinc.**
Amelioration	ameliorated while sitting	Acon., agar., agn., alum., am-c., am-m., anac., ant-t., arn., ars., asaf., aur., bar-c., bell., bor., **Bry.**, cadm., calad., calc., camph., cann-s., canth., caps., carb-an., carb-v., caust., cham., chel., chin., chion., cic., cina., clem., cocc., coff., **Colch.**, coloc., con., croc., cupr., cycl., ferr., gels., glon., graph., guai., hell., hep., hyos., ign., iod., ip., kali-c., kali-n., kreos., laur., led., mag-c., mag-m., mang., meny., merc., mez., mosch., nat-a., nat-m., nit-ac., nux-m., **Nux-v.**, op., par., petr., ph-ac., phos., plb., puls., ran-b., ran-s., rheum., sabin., samb., sars., sec., sel., sil., spig., spong., squil., stann., staph., stram., sul-ac., sulph., sumb., tarax., thuj., valer., verat., zinc.
Amelioration	amelioration of all complaints, during menses	Lach., zinc.
Amelioration	ameliorted from menses	Alum., apis., aran., bell., calc-f., calc., cimic., cycl., kali-bi., kali-c., kali-p., lac-c., **Lach.**, mosch., phos., puls., rhus-t., senec., sep., stann., sulph., ust., verat., zinc.
Amelioration	anal haemorrhoids ameliorated from cold	Aloe., brom.
Amelioration	anal haemorrhoids ameliorated in morning	Alum., coll.
Amelioration	anxiety (feeling of worry) ameliorated by bending forward	Colch.
Amelioration	anxiety ameliorated after eating	Aur., iod., mez., sulph.
Amelioration	anxiety ameliorated after eructations	Kali-c., mag-m.
Amelioration	anxiety Ameliorated after rising on	Carb-an., cast., fl-ac., nux-v., rhus-t., sep.
Amelioration	anxiety ameliorated from breathing deeply	Agar., rhus-t.
Amelioration	anxiety ameliorated from cold drinks	Acon., agar-em., sulph.
Amelioration	anxiety ameliorated from dinner	Sulph.
Amelioration	anxiety ameliorated from exercise	Tarent.
Amelioration	anxiety ameliorated from flatus	Calc.
Amelioration	anxiety ameliorated from menses	Stann., zinc.
Amelioration	anxiety ameliorated from motion	Seneg.
Amelioration	anxiety ameliorated from motion	Acon., act-sp., ars., naja., ph-ac., puls., seneg., sil., tarax.
Amelioration	anxiety ameliorated from rising on	Sil.
Amelioration	anxiety ameliorated from sitting	Iod.
Amelioration	anxiety ameliorated from standing	Calc., phos., tarax.
Amelioration	anxiety ameliorated from stooping	Bar-m.

Body part/Disease	Symptom	Medicines
Amelioration	anxiety ameliorated from straightening up	Chin.
Amelioration	anxiety ameliorated from waking	Sil.
Amelioration	anxiety ameliorated from walking	Iod., kali-i., kali-s., puls., rhus-t.
Amelioration	anxiety ameliorated from warmth	Graph., phos
Amelioration	anxiety ameliorated from weeping	Dig., graph., tab.
Amelioration	anxiety ameliorated in bed	Mag-c.
Amelioration	anxiety ameliorated in evening	Zinc.
Amelioration	anxiety ameliorated in open air	Alum., arund., bry., calc-s., calc., Cann-i., carl., grat., Kali-s., laur., lyc., mag-m., puls., rhus-t., spong., til., valer., verat.
Amelioration	anxiety ameliorated while in house	Ign.
Amelioration	anxiety ameliorated while lying	Mang.
Amelioration	asthma ameliorated after eating	Ambr., graph.
Amelioration	asthma ameliorated by bending head backward	Cham., Spong., verat.
Amelioration	asthma ameliorated from cold air	Bry., carb-v., cham., merc.
Amelioration	asthma ameliorated from expectorations	Hyper.
Amelioration	asthma ameliorated from talking	Ferr.
Amelioration	asthma ameliorated in open air	Am-c.
Amelioration	asthmatic ameliorated from eructations	Carb-v., nux-v.
Amelioration	asthmatic breathing ameliorated by bathing in cold water	Calc-s.
Amelioration	asthmatic respiration ameliorated from cold water	Cham.
Amelioration	barking cogh ameliorated from drinking cold water	Coc-c.
Amelioration	bathing ameliorates affected part	Alum., am-m., ant-t., ars., **Asar.**, bor., bry., caust., cham., chel., euphr., laur., mag-c., mez., mur-ac., nux-v., **Puls.**, rhod., sabad., sep., spig., staph., zinc.
Amelioration	blindness, ameliorated by sleeping	Calc., grat.
Amelioration	blindness, ameliorated in open air	Merc., phos.
Amelioration	boring pain in left scapula ameliorated from motion	Paeon.
Amelioration	boring pain in lumbar ameliorated after walking	Meli.
Amelioration	boring pain in lumbar ameliorated on moving	Kreos., nux-m.
Amelioration	boring pain in lumbar ameliorated while standing	Meli.
Amelioration	boring pain in lumbar region ameliorated from motion	Kreos.
Amelioration	breathing difficult ameliorated from expectoration	Ail., Ant-t., grin., guai., ip., manc., nit-ac., sep., zinc.
Amelioration	breathing difficult ameliorated from expectoration in morning	Sep.
Amelioration	breathing difficult ameliorated after drinking water	Cham.
Amelioration	breathing difficult ameliorated after eating	Cedr., graph., iod., spong.
Amelioration	breathing difficult ameliorated after rising in morning	Led., puls., sulph.
Amelioration	breathing difficult ameliorated after stool	Poth.
Amelioration	breathing difficult ameliorated after talking	Ferr.

Body part/Disease	Symptom	Medicines
Amelioration	breathing difficult ameliorated by walking rapidly	Sep.
Amelioration	breathing difficult ameliorated by walking slowly	Ferr.
Amelioration	breathing difficult ameliorated by while sitting with head bent forward on knees	Coc-c., Kali-c.
Amelioration	breathing difficult ameliorated from rising on	Olnd.
Amelioration	breathing difficult ameliorated from arms outstretched	Psor.
Amelioration	breathing difficult ameliorated from eructations	Aur., Carb-v., nux-v.
Amelioration	breathing difficult ameliorated from hanging down legs	Sul-ac.
Amelioration	breathing difficult ameliorated from head on back	Cact., dig., Ind., kali-i., kalm., nux-v.
Amelioration	breathing difficult ameliorated from motion	Aur., calc., Ferr., nat-m., seneg., sep., sil., sulph.
Amelioration	breathing difficult ameliorated in bed at night	Chel.
Amelioration	breathing difficult ameliorated in bed in evening	Chel.
Amelioration	breathing difficult ameliorated in cold air	Am-c., arg-n., bell., bry., carb-s., carb-v., cham., cist., lac-c., op., puls., ust.
Amelioration	breathing difficult ameliorated in evening	Lyc.
Amelioration	breathing difficult ameliorated in open air	Alum., am-c., Apis., ars-i., bapt., bell., bry., cact., chel., chin-a., cist., dig., fl-ac., gels., ip., kali-i., kali-s., lach., lil-t., Nat-m., nux-v., Puls., stram., Sulph., tub.
Amelioration	breathing difficult ameliorated on lying	Bry., calc-p., chel., dig., euphr., hell., laur., nat-s., nux-v., Psor.
Amelioration	breathing difficult ameliorated on rising in morning	Calc-p., kali-bi.
Amelioration	breathing difficult ameliorated on walking	Brom., bry., dros., ferr., indg., nicc., sep.
Amelioration	breathing difficult ameliorated whie reading	Ferr.
Amelioration	breathing difficult ameliorated while riding	Psor.
Amelioration	breathing difficult ameliorated while writing	Ferr.
Amelioration	breathing difficult ameliorated while yawning	Croc.
Amelioration	bubling sensation in brain ameliorated by leaning back while sitting	Spig.
Amelioration	burning in ear ameliorated by rubbing	Ol-an., phel.
Amelioration	burning in ear ameliorated by scratching	Caust., mag-c., nat-c.
Amelioration	burning pain between scapula ameliorated from rubbing	Phos.
Amelioration	burning pain in back ameliorated after scratching	Rhus-v.
Amelioration	burning pain in back ameliorated from motion	Mag-m., pic-ac., rat.
Amelioration	burning pain in back ameliorated from walking in open air	Kali-n.
Amelioration	burning pain in back in morning on rising ameliorated by motion	Rat.
Amelioration	burning pain in cervical region ameliorated from sleep	Calc.
Amelioration	burning pain in forearm ameliorated from rubbing	Ol-an.
Amelioration	burning pain in hollow of knee ameliorated from walking	Grat.

Body part/Disease	Symptom	Medicines
Amelioration	burning pain in knee ameliorated while walking	Phos.
Amelioration	burning pain in scapula ameliorated from walking	Bar-c.
Amelioration	burning pain in soles ameliorated in bed	Nat-c.
Amelioration	burning pain in soles ameliorated while walking	Ol-an.
Amelioration	burning pain in spine ameliorated from rubbing	Phos.
Amelioration	burning pain in spine stitching ameliorated by motion	Mag-m.
Amelioration	burning pain in thigh ameliorated after scratching	Alum.
Amelioration	burning pain in upper limbs ameliorated after scratching	Jug-c.
Amelioration	burning pain in urethra ameliorated during urination	Berb., bry., cocc.
Amelioration	chill ameliorated after eating	Acon., **Ambr.**, ars., bov., cann-s., chel., cop., cur., ferr., ign., **Iod.**, kali-c., laur., mez., nat-s., petr., phos., rhus-t., sabad., squil., stront.
Amelioration	chill ameliorated after exercise in open air	Alum., **Caps.**, mag-c., mag-m., **Puls.**, spong., staph., sul-ac.
Amelioration	chill ameliorated after motion	Acon., apis., arn., asar., bell., caps., cycl., dros., kreos., mag-m., merc., mez., nit-ac., nux-v., podo., **Puls.**, rhus-t., sep., sil., spig., staph., sul-ac., tarent.
Amelioration	chill ameliorated after sleep	Arn., ars., bry., calad., calc., caps., chin., colch., cupr., ferr., kreos., nux-v., **Phos.**, rhus-t., samb., sep.
Amelioration	chill ameliorated during drinking	Bry., carb-an., **Caust.**, **Cupr.**, graph., ip., mosch., nux-v., olnd., phos., rhus-t., sil., spig., tarax.
Amelioration	chill ameliorated from external warmth	Aesc., arg-m., arn., **Ars.**, bar-c., **Bell.**, canth., **Caps.**, carb-an., caust., chel., chin-a., chin., cic., cimx., cocc., colch., con., cor-r., eup-per., ferr., gels., hell., hep., hyos., **Ign.**, **Kali-c.**, kali-i., lach., lachn., laur., **Meny.**, merl., mez., mosch., nat-c., **Nux-m.**, **Nux-v.**, plat., podo., **Rhus-t.**, **Sabad.**, samb., sep., sil., squil., stram., stront., sulph., tarent., ther.
Amelioration	chill ameliorated from rising from bed	Am-c., ambr., ant-t., arg-m., ars., aur., bell., dros., eupho., ferr., ign., **Iod.**, led., lyc., mag-c., merc-c., merc., nat-c., plat., puls., rhod., rhus-t., sel., sep., stront., sulph., verat.
Amelioration	chill ameliorated from sun shine	Anac., con.
Amelioration	chill ameliorated from uncovering and undressing	Apis., **Camph.**, ip., med., puls., **Sec.**, sep.
Amelioration	chill ameliorated from warm drinks	Bry., eupi.
Amelioration	chill ameliorated from wrapping up followed by severe fever and sweat	Sil.
Amelioration	chill ameliorated in bed	Am-c., bry., canth., **Caust.**, cimx., cocc., con., hell., **Kali-c.**, kali-i., kali-n., lachn., mag-c., **Mag-m.**, mag-s., mez., mosch., nat-c., nit-ac., nux-v., podo., puls., **Pyrog.**, rhus-t., sars., squil., stram., sulph.
Amelioration	chill ameliorated in open air	Acon., alum., ang., ant-c., **Apis.**, arg-m., **Asar.**, **Bry.**, **Caps.**, cocc., graph., **Ip.**, mag-c., mag-m., mez., nat-m., phos., **Puls.**, sabin., staph., **Sul-ac.**

Body part/Disease	Symptom	Medicines
Amelioration	chill ameliorated in warm room	Aesc., agar., am-c., **Ars.**, bar-c., bell., brom., camph., canth., carb-an., carb-v., caust., **Chel.**, chin-a., chin., cic., con., gels., hell., hep., **Ign.**, **Kali-ar.**, kali-bi., **Kali-c.**, kreos., lach., laur., mag-c., mang., **Meny.**, merc-c., merc., mez., nat-a., **Nux-m.**, nux-v., petr., plat., ran-b., rat., rhod., rhus-t., **Sabad.**, sel., sep., sil., spig., sul-ac., sulph., tarent., ther., valer., zinc.
Amelioration	chill ameliorated on bed but not by heat of stove	Kali-i., kreos., podo., tarent.
Amelioration	chill ameliorated on bed but not from external covering	Lachn.
Amelioration	chill ameliorated on rising	Rhus-t.
Amelioration	chill ameliorated on sitting	Ign., nux-v.
Amelioration	chill ameliorated while lying	Arn., asar., bry., canth., colch., kali-n., nat-m., nux-v., sil., zinc.
Amelioration	chilliness in evening ameliorated on lying on bed	Kali-i., kali-n., mag-m., mag-s.
Amelioration	chilliness in forenoon before dinner ameliorated by eating	Ambr.
Amelioration	choking of throat ameliorated by lying on back	Spong.
Amelioration	chorea ameliorated from exercise	Zinc.
Amelioration	chorea ameliorated from loosening clothing	Am-c., arn., asar., bry., **Calc.**, cann-i., caps., carb-v., caust., chel., chin., coff., hep., **Lach.**, **Lyc.**, **Nit-ac.**, **Nux-v.**, olnd., op., puls., ran-b., sanic., sars., sep., spig., spong., stann., sulph.
Amelioration	chorea ameliorated from lying on back	Cupr., ign.
Amelioration	chorea ameliorated from sleep	**Agar.**, hell., ziz.
Amelioration	coldness ameliorated after loosening cloth	Chin-s.
Amelioration	coldness ameliorated from motion	Acon.
Amelioration	coldness in back ameliorated by lying down	Cast., kali-n., sil.
Amelioration	coldness in foot ameliorated while lying	Phos.
Amelioration	coldness in foot ameliorated after menses	Carb-v., chin-s.
Amelioration	coldness in foot ameliorated before menses	Calc., hyper., lyc., nux-m.
Amelioration	coldness in foot ameliorated during menses	Arg-n., calc., cop., crot-h., graph., nat-p., nux-m., phos., sabin., Sil.
Amelioration	coldness in foot ameliorated in cold air	Camph., led.
Amelioration	coldness in foot ameliorated in house	Mang.
Amelioration	coldness in foot ameliorated while sitting	Mang.
Amelioration	coldness in foot in evening ameliorated in bed	Sulph.
Amelioration	coldness in foot while ameliorated walking	Aloe.
Amelioration	coldness in foot with heat of feet ameliorated from bath	Glon.
Amelioration	coldness in hands ameliorated from lying down	Phos.
Amelioration	coldness in leg ameliorated from uncovering	Camph., med., Sec., tub.
Amelioration	coldness in lumbar region ameliorated from warmth of stove	Hell.
Amelioration	coldness in toes ameliorated while walking on	Bry.

Body part/Disease	Symptom	Medicines
Amelioration	coldness of forehead ameliorated from walking	Gins.
Amelioration	coldness of forehead ameliorated on lying	Calc.
Amelioration	coldness of forehead ameliorated when covered	Aur., grat., kali-i., nat-m., sanic.
Amelioration	Coldness of head ameliorated by warmth	Lach.
Amelioration	compression of thigh ameliorated on continued motion	Sabad.
Amelioration	Constriction in brain ameliorated by heat of sun	Stront.
Amelioration	Constriction in brain ameliorated from motion	Op., sulph., valer.
Amelioration	Constriction in brain ameliorated from pressure	Aeth., anac., lach., meny., thuj.
Amelioration	Constriction in brain ameliorated from uncovering head	Carb-v.
Amelioration	Constriction in brain ameliorated from vomitting	Stann.
Amelioration	Constriction in brain ameliorated from walking in open air	Ox-ac.
Amelioration	Constriction in brain ameliorated from warmth	Stront.
Amelioration	Constriction in brain ameliorated in morning	Glon.
Amelioration	Constriction in brain ameliorated in open air	Berb., coloc., kali-i., lach., lyc.
Amelioration	Constriction in brain ameliorated on lying	Nat-m.
Amelioration	Constriction in brain ameliorated on rising	Dig., laur., merc.
Amelioration	constriction in chest ameliorated after eating	Sulph.
Amelioration	constriction in chest ameliorated during deep respiration	Sulph.
Amelioration	constriction in chest ameliorated from bending backwards	Caust.
Amelioration	constriction in chest ameliorated from drawing shoulders back	Calc.
Amelioration	constriction in chest ameliorated from expectoration	Calc., manc.
Amelioration	constriction in chest ameliorated from motion	Seneg.
Amelioration	constriction in chest ameliorated from perspiration	Sulph.
Amelioration	constriction in chest ameliorated from straightening up	Mez.
Amelioration	constriction in chest ameliorated from warmth of bed	Phos.
Amelioration	constriction in chest ameliorated from weeping	Anac.
Amelioration	constriction in chest ameliorated while lying	Calc-p.
Amelioration	constriction in chest ameliorated while lying head high	Ferr.
Amelioration	constriction in chest ameliorated while sitting	Nux-v.
Amelioration	constriction in chest ameliorated while sitting bent	Lach.
Amelioration	constriction in chest ameliorated while standing	Mez.
Amelioration	constriction in chest ameliorated while walking	Ferr.
Amelioration	constriction in chest ameliorated while walking	Ferr.

Body part/Disease	Symptom	Medicines
Amelioration	constriction in chest ameliorated while walking in open air	Alum., chel., dros., puls.
Amelioration	constriction in heart ameliorated by bending chest forward	Lact-ac., lil-t.
Amelioration	constriction in heart ameliorated from drinking water	Phos.
Amelioration	constriction in larynx ameliorated aduring cough	Asar.
Amelioration	constriction in larynx ameliorated from walking	Dros.
Amelioration	constriction in larynx ameliorated in open air	Coloc.
Amelioration	constriction in stomach ameliorated after eating	Rat., sep., thuj.
Amelioration	constriction in throat (the part of the airway and digestive tract between the mouth and both the esophagus and the windpipe) pit ameliorated from eating	Rhus-t.
Amelioration	convulsion ameliorated by bending elbow	Nux-v.
Amelioration	convulsion ameliorated during vomiting	Agar.
Amelioration	convulsion ameliorated from bending head backwards	**Nux-v.**
Amelioration	convulsion ameliorated from cold water	Caust.
Amelioration	convulsion ameliorated from diarrhoea	Lob.
Amelioration	convulsion ameliorated from eructations	Kali-c.
Amelioration	convulsion ameliorated from forceful extension of body	Nux-v., stry.
Amelioration	convulsion ameliorated from riding in carriage	Nit-ac.
Amelioration	convulsion ameliorated from rubbing	Phos., sec.
Amelioration	convulsion ameliorated from stretching limbs	Sec.
Amelioration	convulsion ameliorated from stretching out parts	Sec.
Amelioration	convulsion ameliorated from tight grasp	Nux-v.
Amelioration	convulsion ameliorated from tightly binding the body	Mez.
Amelioration	convulsion ameliorated from vinegar	Stram.
Amelioration	convulsion ameliorated from warm bath	Apis., glon., nat-m., op.
Amelioration	convulsive motion ameliorated when lying on side	Calc-p.
Amelioration	coryza, ameliorated in warm room	Ars., calc-p., coloc., dulc., sabad.
Amelioration	cough aggravated from lying and ameliorated from sitting	Hyos., laur., Puls., rhus-t., sang., Sep.
Amelioration	cough ameliorated after breakfast	Alumn., aspar., bar-c., coc-c., kali-c., lach., murx.
Amelioration	cough ameliorated at daybreak	Syph.
Amelioration	cough ameliorated by developing eruptions of measles	Cupr.
Amelioration	cough ameliorated by diarrhoea	Bufo.
Amelioration	cough ameliorated by expectoration	Ail., alum., alumn., bell., calc., carb-an., caust., guai., hep., iod., ip., kali-n., kreos., lach., lob., meli., mez., phos., phyt., plan., sang., sep., sulph., zinc.

Body part/Disease	Symptom	Medicines
Amelioration	cough ameliorated by lying down in noon	Mang.
Amelioration	cough ameliorated during day time	Bell., caust., con., dulc., euphr., ign., lach., lyc., merc., nit-ac., sep., spong.
Amelioration	cough ameliorated from becoming warm in bed	Cham., kali-bi.
Amelioration	cough ameliorated from bending head forward	Eup-per., spong.
Amelioration	cough ameliorated from cold	Calc-s., coc-c., kali-s.
Amelioration	cough ameliorated from cold milk	Am-caust., bor., brom., caps., Caust., coc-c., Cupr., euphr., glon., iod., ip., kali-c., kali-s., onos., op., sulph., verat.
Amelioration	cough ameliorated from deep breath	Lach., puls., verb.
Amelioration	cough ameliorated from eating	All-s., am-c., ammc., anac., carb-an., euphr., ferr-m., ferr., kali-c., sin-n., Spong., tab.
Amelioration	cough ameliorated from eructations	Sang.
Amelioration	cough ameliorated from frequent stools	Bufo.
Amelioration	cough ameliorated from kneeling with face towards pillow	Eup-per.
Amelioration	cough ameliorated from lying	Mang.
Amelioration	cough ameliorated from motion	Ambr., arg-n., ars., caps., coc-c., dros., dulc., eupho., euphr., grat., hyos., kali-i., mag-c., mag-m., nux-v., ph-ac., phos., psor., puls., rhus-r., rhus-t., sabad., samb., sep., sil., stann., sulph., verb., zinc.
Amelioration	cough ameliorated from passing flatus	Sang.
Amelioration	cough ameliorated from rising	Mag-c., mag-s., rhus-t.
Amelioration	cough ameliorated from sitting bent	Iod.
Amelioration	cough ameliorated from smoking at night	Tarent.
Amelioration	cough ameliorated from sneezing	Osm.
Amelioration	cough ameliorated from standing	Mag-s.
Amelioration	cough ameliorated from sugar	Sulph.
Amelioration	cough ameliorated from swallowing	Apis., eug., spong.
Amelioration	cough ameliorated from turning left to right side	Ars., kali-c., phos., rumx., sep., thuj.
Amelioration	cough ameliorated from vomiting	Mez.
Amelioration	cough ameliorated from warm fluids	Alum., Ars., bry., eupi., Lyc., Nux-v., Rhus-t., Sil., spong., verat.
Amelioration	cough ameliorated from warm food	Spong.
Amelioration	cough ameliorated from wine	Sulph.
Amelioration	cough ameliorated in frosty (very cold) weather	Spong.
Amelioration	cough ameliorated in morning	Agar., coc-c., grat.
Amelioration	cough ameliorated while sitting still	Verat.
Amelioration	cough before menses in evening ameliorated by sitting up in bed	Sulph.
Amelioration	cough short ameliorated from sitting up	Arg-n., cinnb., nat-c.
Amelioration	cough while ameliorated from sitting erect	Ant-t.
Amelioration	cramp in calf ameliorated on motion	Arg-m., bry., ferr., rhus-t.

Body part/Disease	Symptom	Medicines
Amelioration	cramp in hand ameliorated on motion	Acon.
Amelioration	cramp in leg ameliorated from sitting	Cina.
Amelioration	cramp in sole ameliorated while walking	Verb.
Amelioration	cramping pain in abdomen after taking cold	All-c., alumn., Asaf., dulc.
Amelioration	cramping pain in abdomen ameliorated by warm milk	Crot-t., op.
Amelioration	cramping pain in abdomen ameliorated from hot milk	Crot-t.
Amelioration	cramping pain in abdomen ameliorated from kneading abdomen	Nat-s.
Amelioration	cramping pain in abdomen ameliorated from passing flatus	Acon., am-c., cimx., coloc., con., echi., graph., hydr., lyc., mag-c., merc-c., nat-a., nat-m., nux-m., ol-an., psor., rumx., sil., spong., squil., sulph.
Amelioration	cramping pain in abdomen ameliorated while lying	Cupr., ferr.
Amelioration	cramping pain in abdomen ameliorated while lying on the abdomen	Am-c., chion., coloc., dor.
Amelioration	cramps in chest ameliorated on lying down	Sulph.
Amelioration	cutting pain in abdomen ameliorated from passing flatus	Anac., ars-i., bapt., bov., bry., calc-p., Con., eupi., gamb., hydr., laur., plb., psor., sel., sulph., viol-t.
Amelioration	delirium ameliorated from eating	Anac., bell.
Amelioration	diarrhoea ameliorated after acidic food	Arg-n.
Amelioration	diarrhoea ameliorated after breakfast	Bov., nat-s., trom.
Amelioration	diarrhoea ameliorated after eructations	Arg-n., carb-v., grat., hep., lyc.
Amelioration	diarrhoea ameliorated after external heat	Ars., hep.
Amelioration	diarrhoea ameliorated after ice cream	Phos.
Amelioration	diarrhoea ameliorated by cold food	Phos.
Amelioration	diarrhoea ameliorated from cold drinks	Phos.
Amelioration	diarrhoea ameliorated from riding in train	Nit-ac.
Amelioration	diarrhoea ameliorated from wine	Chel., dios.
Amelioration	diarrhoea ameliorated in damp weather	Alum., asar.
Amelioration	diarrhoea ameliorates all symptoms	Zinc.
Amelioration	diarrhoea ameliotated after hot milk	Chel., crot-t.
Amelioration	distension ameliorated by eructation (to expel stomach gases through the mouth)	Carb-v., sep., thuj.
Amelioration	distension of abdomen ameliorated by passing flatus	All-c., am-m., ant-t., bov., bry., carb-v., kali-i., Lyc., mag-c., mang., nat-c., nat-m., ph-ac., sulph.
Amelioration	distension of abdomen ameliorated by passing flatus (Intestinal gas, composed partly of swallowed air and partly of gas produced by bacterial fermentation of intestinal contents. It consists mainly of hydrogen, carbon dioxide, and methane in varying proportionsGas produced in the digestive system usually expelled from the body through the anus)	All-c., am-m., ant-t., bov., bry., carb-v., kali-i., Lyc., mag-c., mang., nat-c., nat-m., ph-ac., sulph.
Amelioration	distension of abdomen ameliorated from stool	Alum., am-m., asaf., calc-p., corn., hyper., nat-m.
Amelioration	distension of abdomen, ameliorated by lying on abdomen	Con.

Body part/Disease	Symptom	Medicines
Amelioration	distension of abdomen, ameliorated from motion	Cedr.
Amelioration	distension of abdomen, ameliorated from stool	Corn.
Amelioration	distension of abdomen, ameliorated from walking	Calad., cedr.
Amelioration	distesion of abdomen, ameliorated after eating	Cedr., rat.
Amelioration	distesion of abdomen, ameliorated after eructations	Arg-n., Carb-v., mag-c., nat-s.
Amelioration	distesion of abdomen, ameliorated after passing flatus	Rat.
Amelioration	distension of abdomen, not ameliorated after eructations	Chin., echi., lyc.
Amelioration	dry cough ameliorated after dinner	Bar-c.
Amelioration	dry cough ameliorated after drinking	Brom., bry., caust., coc-c., iod., kali-c., op., Spong.
Amelioration	dry cough ameliorated by discharge of flatus up and down and must sit up	Sang.
Amelioration	dry cough ameliorated from eating	Spong.
Amelioration	dry cough ameliorated from lying down	Sep.
Amelioration	dry cough ameliorated from open air	Iod., lil-t.
Amelioration	dry cough ameliorated on motion	Kali-c., phos.
Amelioration	dry cough ameliorated while lying	Am-c., Mang., sep., zinc.
Amelioration	dry cough ameliorated while sitting	Arg-n., cinnb., sang.
Amelioration	dry cough at midnight ameliorated from lying on side	Nux-v.
Amelioration	dry cough at night ameliorated from sitting up	Hyos., Puls., sang.
Amelioration	dry cough at night ameliorated from smoking	Tarent.
Amelioration	dry cough in evening ameliorated on lying down	Am-m., zinc.
Amelioration	dryness of throat ameliorated after eating	Cist.
Amelioration	dryness of throat ameliorated from swallowing of saliva	Cist.
Amelioration	dryness of throat not ameliorated by drinking	Sang.
Amelioration	emptyness of abdomen, ameliorated from eructations	Sep.
Amelioration	eructations ameliorated after sleep	Chel., chin.
Amelioration	eructations ameliorated on lying	Aeth., rhus-t.
Amelioration	eructations ameliorated while walking	Lyc.
Amelioration	eruptions burning ameliorated after scratching	Kali-n.
Amelioration	eruptions itching ameliorated from heat of stove	Rumx., tub.
Amelioration	eruptions itching ameliorated in cold air	Kali-bi.
Amelioration	eruptions on face ameliorated from warmth	Ars.
Amelioration	eruptions, in lower limbs ameliorated from cold bathing	Lyc.
Amelioration	excessive flow of blood in brain at night ameliorated in open air	ars., camph., caust., coc-c., grat., hell., mag-m., mosch.
Amelioration	expectoration ameliorated from drinking	Am-c.
Amelioration	expectoration ameliorated in cold air	Calc-s.

Body part/Disease	Symptom	Medicines
Amelioration	expectoration ameliorated in open air	Arg-n., calc-s.
Amelioration	faintness ameliorated from acidic fruit	Naja.
Amelioration	faintness ameliorated from deep breath	Asaf.
Amelioration	faintness ameliorated from taking cold water	Glon.
Amelioration	faintness ameliorated in morning during eating	Nux-v.
Amelioration	faintness ameliorated on moving	Jug-c.
Amelioration	faintness ameliorated while lying	Alumn., dios., merc-i-f., nux-v.
Amelioration	feeling of tightness in abdomen ameliorated by passing flatus	Sil.
Amelioration	feeling of tightness in inguinal ameliorated by stretching	Bov.
Amelioration	feeling relaxed in abdomen, ameliorated by lying on back	Cast-v.
Amelioration	Felon (a pus-filled infection on the skin at the side of a fingernail or toenail) ameliorated from cold application	Apis., fl-ac., led., **Nat-s.**, **Puls.**
Amelioration	fever ameliorated after dinner	**Anac.**, ars., **Chin.**, cur., ferr., ign., iod., nat-c., phos., rhus-t., stront.
Amelioration	fever ameliorated after exertion	Ign., sep., stann.
Amelioration	fever ameliorated after mental exertion	Ferr., nat-m.
Amelioration	fever ameliorated after sleep	**Calad.**, chin., colch., hell., nux-v., phos., sep.
Amelioration	fever ameliorated after walking in open air	Ars., caust., petr., **Ran-s.**, rhus-t., sabin., sep.
Amelioration	fever ameliorated by uncovering	Acon., ars., bov., cham., chin-a., chin., coloc., ferr., ign., led., lyc., mur-ac., nux-v., plat., puls., staph., verat.
Amelioration	fever ameliorated during vomiting	Acon., dig., puls., sec.
Amelioration	fever ameliorated from drinking coffee	Ars.
Amelioration	fever ameliorated from drinking cold water	Bism., **Caust.**, cupr., fl-ac., lob., op., phos., sep.
Amelioration	fever ameliorated from standing	Bell., cann-s., iod., ip., phos., sel.
Amelioration	fever ameliorated from walking in open air	Alum., asar., caps., cic., lyc., mag-c., mosch., phos., puls., sabin., tarax.
Amelioration	fever ameliorated from washing	**Apis.**, bapt., **Fl-ac.**, **Puls.**
Amelioration	fever ameliorated in bed	Agar., bell., canth., caust., cic., cocc., con., hyos., lach., laur., nux-v., sil., squil., staph., stram.
Amelioration	fever ameliorated on motion	Agar., apis., **Caps.**, cycl., ferr., lyc., merc-c., puls., rhus-t., sabad., samb., sel., tarax., valer.
Amelioration	fever ameliorated while eating	**Anac.**, ign., lach., mez., zinc.
Amelioration	fever ameliorated while sitting	Nux-v.
Amelioration	fever at night with perspiration ameliorated on waking	Calad.
Amelioration	fluttering in chest ameliorated in open air	Nat-m., Nat-s.
Amelioration	formication ameliorated from rubbing	Zinc.
Amelioration	formication ameliorated from scratching	Croc., zinc.
Amelioration	formication ameliorated from warmth	Acon.
Amelioration	formication in foot ameliorated from open air	Bor., zinc.

Body part/Disease	Symptom	Medicines
Amelioration	fullness ameliorated after drinking	Rhus-t.
Amelioration	fullness ameliorated on passing flatus	Grat., hell., rhod., sulph.
Amelioration	fullness in chest ameliorated after expectoration	Ail.
Amelioration	fullness of stomach, ameliorated by eructation	Carb-v., euphr., iris., mag-c., nux-v., phos., sil.
Amelioration	fullness of stomach, ameliorated by sleeping	Phos.
Amelioration	fulness in ear, ameliorated by boring in ear	Mez.
Amelioration	hacking cough ameliorated in open air	Lil-t.
Amelioration	hacking cough ameliorated from holding pit of stomach	Con., Croc., dros.
Amelioration	hacking cough ameliorated from rising on	Rhus-t.
Amelioration	hacking cough ameliorated in evening after lying down	Am-m.
Amelioration	haemorrhage from chest ameliorated from walking slowly	Ferr.
Amelioration	hand hot ameliorated in open air	Phos., verat.
Amelioration	head heat , ameliorated from cold water	Apis., con.
Amelioration	head heat ameliorated from cold bath	Euphr., Ind., mez., nat-m., sep.
Amelioration	head heat ameliorated in bed	Euphr., Ind., mez., nat-m., sep.
Amelioration	headache ameliorated while lying in dark room	Acon., Bell., brom., bry., lac-d., podo., sang., sep., Sil.
Amelioration	headache ameliorated after bathing	Lact-ac.
Amelioration	headache ameliorated after closing eyes	Agar., aloe., arn., bell., calc., carb-v., chin-s., eupho., mez., nat-m., sil.
Amelioration	headache ameliorated after rising on	Alum., ars., cham., coc-c., crot-h., graph., hep., ign., jug-c., Kali-i., merc-i-r., murx., nat-m., nit-ac., Nux-v., ph-ac., phos., Rhod.
Amelioration	headache ameliorated after sleep	Agar.
Amelioration	headache ameliorated by eructations	Bry., cinnb., gent-c., lach., sang.
Amelioration	headache ameliorated during diarrhœa	Agar., alum., apis., lachn.
Amelioration	headache ameliorated from binding the head	Apis., arg-m., Arg-n., arn., bell., bry., calc., carb-ac., hep., lac-d., mag-m., nux-v., pic-ac., psor., Puls., rhod., Sil., spig
Amelioration	headache ameliorated from clenching teeth	Sulph.
Amelioration	headache ameliorated from coffee	Cann-i., chin., coloc., glon., hyos., til.
Amelioration	headache ameliorated from cold air	Aloe., arg-n., ars., bufo., caust., cimic., croc., dros., euphr., ferr-p., glon., iod., kali-s., lyc., lyss., Phos., puls., seneg., sin-n.
Amelioration	headache ameliorated from cold applications	Acon., Aloe., alumn., am-c., ant-c., ant-t., ars., asar., aur-m., bell., bism., bry., bufo., calc-p., calc., caust., cedr., cham., chin-s., cinnb., cycl., eupho., euphr., ferr-ar., ferr-p., ferr., glon., Ind., iod., kali-bi., kalm., lac-c., lac-d., lach., led., meny., merc-c., merl., mosch., myric., nat-m., phos., plan., psor., puls., seneg., spig., stram., sulph., zinc.
Amelioration	headache ameliorated from cold drinks	Alumn., bism., kali-c.
Amelioration	headache ameliorated from combing the hair	Form.

Body part/Disease	Symptom	Medicines
Amelioration	headache ameliorated from emmission of flatus	Aeth., cic.
Amelioration	headache ameliorated from hot drinks	Kali-bi.
Amelioration	headache ameliorated from light	Lac-c.
Amelioration	headache ameliorated from profuse urination	Acon., ferr-p., Gels., ign., kalm., meli., sang., sil., ter., verat.
Amelioration	headache ameliorated from strong tea	Carb-ac., glon.
Amelioration	headache ameliorated from tea	Cimic., ferr-p., kali-bi.
Amelioration	headache ameliorated from thinking of pain	Agar., camph., cic., pall., prun-s.
Amelioration	headache ameliorated from urination	Fl-ac.
Amelioration	headache ameliorated from vomiting	Arg-n., asar., calc., cycl., gels., glon., kali-bi., lac-d., lach., manc., op., raph., sang., sep., sil., stann., sul-ac., tab.
Amelioration	headache ameliorated in bed	Mag-c., Nux-v., sulph.
Amelioration	headache ameliorated in darkness	Acon., arn., bell., brom., chin., hipp., lac-d., mag-p., mez., sang., sep., sil., stram., zinc.
Amelioration	headache ameliorated in evening	Bry., calc-f, ham., kali-bi., lach., mang., nat-a., nat-m., phys., pic-ac., sang., spig., ter.
Amelioration	headache ameliorated in night	Bufo., ham., mag-c., sol-t-ae., spira.
Amelioration	headache ameliorated on bending head to one side	Meny., puls., sep., stann.
Amelioration	headache ameliorated on going to bed	Alum., colch., mag-c., rhus-t., sep.
Amelioration	headache on left side of head and face, extending to neck ameliorated by lying on right side	Brom.
Amelioration	hearing impaired ameliorated from blowing nose	Hep., mang., merc., sil., stann.
Amelioration	hearing impaired before menses	Ferr., kreos.
Amelioration	heat of throat ameliorated by cold air	Sang.
Amelioration	heaviness in back ameliorated from motion	Rhod.
Amelioration	heaviness in coccyx ameliorated from standing	Arg-n.
Amelioration	heaviness in extremities ameliorated after rising	Lyc., nat-m.
Amelioration	heaviness in extremities ameliorated after while walking in open air	Carb-v.
Amelioration	heaviness in extremities ameliorated on motion	Caps., cham.
Amelioration	heaviness in extremities ameliorated on rising after sittiing	Merc., nat-m.
Amelioration	heaviness in foot ameliorated during menses	**Cycl.**
Amelioration	heaviness in foot ameliorated from motion	Nicc., zinc.
Amelioration	heaviness in foot ameliorated while walking	Ars-i., **Mag-c.,** nat-m., sulph.
Amelioration	heaviness in hand ameliorated from motion	Cann-s., nicc.
Amelioration	heaviness in hip ameliorated from walking	Ph-ac.
Amelioration	heaviness in left upper limbs ameliorated on motion	Apis., camph., led., rhod.
Amelioration	heaviness in leg ameliorated while walking	Sec.
Amelioration	heaviness in lower limbs ameliorated after walking	Rat., rhod.
Amelioration	heaviness in lower limbs ameliorated on motion	Nat-m., nit-ac.

Body part/Disease	Symptom	Medicines
Amelioration	heaviness in lumbar region ameliorated from lying on left side	Coloc.
Amelioration	heaviness in lumbar region ameliorated from motion	Nat-c.
Amelioration	heaviness in sacral region ameliorated from standing	Arg-n.
Amelioration	heaviness of Head ameliorated after a afternoon rest	Sulph.
Amelioration	heaviness of Head ameliorated after dinner	Carb-an.
Amelioration	heaviness of Head ameliorated after open air	Bov.
Amelioration	heaviness of Head ameliorated after sleep	Laur.
Amelioration	heaviness of Head ameliorated from looking steadily	Sabad.
Amelioration	heaviness of Head ameliorated from motion	Mag-c., mosch., stann.
Amelioration	heaviness of Head ameliorated from pressure	Ail., Cact., camph., cop., mur-ac., nat-m., sabin.
Amelioration	heaviness of Head ameliorated from profuse discharge of urine	Fl-ac., Gels.
Amelioration	heaviness of Head ameliorated from raising head	Bry.
Amelioration	heaviness of Head ameliorated from rising on	Kali-i., mag-s., nat-m., nicc.
Amelioration	heaviness of Head ameliorated from shaking head	Gels.
Amelioration	heaviness of Head ameliorated from strong coffee	Corn.
Amelioration	heaviness of Head ameliorated in open	Ant-t., Apis., Ars., caust., clem., ferr-i., gamb., hell., hydr., mang., mosch., nicc., phos., puls., tab., zinc.
Amelioration	heaviness of Head ameliorated while lying	Manc., nat-m., olnd., rhus-t., tell.
Amelioration	heaviness of Head ameliorated while lying head high	Sulph.
Amelioration	heaviness of Head ameliorated while lying side on	Cact.
Amelioration	heaviness of Head ameliorated while walking	Kali-bi., mag-c.
Amelioration	heaviness of Head ameliorated while walking in open air	Hydr.
Amelioration	heaviness of Occiput ameliorated on lying down on back	Cact.
Amelioration	hysteriacal, ameliorated during menses	Zinc.
Amelioration	impeded, obstructed breath ameliorated while lying on the back	Sumb.
Amelioration	inability to cough from pain ameliorated by pressure of hand on pit of stomach	Dros.
Amelioration	Inflammation of eye ameliorated from cold	Apis., Arg-n., asar., bry., caust., Puls., sep.
Amelioration	inflammation of eye ameliorated from cold applications	Apis., asar., puls.
Amelioration	Inflammation of eye ameliorated from warm covering	Hep.
Amelioration	involuntary urination ameliorated during motion	Rhus-t.
Amelioration	involuntary urination ameliorated while walking	Rhus-t.

Body part/Disease	Symptom	Medicines
Amelioration	irritation in larynx ameliorated from suppressing the cough	Hyos.
Amelioration	itching in eye ameliorated from cold application	Puls.
Amelioration	itching in eye ameliorated from rubbing	Agar., caust., euphr., mag-c., nat-c., nux-v., ol-an., spong., stram., sulph., zinc.
Amelioration	itching in eye ameliorated in open air	Puls.
Amelioration	itching behind ear ameliorated by scratching	Brom., mag-c., mag-m., ruta.
Amelioration	itching below ear ameliorated by scratching	Mag-c.
Amelioration	itching between scapula ameliorated from scratching	Mag-c.
Amelioration	itching in ankle ameliorated from warmth	Cocc.
Amelioration	itching in back ameliorated from scratching	Mag-c., mag-m., mez., nat-c., pall., rat., rhus-v.
Amelioration	itching in back of foot ameliorated from scratching	Mag-m., nat-s., tarax.
Amelioration	itching in back of hand ameliorated from scratching	Alum., camph., merc., ol-an.
Amelioration	itching in buttock ameliorated from cold water	Petr.
Amelioration	itching in buttock ameliorated from scratching	Kali-i., olnd., thuj.
Amelioration	itching in calf ameliorated from rubbing	Paeon.
Amelioration	itching in calf ameliorated from scratching	Laur., mag-c., mag-
Amelioration	itching in chest biting ameliorated from scratching	Nicc.
Amelioration	itching in ear ameliorated by boring with finger	Aeth., agar., bov., coc-c., coloc., fl-ac., lachn., laur., mag-m., mill., ol-an., zinc.
Amelioration	itching in ear not ameliorated by boring with finger	Agar., carb-v., laur., mang.
Amelioration	itching in elbow ameliorated by rubbing	Ol-an.
Amelioration	itching in elbow ameliorated by scratching	Ol-an.
Amelioration	itching in external throat ameliorated by scratching	Mag-c.
Amelioration	itching in extremities ameliorated after scratching	Alum., ant-t., bov., camph., cann-i., chel., chin., coloc., graph., jug-c., kali-c., laur., led., mag-c., mag-m., mang., merc., mill., **Nat-c.**, nat-s., nicc., ol-an., olnd., pall., ph-ac., tarax., thuj.
Amelioration	itching in female genitalia ameliorasted by scrartching	Crot-t.
Amelioration	itching in female genitalia from leucorrhoea ameliorated on lying	Berb.
Amelioration	itching in fifth toe ameliorated from scratching	Nicc.
Amelioration	itching in foot ameliorated from motion	Psor., rhus-v., spig.
Amelioration	itching in foot ameliorated from scratching	Cann-i.
Amelioration	itching in forearm ameliorated after scratching	Mag-c., mill., ol-an.
Amelioration	itching in fourth toe ameliorated from scratching	Nicc.
Amelioration	itching in hand ameliorated from hot water	Rhus-t., rhus-v.
Amelioration	itching in hand ameliorated from motion	Sars.
Amelioration	itching in hand ameliorated from rubbing	Berb., ham.
Amelioration	itching in hand ameliorated from scratching	Alum., anac., camph., merc., ol-an.
Amelioration	itching in Hypogastrium (The part of the front of the abdomen that lies below the navel) ameliorated by scratching	Ph-ac.

Body part/Disease	Symptom	Medicines
Amelioration	itching in inguinal region ameliorated by scratching	Laur., mag-c., mag-s.
Amelioration	itching in inguinal region not ameliorated by scratching	Mag-m.
Amelioration	itching in knee ameliorated from scratching	Bov., mag-m.
Amelioration	itching in knee ameliorated on falling asleep	Mur-ac.
Amelioration	itching in leg ameliorated from rubbing	Cupr-ar.
Amelioration	itching in leg ameliorated from scratching	Laur.
Amelioration	itching in lower limbs ameliorated from motion	Mur-ac., olnd., psor., spig.
Amelioration	itching in lower limbs ameliorated from rubbing	Cupr., paeon.
Amelioration	itching in lower limbs ameliorated from scratching	Alum., bov., cann-i., chin., kali-c., laur., led., mag-c., mag-m., nat-c., nat-s., nicc., olnd., pall., tarax., thuj.
Amelioration	itching in lower limbs ameliorated from warmth	Cocc.
Amelioration	itching in male genitalia ameliorated from friction	Junc., mag-m., rhus-v., staph.
Amelioration	itching in male genitalia ameliorated from scratching	Ign.
Amelioration	itching in male genitalia ameliorated from scratching	Alum., carb-ac., crot-t., viol-t.
Amelioration	itching in palm ameliorated from moving about	Com.
Amelioration	itching in palm ameliorated from rubbing	**Anag.**, mag-s.
Amelioration	itching in palm ameliorated from scratching	Chel., graph., mag-c., mang., ol-an.
Amelioration	itching in scapula ameliorated from rubbing	Grat.
Amelioration	itching in shoulder ameliorated from scratching	Bov., ol-an.
Amelioration	itching in sides of inguinal region ameliorated after scratching	Phos., sars.
Amelioration	itching in sole of foot ameliorated from motion	Mur-ac., olnd.
Amelioration	itching in sole of foot ameliorated from scratching	Chin.
Amelioration	itching in thigh ameliorated from scratching	Alum., led., pall.
Amelioration	itching in third toe ameliorated from scratching	Nicc.
Amelioration	itching in thumb ameliorated from scratching	Chel., olnd.
Amelioration	itching in tip of finger and scratching does not ameliorate	Am-m.
Amelioration	itching in upper arm ameliorated from scratching	Chel., led., mang., pall.
Amelioration	itching in upper limbs ameliorated from hot water	Rhus-t., rhus-v.
Amelioration	itching in upper limbs ameliorated from motion	Com., sars.
Amelioration	itching in upper limbs ameliorated from scratching	Alum., ant-t., bov., camph., chel., coloc., graph., jug-c., led., mag-c., mang., merc., ol-an., olnd., ph-ac.
Amelioration	itching of abdomen ameliorated by scratching	Arn., ferr-ma., mez., sars.
Amelioration	itching of canthi ameliorated in open air	Gamb.
Amelioration	itching of face ameliorated by rubbing	Rhus-v.
Amelioration	itching of face ameliorated by scratching	Apis., grat., nat-c.
Amelioration	itching of Forehead ameliorated by rubbing	Ol-an., samb., tab.
Amelioration	itching of Forehead ameliorated by scratching	Bov., mag-c., squil.
Amelioration	itching of Forehead ameliorated in open air	Gamb.

Body part/Disease	Symptom	Medicines
Amelioration	itching of occiput ameliorated by scratching	Chel., ruta.
Amelioration	itching of Scalp ameliorated by rubbing	Dros., nat-m.
Amelioration	itching of Scalp ameliorated by scratching	Agar., bar-c., caps., caust., mag-c., mez., nat-m., ol-an., olnd., ph-ac., ran-s., sabad., sars., thuj.
Amelioration	itching of Scalp not ameliorated after scratching	Bov., calc., carb-an.
Amelioration	jar amliorated from stepping	Caps.
Amelioration	jerking ameliorated from walking	Valer.
Amelioration	jerking ameliorated on motion	Merc., thuj., valer., zinc.
Amelioration	jerking in leg ameliorated on motion	Carb-v.
Amelioration	jerking in lower limb ameliorated on motion	Hep., thuj., valer.
Amelioration	jerking in right thigh ameliorated from drawing up leg or standing	Meny.
Amelioration	jerking of upper limb ameliorated in warm room	Sulph.
Amelioration	lameness in hip ameliorated while walking	Ars-m.
Amelioration	lameness in thigh ameliorated from motion	Cocc.
Amelioration	lassitude ameliorated from walking in open air	Alum., am-c.
Amelioration	loose cough ameliorated by sitting up	Phos.
Amelioration	loose cough ameliorated from drinking cold water	Coc-c.
Amelioration	menses, copious, ameliorated from walking	Kreos., mag-m.
Amelioration	mental or physical pain ameliorated from open air	Cann-i.
Amelioration	metrorrhagia ameliorated from walking	Sabin.
Amelioration	nausea after cold drinks ameliorated after heated	Bism., phos., puls.
Amelioration	nausea ameliorated after breakfast	Alum.
Amelioration	nausea ameliorated after sleep	Rhus-t.
Amelioration	nausea ameliorated after wine	Coc-c.
Amelioration	nausea ameliorated during eructations	Agar., all-c., am-m., ant-t., camph., carb-s., caust., chel., cinnb., fago., glon., grat., kali-p., lac-c., lyc., mag-m., nicc., ol-an., osm., phos., rhod., rumx., sabad., sul-ac., verat-v.
Amelioration	nausea ameliorated from closing the eyes	Con.
Amelioration	nausea ameliorated from lying on left side	Cann-s.
Amelioration	nausea ameliorated from lying on side	Ant-t., nat-m.
Amelioration	nausea ameliorated from motion	Nit-ac.
Amelioration	nausea ameliorated from rising up in bed	Sabin.
Amelioration	nausea ameliorated from soup	Cast., kali-bi., mag-c.
Amelioration	nausea ameliorated from sour things	Arg-n.
Amelioration	nausea ameliorated from stool	Con., ferr., raph., sang.
Amelioration	nausea ameliorated from warm drinks	Ther.
Amelioration	nausea ameliorated in bed	Nat-c.
Amelioration	nausea ameliorated on lying down	Alum., alumn., arn., echi., nux-v., ph-ac., phos., sep., sil.
Amelioration	nausea ameliorated while bent over	Zinc.
Amelioration	nausea ameliorated while standing	Tarax.

Body part/Disease	Symptom	Medicines
Amelioration	noises in the ear when blowing nose ameliorated by boring into ear	Lach., meny., nicc.
Amelioration	numbness ameliorated from motion	Am-c., anac., aur.
Amelioration	numbness in forearm ameliorated from motion	Cinnb., puls.
Amelioration	numbness in fourth finger ameliorated from rubbing	Nat-c.
Amelioration	numbness in hand ameliorated on wetting	Spig.
Amelioration	numbness in left hand ameliorated from grasping anything	Spig.
Amelioration	numbness in left hand ameliorated on motion	Am-c., apis., cann-s., carb-an., ferr., nat-m., spig., stront.
Amelioration	numbness in leg ameliorated from rubbing	Stram.
Amelioration	numbness in leg ameliorated in open air	Pic-ac.
Amelioration	numbness in sole of foot ameliorated while walking	Puls., zinc.
Amelioration	numbness in upper arm ameliorated from motion	Ambr., apis., aur., dros., merc., rumx., sep., sulph.
Amelioration	numbness in upper arm ameliorated from raising them upright	Ars.
Amelioration	obstruction in nose ameliorated by walking in open air	Kali-c., puls.
Amelioration	obstruction in nose ameliorated from rising from bed	Nux-m.
Amelioration	obstruction in nose, ameliorated in open air	Arg-n., phos., pic-ac., rhod., sulph.
Amelioration	orgasm of blood ameliorated after walking	Mag-m.
Amelioration	orgasm of blood ameliorated from eating	Alum., chin.
Amelioration	orgasm of blood in evening ameliorated from sitting	Thuj.
Amelioration	orgasm of blood in morning ameliorated on rising	Nux-v.
Amelioration	ovaries painful ameliorated by eating	Iod.
Amelioration	ovaries painful ameliorated by extending limbs	Plb.
Amelioration	ovaries painful ameliorated by flexing thighs	Coloc., pall.
Amelioration	ovaries painful ameliorated during menses	Lac-c., lach., mosch., ust., zinc.
Amelioration	ovaries painful ameliorated from lying on left side	Pall.
Amelioration	ovaries painful ameliorated from lying on painful side	Bry.
Amelioration	ovaries painful ameliorated from lying on right side	Apis.
Amelioration	ovaries painful ameliorated from motion	Iod.
Amelioration	ovaries painful ameliorated from pressure	Pall., podo., zinc.
Amelioration	ovaries painful ameliorated from rubbing	Pall.
Amelioration	pain ameliorated in prostate gland on walking	Rhus-t.
Amelioration	pain ameliorated in prostate gland when urine starts	Prun-s.
Amelioration	pain between scapula ameliorated from bending backward	Sil.
Amelioration	pain between scapula ameliorated from lying	Ars.

Body part/Disease	Symptom	Medicines
Amelioration	pain between scapula ameliorated from lying on right side	Kali-n.
Amelioration	pain between scapula ameliorated on moving	Kali-c., laur., ph-ac., sulph.
Amelioration	pain between scapula ameliorated on straightening up	Bov.
Amelioration	pain between scapula ameliorated while walking	Bry., ferr., puls.
Amelioration	pain between scapula ameliorated from bending forward	Nat-a.
Amelioration	pain between scapula ameliorated from warmth	Rhus-t.
Amelioration	pain in abdomen amelioated from lying	Am-c., bry., canth., cupr., dios., gran., merc., nux-v., phys.
Amelioration	pain in abdomen amelioated from lying on abdomen	Aloe., am-c., ars-h., Bell., bry., chin-a., chion., coloc., Ind., phos., plb., rhus-t., stann.
Amelioration	pain in abdomen amelioated from lying on back	Coloc., kalm., mez., onos.
Amelioration	pain in abdomen amelioated from lying on left side	Pall., sec.
Amelioration	pain in abdomen amelioated from lying on right side	Nux-v., phos., phys.
Amelioration	pain in abdomen amelioated from lying on side	Nat-s.
Amelioration	pain in abdomen ameliorated after dinner	Chel., graph., mang.
Amelioration	pain in abdomen ameliorated when flow becomes free	Bell., kali-c., kali-p., lach., lap-a., mosch., sep., sulph.
Amelioration	pain in abdomen ameliorated after bread	Nat-c.
Amelioration	pain in abdomen ameliorated after cold food	Phos.
Amelioration	pain in abdomen ameliorated after eating	Aur-m., bov., chel., iod., mang., mez., nat-c., Nat-s., plan., psor.
Amelioration	pain in abdomen ameliorated after eating	Aesc., agar., anac., aur., brom., cham., chel., chin-a., cina., dios., fago., gamb., Graph., hep., ign., iod., iris., kali-bi., kalm., lach., lith., mag-m., mang., med., mez., nat-c., nat-s., nicc., ox-ac., petr., phos., raph., verat.
Amelioration	pain in abdomen ameliorated after food	Mag-c., ph-ac.
Amelioration	pain in abdomen ameliorated after ice cream	Phos.
Amelioration	pain in abdomen ameliorated after milk	Chel., crot-t., op.
Amelioration	pain in abdomen ameliorated after stool	Chel.
Amelioration	pain in abdomen ameliorated after urination	Carb-an.
Amelioration	pain in abdomen ameliorated after warm drinks	Acon., chel., mag-p., spong.
Amelioration	pain in abdomen ameliorated by drawing up the limbs	Bry., chel.
Amelioration	pain in abdomen ameliorated by knee-elbow position	Con.
Amelioration	pain in abdomen ameliorated by passing flatus	Agar., chel., dig., hep., lact., tarent.
Amelioration	pain in abdomen ameliorated from bending backward	Bell., bism., caust., kali-c.
Amelioration	pain in abdomen ameliorated from bending double	Alumn., carb-v., cham., chel., colch., Coloc., lach., lyc., nux-v., psor., ptel., verat-v.
Amelioration	pain in abdomen ameliorated from heat	Ars., bry., caust., chel., lyc., mag-p., nux-v., sil.

Body part/Disease	Symptom	Medicines
Amelioration	pain in abdomen ameliorated from legs drawn up	Ars., bry., caust., chel., lyc., mag-p., nux-v., sil.
Amelioration	pain in abdomen ameliorated from lying on abdomen	Elaps.
Amelioration	pain in abdomen ameliorated from lying on back	Calc., laur.
Amelioration	pain in abdomen ameliorated from pressure	Alumn., coloc., dios., mag-p., mang., plb., stann.
Amelioration	pain in abdomen ameliorated from rubbing	Lyc.
Amelioration	pain in abdomen ameliorated from sitting bent over	Bry., coloc., ox-ac., staph., sulph.
Amelioration	pain in abdomen ameliorated from sitting erect	Dios.
Amelioration	pain in abdomen ameliorated from stretching	Dios., nat-c.
Amelioration	pain in abdomen ameliorated from warm application	Chel., Mag-p., nux-m., nux-v., sil.
Amelioration	pain in abdomen ameliorated from warm drinks	Alum., ars., bry., graph., mang., nux-m., Nux-v., ph-ac., rhus-t., spong., sulph., verat.
Amelioration	pain in abdomen ameliorated from warm milk	Chel., graph.
Amelioration	pain in abdomen ameliorated from warmth of bed	Carb-v., graph., lyc., Nux-v.
Amelioration	pain in abdomen ameliorated from yawning	Lyc., nat-m.
Amelioration	pain in abdomen ameliorated on bending backward	Bell., dios., lac-c., nux-v., onos.
Amelioration	pain in abdomen ameliorated on motion	Aur-m., bov., cycl., kali-n., petr., phos., ptel., rhus-t., sulph.
Amelioration	pain in abdomen ameliorated when over heated	Alumn., arg-n., calc-s., caust., Phos., puls., tep.
Amelioration	pain in abdomen ameliorated while lying	Am-c., bell., caust., chin., graph., kali-i., lach., lyc., sil., stann.
Amelioration	pain in abdomen during night ameliorated in open air	Naja.
Amelioration	pain in abdomen, violent ameliorated from walking	Nit-ac.
Amelioration	pain in abdomen, violent ameliorated while walking	All-c., bor., bov., dios., elaps., lyc., nat-c., op., stann.
Amelioration	pain in ankle ameliorated from motion	Aur-m-n., dios., nat-s., plan., valer.
Amelioration	pain in ankle ameliorated from warmth	Chel.
Amelioration	pain in ankle ameliorated while walking	Ph-ac., rhus-t., sulph., **Valer.**
Amelioration	pain in ankle in morning ameliorated on walking	Sulph.
Amelioration	pain in anus ameliorated from cold application	Aloe., apis., euphr., kali-c., ter.
Amelioration	pain in arm ameliorated from warmth	Ferr.
Amelioration	pain in arm ameliorated on motion	Arg-m., aur-m-n., cina., cocc., cupr., dulc., kali-bi., meph., ox-ac., paeon., **Rhus-t.**, thuj.
Amelioration	pain in arm ameliorated on slow motion	Ferr.
Amelioration	pain in back ameliorated after eating	Kali-n.
Amelioration	pain in back ameliorated after stool	Nux-v., ox-ac., puls.
Amelioration	pain in back ameliorated after urinating	Lyc., med.
Amelioration	pain in back ameliorated bending backward	Acon., aeth., am-m., bell., cycl., eupi., fl-ac., hura., lach., petr., puls., rhus-t., sabad., sabin., sil.
Amelioration	pain in back ameliorated bending forward	Chel., meny., nat-a., ph-ac., puls., sang., sec., sep., thuj.
Amelioration	pain in back ameliorated from erructation	Sep.
Amelioration	pain in back ameliorated from exertion	Ruta., sep.
Amelioration	pain in back ameliorated from external warmth	Calc-f., caust., cinnb., nux-v., Rhus-t.

Body part/Disease	Symptom	Medicines
Amelioration	pain in back ameliorated from flatus	Berb., coc-c., ruta.
Amelioration	pain in back ameliorated from leaning back against chair	Eupi., sarr., zing.
Amelioration	pain in back ameliorated from lying on abdomen	Acet-ac., chel., mag-c., nit-ac., sel.
Amelioration	pain in back ameliorated from lying on back	Ambr., bufo., chin., cob., colch., equis., ign., kali-c., lach., Nat-m., nux-v., phos., puls., rhus-t., Ruta., sanic., sep., sil.
Amelioration	pain in back ameliorated from lying on pillow	Carb-v., sep.
Amelioration	pain in back ameliorated from lying on right side	Kali-n., nat-s., ust.
Amelioration	pain in back ameliorated from lying on side	Kali-n., nat-c., nux-v., puls., zinc.
Amelioration	pain in back ameliorated from lying on something hard	Am-m., bell., kali-c., lyc., Nat-m., puls., rhus-t., sep., stann.
Amelioration	pain in back ameliorated from pressure	Aur., camph., carb-ac., cimic., dulc., fl-ac., Kali-c., led., mag-m., nat-m., ph-ac., plb., rhus-t., ruta., Sep., verat., vib.
Amelioration	pain in back ameliorated from rubbing	Aeth., kali-n., lach., lil-t., nat-s., Phos., plb., puls., thuj.
Amelioration	pain in back ameliorated from straightening up the back	Bov., laur.
Amelioration	pain in back ameliorated from throwing shoulder backward	Cycl.
Amelioration	pain in back ameliorated in cold air	Kali-s.
Amelioration	pain in back ameliorated in open air	Acon., nux-v., vib.
Amelioration	pain in back ameliorated on gentle motion	Bell., calc-f., ferr., kali-p., Puls.
Amelioration	pain in back ameliorated on motion	Aesc., aloe., alum., am-c., am-m., bry., calc-f., calc-p., cina., coloc., cupr., dios., Dulc., fl-ac., graph., kali-c., kali-n., kali-p., kali-s., kreos., lach., laur., Lyc., mag-c., mag-m., mang., nat-a., nat-c., nat-s., nux-m., ox-ac., ph-ac., phos., puls., rat., rhod., Rhus-t., samb., sep., sin-n., spig., staph., stront., sulph., ust., vib.
Amelioration	pain in back ameliorated on rising	Lach., nat-c., nat-m., nit-ac.
Amelioration	pain in back ameliorated when turning in bed	Nat-m.
Amelioration	pain in back ameliorated while lying	Agar., ars., asar., bry., cob., kali-c., nat-m., nux-v., phos., psor., ruta., sars., sil.
Amelioration	pain in back ameliorated while sitting	Aeth., bor., caust., mag-c., meny., mur-ac., plb., sars., staph.
Amelioration	pain in back ameliorated while standing	Arg-n., bell., mur-ac.
Amelioration	pain in back ameliorated while walking	Am-c., ant-c., ap-g., Arg-m., arg-n., arn., ars-m., asar., bar-c., bell., bry., calc-f., cob., Dulc., ferr., gamb., kali-n., kali-s., kreos., mag-s., merc., nat-a., nat-m., nux-v., ph-ac., phos., puls., Rhus-t., ruta., sep., staph., stront., tell., thuj., vib., zinc.
Amelioration	pain in back of foot ameliorated from warnth of bed	**Caust.**
Amelioration	pain in bladder ameliorated after start of urine	Prun-s.
Amelioration	pain in bladder ameliorated from lying on abdomen	Chel.
Amelioration	pain in Bladder ameliorated in bed in evening	Alum.

Body part/Disease	Symptom	Medicines
Amelioration	pain in bladder with burning ameliorated by walking in open air	Ter.
Amelioration	pain in bones of leg ameliorated from warmth of bed	Agar., merc., mez.
Amelioration	pain in calf ameliorated from drawing feet	Cham.
Amelioration	pain in calf ameliorated from warmth of bed	Nux-v.
Amelioration	pain in calf ameliorated on motion	Agar., am-c., ars-i., cupr., rhus-t.
Amelioration	pain in cervical region ameliorated after stool	Asaf.
Amelioration	pain in cervical region ameliorated from external warmth	Rhus-t.
Amelioration	pain in cervical region ameliorated from motion	Aur-m-n.
Amelioration	pain in cervical region ameliorated from perspiration	Thuj.
Amelioration	pain in chest ameliorated after eating	Chel., rhod.
Amelioration	pain in chest ameliorated after rising in bed	Kali-c.
Amelioration	pain in chest ameliorated by arms near chest	Lact-ac.
Amelioration	pain in chest ameliorated from bending forward	Asc-t., chel., chin-s., Puls.
Amelioration	pain in chest ameliorated from eructations	Bar-c., kali-c., lyc.
Amelioration	pain in chest ameliorated from expectoration (to cough up and spit out phlegm, thus clearing the bronchial passages)	Chel., euon., mag-s.
Amelioration	pain in chest ameliorated from heat	Phos.
Amelioration	pain in chest ameliorated from lieing on painful sides	Ambr., Bry., calad., nux-v., stann.
Amelioration	pain in chest ameliorated from lieing on sides	Alum.
Amelioration	pain in chest ameliorated from lying on back	Ambr., cact.
Amelioration	pain in chest ameliorated from lying on painful side	Ambr., bry., kali-c.
Amelioration	pain in chest ameliorated from motion	Lob., phos., rhus-t., seneg.
Amelioration	pain in chest ameliorated from pressure	Arn., bor., Bry., cimic., Dros., eup-per., kreos., merc., nat-m., nat-s., phos., ran-b., sep.
Amelioration	pain in chest ameliorated from pressure on sides	Bor., bry., cimic., phos.
Amelioration	pain in chest ameliorated from rubbing	Calc., phos.
Amelioration	pain in chest ameliorated from sitting	Alum., am-m., asaf.
Amelioration	pain in chest ameliorated from standing	Chin., graph.
Amelioration	pain in chest ameliorated from warmth	Ars., caust., Phos.
Amelioration	pain in chest ameliorated in open air	Nat-m.
Amelioration	pain in chest ameliorated on motion	Aur-m-n.
Amelioration	pain in chest ameliorated on stretching the arm	Berb.
Amelioration	pain in chest ameliorated while lying	Alum., ox-ac.
Amelioration	pain in chest ameliorated while lying on abdomen	Bry.
Amelioration	pain in chest ameliorated while lying on back	Phos.
Amelioration	pain in chest ameliorated while sitting bent	Chel., ran-b.
Amelioration	pain in chest ameliorated while walking	Chin., dros., mez., nat-m., ph-ac., seneg.

Body part/Disease	Symptom	Medicines
Amelioration	pain in coccyx ameliorated from pressure on abdomen	Merc.
Amelioration	pain in coccyx ameliorated from standing	Arg-n., bell., tarent.
Amelioration	pain in coccyx ameliorated from stretching	Alum.
Amelioration	pain in coccyx ameliorated on rising from a seat	Kreos.
Amelioration	pain in coccyx ameliorated while walking slowly	Bell.
Amelioration	pain in dorsal region in right scapula ameliorated from bending shoulders backward	Conv.
Amelioration	pain in elbow ameliorated from warmth	Caust., **Rhus-t.**
Amelioration	pain in elbow ameliorated on motion	Arg-m., aur-m-n., bism., dulc., lyc., mez., **Rhus-t.**
Amelioration	pain in extremities ameliorated after eating	Nat-c.
Amelioration	pain in extremities ameliorated from applying cold	Apis., guai., lac-c., **Led.**, **Puls.**, **Sec.**, thuj.
Amelioration	pain in extremities ameliorated from coffee	Arg-m.
Amelioration	pain in extremities ameliorated from cold water	Puls.
Amelioration	pain in extremities ameliorated from perspiration	Ars., bry., nux-v., thuj.
Amelioration	pain in extremities ameliorated from pressure	Ars., bry., mag-p., plb.
Amelioration	pain in extremities ameliorated from warmth	Aesc., agar., am-c., ant-c., arg-m., **Ars.**, bry., cact., caust., cham., chin., colch., coloc., graph., **Kali-bi.**, kali-c., **Kali-p.**, kalm., lyc., **Mag-p.**, merc., nux-v., ph-ac., pyrog., **Rhus-t.**, **Sil.**, sulph.
Amelioration	pain in extremities ameliorated from warmth of bed	**Ars.**, kali-bi., nux-v., ph-ac., pyrog., **Rhus-t.**
Amelioration	pain in extremities ameliorated in open air	**Kali-s.**, **Puls.**, sabin.
Amelioration	pain in extremities ameliorated on continued motion	Agar., **Cham.**, **Rhus-t.**
Amelioration	pain in extremities ameliorated on motion	Agar., arg-m., aur., cham., chin., con., dig., dulc., ferr., kali-c., kali-p., **Kali-s.**, lach., lyc., med., merc., mur-ac., nat-s., psor., **Puls.**, **Pyrog.**, rat., **Rhod.**, **Rhus-t.**, ruta., sep., thuj., tub., valer., zinc.
Amelioration	pain in extremities ameliorated on walking	Agar., arg-m., ars., cham., chin., ferr., kali-i., kali-s., lyc., merc., nat-a., phos., puls., rhod., **Rhus-t.**, ruta., seneg., valer., verat.
Amelioration	pain in eye amelioratd from warmth	Ars., aur-m., dulc., ery-a., Hep., kali-ar., lac-d., mag-p., nat-a., nat-c., seneg., sil., spig., thuj.
Amelioration	pain in eye ameliorated by closing	Chel., lac-d., nit-ac., ph-ac., pic-ac., plat., sin-n.
Amelioration	pain in eye ameliorated by covering eyes with hand	Aur-m., thuj.
Amelioration	pain in eye ameliorated by dark	chin., euphr., nux-m., staph.
Amelioration	pain in eye ameliorated from lying on left side	Nat-a.
Amelioration	pain in eye ameliorated from lying on painful side	Lach., zinc.
Amelioration	pain in eye ameliorated from motion of eyes	Dulc., op.
Amelioration	pain in eye ameliorated from pressure	Asaf., bapt., bry., calc., caust., chel., chin-s., cimic., coloc., con., ham., mag-m., mag-p., mur-ac., pic-ac.
Amelioration	pain in eye ameliorated from rest	Berb., pic-ac.
Amelioration	pain in eye ameliorated when lying on	Chel., cimic.
Amelioration	pain in face in left zygoma ameliorated by pressure	Mez.

Body part/Disease	Symptom	Medicines
Amelioration	pain in face in left zygoma ameliorated by touch	Thuj.
Amelioration	pain in fingers ameliorated from cold	Caust., lac-c.
Amelioration	pain in fingers ameliorated from grasping	Lith.
Amelioration	pain in fingers ameliorated from pressure	Lith.
Amelioration	pain in fingers ameliorated from warmth	Agar., ars., bry., calc., **Hep.**, lyc., rhus-t., stram.
Amelioration	pain in fingers ameliorated when moving	Lith.
Amelioration	pain in foot ameliorated after coffee	Calo.
Amelioration	pain in foot ameliorated in warm bed	**Caust.**
Amelioration	pain in foot ameliorated on motion	Abrot., calo., cur., dios., psor., rhod., **Rhus-t.**, verat.
Amelioration	pain in foot ameliorated on motion	Abrot., calo., cur., dios., psor., rhod., **Rhus-t.**, verat.
Amelioration	pain in foot ameliorated while walking	Dig., puls., **Rhus-t.**, verat.
Amelioration	pain in forearm ameliorated from touch	Bism., meny.
Amelioration	pain in forearm ameliorated from warm application	Chel., chin., dulc., ferr., gran., kali-c., kalm., lyc., nit-ac., **Nux-v.**, **Rhus-t.**, sil., zinc.
Amelioration	pain in forearm ameliorated on motion	Alum., aur-m-n., bar-c., bism., camph., cocc., **Rhus-t.**, spig., stront.
Amelioration	pain in hand alternating with head symptoms	Hell.
Amelioration	pain in hand ameliorated from cold	Guai., lac-c., led., puls.
Amelioration	pain in hand ameliorated on motion	Com., dios.
Amelioration	pain in heart ameliorated on moving	Mag-m.
Amelioration	pain in heart ameliorated after urination	Lith., nat-m.
Amelioration	pain in heart ameliorated from lying on back	Cact., psor.
Amelioration	pain in heart ameliorated from pressure of hand	Nat-m.
Amelioration	pain in heart ameliorated while walking	Colch., puls.
Amelioration	pain in heel ameliorated from elevating the feet	Phyt.
Amelioration	pain in heel ameliorated from resting the boots off	Raph., valer.
Amelioration	pain in heel ameliorated from rubbing	Am-m.
Amelioration	pain in heel ameliorated from walking	Laur., **Valer.**
Amelioration	pain in heel ameliorated from warmth	Stram.
Amelioration	pain in hip ameliorated after walking	Am-c.
Amelioration	pain in hip ameliorated from flexing legs	Kali-bi.
Amelioration	pain in hip ameliorated from lying on painful side	Bell., coloc., ferr-ma.
Amelioration	pain in hip ameliorated from walking in open air	Acon., lyc.
Amelioration	pain in hip ameliorated from warmth	Rhus-t., staph.
Amelioration	pain in hip ameliorated on motion	Arg-m., ferr., gels., lil-t., lyc., nat-a., puls., rhus-t., valer.
Amelioration	pain in hip ameliorated on walking	Am-c., ferr., kali-bi., **Kali-s.**, **Lyc.**, **Puls.**, rhus-t., valer.
Amelioration	pain in hip ameliorated when standing	Staph.
Amelioration	pain in hip ameliorated while sitting	Aur., tarent.
Amelioration	pain in joints ameliorated after midnight	Ars., mag-p., plb.
Amelioration	pain in joints ameliorated from pressure	Bry., form.
Amelioration	pain in joints ameliorated from warmth	**Ars.**, bry., caust., lyc., **Nux-v.**, rhus-t., sulph.

Body part/Disease	Symptom	Medicines
Amelioration	pain in joints ameliorated on motion	Arg-m., **Aur.**, caps., cedr., chel., chin., dros., ferr., nat-s., phos., rhod., **Rhus-t.**, sulph., teucr.
Amelioration	pain in joints of upper limb ameliorated on motion	Aur-m-n.
Amelioration	pain in kidney amelioraed from motion	Ter.
Amelioration	pain in kidney ameliorated from standing	Berb.
Amelioration	pain in kidney ameliorated while lying on abdomen	Chel.
Amelioration	pain in kidney ameliorated while lying on back	Nux-v.
Amelioration	pain in kidneys ameliorated after urination	Lyc., med., tarent.
Amelioration	pain in kidneys ameliorated from lying on abdomen	Chel.
Amelioration	pain in kidneys ameliorated from motion	Ter.
Amelioration	pain in kidneys ameliorated from standing	Berb.
Amelioration	pain in knee ameliorated from continued walking	Dios.
Amelioration	pain in knee ameliorated from drawing limbs	Cham.
Amelioration	pain in knee ameliorated from extending limb	Ferr.
Amelioration	pain in knee ameliorated from flexing limb	Ferr.
Amelioration	pain in knee ameliorated from lying	Caj., sulph.
Amelioration	pain in knee ameliorated from pressure	Acon-c., ars.
Amelioration	pain in knee ameliorated from rubbing	Cast., cedr., phos., tarent.
Amelioration	pain in knee ameliorated from stretching	Dros.
Amelioration	pain in knee ameliorated from warmth	Canth.
Amelioration	pain in knee ameliorated in open air	Pic-ac., sumb.
Amelioration	pain in knee ameliorated on continued motion	Jac.
Amelioration	pain in knee ameliorated on motion	Agar., calc., colch., cycl., dios., indg., jac., lob., **Lyc.**, mez., nat-s., pic-ac., **Puls.**, ran-b., rhod., rhus-t., sep., stict., sulph., verat.
Amelioration	pain in knee ameliorated on walking	Agar., grat., kali-s., **Lyc.**, nat-c., nat-s., puls., pyrog., rhod., sulph., valer., verat.
Amelioration	pain in leg ameliorated after sleep	Plan.
Amelioration	pain in leg ameliorated at night	Puls.
Amelioration	pain in leg ameliorated at night in bed	Phos.
Amelioration	pain in leg ameliorated from cold application	Led., puls., syph., thuj.
Amelioration	pain in leg ameliorated from elevating feet	Bar-c., dios.
Amelioration	pain in leg ameliorated from walking	Agar., am-c., dulc., indg., kali-n., **Kali-s.**, **Lyc.**, puls., **Rhus-t.**, tub., valer., **Verat.**
Amelioration	pain in leg ameliorated from warmth of bed	Agar., am-c., ars., **Nux-v.**, ph-ac., pyrog., tub.
Amelioration	pain in leg ameliorated on motion	Agar., coloc., dios., dulc., gels., indg., kali-p., **Kali-s.**, nit-ac., plan., **Puls.**, pyrog., rhod., **Rhus-t.**, tub.
Amelioration	pain in leg ameliorated while sitting	Puls.
Amelioration	pain in liver ameliorated from warm drinks	Graph.
Amelioration	pain in lower chest ameliorated from lying	Chel.
Amelioration	pain in lower chest ameliorated from lying on back	Ambr.
Amelioration	pain in lower chest ameliorated from walking	Chin.

Body part/Disease	Symptom	Medicines
Amelioration	pain in lower chest ameliorated from walking extending transversely (lying or extending crosswise or at right angles to something)	Bism.
Amelioration	pain in lower left side of chest ameliorated from eating	Rhod.
Amelioration	pain in lower limb ameliorated from cold	Apis., coff., guai., lac-c., **Led.**, **Puls.**, **Sec.**
Amelioration	pain in lower limb ameliorated from dancing	Sep.
Amelioration	pain in lower limb ameliorated from lying	Am-m., dios., ham.
Amelioration	pain in lower limb ameliorated from motion	Agar., arg-m., aur-m-n., bell., calc-p., calc., caps., coloc., cupr., eupho., **Ferr.**, gels., indg., kali-bi., kali-p., **Kali-s.**, **Lyc.**, merc-i-r., merc., mur-ac., nat-s., ph-ac., plan., **Puls.**, rat., **Rhod.**, **Rhus-t.**, ruta., sep., stront., sulph., tarax., **Tub.**, valer., zinc.
Amelioration	pain in lower limb ameliorated from perspiration	Gels.
Amelioration	pain in lower limb ameliorated from pressure	Ars., **Mag-p.**
Amelioration	pain in lower limb ameliorated from pressure	Ars., coff., coloc., **Mag-p.**, meny., phyt., rhus-t.
Amelioration	pain in lower limb ameliorated from sitting	Gnaph., guai., kali-i.
Amelioration	pain in lower limb ameliorated from standing	Bell., mag-p., meny., staph.
Amelioration	pain in lower limb ameliorated from urination	Tell.
Amelioration	pain in lower limb ameliorated from walking	Agar., am-c., am-m., arg-m., ars., bell., caps., chin., coc-c., dig., dulc., **Ferr.**, indg., kali-bi., kali-i., kali-p., kali-s., **Lyc.**, ph-ac., puls., **Pyrog.**, **Rhus-t.**, ruta., seneg., sep., syph., tub., valer., verat.
Amelioration	pain in lower limb ameliorated from warmth	**Ars.**, bell., caust., coloc., kali-c., kali-p., **Lyc.**, **Mag-p.**, nat-m., nux-v., pall., phos., **Rhus-t.**, sil., staph., thuj.
Amelioration	pain in lower limb ameliorated from warmth of bed	Ars., caust., **Lyc.**, mag-p., nux-v., phos., sil.
Amelioration	pain in lower limb ameliorated from warmth of bed	Agar., ars., bell., caust., dulc., **Lyc.**, mag-p., **Nux-v.**, ph-ac., phos., **Pyrog.**, **Rhus-t.**
Amelioration	pain in lower limb ameliorated in morning	Aur., colch., merc., mez., nux-v., syph.
Amelioration	pain in lower limb ameliorated in morning on rising	**Rhus-t.**, stann.
Amelioration	pain in lower limb ameliorated in wet weather	Asar.
Amelioration	pain in lower limb ameliorated when warm	Ars., bar-c., caust., graph., lyc., nat-c., ph-ac., phos., stront., sulph.
Amelioration	pain in lumbar (lower back) region ameliorated while lying	Bry., cob., colch., cop., kali-c., nat-m., nux-v., ruta., sars.
Amelioration	pain in lumbar region ameliorated after rising from bed	Cocc., form., kali-p., staph.
Amelioration	pain in lumbar region ameliorated after stool	Ox-ac.
Amelioration	pain in lumbar region ameliorated after urinating	Lyc., med.
Amelioration	pain in lumbar region ameliorated from bending backward	Acon., am-m., fl-ac., hura., sabad., sabin.
Amelioration	pain in lumbar region ameliorated from bending forward while sitting	Chel.
Amelioration	pain in lumbar region ameliorated from flatus passing	Am-m., bar-c., coc-c., kali-c., Lyc., pic-ac., ruta.

Body part/Disease	Symptom	Medicines
Amelioration	pain in lumbar region ameliorated from motion	Aesc., alum., am-c., bry., calc-f., calc., cupr., dios., ferr., fl-ac., graph., kali-c., kali-n., kali-p., kreos., nat-a., nat-s., nux-m., nux-v., ox-ac., ph-ac., phos., podo., puls., rat., rhod., Rhus-t., ruta., staph., stront., vib.
Amelioration	pain in lumbar region ameliorated from pressure	Aesc., arg-m., aur., carb-ac., dig., dulc., fl-ac., led., nat-m., ph-ac., plb., rhus-t., ruta., sabad., sep., vib.
Amelioration	pain in lumbar region ameliorated from rising from seat	Com., ferr., ptel., ruta., sulph.
Amelioration	pain in lumbar region ameliorated from rubbing	Kali-c., kali-n., lil-t., nat-s., Phos., plb.
Amelioration	pain in lumbar region ameliorated from sitting	Aeth., bor., caust., mag-c., meny., ph-ac., plb., sars.
Amelioration	pain in lumbar region ameliorated from sitting bent	Chel., ran-b.
Amelioration	pain in lumbar region ameliorated from standing	Arg-n., kreos., meli.
Amelioration	pain in lumbar region ameliorated from stool	Indg.
Amelioration	pain in lumbar region Ameliorated from stooping	Chel., meny., ph-ac., puls., sang.
Amelioration	pain in lumbar region ameliorated from walking slowly	Ferr., puls.
Amelioration	pain in lumbar region ameliorated from warmth	Calc-f., caust., rhus-t.
Amelioration	pain in lumbar region ameliorated lying bent backward	Cahin.
Amelioration	pain in lumbar region ameliorated while lying on abdomen	Chel., nit-ac., sel.
Amelioration	pain in lumbar region ameliorated while lying on back	Ambr., cob., colch., kali-c., nat-m.
Amelioration	pain in lumbar region ameliorated while lying on something hard	Nat-m., Rhus-t.
Amelioration	pain in lumbar region ameliorated while walking	Am-c., ant-c., apoc., Arg-m., arg-n., ars-m., asaf., cob., dulc., gamb., kali-n., mag-c., meli., nat-a., ph-ac., phel., phos., puls., ruta., sabad., Sep., staph., sulph., thuj., vib., zinc.
Amelioration	pain in middle of mammae ameliorated from motion	Seneg.
Amelioration	pain in nail of toes ameliorated by cold application	Sabin.
Amelioration	pain in nail of toes ameliorated from lying	Puls.
Amelioration	pain in nail of toes ameliorated from motion	Ind.
Amelioration	pain in nose ameliorated from lying down	Cupr.
Amelioration	pain in nose ameliorated from pressure	Agn.
Amelioration	pain in nose ameliorated from rubbing	Bell., nat-c.
Amelioration	pain in region of heart ameliorated from eructations	Lyc.
Amelioration	pain in region of heart ameliorated from inspirations	Merc.
Amelioration	pain in region of heart ameliorated from motion	Seneg.
Amelioration	pain in right scapula ameliorated from bending shoulders backward	Conv.
Amelioration	pain in right testes ameliorated after urination	Cob.
Amelioration	pain in sacral region ameliorated after stool	Berb., indg.
Amelioration	pain in sacral region ameliorated during gentle motion	Puls.

Body part/Disease	Symptom	Medicines
Amelioration	pain in sacral region ameliorated during motion	Aloe., ang., coloc., fl-ac., lac-c., lyc., Nux-m., psor., Puls., Rhus-t., thuj.
Amelioration	pain in sacral region ameliorated from turning left in bed	Agar.
Amelioration	pain in sacral region ameliorated from lying on face	Bapt.
Amelioration	pain in sacral region ameliorated from lying on side	Puls.
Amelioration	pain in sacral region ameliorated from passing flatus	Pic-ac.
Amelioration	pain in sacral region ameliorated from pressure	Kali-c., led., mag-m., sep.
Amelioration	pain in sacral region ameliorated from stretching	Alum.
Amelioration	pain in sacral region ameliorated in evening	Lil-t.
Amelioration	pain in sacral region ameliorated on bending backward	Lac-c., puls.
Amelioration	pain in sacral region ameliorated on bending forward	Sang.
Amelioration	pain in sacral region ameliorated while lying on the back	Agar., calc-p., puls.
Amelioration	pain in sacral region ameliorated while lying with body bent forward	Bry.
Amelioration	pain in sacral region ameliorated while standing	Arg-n., bell.
Amelioration	pain in sacral region ameliorated while walking	Ang., arg-m., arg-n., lyc., merc., nat-a., psor., staph., tell., thuj.
Amelioration	pain in sacral region ameliorated while walking in open air	Ruta., tell.
Amelioration	pain in sacral region ameliorated while walking slow	Bell., Puls.
Amelioration	pain in shouder ameliorated from motion of shoulder	Ph-ac.
Amelioration	pain in shoulder ameliorated from cold air	Thuj.
Amelioration	pain in shoulder ameliorated from hanging down the arm	Phos.
Amelioration	pain in shoulder ameliorated from lying quite	Sang.
Amelioration	pain in shoulder ameliorated from lying quite on painful side	Coc-c., kali-bi., lyc., nux-v., puls.
Amelioration	pain in shoulder ameliorated from perspiration	Thuj.
Amelioration	pain in shoulder ameliorated from pressure	Coc-c., nat-c.
Amelioration	pain in shoulder ameliorated from raising the arm	Ph-ac.
Amelioration	pain in shoulder ameliorated on motion	Alumn., arg-m., bapt., calc., cham., colch., dios., dros., eupho., ferr-p., **Ferr.**, kali-p., lyc., mez., mur-ac., ph-ac., **Rhus-t.**, sep., stann., verb.
Amelioration	pain in shoulder ameliorated on motion of arm	Asar., bell., calc., cann-s., caust., chel., croc., ferr., iris., kali-bi., kali-c., kali-n., kreos., lach., lact-ac., led., mag-c., med., merc., mur-ac., nat-a., olnd., petr., phyt., puls., rhod., ruta., sang., sep.
Amelioration	pain in shoulder ameliorated on motion of arm backwards	Berb., dros., ign., kali-bi., laur., puls., sep., zinc.

Body part/Disease	Symptom	Medicines
Amelioration	pain in shoulder at night ameliorated from warm wrapping	Sil.
Amelioration	pain in soles of foot ameliorated from motion	Aloe., coloc., puls.
Amelioration	pain in soles of foot ameliorated while standing	Eupho.
Amelioration	pain in spine ameliorated from pressure	Verat.
Amelioration	pain in spine ameliorated on motion	Euphr., ph-ac.
Amelioration	pain in spine ameliorated on walking	Ph-ac.
Amelioration	pain in spine ameliorated while sitting	Mur-ac.
Amelioration	pain in spine ameliorated while standing	Mur-ac.
Amelioration	pain in spleen ameliorated while lying on left side	Phyt., squil.
Amelioration	pain in sternum ameliorated from sitting erect	Kalm.
Amelioration	pain in teeth ameliorated by picking teeth	All-c., bell., ph-ac., sanic.
Amelioration	pain in teeth ameliorated after dinner	Am-c., ambr., arn., calc., carb-v., ip., ph-ac., Rhod., rhus-t., sil.
Amelioration	pain in teeth ameliorated at night from cold air	Chel., clem., kali-s., mag-m., mez., nat-s., nux-v., Puls., sars., sel., thuj.
Amelioration	pain in teeth ameliorated from bleeding of gums	Bell., caust., sanic., sars., sel.
Amelioration	pain in teeth ameliorated from cold water	Aesc., all-c., ambr., ap-g., bell., bism., Bry., camph., caust., cham., chel., chim., clem., Coff., ferr-p., ferr., fl-ac., lac-c., laur., mag-c., mag-m., merc., nat-s., nux-v., phos., Puls., rhus-t., sel., sep., sulph., thuj.
Amelioration	pain in teeth ameliorated from cold water	All-c., asar., bell., bry., cham., clem., kali-c., laur., puls.
Amelioration	pain in teeth ameliorated from lying on painful side	Bry., chin-s., hyper., ign., mag-c., puls.
Amelioration	pain in teeth ameliorated from lying on painless side	Nux-v.
Amelioration	pain in teeth ameliorated from masticating	Bry., rhod., seneg.
Amelioration	pain in teeth ameliorated from motion	Mag-c., phos., puls., rhus-t.
Amelioration	pain in teeth ameliorated from rubbing cheek	Merc., phos.
Amelioration	pain in teeth ameliorated from salt	Mag-c.
Amelioration	pain in teeth ameliorated from salt food	Carb-an.
Amelioration	pain in teeth ameliorated from sour things	Puls.
Amelioration	pain in teeth ameliorated from sucking teeth	All-c., bov., caust., clem., mang., sep.
Amelioration	pain in teeth ameliorated from tobacco chewing	Bry.
Amelioration	pain in teeth ameliorated from warm drinks	Ars., bry., cast., lyc., mag-p., nux-m., nux-v., puls., rhus-t., sang., sil., staph., sul-ac., sulph., trom.
Amelioration	pain in teeth ameliorated from warmth of bed	Lyc., mag-s., nux-v., sil., spig., vinc.
Amelioration	pain in teeth ameliorated from wrapping up head	Nux-v., phos., Sil.
Amelioration	pain in teeth ameliorated in open air at night	All-c., ant-c., bov., bry., hep., mag-m., puls., sep., stann., sulph., thuj.
Amelioration	pain in teeth ameliorated while ltying	Alum., am-m., bry., lyc., nat-c., nux-v., spig.
Amelioration	pain in thigh ameliorated after sleep	Sep.
Amelioration	pain in thigh ameliorated from flexing knee	Ars.
Amelioration	pain in thigh ameliorated from rubbing	Tarent.
Amelioration	pain in thigh ameliorated from stretching limb	Agar., dros., ferr.

Body part/Disease	Symptom	Medicines
Amelioration	pain in thigh ameliorated from turning side to side	Merc-i-f., **Rhod.**, **Rhus-t.**
Amelioration	pain in thigh ameliorated from walking	Agar., bell., dulc., ferr., indg., **Kali-s.**, **Lyc.**, merc., puls., **Rhod.**, **Rhus-t.**
Amelioration	pain in thigh ameliorated on motion	Aeth., agar., caps., cham., con., dulc., **Ferr.**, hyos., indg., kreos., lyc., merc-i-f., mosch., **Puls.**, rhod., **Rhus-t.**, sabin.
Amelioration	pain in thigh ameliorated while sitting	Aur.
Amelioration	pain in thigh ameliorated while standing	Eupho.
Amelioration	pain in throat ameliorated after drinking	Bry., ign., tell.
Amelioration	pain in throat ameliorated from cold drinks	Apis., coc-c., Ind., lac-c., lach., lyc., merc-i-f., onos., phyt.
Amelioration	pain in throat ameliorated from sitting	Spong.
Amelioration	pain in throat ameliorated when yawning	Manc.
Amelioration	pain in throat ameliorated while eating	Acon., apis., benz-ac., carb-an., lach., onos., pic-ac., tell.
Amelioration	pain in throat ameliorated while lying	Canth.
Amelioration	pain in thumb ameliorated from pressure	Tarent.
Amelioration	pain in tibia ameliorated while standing	**Agar.**, aur-m-n., dulc., tub., verat.
Amelioration	pain in tibia ameliorated from crossing legs	Aur., bar-c.
Amelioration	pain in tibia ameliorated on motion	Agar., arg-m., aur-m-n., dulc., psor., rhus-t., verat.
Amelioration	pain in upper limb ameliorated during cold weather	Thuj.
Amelioration	pain in upper limb ameliorated from perspiration	Thuj.
Amelioration	pain in upper limb ameliorated from taking hold of anything	Lith.
Amelioration	pain in upper limb ameliorated from turning	Spig.
Amelioration	pain in upper limb ameliorated from warmth	**Ars.**, cinnb., graph., mag-p., sil.
Amelioration	pain in upper limb ameliorated in slow motion	Ferr.
Amelioration	pain in upper limb ameliorated on extending them	Merc.
Amelioration	pain in upper limb ameliorated on motion	Abrot., acon., agar., aur-m-n., camph., cina., cupr., cycl., dulc., kali-p., lyc., meph., phos., puls., rhod., **Rhus-t.**, spig., stel., thuj.
Amelioration	pain in upper limb ameliorated when bending arm	Ferr.
Amelioration	pain in upper limb ameliorated when lifting a load	Spig.
Amelioration	pain in upper limb ameliorated when lying on it	Acon., **Ars.**, calc., carb-v., cocc., dros., graph., ign., iod., **Kali-c.**, spig., urt-u.
Amelioration	pain in upper limb ameliorated while walking	Daph., valer., verat.
Amelioration	pain in upper limb ameliorated while walking slow	Ferr.
Amelioration	pain in ureters ameliorated during urination	Lyc., tarent.
Amelioration	pain in uterus ameliorated by bending double	Acon., cimic., coloc., nux-v.
Amelioration	pain in uterus ameliorated by flow of blood	Arg-n., bell., kali-c., Lach., mosch., sep., sulph., ust., vib.
Amelioration	pain in uterus ameliorated during menses	Bell., lach., mosch., sep., sulph., zinc.
Amelioration	pain in uterus ameliorated from lying on back	Onos.
Amelioration	pain in uterus ameliorated from lying on right side	Sep.

Body part/Disease	Symptom	Medicines
Amelioration	pain in uterus ameliorated from pressure	Ign., lil-t., mag-p., sep.
Amelioration	pain in uterus ameliorated from pressure on back	Mag-m.
Amelioration	pain in uvula ameliorated after cold drinks	Apis.
Amelioration	pain in uvula ameliorated after eating	Mez.
Amelioration	pain in uvula ameliorated from sleep	Crot-t.
Amelioration	pain in uvula ameliorated from warm drinks	Alum., ars., calc-f., hep.
Amelioration	pain in wrist ameliorated on motion	Arg-m., aur-m-n., bism., hyos., nat-s., prun-s., rhod., **Rhus-t.**, sulph.
Amelioration	pain of ear ameliorated from cold drinks	Bar-m.
Amelioration	pain of ear ameliorated from opening the mouth	Nat-c.
Amelioration	pain of ear ameliorated from pressure	Alum., bism., carb-an., caust., ham.
Amelioration	pain of ear ameliorated from sleep	Sep.
Amelioration	pain of ear ameliorated from swallowing	Rhus-t.
Amelioration	pain of ear ameliorated in open air	Am-m.
Amelioration	pain of ear ameliorated in warm room	Sep.
Amelioration	pain of eyes ameliorated by cold water	Acon., apis., asar., aur., form., lac-d., nat-a., nit-ac., phos., pic-ac., puls.
Amelioration	pain of eyes ameliorated from profuse urination	Acon., ferr-p., gels., ign., kalm., sang., sil., ter., verat.
Amelioration	pain of face ameliorated from hard pressure	Bell., bry., chin-s., chin., rhus-t., spig.
Amelioration	pain of face ameliorated from pressure	Ail., bry., coloc., cupr., dig., guai., lepi., mag-c., Mag-p., mez., sang., sep., spig., stann., staph., syph.
Amelioration	pain of face ameliorated after eating	Chin., kali-p., kalm., spig.
Amelioration	pain of face ameliorated by chewing	Cupr.
Amelioration	pain of face ameliorated by chewing	All-c., Kali-s., nicc., puls.
Amelioration	pain of face ameliorated by cold application	Apis., arg-m., ars-m., asar., bism., bry., caust., chin., coff., ferr-p., fl-ac., kali-p., lac-c., nicc., puls., sabad., sep.
Amelioration	pain of face ameliorated from excitement	Kali-p., pip-m.
Amelioration	pain of face ameliorated from motion	Agar., bism., ferr., iris., kali-p., lyc., mag-c., mag-p., meny., plat., puls., rhod., Rhus-t., ruta., valer.
Amelioration	pain of face ameliorated from profuse urination	Acon., ferr-p., Gels., ign., kalm., sang., sil., ter., verat.
Amelioration	pain of face ameliorated from rubbing	Ant-c., caust., Phos., plat., plb., rhus-t., valer.
Amelioration	pain of face ameliorated from sleep	Mag-p., Phos., sep.
Amelioration	pain of face ameliorated from talking	Kali-p.
Amelioration	pain of face ameliorated from touch	Am-c., am-m., asaf., chin., euphr., kali-p., olnd., thuj.
Amelioration	pain of face ameliorated from warmth	Ars., calc-p., calc., caust., cham., chin-s., coloc., cupr., Hep., kali-p., lach., Mag-p., mez., phos., rhod., rhus-t., sanic., Sil., spig., sul-ac., sulph.
Amelioration	pain of face ameliorated in open air	All-c., am-m., Asar., coloc., hep., kali-bi., kali-i., kali-s., lac-c., mag-c. nat-m., nat-s., puls., sulph.
Amelioration	pain of face ameliorated while eating	Caj., rhod.
Amelioration	pain of face ameliorated while lying	Cact., calc-p., chin-s., coff., nux-v., sep., spig.
Amelioration	pain of face ameliorated while lying on affected side	Bry., cupr., ign., sul-ac.

Body part/Disease	Symptom	Medicines
Amelioration	pain under left scapula ameliorated from sitting bent	Merc.
Amelioration	pain under left scapula ameliorated from lying with shoulder on something hard	Agar., kreos.
Amelioration	pain under left scapula ameliorated from pressure	Kreos.
Amelioration	pain under left scapula ameliorated on moving	Am-m., sabin.
Amelioration	pain, cutting in bladder ameliorated in open air	Ter.
Amelioration	pain, stitching in kidneys ameliorated from lying on face	Chel.
Amelioration	pain, stitching in kidneys ameliorated in warm bed	Staph.
Amelioration	pain, stitching in kidneys ameliorated while standing	Berb.
Amelioration	palpitation of heart ameliorated by pressure of hands	Arg-n.
Amelioration	palpitation of heart ameliorated during menses	Eupi.
Amelioration	palpitation of heart ameliorated from cold bathing	Iod.
Amelioration	palpitation of heart ameliorated from deep respiration	Carb-v.
Amelioration	palpitation of heart ameliorated from eructations	Aur., bar-c., carb-v.
Amelioration	palpitation of heart ameliorated from exertion	Mag-m.
Amelioration	palpitation of heart ameliorated from motion	Arg-m., arg-n., glon., mag-m., par., phos., rhus-t.
Amelioration	palpitation of heart ameliorated from warm drinks	Nux-m.
Amelioration	palpitation of heart ameliorated from washing hands in cold water	Tarent.
Amelioration	palpitation of heart ameliorated while lying	Arg-n., colch., lach., laur., phos., psor.
Amelioration	palpitation of heart ameliorated while lying long in one position	Alumn.
Amelioration	palpitation of heart ameliorated while lying on back	Kalm., lil-t.
Amelioration	palpitation of heart ameliorated while lying on right side	Glon., lach., Phos., Psor., tab.
Amelioration	palpitation of heart ameliorated while sitting	Lach.
Amelioration	palpitation of heart in morning ameliorated after breakfast	Kali-c.
Amelioration	paralysis of upper limb ameliorated during motion	Dulc.
Amelioration	paroxysmal cough ameliorated at at day time	Bell., ign., lyc., spong.
Amelioration	paroxysmal cough ameliorated from lying hand on pit of stomach	Croc.
Amelioration	paroxysmal cough ameliorated from rinsing mouth with cold water	Coc-c.
Amelioration	paroxysmal cough ameliorated from sitting up	Cinnb.
Amelioration	paroxysmal cough at midnight ameliorated by swallowing mucous	Apis.
Amelioration	paroxysmal cough in morning ameliorated by eating	Ferr.
Amelioration	paroxysmal pain in arm ameliorated from perspiration	Thuj.

Body part/Disease	Symptom	Medicines
Amelioration	persistent cough at midnight aggravated from lying on back and ameliorated from lying on side	Nux-v.
Amelioration	perspiration ameliorated after drinking	Caust., chin-s., cupr., nux-v., phos., sil., thuj.
Amelioration	perspiration ameliorated after eating	Alum., anac., chin., cur., ferr., **Lach.**, nat-c., phos., rhus-t., sep., verat.
Amelioration	perspiration ameliorated after exertion	Agar., bry., polyg-h., sep.
Amelioration	perspiration ameliorated after mental exertion	Ferr., nat-c.
Amelioration	perspiration ameliorated after waking	Ant-c., ars., bell., cham., **Chel.**, chin., cycl., euphr., hell., **Nux-v.**, op., **Phos.**, plat., **Puls.**, sel., sep., sil., stram., sulph., **Thuj.**
Amelioration	perspiration ameliorated during sleep	Ars., bell., bry., carb-an., chin., hep., merc., nux-v., ph-ac., phos., puls., **Samb.**
Amelioration	perspiration ameliorated from cold	Nux-v.
Amelioration	perspiration ameliorated from getting out of bed	Ars., bell., calc., camph., hell., hep., lach., lyc., merc., puls., **Rhus-t.**, sep., sulph., **Verat.**
Amelioration	perspiration ameliorated from uncovering	Acon., bell., calc., camph., **Cham.**, chin., led., **Lyc.**, nit-ac., puls., spig., staph., sulph., thuj., verat.
Amelioration	perspiration ameliorated from wine	Acon., apis., con., lach., op., sul-ac., thuj.
Amelioration	perspiration ameliorated in cold air	Ars., **Bry.**, **Calc.**, carb-an., lyc., sep., verat.
Amelioration	perspiration ameliorated in the open air	Alum., graph.
Amelioration	perspiration ameliorated on motion	Ars., **Caps.**, con., ferr., **Merc.**, puls., **Rhus-t.**, sabad., **Samb.**, sep., sul-ac., sulph., thuj., valer., verat.
Amelioration	perspiration ameliorated when going to sleep	Bry., merc., nux-m., ph-ac., phos., **Samb.**, sep.
Amelioration	perspiration ameliorated while eating	Anac., ign., lach., mez., **Phos.**, zinc.
Amelioration	perspiration ameliorated while walking	Cham., chel., puls., thuj.
Amelioration	perspiration ameliorated while walking in open air	Alum., **Ars.**, bry., graph., puls., thuj.
Amelioration	perspiration in cervical region ameliorated in sleep	Samb.
Amelioration	pulsation ameliorated from motion	Kreos., nat-m.
Amelioration	pulsation ameliorated in open air	Aur.
Amelioration	pulsation in cervical region ameliorated from holding head backward	Lyss., manc.
Amelioration	pulsation in head ameliorated from lying	Anac., calc., kali-bi.
Amelioration	pulsation in head ameliorated from motion	Aloe., lact.
Amelioration	pulsation in head ameliorated from resting head	Kali-bi.
Amelioration	pulsation in head ameliorated from sweating	Nat-m.
Amelioration	pulsation in head ameliorated from thinking of it	Ant-c.
Amelioration	pulsation in head ameliorated from warm tea	Glon.
Amelioration	pulsation in head ameliorated from wrapping head up warmly	Sil.
Amelioration	pulsation in head ameliorated in darkness	Sep.
Amelioration	pulsation in head ameliorated in open air	Ars., eup-pur., guai.
Amelioration	pulsation in head ameliorated lying on side	Nat-m., sep.
Amelioration	pulsation in lumbar region ameliorated from motion	Am-c., bar-c.

Body part/Disease	Symptom	Medicines
Amelioration	pulsation on back ameliorated during motion	Bar-c.
Amelioration	pulsation sensation ameliorated from cold	Ars., Ind., phos.
Amelioration	Pulsation sensation ameliorated after sleep	Cast.
Amelioration	redness of eyes ameliorated in open air	Arg-n.
Amelioration	remitent fever ameliorated while riding in a carriage	Kali-n., nit-ac.
Amelioration	respiration arreasted ameliorated from rubbing	Mur-ac.
Amelioration	respiration arreasted ameliorated while lying	Psor.
Amelioration	restlessness ameliorated during mental labor	Nat-c.
Amelioration	restlessness ameliorated from mental exertion	Nat-c.
Amelioration	restlessness ameliorated from motion	Fago.
Amelioration	restlessness ameliorated from music	**Tarent.**
Amelioration	restlessness ameliorated from walking in open air	Sumb.
Amelioration	restlessness ameliorated in open air	Aur-m., graph., lach., laur., lyc., valer.
Amelioration	restlessness ameliorated on lying on side	Calc-p.
Amelioration	restlessness ameliorated on stretching backward	Bor.
Amelioration	restlessness ameliorated while walking	Dios., nat-m., nicc.
Amelioration	restlessness ameliorated while walking in open air	Aur-m., graph., Lyc., Puls.
Amelioration	restlessness in lumbar region ameliorated from passing flatus	Bar-c., calc-f., cedr., chin-s.
Amelioration	retching ameliorated after eating	Ign., nat-c.
Amelioration	retching ameliorated from warm drinks	Ther.
Amelioration	retention of urine painful ameliorated by sitting bent backwards	Zinc.
Amelioration	rheumatic pain in extremities ameliorated after a cold	Guai., lac-c., **Led.**, **Puls.**, **Sec.**
Amelioration	rheumatic pain in joints ameliorated after walking	Sul-ac.
Amelioration	rheumatic pain in shoulder ameliorated from external warmth	Echi., ferr., **Hep.**, lyc., **Rhus-t.**, sil., thuj.
Amelioration	rheumatic pain in shoulder ameliorated while walking	Ferr.
Amelioration	rheumatic pain in shoulder on waking ameliorated while walking	Calc-s., eupho., rhod., **Rhus-t.**
Amelioration	rheumatic swelling of knee ameliorated from cold application	Lac-c., **Led.**, puls.
Amelioration	sadness ameliorated from sad music	Mang.
Amelioration	sadness ameliorated from urination	Eug., hyos.
Amelioration	scales ameliorated by washing	Graph.
Amelioration	sciatic pain in lower limb ameliorated at night	Staph.
Amelioration	sciatic pain in lower limb ameliorated from flexing legs	Ars., coloc., guai., kali-bi., kali-i., tell., valer.
Amelioration	sciatic pain in lower limb ameliorated from lying	**Am-m.**, bar-c., bry., dios., lach.
Amelioration	sciatic pain in lower limb ameliorated from lying on back	Phos.

Body part/Disease	Symptom	Medicines
Amelioration	sciatic pain in lower limb ameliorated from lying on on painful side	**Bry.**, coloc.
Amelioration	sciatic pain in lower limb ameliorated from lying on on right side	Phos.
Amelioration	sciatic pain in lower limb ameliorated from motion	Acon., agar., arg-m., caps., cham., coc-c., dulc., eupho., **Ferr.**, gels., indg., kali-bi., kali-i., kali-p., kreos., lac-c., lyc., meny., nat-s., puls., rhod., **Rhus-t.**, ruta, sep., sil., sulph., ter., valer.
Amelioration	sciatic pain in lower limb ameliorated from slow motion	Ferr., kali-p., puls.
Amelioration	sciatic pain in lower limb ameliorated in open air	**Kali-i.**, mez., **Puls.**, thuj.
Amelioration	sensation as if cold air passed over brain ameliorated in open air	Laur., sep.
Amelioration	sensation of bread crumbs in throat ameliorated from hawking	Lach.
Amelioration	sensation of lump in abdomen ameliorated after eructation	Bar-c.
Amelioration	sensation of lump in oesophagus ameliorated after swallowing	Phos.
Amelioration	sensation of paralysis in fourth finger ameliorated on rest	Hell.
Amelioration	sensation of paralysis in hand ameliorated during sleep	Plat.
Amelioration	sensation of paralysis in hand ameliorated from motion	Acon.
Amelioration	sensation of paralysis in hand ameliorated from rubbing	Chel.
Amelioration	sensation of paralysis in hip ameliorated from lying	Phos.
Amelioration	sensation of paralysis in hip ameliorated from sitting	Phos.
Amelioration	sensation of paralysis in hip ameliorated while walking	Ph-ac.
Amelioration	sensation of paralysis in knees ameliorated while walking	Lach.
Amelioration	sensation of suffocation in throat ameliorated from warm drinks	Calc-f.
Amelioration	shaking chill in evening ameliorated in bed	Mag-m., mag-s.
Amelioration	shaking chill in the open air not ameliorated by covering	Rhus-t.
Amelioration	shuddering knee ameliorated while walking	Nat-m.
Amelioration	skin, burning ameliorated in cold air	Kali-bi.
Amelioration	skin, crawling ameliorated from heat of stove	Rumx., **Tub.**
Amelioration	skin, crawling ameliorated from lying	Urt-u.
Amelioration	skin, itching ameliorated from scratching	Agar., agn., alum., am-c., am-m., ambr., anac., ant-c., ant-t., apis., am., ars., **Asaf.**, bell., bor., bov., brom., bry., cadm., calc-s., **Calc.**, camph., cann-s., canth., caps., carb-an., caust., chel., chin., cic., cina., clem., coloc., com., con., crot-t., **Cycl.**, dig., dros., form., guai., hep., hydr., ign., jug-c., kali-ar., kali-c., kali-n., kali-s., kreos., laur., led., mag-c., mag-m., mang., meny., merc., mez., mosch., **Mur-ac.**, **Nat-c.**, nat-p., nit-ac., nux-v., olnd., ph-ac., **Phos.**, plat., plb., prun-s., ran-b., rhus-t., ruta., sabad., sabin., sal-ac., samb., sars., sec., sel., seneg., sep., spig., spong., squil., stann., staph., sul-ac., sulph., tarax., thuj., valer., viol-t., zinc.

Body part/Disease	Symptom	Medicines
Amelioration	skin, itching ameliorated in evening	Cact.
Amelioration	skin, itching at night ameliorated from bathing	Clem.
Amelioration	slow breath ameliorated on walking	Ferr.
Amelioration	sneezing, ameliorated in cold air	All-c., calc-i., calc-s., phos., puls.
Amelioration	sneezing, ameliorated from lying	Merc.
Amelioration	spasmodic yawning ameliorated after wine	Nat-m.
Amelioration	stiffness ameliorated after walking	**Rhus-t.**
Amelioration	stiffness ameliorated while walking	Calc., carb-v., lyc., rhus-t.
Amelioration	stiffness in back ameliorated from sitting bent	Anac.
Amelioration	stiffness in back ameliorated from walking	Bry., calc-s., cop., Rhus-t., sep., sulph.
Amelioration	stiffness in back ameliorated on moving	Rhus-t., sul-ac.
Amelioration	stiffness in back in morning ameliorated on rising in bed	Anac.
Amelioration	stiffness in cervical region ameliorated from violent motion	Rat.
Amelioration	stiffness in foot ameliorated after rising from sitting	Alum.
Amelioration	stiffness in foot ameliorated while walking	Alum., laur.
Amelioration	stiffness in fourth finger ameliorated at rest	Hell.
Amelioration	stiffness in fourth finger ameliorated at rest	Hell.
Amelioration	stiffness in hand ameliorated from walking	Alum.
Amelioration	stiffness in hip ameliorated from walking	Ph-ac.
Amelioration	stiffness in joints ameliorated after applying cold water	Led.
Amelioration	stiffness in lower limbs ameliorated from stretching	Stram.
Amelioration	stiffness in lower limbs ameliorated in evening on rising	Mang.
Amelioration	stiffness in lower limbs ameliorated on rubbing	Stram.
Amelioration	stiffness in lower limbs ameliorated while walking	Carb-v., dig.
Amelioration	stiffness in morning ameliorated from cold bathing	Led.
Amelioration	stiffness in shoulder ameliorated after walking	Calc-s.
Amelioration	stiffness in shoulder ameliorated after walking in open air	Lyc.
Amelioration	stiffness in wrist ameliorated in evening	Arg-n.
Amelioration	stiffness of ankle ameliorated from exercise	Dios., sulph.
Amelioration	stinging after itching ameliorated from scratching	Anac.
Amelioration	stitching pain in chest ameliorated from pressure of hand	Aur-m., puls.
Amelioration	stitching pain in chest ameliorated from scratching	Plat.
Amelioration	stitching pain in chest extending to back ameliorated from lying on right side	Kali-c.
Amelioration	stitching sensation in chest ameliorated from bending forward	Chel., chin.
Amelioration	stitching sensation in chest ameliorated from rubbing	Calc., phos.

Body part/Disease	Symptom	Medicines
Amelioration	sudden stinging after itching ameliorated from scratching	Ph-ac.
Amelioration	suicidal disposition ameliorated from weeping	Phos.
Amelioration	swelling in foot ameliorated in evening	Dig., sil.
Amelioration	swelling in foot ameliorated when out of bed	Sulph.
Amelioration	swelling in leg ameliorated from walking	Aur., sep.
Amelioration	swelling in nose ameliorated in evening	Caust.
Amelioration	swelling in upper limbs ameliorated from uncovering	Chin.
Amelioration	symptoms ameliorated while sweating	Acon., aesc., aeth., apis., ars., bapt., bell., bov., **Bry.**, calad., camph., canth., cham., chin-s., cimx., **Cupr.**, elat., eup-per., **Gels.**, graph., hep., lach., lyc., **Nat-m.**, psor., **Rhus-t.**, samb., sec., stront., thuj., verat.
Amelioration	symptoms ameliorated while sweating except the headache	Nat-m.
Amelioration	symptoms ameliorated while sweating except the headache which is made worse	Ars., chin-s., **Eup-per.**
Amelioration	tension in cervical region ameliorated from becoming warm	Mosch.
Amelioration	tension in cervical region ameliorated from stretching out	Sulph.
Amelioration	tension in cervical region ameliorated on motion	Con., rhod., rhus-t.
Amelioration	tension in cervical region ameliorated while walking	Mag-s., rhod., rhus-t., sulph.
Amelioration	tension in dorsal region ameliorated from walking	Mag-s.
Amelioration	tension in lumbar region ameliorated from bending backward	Acon.
Amelioration	tension in muscles of back ameliorated during motion	Am-m.
Amelioration	tingling in hand ameliorated on motion	Am-c., carb-an., sep.
Amelioration	trembling ameliorated after breakfast	Calc., con., nat-m., nux-v., staph.
Amelioration	trembling ameliorated from cold drinks	Phos.
Amelioration	trembling ameliorated from resting against anything	Plb.
Amelioration	trembling ameliorated in open air	Clem.
Amelioration	trembling ameliorated on motion	Merc., plat.
Amelioration	trembling in foot ameliorated during motion	Mag-m.
Amelioration	trembling in foot ameliorated while sitting	Ol-an.
Amelioration	trembling in foot ameliorated while walking in open air	Bor.
Amelioration	trembling in hand ameliorated from motion	Crot-h., zinc.
Amelioration	trembling in hand ameliorated from rubbing	Nat-m.
Amelioration	trembling in knee ameliorated while walking	Chin.
Amelioration	trembling in knee ameliorated while walking in open air	Hep., laur.
Amelioration	trembling in knee ameliorated while sitting	Laur.

Body part/Disease	Symptom	Medicines
Amelioration	trembling in leg ameliorated in room	Caust.
Amelioration	trembling in lower limbs ameliorated after motion	**Rhus-t.**
Amelioration	trembling in lower limbs ameliorated while being alone	Ambr.
Amelioration	trembling in lower limbs ameliorated while walking	Nat-m.
Amelioration	trembling in upper arm ameliorated from motion	Asaf.
Amelioration	trembling in upper limbs ameliorated after brandy	Plb.
Amelioration	twitching ameliorated from mannual labour	Agar.
Amelioration	twitching ameliorated from motion	Ars., cop., phos., valer.
Amelioration	twitching in elbow ameliorated from motion	Agn., arg-m.
Amelioration	twitching in elbow ameliorated from sretching arm	Nat-m.
Amelioration	twitching in foot ameliorated when ltying on painless side	Nux-v.
Amelioration	twitching in hip ameliorated on motion	Sulph.
Amelioration	twitching in hollow of knee ameliorated from touch	Dig.
Amelioration	twitching in knee ameliorated from motion	Meny.
Amelioration	twitching in leg ameliorated on motion	Valer.
Amelioration	twitching in lower limbs ameliorated after walking	Valer., verat.
Amelioration	twitching in lower limbs ameliorated while sitting and letting limbs hang out of bed	Verat.
Amelioration	twitching in upper arm ameliorated from motion	Ph-ac., stann.
Amelioration	twitching in upper limbs ameliorated from working hard with hands	Agar.
Amelioration	ulcer in mouth ameliorated from cold water	Dulc.
Amelioration	ulcer in skin ameliorated from cold application	Led.
Amelioration	ulcer in skin ameliorated from warmth	Ars., **Lach.**, **Sil.**, syph.
Amelioration	ulcerative pain in upper limb ameliorated from turning	Berb., thuj.
Amelioration	ulcerative pain in upper limb ameliorated from uncovering	Lac-c., **Led.**, **Puls.**, sulph.
Amelioration	ulcer with cold feeling ameliorated in air	Dros., **Led.**, **Puls.**
Amelioration	ulcer with pain ameliorated from cold application	Cham., fl-ac., **Led.**, lyc., **Puls.**
Amelioration	unconsciousness ameliorated by cold water poured over head	Tab.
Amelioration	unconsciousness ameliorated from rubbing soles of feet	Chel.
Amelioration	urticaria ameliorated from lying	Urt-u.
Amelioration	urticaria ameliorated from warmth & exercise	Hep., sep.
Amelioration	urticaria ameliorated in cold air	Calc., dulc.
Amelioration	vertigo ameliorated after coryza	Aloe.
Amelioration	vertigo ameliorated after eating	Alum., arg-n., cinnb., cocc., dulc., sabad.
Amelioration	vertigo ameliorated after stool	Cupr.
Amelioration	vertigo ameliorated after tea	Glon.
Amelioration	vertigo ameliorated after vomitting	Op.

Body part/Disease	Symptom	Medicines
Amelioration	vertigo ameliorated after wine	Arg-n., coca., gels., phos.
Amelioration	vertigo ameliorated from closing eyes	Alum., con., dig., ferr., gels., graph., phel., pip-m., sel., sulph., tab., verat-v.
Amelioration	vertigo ameliorated from going to sleep	Bell., ferr., grat., pall.
Amelioration	vertigo ameliorated from meditation	Phos.
Amelioration	vertigo ameliorated from rest	Cann-i., coca., con., eupi., nat-m., nux-m., nux-v.
Amelioration	vertigo ameliorated from resting head on table	Sabad.
Amelioration	vertigo ameliorated from rubbing the eyes	Alum.
Amelioration	vertigo ameliorated from sitting	Acon., aur., bry., cycl., form., lach., puls., sil.
Amelioration	vertigo ameliorated from thinking some thing else	Agar., pip-m., sep.
Amelioration	vertigo ameliorated from warm bed	Cocc.
Amelioration	vertigo ameliorated in open air	Carb-ac., crot-h., kali-c., mag-c., mag-m., nat-c., par., puls., rhod.
Amelioration	vertigo ameliorated on elevation (on being raised)	Sulph.
Amelioration	vertigo ameliorated on walking	Acon., am-c., bry., lil-t., mag-c., sil., staph., sulph., zinc.
Amelioration	vertigo ameliorated on wiping eyes	Alum.
Amelioration	vertigo ameliorated when feet become warm	Lach.
Amelioration	vertigo ameliorated while lying on back	Stram.
Amelioration	vertigo ameliorated while lying on side	Merc.
Amelioration	vertigo ameliorated while lying with head high	Nat-m., petr.
Amelioration	vesicles ameliorates by cold things	Nat-s.
Amelioration	vision blurred ameliorated on closing eyes	Calc-f.
Amelioration	vision, dimness ameliorated by looking steadily	Aur., mang.
Amelioration	vision, dimness ameliorated by rubbing	Cina., puls., sulph.
Amelioration	vision, dimness ameliorated by washing	Caust.
Amelioration	vision, dimness ameliorated from lying down	Sep.
Amelioration	vision, dimness ameliorated from twilight	Phos.
Amelioration	vision, dimness ameliorated from urination	Gels.
Amelioration	vision, dimness ameliorated from wiping eyes	Alum., arg-n., carl., cina., croc., euphr., lyc., nat-a., nat-c., puls., sil.
Amelioration	vision, dimness ameliorated in dark day	Eupho., sep.
Amelioration	vision, dimness ameliorated in room	Alum., con.
Amelioration	vision, foggy ameliorated by rubbing	Puls.
Amelioration	vomiting ameliorated from cold water	Cupr., phos., puls.
Amelioration	vomiting ameliorated from wine	Kalm.
Amelioration	vomitting ameliorated from closing eyes	Tab.
Amelioration	weakness ameliorated after beer	Thea.
Amelioration	weakness ameliorated after breakfast	Calc., Coca., con., nat-m., nux-v., staph.
Amelioration	weakness ameliorated after dinner	Ambr.
Amelioration	weakness ameliorated after eating	Aster., Paeon., petr., sil.
Amelioration	weakness ameliorated after sleep	Mez., ph-ac., phos.
Amelioration	weakness ameliorated after urination	Spira.

Body part/Disease	Symptom	Medicines
Amelioration	weakness ameliorated at appearance of menses	Cycl., mag-m.
Amelioration	weakness ameliorated during menses	**Sep.**
Amelioration	weakness ameliorated during motion	Caps., cham., lyc., phos., **Rhus-t.**
Amelioration	weakness ameliorated from alcoholic drinks	Canth.
Amelioration	weakness ameliorated from exertion	Ferr., kali-n.
Amelioration	weakness ameliorated from gentle motion	Kali-n.
Amelioration	weakness ameliorated from leaning towards left during menses	Phel.
Amelioration	weakness ameliorated from lying	Acon-f., ars., lach., mag-c., psor., sep.
Amelioration	weakness ameliorated from lying on back	Cast.
Amelioration	weakness ameliorated from mental occupation	Croc.
Amelioration	weakness ameliorated from motion	Colch., coloc., cycl., gels., kreos., lyc., mosch., pip-m., plat., plb., rhod.
Amelioration	weakness ameliorated from resting head on something and closing eyes	Anac.
Amelioration	weakness ameliorated from sitting	Bry., glon., nux-v.
Amelioration	weakness ameliorated from stimulants	Phos.
Amelioration	weakness ameliorated from walking at day time	Ph-ac.
Amelioration	weakness ameliorated from walking in open air	Agar., am-c., caust., fl-ac., kali-i., ox-ac., sulph.
Amelioration	weakness ameliorated from walking rapidly	Stann.
Amelioration	weakness ameliorated from walking	Anac., coloc., merc., nat-m., **Rhus-t.**, ruta., **Sulph.**
Amelioration	weakness ameliorated from wine	Ars., lyc., phos., thuj.
Amelioration	weakness ameliorated in evening	Asc-t., calc-s., colch., nit-ac.
Amelioration	weakness ameliorated in fresh air	Calc.
Amelioration	weakness ameliorated in interesting meeting	Pip-m.
Amelioration	weakness ameliorated in noon	Hyper.
Amelioration	weakness ameliorated in open air	Chel., colch., **Con.**, croc., gels., grat., naja., nat-m., pic-ac., sabad.
Amelioration	weakness ameliorated on rising from bed	Arg-m., lyc., nat-m.
Amelioration	weakness ameliorated on rising	Acon., carb-v., caust., con., kali-c., mag-c., nat-c., nat-m., phos., puls.
Amelioration	weakness ameliorated on walking	Gins., phos., sulph.
Amelioration	weakness ameliorated slowly	*Ferr.*
Amelioration	weakness ameliorated while walking in open air	Am-c., cham., clem.
Amelioration	weakness from sleepiness in afternoon ameliorated from walking	Ruta.
Amelioration	weakness in ankle ameliorated while walking	Caust.
Amelioration	weakness in back ameliorated from lying down	Casc., nat-m.
Amelioration	weakness in back ameliorated while walking	Hydr.
Amelioration	weakness in calf ameliorated while sitting	Nicc.
Amelioration	weakness in calf ameliorated while walking	Plb.
Amelioration	weakness in chest ameliorated from bending forward	Nux-v.
Amelioration	weakness in chest ameliorated from lying	Alum.

Body part/Disease	Symptom	Medicines
Amelioration	weakness in chest ameliorated from walking	Ph-ac.
Amelioration	weakness in dorsal region between scapula ameliorated from leaning on something	Sarr.
Amelioration	weakness in dorsal region in scapula ameliorated from stooping	Alumn.
Amelioration	weakness in foot ameliorated from lying	Mag-c., nat-m.
Amelioration	weakness in foot ameliorated when riding	Nat-m.
Amelioration	weakness in foot ameliorated while sitting	Nat-m.
Amelioration	weakness in foot ameliorated while walking	Laur., nat-m., zinc.
Amelioration	weakness in hand ameliorated when lying on table	Mag-c.
Amelioration	weakness in hip ameliorated from continued walking	Sep.
Amelioration	weakness in joints ameliorated after walking	Bor.
Amelioration	weakness in joints ameliorated on rising	Carb-v.
Amelioration	weakness in knee ameliorated from extending & flexing knee	Ferr.
Amelioration	weakness in knee ameliorated from rest	**Bry.**
Amelioration	weakness in knee ameliorated on motion	Chin., phos.
Amelioration	weakness in knee ameliorated while sitting	Staph.
Amelioration	weakness in knee ameliorated while walking	Cham., dios., petr., phos.
Amelioration	weakness in leg ameliorated after rising from a seat	Caust.
Amelioration	weakness in leg ameliorated during motion	Aur-m-n., cham., dios., nat-s., stront.
Amelioration	weakness in leg ameliorated in a room	Grat.
Amelioration	weakness in leg ameliorated while sitting	Valer.
Amelioration	weakness in leg ameliorated while sleep	Tell.
Amelioration	weakness in lower limbs ameliorated after continued walking	Zinc.
Amelioration	weakness in lower limbs ameliorated after walking	Cann-s., nat-m., zinc.
Amelioration	weakness in lumbar region ameliorated while lying on back	Nat-m.
Amelioration	weakness in thigh ameliorated on waking	Sep.
Amelioration	weakness in thigh ameliorated while walking	Mag-m., rat.
Amelioration	weakness in upper arm ameliorated on motion	Arg-m.
Amelioration	weakness in upper limbs ameliorated after hanging it down	Asar.
Amelioration	weakness in upper limbs ameliorated on motion	Acon., lyc., plat., rhod., stront.
Amelioration	weakness in wrist ameliorated on motion	Rhod.
Amelioration	Weeping ameliorates symptoms	Anac., colch., cycl., dig., graph., ign., lyc., med., merc., nit-ac., phos., plat., sep., tab.
Amelioration	wheezing breath ameliorated on expectoration	Ip.
Amelioration	whitlow (a pus-filled infection on the skin at the side of a fingernail or toenail) ameliorated from cold application	Apis., fl-ac., led., **Nat-s., Puls.**
Amenorrhoea	pain in joints with amenorrhoea (the suppression or unusual absence of menstruation)	Lach.

Body part/Disease	Symptom	Medicines
Amenorrhoea	urine copious during menses	Canth., cham., hyos., kali-bi., lac-c., Ph-ac., phyt., sulph., vib.
Amenorrhoea	urine copious with amenorrhoea after epilepsy	Cupr.
Amenorrhoea	urine copious with amenorrhoea (Absence of menses)	Alum., am-c., caul., cham., gels., nat-m., sulph.
Amenorrhoea	urine copious with amenorrhoea after coffee	Cahin., olnd.
Amenorrhoea	urine copious with amenorrhoea after eating	Puls.
Amenorrhoea	urine copious with amenorrhoea after headache	Asc-c., iris.
Amenorrhoea	urine copious with amenorrhoea before menses	Cinnb., hyos.
Amenorrhoea	urine copious with amenorrhoea during fever	Ant-c., arg-m., ars., aur-m-n., cedr., cham., colch., dulc., eup-pur., lyc., med., mur-ac., ph-ac., phos., squil., Stram.
Amenorrhoea	urine copious with amenorrhoea with chill	Lec.
Amenorrhoea	urine copious with amenorrhoea with coryza	All-c., calc., verat.
Amenorrhoea	urine copious with amenorrhoea with headache	Acon., bell., bov., canth., chin-s., cinnb., coloc., cupr., eug., ferr-p., gels., glon., ign., iris., kalm., lac-c., Lac-d., lil-t., mosch., ol-an., sang., sel., sep., sil., uran., verat., vib., vip.
Amenorrhoea	urine inadequate with amenorrhoea	Acon., apis., chin., cocc., ham., hell., laur., lil-t., nux-m., xan.
Ammoniacal	urine offensive, ammoniacal (a colorless pungent gas that is highly soluble in water)	Aloe., am-caust., am-m., Asaf., aur., bell., bor., brom., bufo., cahin., calc., carb-ac., carb-v., chel., chin-s., coc-c., dig., dulc., equis., ferr-p., ferr., graph., Iod., kreos., lach., lyc., merc., Mosch., nit-ac., pareir., petr., phos., puls., rhod., sil., stront., sumb., tab., tub., viol-t.
Ammoniacal	urine offensive, ammoniacal in infants	Iod.
Amputation	pain in fingers of amputed (cut off part of body) stump (leg)	Phos., staph.
Anaemia	Anaemia (a blood condition in which there are too few red blood cells or the red blood cells are deficient in hemoglobin, resulting in poor health. Common causes include a lack of dietary iron, heavy blood loss, or the production of too few red blood cells due to disorders such as leukemia) of brain	Alum., ambr., calc-p., calc-s., calc., chin-s., chin., con., dulc., Ferr., fl-ac., hell., kali-c., lyc., mag-c., mosch., mur-ac., nat-c., nat-m., nit-ac., nux-v., petr., Ph-ac., Phos., sang., sel., sep., sil., stry., sulph., zinc.
Anaemia	anaemia after haemorrhage	Calc., carb-v., **Chin., Ferr.,** lach., nat-m., nux-v., ph-ac., phos., sulph.
Anaemia	Anaemia of cojunctiva (a delicate mucous membrane that covers the internal part of the eyelid and is attached to the cornea)	Dig., plb.
Anaemia	Anaemia of retina (a light-sensitive membrane in the back of the eye containing rods and cones that receive an image from the lens and send it to the brain through the optic nerve)	Agar., chin., dig., lith.
Anaemia	chlorosis (iron-deficiency anemia)	Acet-ac., alet., alum., alumn., am-c., ant-c., arg-m., arg-n., ars-i., **Ars.,** bar-c., **Bell., Calc-p., Calc.,** carb-an., **Carb-s.,** carb-v., caust., chin-a., chin., **Cocc.,** con., cupr., cycl., dig., **Ferr-ar.,** ferr-i., **Ferr-m.,** ferr-p., **Ferr., Graph.,** hell., helon., hep., ign., kali-ar., kali-c., kali-fer., kali-p., kali-s., **Lyc.,** lyss., **Mang.,** merc., nat-c., **Nat-m.,** nat-p., **Nit-ac.,** nux-v., olnd., petr., ph-ac., **Phos.,** pic-ac., **Plat.,** plb., **Puls.,** sabin., **Senec., Sep.,** spig., staph., sul-ac., **Sulph.,** thuj., ust., valer., zinc.

Body part/Disease	Symptom	Medicines
Anaemia	chlorosis in winter	Ferr.
Anaemia	white discharge from urethra in anæmic subjects	Calc-p.
Anaesthesia	analgesia (unawareness of pain) in affected parts	Anac., asaf., cocc., con., lyc., olnd., **Plat.**, puls., rhus-t.
Aneurism	aneurism (a bulge in artery or a fluid-filled sac in the wall of an artery that can weaken the wall) in heart	Cact., carb-v.
Aneurism	aneurism in abdomen	Bar-m., sec.
Aneurism	aneurism of large arteries	Bar-c., calc., carb-v., lyc., lycps., ran-s., spong.
Anger	anger about past events	Calc., carb-an., sep.
Anger	anger alternating with cheerfulness	Aur., caps., croc., ign., stram.
Anger	anger before convulsion	Bufo.
Anger	anger from cough	Acon., ant-t., arn., bell., cham.
Anger	anger from interruption	Cham., cocc., nux-v.
Anger	anger from voices of people	Con., teucr., zinc.
Anger	anger when touched	Ant-c., iod., Tarent.
Anger	anger with indignation (unfair or unreasonable)	Aur., Coloc., ip., lyc., merc., mur-ac., nat-m., nux-v., plat., Staph.
Anger	anger with silent grief	Alum., ars., aur., bell., cocc., coloc., hyos., Ign., Lyc., nat-c., nat-m., nux-v., ph-ac., phos., plat., puls., Staph., verat.
Anger	anger with trembling	Ambr., arg-n., aur., chel., cop., daph., ferr-p., nit-ac., pall., phos., sep.
Anger	angery, throws things away	Staph.
Anger	angry at absent persons	Aur., kali-c., lyc.
Anger	angry over his mistakes	Nit-ac., staph., sulph.
Anger	angry when consoled	Ars., cham., nat-m.
Anger	angry when misunderstood	Bufo.
Anger	asthmatic after anger	Ars., Cham.
Ankle	ankles hot	Ang., hyos., kali-bi., laur., lyc., osm., rat.
Ankle	burning pain in ankle	Agar., berb., eupho., kreos., laur., manc., nat-c., plat., puls., sulph., zinc.
Ankle	burning pain in ankle aggravated from rubbing	Sulph.
Ankle	burning pain in ankle extending over the soles to the toes	Kreos.
Ankle	burning pain in ankle in evening	Sulph.
Ankle	burning pain in ankle while walking	Agar.
Ankle	burning pain in thigh extending to ankles	Apis., arund.
Ankle	caries of ankle bones , internal malleolus (either of the hammer-shaped bony protuberances at the sides of the ankle joint that project from the lower end of the tibia and fibula)	Sil.
Ankle	caries of ankle bones	Asaf., calc., guai., plat-m., puls., sil.
Ankle	caries of fibula (the outer and narrower of the two bones in the human lower leg between the knee and ankle)	Sil.

Body part/Disease	Symptom	Medicines
Ankle	chill beginning in and extending from ankles	Chin., lach., puls.
Ankle	chronic ulcer on ankle	Carb-ac.
Ankle	coldness in ankles	Acon., agar., berb., caust., chin., lach.
Ankle	coldness in ankles while walking in open air	Chin.
Ankle	compression (reduction in size) of ankle	Chlf., led., nat-m., nat-s., sep., thuj.
Ankle	compression of ankle after walking in open air	Sep.
Ankle	constrictions in ankles (joint between foot and leg)	Acon., cham., graph., helod., plat.
Ankle	constrictions in ankles as if tied with string	Acon., am-br.
Ankle	cracking in ankle from bending side to side	Caust.
Ankle	cracking in ankle from bending	Ant-c.
Ankle	cracking in ankle from false step	Caust.
Ankle	cracking in ankle in evening	Am-c.
Ankle	cracking in ankle on stretching	Ant-c., thuj.
Ankle	cracking in ankle while walking	Carb-s., nit-ac., nux-v., sulph.
Ankle	cracking in ankle	Am-c., ant-c., aster., camph., Canth., carb-s., caust., hep., kali-bi., mag-s., nit-ac., nux-v., petr., ph-ac., sep., sulph., thuj.
Ankle	cramp in ankle	Agar., calc-p., carl., cupr., plat., sel.
Ankle	cramp in ankle extending over heel	Agar.
Ankle	cramp in ankle extending to calf	Cupr.
Ankle	cramp in ankle feeling as if extremities were going to sleep	Plat.
Ankle	cramp in ankle in evening	Sel.
Ankle	cramp in ankle in evening while lying	Sel.
Ankle	discoloration of ankle joints with redness	Lyc., mang., stann.
Ankle	discoloration of ankle with redness	Agar., apis., calc., carb-s., carb-v., graph., hyos., lach., nat-c., phos., puls., rhus-t., sars., sep., sil., stann., thuj., vesp., vip., zinc.
Ankle	discoloration of ankle with redness in evening	Apis.
Ankle	discoloration of ankle with redness in spots	Apis., ars., bry., chin., elaps., lach., led., lyc., mang., phyt., thuj.
Ankle	discoloration of ankle with white spots	Apis.
Ankle	discoloration of ankle yellow grayish	Vip.
Ankle	discoloration of back of ankle blue	Vip.
Ankle	discoloration of back of ankle with red spots	Carb-o., puls., thuj.
Ankle	discoloration of back of ankle with redness	Rhus-t., thuj.
Ankle	discoloration of ball of ankle with redness	Rhus-t.
Ankle	discoloration purple on ankle	Arn., lach.
Ankle	discoloration with blue spots on ankles	Sul-ac.
Ankle	discoloration with purple spots on ankle	**Sul-ac.**
Ankle	dislocated feeling in ankle	Bry., calc-p., kali-bi., verat-v.
Ankle	dislocation of ankle	Bry., nat-c., nux-v., ruta., sulph.

Body part/Disease	Symptom	Medicines
Ankle	dislocation of left ankle	Kali-bi.
Ankle	eruption, boils in ankle	Merc.
Ankle	eruption, dry in ankle	Cact.
Ankle	eruption, eczema in ankle	Chel., nat-p., psor.
Ankle	eruption, herpes in ankle	Cact., cycl., kreos., nat-c., nat-m., petr., sulph.
Ankle	eruption, in ankle	Cact., calc-p., calc., chel., osm., psor., puls., rhus-v., sel., sep., stront., tep.
Ankle	eruption, malleolus (either of the hammer-shaped bony protuberances at the sides of the ankle joint) in ankle	Cact.
Ankle	eruption, moistness in ankle	Chel.
Ankle	eruption, patches in ankle	Calc.
Ankle	eruption, pimples in ankle	Calc-p., sep., stront.
Ankle	eruption, pustules in ankle	Cupr-ar., lach.
Ankle	eruption, rash in ankle	Osm., tep.
Ankle	eruption, red in ankle	Calc., chel., sars.
Ankle	eruption, spots in ankle	Puls.
Ankle	eruption, urticaria in ankle	Nat-m.
Ankle	eruption, vesicles in ankle	Aster., rhus-v., sel.
Ankle	erysipelatous inflammation in ankle	Lach., rhus-t., tep.
Ankle	fistulous openings in ankle	Calc-p.
Ankle	fistulous ulcer on ankle	Calc-p., sil.
Ankle	formication in ankles	Ars-i., meph., pall., rhus-v.
Ankle	heaviness in ankles	Cupr.
Ankle	inflammation in ankle (joint between foot and leg)	Arn., mang., phyt.
Ankle	injuries in ankle	Ars., calc., rhus-t., ruta., stront.
Ankle	itching in ankle	Apis., berb., bov., cact., calc., carb-ac., chel., cocc., com., dios., hep., jug-c., kali-c., lach., **Led.**, lith., lyc., nat-p., olnd., osm., pall., ran-b., rhus-t., rhus-v., sel., sep., sulph., thea., vinc.
Ankle	itching in ankle aggravated from scratching	Led.
Ankle	itching in ankle aggravated from warmth	**Led.**, rhus-v.
Ankle	itching in ankle ameliorated from warmth	Cocc.
Ankle	itching in ankle at night	Hep.
Ankle	itching in ankle in evening	Rhus-v., sel., sep., sulph.
Ankle	itching in ankle in morning	Sep.
Ankle	itching in ankle in morning in bed	Kali-c.
Ankle	itching in ankle in spots	Vinc.
Ankle	itching in ankle while walking	Cocc., dios.
Ankle	itching in ankle with biting	Berb.
Ankle	itching in ankle with burning	Berb., lith.
Ankle	itching in ankle with tingling	Com.

Body part/Disease	Symptom	Medicines
Ankle	jerking in Ankle	Calc.
Ankle	lameness in ankles	Abrot., aesc., arn., bry., caps., cedr., com., dios., fl-ac., laur., lil-t., lyss., plb., **Ruta.**
Ankle	lameness in ankles after sprain	Rhus-t., **Ruta.**
Ankle	lameness in ankles in evening while walking	Fl-ac.
Ankle	lameness in ankles in morning	Dios., plb.
Ankle	lameness in ankles in morning after rising	Caps.
Ankle	lameness in ankles while sitting	Nat-m.
Ankle	lameness in ankles while walking	Nat-m.
Ankle	lameness in ankles while walking in open air	Com.
Ankle	malleolus (either of the hammer-shaped bony protuberances at the sides of the ankle joint that project from the lower end of the tibia and fibula) ankle	Calc-p.
Ankle	malleolus pain in ankle extending to toes	Bry., calc., coloc., plb., sulph., verat-v.
Ankle	numbness in ankle	Caust., glon., hep., lac-c., nat-m., rhus-t., sulph.
Ankle	numbness in ankle at night	Sulph.
Ankle	pain in ankle after menses	Nat-p.
Ankle	pain in ankle after suppressed gonorrhoea	Med., thuj.
Ankle	pain in ankle aggravated from warmth	Guai., lac-c., **Led., Puls.**
Ankle	pain in ankle ameliorated from motion	Aur-m-n., dios., nat-s., plan., valer.
Ankle	pain in ankle ameliorated from warmth	Chel.
Ankle	pain in ankle ameliorated while walking	Ph-ac., rhus-t., sulph., **Valer.**
Ankle	pain in ankle as if dislocated	Bry., calc-p.
Ankle	pain in ankle at night	Sulph.
Ankle	pain in ankle extending to soles	Stann.
Ankle	pain in ankle extending to toes	Lil-t.
Ankle	pain in ankle from a false step	Caust., chel., coloc., **Led.**
Ankle	pain in ankle from ascending stairs	Alumn., plb.
Ankle	pain in ankle from motion	Arn., bol., bry., bufo., cham., chel., cocc., guai., kalm., led., lil-t., sulph., zinc.
Ankle	pain in ankle from sitting	Arg-n., aur-m-n., bry., caust., led., nat-s., **Valer.**
Ankle	pain in ankle from standing	Cycl., rhus-v., stront., sulph., **Valer.**
Ankle	pain in ankle from touch	Ars., lyc., nat-m., sep.
Ankle	pain in ankle in afternoon	Dios., rhus-v., verat.
Ankle	pain in ankle in evening	Dios., led., nat-c., nat-s., plan.
Ankle	pain in ankle in evening while lying	Nat-s., plan.
Ankle	pain in ankle in morning	All-c., alumn., carb-ac., carb-s., dios., led., mez., sep., sulph.
Ankle	pain in ankle in morning ameliorated on walking	Sulph.
Ankle	pain in ankle in morning on walking	Alumn., mez., plb., psor.
Ankle	pain in ankle when stepping	Bry., **Led.,** mez., nat-m., rhus-t., sil.

Body part/Disease	Symptom	Medicines
Ankle	pain in ankle while running	Mez.
Ankle	pain in ankle while walking	Alumn., aster., bry., calc-p., caust., chel., cycl., dros., fl-ac., kali-n., kalm., led., lith., mez., nit-ac., phos., puls., rhus-v., ruta., stront., stry., sulph.
Ankle	pain in left wrist and right ankle	Lach.
Ankle	pain in leg extending to ankle	Kali-bi., ptel.
Ankle	pain in thigh extending to ankles	Nat-a.
Ankle	painful swelling of ankle	Led., plb.
Ankle	painful ulcer on ankle	Lach., rhus-t.
Ankle	painless ulcer on ankle	Calc.
Ankle	paralysis of ankles	Abrot., ang., nat-m., ruta.
Ankle	paralysis of ankles while sitting	Nat-m.
Ankle	paralysis of ankles while walking	Nat-m.
Ankle	paralysis of right wrist & left ankle	Nat-p.
Ankle	rheumatic swelling of ankle	Cact., chel., kalm., lach.
Ankle	sciatic pain in lower limb beginning at ankle	Ars., cimic., plat.
Ankle	sensation as if ankles bandaged	Acon., calc., helod., petr.
Ankle	sensation of paralysis in ankles	Dros., nat-m.
Ankle	sensation of paralysis in ankles while walking	Dros.
Ankle	sensitive ankle	Ars-h., graph., sars.
Ankle	shuddering ankle	Lyc.
Ankle	spreading ulcer on ankle	Merc.
Ankle	stiffness of ankle ameliorated from exercise	Dios., sulph.
Ankle	stiffness of ankle in evening	Sep.
Ankle	stiffness of ankle on rising in morning	Carb-an.
Ankle	stiffness of ankle while walking	Led., sul-ac., sumb.
Ankle	sudden swelling of ankle	Stann.
Ankle	suppuration of ankle	Arn., hep.
Ankle	swelling in ankle during menses	Eup-per.
Ankle	swelling in ankle in evening	Sep., stann.
Ankle	swelling in ankle in evening while walking	Merc.
Ankle	swelling in ankle with dyspnoea	Hep.
Ankle	swelling in bones of ankle	Merc., staph.
Ankle	swelling in veins of ankle	Lac-c., lyc., sars.
Ankle	tingling in ankle on waking at night	Bar-c.
Ankle	tumours on ankle	Cupr-ar.
Ankle	twitching in ankle	Agar., asaf., carb-s., mag-m., mez.
Ankle	ulcer in ankle	Calc-p., carb-ac., cist., hydr., merc-i-f., merc-sul., puls., rhus-t., sars., sil., sulph., syph.
Ankle	weakness in ankle after warm bath	Calc.
Ankle	weakness in ankle ameliorated while walking	Caust.

Body part/Disease	Symptom	Medicines
Ankle	weakness in ankle at night	Sulph.
Ankle	weakness in ankle in children learning to walk	**Carb-an.**, nat-p.
Ankle	weakness in ankle in morning	Agn., coca.
Ankle	weakness in ankle in morning while walking	Agn., valer.
Ankle	weakness in ankle on motion	Laur., nux-v.
Ankle	weakness in ankle while running	Mez.
Ankle	weakness in ankle while sitting	Paeon.
Ankle	weakness in ankle while sitting after walking	Caust.
Ankle	weakness in ankle while standing	Calc.
Ankle	weakness in ankle while walking	Agn., aloe., carb-an., com., med., nat-c., **Nit-ac.**, nux-v., plb.
Ankle	weakness in right wrist and left ankle	Nat-p.
Ankle	abscess in ankle joint (joint that connects the leg bones with the highest bone in the foot)	Ang., guai., ol-j., sil.
Answers	answers abruptly, shortly , curtly	Ars-h., ars., cic., coff., gels., hyos., jatr., mur-ac., ph-ac., phos., plb., rhus-t., sec., sin-a., stann., sulph., tarent.
Answers	answers but repeats the question first	Ambr., caust., kali-br., sulph., zinc.
Answers	Answers confusedly as though thinking of something else	Bar-m., hell., mosch.
Answers	answers foolish	Ars., bell.
Answers	answers hastily	Ars., bell., bry., cimic., cocc., hep., lach., lyc., rhus-t., stry.
Answers	answers incoherently (not clearly expressed)	Bell., cann-i., chlol., coff-t., cycl., hyos., phos., valer
Answers	answers incorrectly	Bell., carb-v., cham., hyos., merc., nux-v., ph-ac., phos.
Answers	answers irrelevantly	Bell., carb-v., cimic., hyos., led., lyss., nux-m., nux-v., petr., ph-ac., Phos., sabad., sec., stram., sul-ac., Sulph., tarent., valer.
Answers	Answers loquacious (talkative) at other times	Cimic.
Answers	answers monosyllable (a word or sentence consisting of only one syllable, e.g. "Yes" or "Me")	Carb-h., carb-s., gels., kali-br., ph-ac., plb., puls., sep.
Answers	answers no to all Questions	Crot-c., hyos., kali-br.
Answers	answers unintelligibly	Chin., coff-t., hyos., phos.
Answers	answers Which has no connection with question	Coff., crot-h., kali-br., phos., stram., stry.
Anus	anal haemorrhoids aggravated at night	Aesc., aloe., alum., am-c., ant-c., ars., carb-an., carb-v., coll., euphr., ferr., graph., merc., phys., puls., rhus-t., Sulph.
Anus	anal haemorrhoids aggravated during wiping after stool	Aesc., Graph., Mur-ac., Paeon., puls., sulph.
Anus	anal haemorrhoids aggravated from milk	Sep.
Anus	anal haemorrhoids aggravated from touch	Abrot., Bell., berb., calc., carb-an., carb-s., Caust., graph., hep., kali-c., lil-t., lyc., merc., Mur-ac., nit-ac., nux-v., phos., Rat., sep., sil., sul-ac., Sulph., syph., Thuj.
Anus	anal haemorrhoids aggravated in bed	Graph., rumx.
Anus	anal haemorrhoids aggravated in morning	Aloe., Dios., mur-ac., sabin., sulph., sumb., thuj.
Anus	anal haemorrhoids ameliorated from cold	Aloe., brom.

Body part/Disease	Symptom	Medicines
Anus	anal haemorrhoids ameliorated in morning	Alum., coll.
Anus	anal haemorrhoids as soon as the rheumatism is better	Abrot.
Anus	boils in anus	Calc-p., carb-an., caust., petr.
Anus	boils near anus	Caust.
Anus	burning about anus	Ars., calc.
Anus	cracking of lumbar region extending to anus	Sulph.
Anus	crusts about anus	Berb.
Anus	cutting pain in abdomen extending to anus	Coloc.
Anus	cutting pain in abdomen like electric shock darting through the anus	Coloc.
Anus	fissure (a break in the skin lining the anal canal, usually causing pain during bowel movements and sometimes bleeding. Anal fissures occur as a consequence of constipation or sometimes of diarrhoea) in Anus	Aesc., agn., all-c., alum., ant-c., arg-m., arum-t., berb., calc-f., calc-p., calc., carb-an., caust., Cham., cund., cur., fl-ac., Graph., grat., hydr., ign., kali-c., lach., med., merc-i-r., merc., mez., mur-ac., nat-m., Nit-ac., nux-v., paeon., petr., phos., phyt., plat., plb., Rat., rhus-t., Sep., sil., sulph., syph., Thuj.
Anus	fistula (an anal fistula may develop after an abscess in the rectum has burst , creating an opening between the anal canal and the surface of the skin) in inguinal (Groin) glands	Hep., lach., phos., sil., sulph.
Anus	fistula (an opening or passage between two organs or between an organ and the skin, caused by disease, injury, or congenital malformation)	Aloe., alum., ant-c., Aur-m., aur., bell., Berb., bry., cact., Calc-p., calc-s., Calc., carb-s., Carb-v., Caust., fl-ac., graph., hep., hydr., ign., Kali-c., kreos., lach., lyc., merc., Nit-ac., petr., phos., puls., sep., Sil., staph., sulph., syph., thuj.
Anus	formication near anus at night	Nux-v.
Anus	growth resembling a wart at anus	Nit-ac.
Anus	haemorrhage from anus after stool	Puls.
Anus	haemorrhage, black from anus	Alumn., ant-c., colch., crot-h., ham., merc-c., sec.
Anus	herpetic eruptions about anus	Berb., graph., lyc., nat-m., Petr.
Anus	itching about anus	Ars., cinnb., lyc., Petr., staph., sulph.
Anus	itching about anus after dinner	Caust.
Anus	itching about anus aggravated by rubbing	Alum., petr.
Anus	itching about anus at night	Agar., aloe., alum., alumn., ant-c., calc-f., carb-s., ferr., fl-ac., ign., nat-p., petr., phos., rhus-v., sulph.
Anus	itching about anus ending in pain	Zinc.
Anus	itching about anus from ascarides	Calc-f., calc., chin., ferr., ign., nat-p., sabad., sin-a., teucr., urt-u.
Anus	itching about anus in bed in evening	Ant-c., cahin., calc-p., cinnb., ign., lyc., nat-m., petr., plat., sulph., teucr.
Anus	itching around anus	Agn., berb., bry., bufo-s., fl-ac., lyc., mez., nat-s., nux-v., op., Petr., serp., Sulph., tarax.
Anus	itching in ear at night alternating with anus	Sabad.
Anus	leucorrhoea like serum from anus and vagina	Lob.
Anus	numbness of anus	Acon., carb-ac., phos.

Body part/Disease	Symptom	Medicines
Anus	pain in anus aggravated from warm bathing	Brom.
Anus	pain in anus ameliorated from cold application	Aloe., apis., euphr., kali-c., ter.
Anus	pain in anus on passing flatus	Camph., carb-v.
Anus	pain in back ascends with constriction of anus	Coloc.
Anus	pain in fissure of anus	Graph.
Anus	pain in kidneys extending from genitals , anus and thighs	Kreos.
Anus	pain in lumbar region to the perineum (the region of the abdomen surrounding the urogenital and anal openings)	Canth.
Anus	pimples about anus	Agar., brom., carb-v., cinnb., kali-c., kali-i., nit-ac., staph.
Anus	prolapsus of anus after hæmorrhage of rectum	Ars.
Anus	prolapsus of anus after stool	Aloe., alumn., apis., berb., caps., lach., manc., sang., seneg., sulph.
Anus	prolapsus of anus during diarrhoea	Calc., Dulc., gamb., mag-m., Merc., mur-ac., Podo.
Anus	prolapsus of anus during stool	Nat-m.
Anus	prolapsus of anus in children	Ferr., hydr., nux-v., Podo.
Anus	prolapsus of anus painful	Ars., ther.
Anus	prolapsus of anus when passing flatus	Valer.
Anus	prolapsus of anus when vomiting	Mur-ac., podo.
Anus	prolapsus of anus without straining	Graph., ruta.
Anus	pustules about anus	Am-m., calc., caust.
Anus	rectum, aphthous condition of anus	Bapt., bor., bry., kali-chl., merc-c., merc., mur-ac., nit-ac., Sul-ac., sulph.
Anus	redness of anus	Aloe., ars., cham., nat-m., petr., Sulph., valer., zing.
Anus	swelling in anus	Aesc., apis., aur., bell., bor., bufo., coll., crot-t., cur., graph., hep., ign., kali-i., lach., led., mur-ac., nux-v., paeon., phys., podo., sarr., sulph., teucr.
Anus	tension in muscles of back extending to anus while lying and sitting	Nat-c.
Anus	ulceration in anus	Alumn., calc., caust., Cham., cub., hep., hydr., kali-c., kali-i., nat-s., paeon., petr., phos., phyt., puls., sars., Sil., staph., syph.
Anus	ulcerous about anus	Kali-c.
Apoplexy	want of speech after apoplexy (fit of anger)	Bar-c., crot-c., crot-h., ip., laur., Nux-v.
Appendicitis	appendicitis (inflammation of appendix which is small, occurs in the lower right-hand part of the abdomen, and contains cells of the immune system)	Bell., Bry., cadm., calc-s., chel., chin., cocc., con., crot-c., dulc., echi., graph., hep., lach., lyc., Merc-c., merc., nit-ac., Phos., plb., Sil., ter.
Appetite	appetite increased, eating increases the hunger	Lyc.
Appetite	appetite, changeable	Alum., anac., berb., Cina., cur., lach., mag-m., nit-ac., phos., podo.
Appetite	appetite, constant	Bov., fl-ac., gran., kali-bi., kali-p., merc., myric., nat-c., nat-m., rat., tab.
Appetite	appetite, diminished during menses	Mag-c.

Body part/Disease	Symptom	Medicines
Appetite	appetite, diminished when time for eating	Chin., ign.
Appetite	appetite, increased after beer	Ars.
Appetite	appetite, increased after drinking	Nat-m.
Appetite	appetite, increased after eating	Lyc.
Appetite	appetite, increased after headache	Iod.
Appetite	appetite, increased after nausea	Bry.
Appetite	appetite, increased after siesta (afternoon rest)	Onos.
Appetite	appetite, increased after stool	Aloe., fl-ac., Petr.
Appetite	appetite, increased after thinking of food	Calc-p.
Appetite	appetite, increased after vomiting	Cina., colch., olnd., podo., tab.
Appetite	appetite, increased after wine	Nat-m.
Appetite	appetite, increased at sight of food	Alum., caust., colch., crot-c., kali-p., merc-i-f., phos., Sulph.
Appetite	appetite, increased at unusual time	Chin., Cina., coc-c., gins.
Appetite	appetite, increased before attack of fever	Eup-per., staph.
Appetite	appetite, increased before headache	Phos., Psor.
Appetite	appetite, increased before menses	Mag-c., spong.
Appetite	appetite, increased during apyrexia (a period during which a patient experiences no fever)	Staph.
Appetite	appetite, increased during beer	Ail., Ars., chin-s., eup-per., lec., nux-v., phos., Sil., staph.
Appetite	appetite, increased during fever	Chin., cina., cur., eup-pur., hell., Phos.
Appetite	appetite, increased during menses	Kali-p.
Appetite	appetite, increased during perspiration	Cimx., cina., sanic.
Appetite	appetite, increased from smell of food	Carb-an., caust., Colch.
Appetite	appetite, increased in dysentry	Nux-v.
Appetite	appetite, increased on waking	Chin., dig., ptel.
Appetite	appetite, increased with diarrhoea	Aloe., asaf., calc., coch., fl-ac., iod., lyc., olnd., Petr., stram., sulph., verat., zinc.
Appetite	appetite, increased with emaciation	Abrot., Calc., Iod., Nat-m., Petr., phos., psor., sulph., tub.
Appetite	appetite, increased with headache	Ars., crot-h., elaps., kali-c., kali-p., lac-d., lyc., Phos., Psor., ptel., sang., sep., sil., sulph., thuj.
Appetite	appetite, increased with marasmus.	Abrot., ars-i., bar-c., bar-i., calc-p., Calc., caust., chin., Cina., Iod., lyc., mag-c., Nat-m., nux-v., petr., sil., sulph.
Appetite	appetite, increased with neuralgia	Dulc.
Appetite	appetite, increased with pain in stomach	Lach., lyc., puls., sil.
Appetite	appetite, increased with thirst	Am-c., ant-t., ars., bor., calc., colch., coloc., kali-n., kreos., nux-v., ox-ac., phos., psor., rhus-t., seneg., sep., sil., spig., Sulph., zinc.
Appetite	appetite, insatiable (impossible to satisfy)	Ant-c., arg-m., arg-n., arum-t., asc-t., aur., bar-c., ferr-i., ferr., Iod., Lyc., petr., puls-n., sec., sep., spong., squil., stann., staph., zinc.
Appetite	appetite, insatiable before attack of fever	Eup-per., staph.

Body part/Disease	Symptom	Medicines
Appetite	appetite, returns after eating a mouthful	Anac., calc., Chin., mag-c., sabad.
Appetite	appetite, vanishes at sight of food	Caust., crot-c., kali-p., merc-i-f., phos., Sulph.
Appetite	appetite, vanishes on attempting to eat	Sil.
Arm	faintness from raising arms above head	Lac-d., lach., spong.
Arm	fever with dry heat at night without thirst with swollen veins of arms and hands	**Chin.**, sumb.
Arm	fluttering in chest on raising arms	Dig., sulph.
Arm	hypertrophy of heart with numbness in left arm and fingers	Acon., Rhus-t.
Arm	impeded, obstructed breath with pain from raising the arm	Berb.
Arm	inflammation of lymphatics (body fluid containing white cells) of arm	**Bufo.**
Arm	intermittent pain in arm	Asaf., led., sars.
Arm	involuntary motion of one arm and leg	Apoc., cocc., hell.
Arm	irregular motion of left arm	Cimic.
Arm	jerking extending to both arms in chorea	Cupr.
Arm	jerking in chest when moving the arm	Anac.
Arm	jerking in paralyzed arm	Arg-n., merc., nux-v., phos., sec.
Arm	jerking of one leg and arm	Apis., apoc., hell., stram.
Arm	jerking pain in arm	Anac., chin., kali-bi., lact., puls., ran-b., rhus-t., ruta., sil., tarax., valer.
Arm	jumping sensation as something alive in arms	Croc.
Arm	lameness of left arm and foot after fright	Stann.
Arm	neuralgic pain in arm (limb attached to the shoulder)	Hyper.
Arm	numbnes in left arm and right leg	Tarent.
Arm	numbnes in right arm and left leg	Ars., kali-c.
Arm	numbness alternating arms & legs	Phos.
Arm	numbness in first finger up radial (radius bone of the forearm) side of arm	Anac., carb-an., phos.
Arm	numbness in hand extending to arm	Agar., aster., dios., fl-ac.
Arm	pain alternately in arms and legs	Merc-i-r.
Arm	pain as of splinter in arm (limb attached to the shoulder of the human body)	Agar., nit-ac.
Arm	pain between scapula extending down arms	Echi.
Arm	pain from extending arm	Phyt.
Arm	pain in abdomen from raising arm high	Arg-n.
Arm	pain in arm after chill	Ars-h.
Arm	pain in arm after lifting	Berb.
Arm	pain in arm aggravated from touch	Agn., arg-m., chin., sabin., staph.
Arm	pain in arm aggravated from turning in bed	Sang.
Arm	pain in arm ameliorated from warmth	Ferr.

Body part/Disease	Symptom	Medicines
Arm	pain in arm ameliorated on motion	Arg-m., aur-m-n., cina., cocc., cupr., dulc., kali-bi., meph., ox-ac., paeon., **Rhus-t.**, thuj.
Arm	pain in arm ameliorated on slow motion	Ferr.
Arm	pain in arm as from a blow	Anac.
Arm	pain in arm during menses	Berb.
Arm	pain in arm extending downward	Agar., berb., carb-v., dros., kali-bi., lach., lyc., sulph.
Arm	pain in arm extending into hand and thumb	Kali-bi., puls.
Arm	pain in arm extending to finger	Chel.
Arm	pain in arm extending to neck during menses	Berb.
Arm	pain in arm from cold air	Kalm.
Arm	pain in arm from excitement	Coloc.
Arm	pain in arm from lying on painful side	Mang.
Arm	pain in arm from putting it across the back	Calc.
Arm	pain in arm from raising arm	Agar., bar-c., bry., bufo., calc-p., calc., cocc., colch., ferr., nat-c., nat-m., olnd., phos., plb., rhus-t., sang., syph., teucr., zinc.
Arm	pain in arm in damp weather	Phyt., rhod., rhus-t., sanic.
Arm	pain in arm in heart affections	Cact.
Arm	pain in arm like electric shocks	Tarax.
Arm	pain in arm on motion	Anag., berb., bry., bufo., calc., cocc., colch., crot-t., eupho., ferr-p., ferr., fl-ac., iris., kalm., lac-c., led., mag-c., merc., nux-v., phyt., sabad., sabin., staph.
Arm	pain in arm when lying on it	Carb-an., nat-m.
Arm	pain in arm while walking	Arg-n., merc-c.
Arm	pain in arm while writing	Ars-i., cycl., fl-ac., valer.
Arm	pain in arm worse on going to sleep	Kali-c., kalm.
Arm	pain in axilla extending down arms	Jug-c., nat-a.
Arm	pain in back extending to arms	Calc-ar., calc.
Arm	pain in back from raising arms	Graph.
Arm	pain in cervical region extending arm	Nat-m., nux-v.
Arm	pain in cervical region extending arm and fingers	Kalm., nux-v., par.
Arm	pain in cervical region extending left arm	Kalm., lach., par.
Arm	pain in cervical region from raising arms	Ang., ant-c., graph.
Arm	pain in chest aggravated by arms near chest	Psor.
Arm	pain in chest ameliorated by arms near chest	Lact-ac.
Arm	pain in chest ameliorated on stretching the arm	Berb.
Arm	pain in chest from motion of arms	Carb-an., card-m., caust., nux-m., seneg., sulph.
Arm	pain in chest on stretching the arm	Ran-b.
Arm	pain in dorsal region extending to arms & legs	Calc.
Arm	pain in dorsal region from motion of arm	Ail., con., ruta.
Arm	pain in dorsal region from motion of right arm	Chel.
Arm	pain in elbow when bending arm	All-s., chel., dulc., mag-c., mur-ac., puls.

Body part/Disease	Symptom	Medicines
Arm	pain in elbow when stretching arm	Hep., kali-c., puls., ruta.
Arm	pain in eye alternates with pain in left arm	Plb.
Arm	pain in eye extending to arm	Rumx.
Arm	pain in heart extending to right arm	Phyt., spig.
Arm	pain in ilium extending to arms	Rhod.
Arm	pain in left arm at night on lying on it	Nat-m.
Arm	pain in left arm from bending arms backwards	**Rhus-t.**
Arm	pain in left arm in afternoon	Abrot., fl-ac., phos., stry.
Arm	pain in left arm in afternoon at 1.00 p.m. while riding	Hydr.
Arm	pain in left arm in afternoon at 2.00 p.m.	**Rhus-t.**
Arm	pain in left arm in afternoon at 3.00 p.m.	Dios., phos., **Rhus-t.**, sarr.
Arm	pain in left arm in bed	Dulc., led., rhus-t.
Arm	pain in left arm in evening in bed	Dulc., led.
Arm	pain in left arm in forenoon	Agar., bov., com.
Arm	pain in left arm in morning after rising	Dulc.
Arm	pain in left arm in morning on waking	Ars-s-r., mez.
Arm	pain in left arm in morning	Ars-i., chel., eupho., lyc., mez., rhus-t.
Arm	pain in left arm in noon after lying down	Rhus-t.
Arm	pain in lumbar region from motion of arms	Kreos.
Arm	pain in mammae when raising arm	Bry.
Arm	pain in right left arm from bending arms	Ant-c.
Arm	pain in right left arm in evening	Anac., chin., colch., kali-bi., ox-ac., stry., sulph., zinc.
Arm	pain in right left arm in noon	Sulph.
Arm	pain in right scapula from motion of right arm	Chel.
Arm	pain in sacral region on moving arm	Chel.
Arm	pain in shoulder aggravated from pulling arm	Chel.
Arm	pain in shoulder aggravated from putting the arm behind him	**Ferr.**, rhus-t., **Sanic.**
Arm	pain in shoulder aggravated from raising the arm	Alum., bar-c., bry., calc., card-m., chel., cocc., dros., ferr., hep., ign., iris., kali-bi., kali-n., kreos., lac-c., led., lyc., mag-c., mag-m., nat-c., nat-m., nit-ac., petr., phos., phyt., prun-s., puls., rhus-t., **Sang.**, sanic., sep., sul-ac., sulph., syph., thuj., zinc.
Arm	pain in shoulder ameliorated from hanging down the arm	Phos.
Arm	pain in shoulder ameliorated from raising the arm	Ph-ac.
Arm	pain in shoulder ameliorated on motion of arm	Asar., bell., calc., cann-s., caust., chel., croc., ferr., iris., kali-bi., kali-c., kali-n., kreos., lach., lact-ac., led., mag-c., med., merc., mur-ac., nat-a., olnd., petr., phyt., puls., rhod., ruta., sang., sep.
Arm	pain in shoulder ameliorated on motion of arm backwards	Berb., dros., ign., kali-bi., laur., puls., sep., zinc.
Arm	pain in shoulder extending to arm	Ars., bapt., brom., bry., cimx., glon., Ind.

Body part/Disease	Symptom	Medicines
Arm	pain in shoulder from hanging down the arm	Mez., nux-v., ruta., thuj.
Arm	pain in sternum from raising arm	Chin.
Arm	pain in upper limb ameliorated when bending arm	Ferr.
Arm	pain in upper limb from raising arm	Apis., caj., calc., cocc., eup-pur., **Ferr.,** kali-p., lac-c., olnd., phyt., sang., sulph., syph., tab., zinc.
Arm	pain in upper limb when bending arm	Aeth.
Arm	pain of face extending to arms	Kalm.
Arm	pain under left scapula extending to arm	Aeth., coc-c.
Arm	pain under left scapula from bending arm	Carb-v.
Arm	pain under left scapula from hanging down arm	Ign.
Arm	pain under left scapula on moving arm	Chel., ign.
Arm	palpitation of heart aggravated from motion of arms	Acon., am-m., bor., bry., camph., chel., dig., ferr., led., naja., puls., rhus-t., seneg., spig., spong., Sulph., thuj.
Arm	palpitation of heart on raising arms	Dig., spig., sulph.
Arm	paralysis of lower limb with spasms of the arms	Agar.
Arm	paralysis of right arm & left leg	Ter.
Arm	paralytic pain in arm	Aloe., alum., arg-m., arg-n., bell., bry., cham., chel., chin., cina., cocc., con., ferr., kali-bi., mur-ac., nit-ac., phos., sep., staph., thuj.
Arm	paroxysmal pain in arm	Gels., mur-ac.
Arm	paroxysmal pain in arm ameliorated from perspiration	Thuj.
Arm	paroxysmal pain in arm on pressure	Berb., calc., phyt., sil.
Arm	perspiration in left arm and left leg	Lac-d.
Arm	pulsation pain in arm	Ign., **Kali-c.,** mur-ac., nat-m.
Arm	rheumatic pain in arm (limb attached to the shoulder) from raising arm	Alumn., ars., aspar., bry., calc-p., calc., carb-s., chel., chim., coff., colch., crot-t., dulc., ferr-i., ferr-p., **Ferr.,** fl-ac., hyos., iod., iris., kalm., merc., nat-m., phos., phyt., ptel., rhod., **Rhus-t., Sang.,** urt-u., verat., zinc.
Arm	rheumatic pain in arm when singing	Stann.
Arm	rigidly extended arms	Merc.
Arm	sensation of electrical current in arms	Bol., dor., gels.
Arm	sensation of paralysis in elbow from raising the arm	Mez.
Arm	Sensation of paralysis in left arm & right foot	Hyper., stann.
Arm	sleeplessness from heavy feelings in arm	Alum.
Arm	sleeps on abdomen with one arm under the head	Cocc.
Arm	sleeps with arm on abdomen	Cocc., **Puls.**
Arm	sleeps with arm under head	Acon., ambr., ant-t., ars., bell., cocc., coloc., ign., meny., nux-v., plat., puls., rhus-t., sabad., spig., viol-o.
Arm	spasmodic pain in arm	Agar., lact., mosch., olnd., valer.
Arm	stitching pain in chest extending to arms	Brom., nat-m.
Arm	stitching pain in chest with numbness and lameness of left arm	Rhus-t.

Body part/Disease	Symptom	Medicines
Arm	tension in dorsal region below scapula from raising arm	Con.
Arm	tension in muscles of back from moving arm	Sulph.
Arm	tingling in right arm & left leg at night	Kali-c.
Arm	tingling in tips of fingers when hanging down the arms	Sulph.
Arm	twitching in elbow ameliorated from sretching arm	Nat-m.
Arm	twitching in one arm & one leg	Apis., apoc., hell., stram., tub.
Arm	twitching in right upper arm	Am-c.
Arm	upper arm hot	Calc-p., cic., nat-m.
Arm	wandering pain in arm while walking	Phyt.
Arm	waving motion of left arm and leg with sighing	Bry.
Arm	weakness in back on motion of arms	Clem., par., sil.
Arm	weakness on moving arms	Nat-m.
Arm pit	abscess in axilla (Arm pit)	Am-c., apis., ars., bell., bufo., cadm., calc-s., calc., cedr., coloc., crot-h., Hep., kali-bi., kali-c., lac-c., merc-i-r., Merc., nat-m., nat-s., Nit-ac., petr., ph-ac., prun-s., Rhus-t., sep., Sil., sulph., thuj.
Arm pit	boils in axila (armpit)	Bor., Hep., lyc., merc., nat-s., petr., ph-ac., phos., sep., sil., sulph., thuj.
Arm pit	boils in right axila (armpit)	Thuj.
Arm pit	bubbling in axilla	Colch.
Arm pit	bubo (swelling and inflammation of a lymph node, especially in the area of the armpit or groin) in arm pit	Alum., ars-i., ars., aur-m-n., aur-m., aur., bad., bar-m., bell., Bufo., carb-an., chel., Cinnb., clem., crot-h., Hep., iod., kali-chl., kali-i., lac-c., lach., lyc., merc., nit-ac., phyt., sil., sulph., tarent-c., zinc.
Arm pit	burning boils in axila	Merc.
Arm pit	cancer of axilla	Aster.
Arm pit	cracks in axilla	Hep.
Arm pit	cramps in axilla	Com., hura., iod.
Arm pit	crusts in axilla	Anac., jug-r., Nat-m.
Arm pit	dryness of axilla	Hep.
Arm pit	eczema in axilla	Hep., jug-r., merc., nat-m., petr., Psor., sep.
Arm pit	fistulous openings in axilla	Calc., sulph.
Arm pit	formication in axilla	Berb., con.
Arm pit	herpes in axilla	Carb-an., elaps., lac-c., lyc., mez., nat-m., rhus-t., sep.
Arm pit	inflammation of axillary glands	Nit-ac., petr., phos.
Arm pit	itching in axilla	Elaps., hep., psor.
Arm pit	itching in axilla aggravated from perspiration	Jug-r.
Arm pit	itching in axilla before menses	Sang.
Arm pit	itching in axilla in morning	Form.
Arm pit	itching in axilla when body becomes heated	Arg-n., hep.
Arm pit	itching in back ameliorated from scratching	Mag-c., mag-m., mez., nat-c., pall., rat., rhus-v.

Body part/Disease	Symptom	Medicines
Arm pit	moistness in axilla	Brom., carb-v., jug-r., nat-m., sep., sulph.
Arm pit	moisture from axilla	Carb-v., sulph.
Arm pit	nodules in axilla	Mag-c.
Arm pit	pain in axilla before menses	Calc.
Arm pit	pain in axilla extending down arms	Jug-c., nat-a.
Arm pit	pain in axilla extending down to little finger	Nat-a.
Arm pit	pain in axilla extending to pectoral (chest muscle) muscles	Brach.
Arm pit	pain in axilla from right to left	Elaps.
Arm pit	pain in heart extending to axilla	Ferr-i., lat-m.
Arm pit	pain in region of axilla in morning	Ran-b.
Arm pit	pain in upper limb extending from axilla to little finger	Nat-a.
Arm pit	painless swelling in gland of armpit	Lach.
Arm pit	perspiration in axilla (armpit) during menses	Stram., tell.
Arm pit	perspiration in axilla between menses	Sep.
Arm pit	perspiration in axilla copious (abundant)	Sanic., sel.
Arm pit	perspiration in axilla during coldness	Tab.
Arm pit	perspiration in axilla in cold air	Bov.
Arm pit	perspiration in axilla yellow	Lac-c.
Arm pit	pimples in axilla	Cocc., phos.
Arm pit	pustules in axilla	Crot-c., viol-t.
Arm pit	rash in axilla	Hep., sulph.
Arm pit	recurrent boils in axila	Lyc.
Arm pit	scaly axilla	Jug-r.
Arm pit	small painful boils in axila	Sep.
Arm pit	swelling in gland of armpit (axillary) before menses	Aur.
Arm pit	tubercles in axilla	Nit-ac., phos.
Arm pit	tumour in axilla	Ars-i., bar-c., petr.
Arm pit	twitching in posterior margin of axilla	Arg-m.
Arm pit	ulcer in axilla	Bor.
Armpit	excoriation of axilla	Ars., aur., carb-v., con., graph., mez., sanic., sep., sulph., zinc.
Armpit	induration of axillary glands	Am-c., bufo., calc., Carb-an., clem., Iod., kali-c., lac-c., Sil.
Armpit	pain in upper limb with swollen axillary glands	**Bar-c.**
Armpit	ulcer in incised buboes	Carb-an., chel.
Artery	aneurism of large arteries	Bar-c., calc., carb-v., lyc., lycps., ran-s., spong.
Artery	bubbles starts from heart and passes through the arteries	Nat-p.
Artery	hardening of Arteries (A blood vessel that is part of the system carrying blood under pressure from the heart to the rest of the body)	Bar.Mur 3X

Body part/Disease	Symptom	Medicines
Artery	protrusion, exophthalmus (bulge in artery)	Aml-n., ars., aur., bad., bar-c., bell., cact., calc., con., crot-h., dig., Ferr-i., Ferr., ign., Iod., lycps., nat-m., phos., Sec., spong.
Artery	sensation of shot rolling through the arteries	Nat-p.
Artery	tumours atheroma (fatty deposit in artery like cholesterol)	Bar-c.
Arthritis	arthritic (joint or joints, causing pain, swelling, and stiffness) nodosities (a lump, knob, knot, or other kind of swelling that sticks out) on condyles (rounded end of bone.The ball part of a ball-and-socket joint such as the hip or shoulder joint is a condyle) painful	Led.
Arthritis	arthritic nodosities on condyles	Calc-p.
Arthritis	arthritic nodosities on condyles above elbow	Mag-c.
Arthritis	arthritic nodosities on condyles above elbow with stiffness	Lyc.
Arthritis	arthritic nodosities on condyles on back of wrist	Petr.
Arthritis	arthritic nodosities on condyles on finger joints	Aesc., agn., ant-c., Apis., Benz-ac., calc-f., calc-p., Calc., Caust., clem., colch., dig., Graph., hep., Led., Lith., Lyc., ox-ac., ran-s., rhod., sil., staph., sulph., urt-u.
Arthritis	arthritic nodosities on condyles on first toe	Rhod.
Arthritis	arthritic nodosities on condyles on foot	Bufo., kali-i., Led., nat-s.
Arthritis	arthritic nodosities on condyles on forearm	Am-c.
Arthritis	arthritic nodosities on condyles on hands	Ant-c., benz-ac., calc., carb-s., hep., led., plb.
Arthritis	arthritic nodosities on condyles on knee	Bufo., calc., led., nux-v.
Arthritis	arthritic nodosities on condyles on olecranon (the upper end of the ulna bone that extends beyond the joint of the elbow to form the elbow's hard projecting point)	Still.
Arthritis	arthritic nodosities on condyles on shoulder	Calc., kali-i.
Arthritis	arthritic nodosities on condyles on toes	Asaf., caust., graph., ran-s., sabin., sulph., thuj.
Arthritis	arthritic nodosities on condyles on wrist	Benz-ac., calc., led., lyc., petr., rhod.
Arthritis	arthritic nodosities on condyles pinching & cracking on motion	Led.
Arthritis	arthritic nodosities on condyles pinching & cracking on motion in skin over joints	Led.
Arthritis	arthritic nodositieson condyles on finger joints with stiffness	Carb-an., graph., Lyc.
Asthma	asthma aggravated from cold air	Lob., nux-v., petr.
Asthma	asthma aggravated from cold water	Meph.
Asthma	asthma aggravated from coughing	Meph.
Asthma	asthma aggravated from music	Ambr.
Asthma	asthma aggravated from talking	Dros.
Asthma	asthma aggravated from warm food	Cham., lob.
Asthma	asthma aggravated in draught (current of cold air) of air	Sil.

Body part/Disease	Symptom	Medicines
Asthma	asthma aggravated in warm room	Am-c., carb-v., kali-s.
Asthma	asthma alternating with eruptions	Calad., crot-t., hep., kalm., lach., mez., rhus-t., sulph.
Asthma	asthma alternating with gout	Benz-ac., lyc., sulph.
Asthma	asthma alternating with headache	Ang., glon., kali-br.
Asthma	asthma alternating with nocturnal diarrhoea	Kali-c.
Asthma	asthma alternating with urticaria	Calad.
Asthma	asthma ameliorated after eating	Ambr., graph.
Asthma	asthma ameliorated by bending head backward	Cham., Spong., verat.
Asthma	asthma ameliorated from cold air	Bry., carb-v., cham., merc.
Asthma	asthma ameliorated from expectorations	Hyper.
Asthma	asthma ameliorated from stool	Poth.
Asthma	asthma ameliorated from talking	Ferr.
Asthma	asthma ameliorated in open air	Am-c.
Asthma	asthma catching after cough	Arn., ars., bry., hep., nat-m., puls.
Asthma	asthma catching after dancing	Spong.
Asthma	asthma catching at night	Sil.
Asthma	asthma catching before menses	Bor.
Asthma	asthma catching during fever	Sil.
Asthma	asthma catching during sleep	Lyc.
Asthma	asthma catching from cough	Bry., cina.
Asthma	asthma catching in morning	Sars.
Asthma	asthma catching on bending	Calc.
Asthma	asthma croaking	Cham., lach.
Asthma	asthma from inhaling dusts	Poth.
Asthma	asthma in old people	Ambr., Ars., bar-c., carb-v., con., phel., sulph.
Asthma	asthmatic (a disease of the respiratory system, sometimes caused by allergies, with symptoms including coughing, sudden difficulty in breathing, and a tight feeling in the chest) after emotions	Acon., ambr., cham., coff., cupr., gels., ign., nux-v., pall., verat.
Asthma	asthmatic after anger	Ars., Cham.
Asthma	asthmatic after coition	Asaf., cedr., kali-bi.
Asthma	asthmatic after dinner	Thuj.
Asthma	asthmatic after eating	Kali-p., nux-v., puls.
Asthma	asthmatic after injury of spine	Hyper.
Asthma	asthmatic after lying down	Aral., ars., cist., meph.
Asthma	asthmatic after measles	Brom., carb-v.
Asthma	asthmatic after menses	Puls., spong.
Asthma	asthmatic after mercury	Aur.
Asthma	asthmatic after midnight	Ars., calc-ar., carb-v., ferr-ar., ferr., graph., lach., Samb.
Asthma	asthmatic after midnight must spring out of bed	Ars., graph., Samb.
Asthma	asthmatic after suppressed eruptions	Apis., ars., carb-v., dulc., ferr., hep., ip., psor., Puls., sec., sulph.

Body part/Disease	Symptom	Medicines
Asthma	asthmatic after suppression of acute rash (skin eruption often reddish and itchy)	Acon., apis., puls.
Asthma	asthmatic after vaccination	Thuj.
Asthma	asthmatic ameliorated from eructations	Carb-v., nux-v.
Asthma	asthmatic at 2 to 3 a.m	Kali-ar., Kali-c.
Asthma	asthmatic at 3 a.m	Chin., cupr., Kali-c., Kali-n.
Asthma	asthmatic at 4 to 5 a.m.	Nat-s., stann.
Asthma	asthmatic at 5 a.m	Kali-i.
Asthma	asthmatic at 9 p.m.	Bry.
Asthma	asthmatic at night	Am-m., ant-t., Ars., aur., brom., bry., carb-v., Chel., chlol., cist., coff., coloc., daph., dig., ferr-ar., ferr., ip., kali-ar., kali-c., lach., meph., nux-v., op., phos., Puls., sang., sep., sulph., syph., thuj., zinc.
Asthma	asthmatic attacks in winter	Carb-v., nux-v., phel.
Asthma	asthmatic before menses	Sulph.
Asthma	asthmatic breathing ameliorated by bathing in cold water	Calc-s.
Asthma	asthmatic breathing from nose	Ars-i., ars., bad., carb-v., dulc., euphr., Iod., kali-i., lach., naja., nat-s., nux-v., sabad., sang., sil., sin-n., stict.
Asthma	asthmatic deep at midnight on waking	Cann-i.
Asthma	asthmatic deep from heaviness of heart	Croc.
Asthma	asthmatic deep from waking	Alumn., cann-s.
Asthma	asthmatic desires to breathe deep during chill	Cimx.
Asthma	asthmatic desires to breathe deep while lying	Ind.
Asthma	asthmatic during coition	Aeth., ambr.
Asthma	asthmatic during menses	Kali-c.
Asthma	asthmatic during sleep coming on	Acon., ars., carb-v., hep., kali-c., lach., meph., nat-s., op., sep., sulph.
Asthma	asthmatic every 8 days	Sulph.
Asthma	asthmatic from excitements	Ambr.
Asthma	asthmatic from fatty degeneration of heart	Arn.
Asthma	asthmatic from flatulance	Carb-v., cham., chin., lyc., mag-p., nux-v., op., phos., sulph., zinc.
Asthma	asthmatic from leaning backward	Psor.
Asthma	asthmatic from taking cold	Acon., dulc., lob., podo., puls., sil., Spong., stann.
Asthma	asthmatic from walking against wind	Cupr.
Asthma	asthmatic in autumn	Chin.
Asthma	asthmatic in change of weather	Ars., chel., dulc.
Asthma	asthmatic in children	Acon., ambr., Cham., Ip., kali-br., kali-i., mosch., Nat-s., nux-v., psor., Puls., Samb., stram., sulph.
Asthma	asthmatic in children after vaccination	Thuj.
Asthma	asthmatic in damp weather	Dulc., med., nat-s.
Asthma	asthmatic in drunkards	Meph.

Body part/Disease	Symptom	Medicines
Asthma	asthmatic in evening	Bell., cist., ferr., nux-v., phos., Puls., stann., sulph., zinc.
Asthma	asthmatic in evening in bed	Am-c., graph., sep.
Asthma	asthmatic in morning	Aur., calc., carb-an., carb-v., coff., con., dig., Kali-c., meph., phos., verat., zing.
Asthma	asthmatic in morning in bed	Alum., con.
Asthma	asthmatic in noon	Lob.
Asthma	asthmatic in piles	Sulph.
Asthma	asthmatic in sailors as soon as they go ashore	Brom.
Asthma	asthmatic in summer	Ars.
Asthma	asthmatic in warm wet weather	Bell., carb-v.
Asthma	asthmatic in wet weather	Aur., chin., con., dulc., nat-s., sil., verat.
Asthma	asthmatic on walking	Alum., con., sep.
Asthma	asthmatic periodic	All-s., alum., ant-t., Ars., asaf., carb-v., chel., hydr-ac., nux-v., phos., plb., seneg., sulph., tab., thuj.
Asthma	asthmatic respiration aggravation from riding	Meph.
Asthma	asthmatic respiration ameliorated from cold water	Cham.
Asthma	asthmatic respiration catching while working	Sars.
Asthma	asthmatic respiration from hay asthma	Ambr., ars-i., ars., bad., carb-v., dulc., euphr., Iod., kali-i., lach., naja., nat-s., nux-v., op., sabad., sil., sin-n., stict.
Asthma	asthmatic when heated	Sil.
Asthma	asthmatic with face ache and disappearance of tetter (eruption) on face	Dulc.
Asthma	asthmatic with intermittent fever	Mez.
Asthma	asthmatic with stitching in abdomen to back	Calc.
Asthma	Cardiac Asthma, (asthma arising from heart)	Aspidosperma
Asthma	constriction in chest asthmatic	Ang., coff., led., mez., naja., nux-v., sulph.
Asthma	discoloration, blue on upper limbs with asthma	Kali-c.
Asthma	discolouration of face blue in asthma	Stram., tab.
Asthma	dropsy of chest with asthma	Psor.
Asthma	eruption, pimples in forearm alternating with asthma	Calad.
Asthma	eruption, rash alternating with asthma in upper limbs	Calad., mez.
Asthma	eruption, rash in forearm alternating with asthma	Calad.
Asthma	eruptions on skin alternating with asthma	Calad., mez., rhus-t., sulph.
Asthma	eruption, rash from tightness of chest alternating with asthma	Calad.
Asthma	gouty pain in joints alternates with asthma	Sulph.
Asthma	headache alternating with asthma	Ang., glon., kali-br.
Asthma	inflammation of pleura in phthisical (a disease of the respiratory system, especially asthma or tuberculosis. A wasting disease) patients	Arg-n., calc., seneg.
Asthma	menses, copious, phthisical (disease of the respiratory system, especially asthma or tuberculosis)	Calc., kali-c., phos., sang., senec., stann.

Body part/Disease	Symptom	Medicines
Asthma	rash alternating with asthma on chest	Calad.
Asthma	sneezing, with hay asthma	Ars., carb-v., dulc., euphr., lach., naja., nat-s., nux-v., sin-n., stict.
Asthma	sudden attack of asthmatic	Cupr., ip.
Asthma	urticaria alternating with asthma	Calad.
Asthma	urticaria in asthmatic troubles	Apis.
Atrophy	atrophy (shrinking in size of some part or organ of the body, usually caused by injury, disease, or lack of use) of gums	Kali-c., merc., plb.
Atrophy	atrophy of glands	Anan., ars., aur., bar-c., carb-an., cham., chin., **Con., Iod.,** kali-ar., kali-c., **Kali-i.,** kali-p., kreos., lac-d., nit-ac., nux-m., ph-ac., plb., sars., sec., sil., staph., verat.
Atrophy	atrophy of liver	Arg-n., ars., Aur., bry., Calc., carb-v., card-m., chel., chin., chion., cupr., hydr., iod., lach., lept., lyc., mag-m., merc., mur-ac., nat-m., nat-s., nit-ac., nux-v., Phos., plb., puls., sep., sulph.
Atrophy	atrophy of mammae	Anan., ars., bar-c., chim., Con., Iod., Kali-i., kreos., lac-d., nat-m., nit-ac., nux-m., plb., sacc., sars., sec.
Atrophy	atrophy of nipples	Iod., sars.
Atrophy	atrophy of optic nerve	Nux-v., Phos., tab.
Atrophy	atrophy of optic nerve from tobacco	Ars.
Atrophy	atrophy of tongue	Mur-ac.
Aversion	aversion to being approached	Aur., caj., hell., helon., hipp., iod., lil-t., Lyc., sulph.
Aversion	aversion to members of family	Calc., crot-h., fl-ac., nat-c., Sep.
Aversion	aversion to acids	Abies-c., bell., cocc., ferr-m., ferr., ign., nux-v., ph-ac., sabad., sulph.
Aversion	aversion to alcoholic drinks	Ferr., Nux-v.
Aversion	aversion to Amusement (the act of keeping somebody occupied or entertained)	Bar-c., lil-t., meny., olnd., sulph.
Aversion	aversion to apples	Lyss.
Aversion	aversion to bananas	Elaps.
Aversion	aversion to bed	Acon., ars., bapt., calc., camph., cann-s., canth., caust., cedr., cench., cupr., kali-ar., lach., lyc., merc., nat-c., squil.
Aversion	aversion to beer	Alum., asaf., atro., bell., bry., calc., cham., Chin., clem., cocc., crot-t., cycl., ferr., nat-m., nat-s., Nux-v., pall., ph-ac., phos., rhus-t., sep., spig., spong., stann., sulph.
Aversion	aversion to Black or dark colour	Rob., stram., tarent.
Aversion	aversion to brandy	Ign., merc., rhus-t., zinc.
Aversion	aversion to brandy in brandy drinkers	Arn.
Aversion	aversion to bread	Agar., Chin., con., cur., cycl., elaps., ign., kali-c., kali-p., kali-s., lach., lact., lil-t., lyc., mag-c., manc., meny., Nat-m., nat-p., nat-s., nit-ac., nux-v., ol-an., ph-ac., phos., puls., rhus-t., sep., sulph., tarent.
Aversion	aversion to bread and butter	Cycl., mag-c., meny., nat-p.

Body part/Disease	Symptom	Medicines
Aversion	aversion to bringing objects near the eyes	Fl-ac., mang.
Aversion	aversion to Business	Agar., am-c., anac., ars-h., ars., aur-m., brom., chin-s., cimic., con., cop., fl-ac., graph., hipp., kali-ar., kali-bi., kali-br., kali-c., kali-i., kali-s., lach., lact-ac., laur., lil-t., mag-s., ph-ac., phyt., puls., Sep., sulph.
Aversion	aversion to butter	Ars., carb-v., Chin., cycl., mag-c., meny., merc., petr., phos., ptel., Puls., sang.
Aversion	aversion to cereals	Ars., phos.
Aversion	aversion to certain persons	Am-m., aur., calc., crot-h., Nat-c., sel., stann.
Aversion	aversion to cheese	Chel., olnd.
Aversion	aversion to children	Plat.
Aversion	aversion to chocolate	Osm., tarent.
Aversion	aversion to coffee	Bell., bry., calc-s., Calc., carb-v., cham., chel., chin., coc-c., coff., dulc., fl-ac., kali-br., kali-n., lil-t., lyc., mag-p., merc., nat-c., nat-m., Nux-v., osm., ox-ac., ph-ac., phos., phys., rheum., rhus-t., sabad., spig., sul-ac.
Aversion	aversion to cold drinks	Calad., phys.
Aversion	aversion to cold water	Bell., brom., bry., calad., canth., caust., chel., chin-a., chin., lyss., nat-m., nux-v., phel., phys., stram., tab.
Aversion	aversion to company in forenoon	Alum.
Aversion	aversion to company in morning	Alum.
Aversion	aversion to eggs	Ferr., kali-s., nit-ac., sulph.
Aversion	aversion to every thing	Alumn., am-m., calc., caps., cupr., hyos., ip., merc., mez., puls., sulph., thuj
Aversion	aversion to fat & rich food	Ang., ars., bell., bry., calc., carb-an., carb-s., carb-v., chin-a., Chin., colch., croc., cycl., dros., grat., guare., hell., hep., lyss., meny., merc., nat-a., nat-c., nat-m., Petr., phos., Ptel., Puls., rheum., rhus-t., sang., sec., sep., sulph.
Aversion	aversion to fish	Colch., Graph., guare., nat-m., phos., sulph., zinc.
Aversion	aversion to flour	Ars., ph-ac., phos.
Aversion	aversion to food containing starch	Ars., phos.
Aversion	aversion to friends	Cedr., ferr., led.
Aversion	aversion to fruit	Bar-c., ign.
Aversion	aversion to garlic	Sabad.
Aversion	aversion to her usual house work	Cit-ac.
Aversion	aversion to hot drinks	Ferr., kali-s.
Aversion	aversion to Husband	Glon., kali-p., nat-c., nat-m., Sep., verat.
Aversion	aversion to meat of calf	Phel., zinc.
Aversion	aversion to milk	Aeth., am-c., ant-t., arn., bell., bry., calad., calc-s., calc., carb-s., carb-v., cina., ferr-p., guai., guare., ign., Lac-d., lec., mag-c., Nat-c., nat-p., nat-s., nux-v., phos., puls., rheum., sep., sil., stann., sulph.
Aversion	aversion to mother's milk	Ant-c., cina., lach., merc., Sil., stann., stram.

Body part/Disease	Symptom	Medicines
Aversion	aversion to motion	**Acon.**, alum., am-c., ambr., anac., ant-c., ant-t., arn., **Ars.**, asar., bar-c., **Bell.**, bor., **Bry.**, cadm., **Calad.**, **Calc-s.**, **Calc.**, canth., caps., carb-an., carb-s., carb-v., caust., cham., chel., chin-a., chin., cina., cocc., coff., con., croc., cupr., cycl., dig., dros., dulc., ferr-i., ferr., gels., graph., **Guai.**, hyos., ign., ip., kali-ar., kali-bi., kali-c., kali-p., **Lach.**, led., lyc., mag-c., mag-m., merc., mez., mur-ac., nat-a., nat-c., nat-m., nit-ac., **Nux-v.**, op., petr., ph-ac., phos., psor., puls., **Ruta.**, sang., sep., **Sil.**, stann., stront., **Sulph.**, tarax., teucr., thuj., zinc.
Aversion	aversion to mutton	Ov.
Aversion	aversion to oatmeal	Ars., calc.
Aversion	aversion to onions	Sabad.
Aversion	aversion to open air	Agar., alum., **Am-c.**, am-m., ambr., anac., **Bapt.**, bell., bry., **Calc-p.**, **Calc.**, camph., canth., caps., carb-an., carb-v., caust., **Cham.**, chel., chin., cina., cist., **Cocc.**, **Coff.**, coloc., con., cycl., dig., ferr-ar., ferr., graph., guai., helon., hep., **Ign.**, ip., kali-ar., **Kali-c.**, kali-n., kali-p., kreos., lach., laur., lyc., lyss., mang., meny., merc-c., merc., mosch., **Nat-c.**, nat-m., nat-p., nit-ac., nux-m., **Nux-v.**, op., **Petr.**, ph-ac., phos., plb., psor., rhod., rhus-t., **Rumx.**, sel., seneg., sep., **Sil.**, spig., stront., sul-ac., **Sulph.**, teucr., thuj., valer., verb., viol-t.
Aversion	aversion to opposite sex	Lyc., puls., sulph.
Aversion	aversion to pickles	Abies-c.
Aversion	aversion to plum	Bar-c.
Aversion	aversion to pork (pig's meat)	Ang., colch., dros., psor., puls.
Aversion	aversion to potatoes	Alum., camph., thuj.
Aversion	aversion to puddings	Ars., phos., ptel.
Aversion	aversion to red , black , yellow or green	Tarent.
Aversion	aversion to salt foods	Acet-ac., carb-v., card-m., Cor-r., Graph., nat-m., sel., sep., sil.
Aversion	aversion to sexual intercourse	Agar., agn., alum., am-c., arund., bov., cann-s., carb-an., carb-s., caust., clem., coff., cub., ferr-ma., ferr-p., fl-ac., graph., hell., ign., kali-br., kali-c., kali-n., kali-p., kali-s., lach., lyc., mag-c., med., Nat-m., onos., op., petr., phos., plat., plb., psor., ran-s., rhod., Sep., stann., staph., stram., sul-ac., sulph., tarent., ther., thuj.
Aversion	aversion to sexual intercourse after menses	Berb., caust., kali-c., nat-m., phos., sep., sul-ac.
Aversion	aversion to sexual intercourse with absent enjoyment	Alum., berb., brom., calc., cann-s., Caust., ferr-m., ferr., graph., kali-br., lyss., med., nat-m., onos., phos., plat., puls., Sep.
Aversion	aversion to sexual intercourse with delayed orgasm	Berb., brom.
Aversion	aversion to sexual intercourse with painful enjoyment	Nat-m.
Aversion	aversion to sitting	Iod., lach.
Aversion	aversion to smell of milk	Bell.

Body part/Disease	Symptom	Medicines
Aversion	aversion to smoking	Alum., arg-m., arn., asar., bor., brom., bry., calc-p., calc., camph., carb-an., clem., coc-c., coff., euphr., grat., Ign., kali-bi., kali-n., lach., lyc., mag-s., nat-a., nat-m., nat-s., nicc., olnd., op., ox-ac., phos., psor., puls., sep., spig., sulph., tarax., tell.
Aversion	aversion to solid foods	Ang., ferr., lyc., merc., staph.
Aversion	aversion to soup	Arn., ars., bell., cham., graph., kali-i., rhus-t.
Aversion	aversion to sweets	Ars., bar-c., caust., Graph., hipp., lac-c., merc., nit-ac., phos., sin-n., sulph., zinc.
Aversion	aversion to tea	Carb-ac., phos., thea.
Aversion	aversion to the every thing	Alum., am-m., bov., caps., cupr., grat., hyos., ip., lyc., merc., mez., nux-v., plat., puls., rheum., rhod., sars., sep., sulph., thea., ther., thuj.
Aversion	aversion to the odor of eggs	Colch.
Aversion	aversion to those around	Ars.
Aversion	aversion to tobacco	Acon., ant-t., arn., bov., brom., bry., Calc., camph., canth., carb-an., chlor., cimic., cocc., con., ign., lach., lyc., mag-s., meph., nat-m., Nux-v., op., phos., psor., puls., spig., sulph., tarax., thuj., til., valer., zing.
Aversion	aversion to uncovering during perspiration	Acon., aeth., arn., ars., aur., bar-c., calc., carb-an., chin., clem., colch., con., eup-per., gels., hell., hep., mag-m., nat-a., nat-c., nux-m., **Nux-v.**, **Rhus-t.**, **Samb.**, sil., squil., stram., stront., tub.
Aversion	aversion to vegetables	Bell., hell., hydr., mag-c., ruta.
Aversion	aversion to warm drinks	Cham., Phos., Puls.
Aversion	aversion to water	Apis., bell., brom., bry., calad., cann-i., canth., carl., caust., cedr., chin., coc-c., coloc., elaps., ham., hell., Hyos., kali-bi., lyc., lyss., manc., merc-c., nat-m., Nux-v., onos., ox-ac., phel., phys., puls., Stram., thea., zinc.
Aversion	aversion to wine	Agar., ars-m., fl-ac., ign., jatr., jug-r., lach., manc., merc., nat-m., ph-ac., rhus-t., Sabad., sulph., zinc.
Aversion	avoids the sight of people	Acon., Cic., cupr., ferr., gels., iod., led., nat-c., sep., thuj.

Body part/Disease	Symptom	Medicines
Back	Aching in back after confinement (the period of time or the process of giving birth, beginning when a woman goes into labor and ending when a child is born)	Hyper.
Back	Aching in back after continued writing	Lyc., mur-ac., sep.
Back	Aching in back after dinner	Agar., cob.
Back	Aching in back after eating	Agar., ant-t.
Back	Aching in back after emission	Ant-c., cob., kali-br., ph-ac., sars., staph.
Back	Aching in back after long sitting	Lith-m., phos., Puls.
Back	Aching in back after menses	Berb., kali-c., mag-c., verat.
Back	Aching in back after midnight worse when inspiring (to inhale air or a gas into the lungs)	Nit-ac.
Back	Aching in back after riding in carriage	Nux-m.
Back	Aching in back after rising from a seat	Aesc., ars., bell., calc.
Back	Aching in back after stool	Rheum.
Back	Aching in back after stooping	Aesc., agar., chel.
Back	Aching in back after supper	Sulph.
Back	Aching in back after taking cold	Nit-ac.
Back	Aching in back after walking	Nat-c., phos., stry.
Back	Aching in back aggravated from coffee	Cham.
Back	Aching in back ameliorated from lying on back	Equis., nat-m.
Back	Aching in back ameliorated from bending backward	Aeth.
Back	Aching in back ameliorated from leaning against something	Eupi., zing.
Back	Aching in back ameliorated from lying on abdomen	Nit-ac.
Back	Aching in back ameliorated from pressure	Kali-c., nat-m., sep.
Back	Aching in back ameliorated from urinating	Lyc.
Back	Aching in back ameliorated from washing	Vesp.
Back	Aching in back ameliorated on motion	Graph.
Back	Aching in back arresting breathing	Cann-s.
Back	Aching in back at night	Agar., aloe., am-m., arg-n., berb., helon., lycps., mag-c., mag-m., nat-c., phys., senec., Sulph.
Back	Aching in back at night after sleep	Am-m.
Back	Aching in back at night during menses	Am-m.
Back	Aching in back before chill	Carb-v., daph., dios., Eup-per., ip., Podo., rhus-t.
Back	Aching in back before menses	Berb., brom., calc., caust., eupi., gels., hyos., hyper., nux-v., Puls., spong.

Body part/Disease	Symptom	Medicines
Back	Aching in back confines him to bed	Ars-s-f.
Back	Aching in back during chill	Ant-t., eup-per., ip.
Back	Aching in back during difficult stool	Puls.
Back	Aching in back during dysuria (pain or difficulty in urinating)	Vesp.
Back	Aching in back during fever	Eug., ziz.
Back	Aching in back during menses	Acon., agar., am-m., bell., berb., bry., calc-p., caul., cimic., crot-h., eupi., ferr., graph., inul., kali-c., nat-c., nat-h., nat-p., phos., phys., rhus-t.
Back	Aching in back during stool	Manc.
Back	Aching in back from lying	Berb., cur.
Back	Aching in back from lying on back	Carb-an., nit-ac.
Back	Aching in back from motion of shoulders	Cocc.
Back	Aching in back from suppressed menses	Aesc., kali-c., sep., sil.
Back	Aching in back in afternoon	Abrot., agar., cham., chel., equis., glon., hyos., pall., plb., ptel., rumx., sep., zing.
Back	Aching in back in cool air	Kali-s.
Back	Aching in back in evening	Acon., agar., alumn., ars., cham., cist., ferr-i., kali-s., led., lil-t., phys., sarr.
Back	Aching in back in evening ameliorated after exertion	Ruta.
Back	Aching in back in forenoon	Equis., ptel.
Back	Aching in back in morning	Berb., dios., equis., eug., eupho., eupi., mag-s., phyt., rhod., thuj.
Back	Aching in back in morning in bed	Ang., berb., eupho., kali-n., mag-s., petr.
Back	Aching in back in morning in on waking	Berb., cham., ptel.
Back	Aching in back in morning on rising	Caust., cedr., graph., hep., ran-b.
Back	Aching in back in open air	Nux-v.
Back	Aching in back in warm room	Kali-s.
Back	Aching in back on coughing	Am-c., kali-n., merc., puls., sep.
Back	Aching in back on false step	Sulph.
Back	Aching in back on motion	Aesc., agar., am-c., equis., ferr., gent-l., ox-ac., petr., sil., stry.
Back	Aching in back on standing	Lyc., tus-p.
Back	Aching in back on stooping	Agar., bor., bov., caps., cham., kali-n., sulph.
Back	Aching in back on swallowing	Kali-c., raph.
Back	Aching in back on turning, must sit up to turn over in bed	Nux-v.
Back	Aching in back on waking	Hep., myric., ptel.
Back	Aching in back rheumatic (a painful condition of the joints or muscles in which neither infection nor injury is a contributing cause)	Arn., Ind., kali-c., plb., stram., stry.
Back	Aching in back when breathing	Inul., raph.
Back	Aching in back when breathing deep	Nat-c.
Back	Aching in back when carrying basket	Phos.

Body part/Disease	Symptom	Medicines
Back	Aching in back when sitting down	Cob.
Back	Aching in back while bent over	Sep.
Back	Aching in back while eating	Crot-c.
Back	Aching in back while fasting	Kali-n.
Back	Aching in back while sitting	Berb., bism., bor., cann-i., cham., cob., cocc., equis., euphr., helon., nat-c., nux-v., ox-ac., pic-ac., plb., podo., puls., Sep., thuj., Zinc.
Back	Aching in back while walking	Aesc., bapt., bor., cham., euphr., iris., Kali-c., lyc., Psor., sep.
Back	Aching in cervical region extending to small of back on going to stool	Verat.
Back	Aching in dorsal (back of the body) region	Aesc., bol., calc-ar., calc., cann-s., pic-ac., rhus-t., tep.
Back	Aching in dorsal region at latter part of night	Calc-p.
Back	Aching in dorsal region in afternoon	Calc-s., erig.
Back	Aching in dorsal region in evening	Calc-s., erig.
Back	Aching in dorsal region in morning	Calc-p.
Back	Aching in dorsal region while writing	Mur-ac., petr.
Back	Aching in left side of back	Bism., carb-an., cocc., mez., tarent.
Back	Aching in lumbo (back) sacral (triangular bone at the base of the spine that joins to a hip bone on each side and forms part of the pelvis) region	Aesc., asc-t., aspar., cimic., colch., dios., gels., hura., lil-t., Onos., phos., sil.
Back	Aching in lumbo sacral region	Aesc., asc-t., aspar., cimic., colch., dios., gels., hura., lil-t., Onos., phos., sil.
Back	Aching in right side of back	Asaf., bar-c., bell., benz-ac., blatta., dios., lyc., merc-i-f.
Back	aggravated from carrying on the back	Alum.
Back	aggravated from lying on back	Acet-ac., acon., aloe., alum., am-c., am-m., arg-m., arn., ars., aur-m., bar-c., bell., bor., bry., bufo., calc., canth., caust., cham., chin., cina., clem., coloc., cupr., dulc., eup-per., eupho., hyper., iod., kali-c., lach., merc., nat-c., nat-m., nat-s., **Nux-v.**, op., par, **Phos.**, plat., ran-b., rhus-t., sep., sil., spig., spong., stront., sulph., thuj.
Back	ameliorated from lying on back	Acon., aeth., am-c., **Am-m.**, anac., apis., arn., bar-c., bell., bor., **Bry.**, cact., calad., **Calc.**, canth., carb-an., caust., chin., cimic., cina., clem., colch., con., conv., ferr., grat., hell., ign., ip., kali-c., kalm., kreos., lach., lyc., **Merc-c.**, merc., mosch., nat-c., nat-m., nat-s., nux-v., ox-ac., par., phos., plat., **Puls.**, ran-b., **Rhus-t.**, sabad., sang., senec., seneg., sep., sil., spig., spong., stann., sulph., thuj., verat., viol-t.
Back	asthmatic with stitching in abdomen to back	Calc.
Back	bluish right side of back	Vip.
Back	boring pain in back as with a gimlet (tool for boring holes in wood)	Lyc.
Back	boring pain in dorsal (relating to or situated on the back of the body) region	Lil-t.
Back	boring pain in spots of back	Thuj.

Body part/Disease	Symptom	Medicines
Back	burning pain between scapula extending down the back	Merc.
Back	burning pain in back after coition	Mag-m.
Back	burning pain in back after emission	Merc., phos.
Back	burning pain in back after grief	Naja.
Back	burning pain in back after scratching	Mag-c.
Back	burning pain in back ameliorated after scratching	Rhus-v.
Back	burning pain in back ameliorated from motion	Mag-m., pic-ac., rat.
Back	burning pain in back ameliorated from walking in open air	Kali-n.
Back	burning pain in back at night	Helon., ph-ac.
Back	burning pain in back before menses	Kreos.
Back	burning pain in back from mental exertion	Pic-ac., sil.
Back	burning pain in back from walking in open air	Arn., kali-c., sil.
Back	burning pain in back in forenoon	Kali-bi.
Back	burning pain in back in morning	Mag-m., zinc.
Back	burning pain in back in morning after coition aggravated by rest ameliorated by motion	Mag-m.
Back	burning pain in back in morning on rising ameliorated by motion	Rat.
Back	burning pain in back in noon	Rhus-t.
Back	burning pain in back in spots	Nit-ac., ph-ac., Phos., zinc.
Back	burning pain in back when getting warm in bed	Sil.
Back	burning pain in back while lying	Lyc.
Back	burning pain in back while lying on back	Ars.
Back	burning pain in back while sitting	Ars., asar., bor., Zinc.
Back	burning pain in cervical region extending down back	Med.
Back	burning pain in dorsal region from needle work or writing	Ran-b., sep.
Back	burning pain in dorsal region	Caps., dios., mang., zinc.
Back	burning pain in spine above small of back	Zinc.
Back	carbuncle in dorsal region	Hep., lach., tarent.
Back	chill as if water running down the back	Agar., alumn., ars.
Back	chilliness in right upper limb extending to back and legs	Mez.
Back	coldness in back after afternoon rest	Cycl.
Back	coldness in back after dinner	Cedr., cycl.
Back	coldness in back after eating	Crot-c., sil.
Back	coldness in back after menses	Kali-c.
Back	coldness in back after stool	Fago., puls., sumb.
Back	coldness in back after urination	Sars.

Body part/Disease	Symptom	Medicines
Back	coldness in back aggravated from warmth	Apis.
Back	coldness in back ameliorated by lying down	Cast., kali-n., sil.
Back	coldness in back as if cold water has been sprayed with force	Caust., lyc., Puls.
Back	coldness in back at night	Ars., arum-t., chin-a., chin-s., chin., coc-c., lil-t., lyc., nat-a., nat-m., puls., stront., thuj.
Back	coldness in back at night on going to bed	Coc-c., lil-t.
Back	coldness in back before stool	Ars.
Back	coldness in back during eating	Raph.
Back	coldness in back during menses	Bell., kreos.
Back	coldness in back during stool	Colch., trom.
Back	coldness in back extending down as if cold water were flowing down in thin stream	Ars., caps., caust.
Back	coldness in back extending down as if cold water were poured down	Agar., alumn., anac., ars., lil-t., lyc., Puls., sabad., stram., vario., zinc.
Back	coldness in back extending down limbs	Gins.
Back	coldness in back extending down on motion	Rumx.
Back	coldness in back extending down lower limbs	Acon., ferr., ham.
Back	coldness in back extending down to feet	Croc.
Back	coldness in back extending down to feet	Croc.
Back	coldness in back extending into arms	Gins., verat.
Back	coldness in back extending over whole body	Amyg., bell., lyc.
Back	coldness in back extending to abdomen	Crot-t., phos., sec., spig.
Back	coldness in back from motion	Asaf., eup-pur., phys., sulph., thuj.
Back	coldness in back in afternoon	Alum., apis., asaf., cast., cic., cimic., cocc., fago., guai., hyos., lyc., nat-a., rumx., stram., thuj.
Back	coldness in back in evening	Ars., bapt., berb., caps., cast., cimic., cocc., coff., dulc., kreos., lyc., mur-ac., nat-m., nux-v., Puls., rhus-t., sang., sep., stann., Sulph., tab., thuj.
Back	coldness in back in forenoon	Ang., asaf., berb., cham., con., hydr., lyc.
Back	coldness in back in forenoon while walking in a room	Ang.
Back	coldness in back in forenoon while walking in open air	Hydr.
Back	coldness in back in morning	Arn., bry., con., ferr., mez., nit-s-d., Nux-v., sumb.
Back	coldness in back in morning after menses	Kali-c.
Back	coldness in back in noon	Arg-n., rhus-t.
Back	coldness in back near warm stove	Jug-c.
Back	coldness in back of hands with heat of palms	Anac., coff.
Back	coldness in back on waking	Dig.
Back	coldness in back when dressing	Anth.
Back	coldness in back while sitting	Brom.
Back	coldness in back while walking	Asaf., hyos., nit-s-d.
Back	coldness in back while walking in open air	Chin.

Body part/Disease	Symptom	Medicines
Back	coldness in dorsal region	Agar., croc., sil., spong., thuj.
Back	coldness in lumbar region after stool	Puls.
Back	coldness in shoulder in epilepsy extending to small of back	Kreos.
Back	constriction in heart extending to back	Lil-t.
Back	contraction of muscles & tendons of shoulder extending to back	Mag-c.
Back	contraction of muscles & tendons of shoulder extending to back in morning	Mag-c.
Back	convulsion begin in back	Sulph.
Back	cough following difficult labour or abortion, with backache and sweat	Kali-c.
Back	cramp in back	Bell., calc-p., iod., kali-bi., lyc., naja., nux-v., plb.
Back	cramp in back of hand at night in bed	Anac.
Back	curvature of dorsal bone	Bar-c., bufo., calc-s., calc., con., lyc., plb., puls., rhus-t., sil., sulph., syph., thuj.
Back	dysuria (difficult or painful urination. This is usually associated with urgency and frequency of urination if due to cystitis or urethritis. The pain is burning in nature and is relieved by curing the underlying cause. A high fluid intake usually helps) with aching in back	Vesp.
Back	dysuria with aching in back	Vesp.
Back	dysuria with aching in back	Vesp.
Back	electric like shocks in dorsal region	Bell., cic.
Back	emaciation of back	Tab.
Back	emaciation of dorsal region	Plb.
Back	emaciation of lumbar region	Plb., sel.
Back	eruptions around lumbar region	Arund., rhus-t.
Back	fever with dry heat in evening in bed with chilliness in back	Coff.
Back	fistula (an opening or passage between two organs or between an organ and the skin, caused by disease, injury, or congenital malformation) on back	Calc-p., hep., ph-ac., Phos., Sil., Sulph.
Back	flushes of heat in back	Acon., bapt., brom., clem., dig., mang., merl., Sumb.
Back	flushes of heat in back after stool	Podo.
Back	flushes of heat in back extending to body	Sumb.
Back	flushes of heat in back in during stool	Podo.
Back	flushes of heat in back in evening	Ph-ac., sol-n.
Back	flushes of heat in back in evening after stool	Podo.
Back	flushes of heat in back in evening after supper	Spig.
Back	flushes of heat in back in evening on continued walking	Glon.
Back	flushes of heat in back in morning	Lil-t.
Back	flushes of heat in lumbar region	Calc-p., sumb.

Body part/Disease	Symptom	Medicines
Back	formication down the back	Carl.
Back	formication in back at night	Bar-c., bov., zinc.
Back	formication in back extending to fingers and toes	Sec.
Back	formication in back extending to limbs	Phos.
Back	formication in back in afternoon	Asaf., mag-s.
Back	formication in back in evening	Lyc., mag-s., osm.
Back	formication in back in morning	Ars-m.
Back	formication in dorsum (the back or upper surface of a part of the body such as the hand or foot)	Con.
Back	formication up and down the back	Crot-h., lach., manc.
Back	headache alternating with back pain	Aloe., brom., meli.
Back	headache alternating with pain in back	Aloe., brom., meli.
Back	headache with pains in back	Ail., benz-ac., cina., cob., daph., fl-ac., graph., hydr., menis., merc., myric., ol-an., op., sabad., sabin., sil., verat., ziz.
Back	heat in back after eating	Staph.
Back	heat in back after excitement	Pic-ac.
Back	heat in back after wine	Gins., zinc.
Back	heat in back alternating with cold	Carl., cham., verat.
Back	heat in back alternating with cold with shivering	Cham.
Back	heat in back extending down	Coff., con., laur., par., phys., sulph.
Back	heat in back extending up	Ars., cann-i., hyos., lyc., Phos., podo., sarr., verat.
Back	heat in back extending up during menses	Phos.
Back	heat in back extending up during stool	Podo.
Back	heat in back from mental exertion	Pic-ac., sil.
Back	heat in back from warmth of bed	Pic-ac.
Back	heat in back in evening	Cham., phys.
Back	heat in back in forenoon	Hell.
Back	heat in back in morning on waking	Con.
Back	heat in back while reading exciting news	Gels.
Back	heat in back while sitting	Meny., zinc.
Back	heat in back while walking	Verat.
Back	heat in back while walking in open air	Merc., ph-ac., sil., sol-n.
Back	heat in cervical region extending down back	Glon., par.
Back	heat in cervical region extending up back	Calc., fl-ac., glon.
Back	heat in dorsal region	Merc., phos., Pic-ac.
Back	heaviness in back aggravated from rising	Ant-t.
Back	heaviness in back ameliorated from motion	Rhod.
Back	heaviness in back at night	Carb-v.
Back	heaviness in back in forenoon	Sulph.
Back	heaviness in back in forenoon while sitting	Nat-c.
Back	heaviness in back in morning in bed	Ant-t., euphr., pic-ac., sep., sulph.

Body part/Disease	Symptom	Medicines
Back	heaviness in back in morning on rising	Ant-t., euphr.
Back	heaviness in back while lying	Phos.
Back	heaviness in dorsal region	Carb-s., phyt., sil.
Back	icy coldness running down back before epilepsy	Ars.
Back	itching in back after scratching	Mez.
Back	itching in back at night	Agar., ail., apoc., ars., asc-t., fl-ac., mez., phos., rhus-v.
Back	itching in back at night from lying down	Mag-c.
Back	itching in back at night in bed from warmth of bed	Nat-a., rhus-v., sulph.
Back	itching in back changes place after scratching	Mez., pall.
Back	itching in back in afternoon	Fago., sars.
Back	itching in back in cold air	Rhus-v.
Back	itching in back in evening	Con., fago., fl-ac., lyc., rat., sulph., thuj.
Back	itching in back in evening in bed	Calc., lyc., merc., nat-m.
Back	itching in back in forenoon	Fl-ac.
Back	itching in back in morning	Asc-t., lyc.
Back	itching in back in morning in bed	Rhus-t.
Back	itching in back while undressing	Cocc., hyper., mag-m., nat-c., nat-s., osm., puls.
Back	itching in back, pain after scratching	Nit-ac.
Back	itching in evening and night on back	Sep.
Back	itching in evening on back	Fago.
Back	itching in pimples on back	Arg-n., asc-t., calc., cann-s., carb-an., crot-t., fl-ac., led., mag-m., mill., rat., rhus-t., sel.
Back	itching on back when warm	Cocc.
Back	itching, ending in coldness in back	Am-m.
Back	jerking in lower limb while lying on back	Nat-s.
Back	miliary rash on back	Bry., Rhus-r., rhus-t., sars., sil.
Back	miliary spots on back	Ant-c., ant-t., bry., caust., Chel., cocc., hydrc., nat-a., ph-ac., prun-s., psor., sec., sumb., valer.
Back	nausea during backache	Coloc., phys., zing.
Back	nausea from pain in back	Sep.
Back	nausea on lying on back	Merc.
Back	numbness in back	Acon., agar., berb., calc-p., calc., cocc., cupr-ar., nux-v., ox-ac., phys., sec., sil.
Back	numbness in left leg while lying on back	Nicc.
Back	ovaries painful extending to small of back	Aesc., merc., plat., podo., syph.
Back	pain in abdomen amelioated from lying on back	Coloc., kalm., mez., onos.
Back	pain in abdomen extendimg to back	Absin., aloe, bell., bor., chel., con., cycl., ferr., hep., ign., indg., mag-m., nat-m., ph-ac., phos., puls., sulph., ter.
Back	pain in abdomen extendimg to back between shoulders	Bell.
Back	pain in arm from putting it across the back	Calc.
Back	pain in back after acid	Lach.

Body part/Disease	Symptom	Medicines
Back	pain in back after anxiety	Nux-v.
Back	pain in back after coition (sexual inter course)	Cann-i., Nit-ac., sabal.
Back	pain in back after falling into sound sleep	Am-m., kalm., lach.
Back	pain in back after injury	Calc., con., Hyper., kali-c., nat-s., rhus-t., thuj.
Back	pain in back after menses	Berb., bor., calc-p., kali-c., mag-c., puls., verat.
Back	pain in back after midnight	Mag-s.
Back	pain in back after sitting long	Aloe., asaf., berb., calc., cupr-ar., led., lith., ph-ac., phos., Puls., rhod., rhus-t., thuj., valer.
Back	pain in back after stool	Aesc., aloe., alum., asaf., berb., caps., colch., dig., dros., ferr., mag-m., nat-m., podo., puls., rheum., tab.
Back	pain in back after supper	Sulph.
Back	pain in back after urinating	Caust., syph.
Back	pain in back after walking	Alum., nat-c., phos., stry.
Back	pain in back aggravated bending backward	Arg-m., bar-c., calc-p., calc., chel., cimic., con., dios., kali-c., lam., mang., plat., puls., sel., stann.
Back	pain in back aggravated bending forward	Pic-ac.
Back	pain in back aggravated during thunderstorm	Agar., rhod.
Back	pain in back aggravated from coffee	Cham.
Back	pain in back aggravated from jarrying (to have an irritating, unsettling, or unpleasantly disturbing effect on somebody or something)	Acon., Bell., carb-ac., carb-an., Graph., podo., seneg., sep., Sil., sulph., ther., thuj.
Back	pain in back aggravated from laughing	Cann-i., phos., plb., tell.
Back	pain in back aggravated from leaning back against chair	Agar., ther.
Back	pain in back aggravated from lying on left side	Ph-ac.
Back	pain in back aggravated from lying on side	Cina., ign., nat-s., puls., staph.
Back	pain in back aggravated from noise	
Back	pain in back aggravated from noise of running water	Lyss.
Back	pain in back aggravated from pulling	Dios.
Back	pain in back aggravated from warmth of bed	Lil-t., sulph.
Back	pain in back aggravated in warm room	Gels., kali-s.
Back	pain in back alternating with headache	Aloe., brom., meli.
Back	pain in back ameliorated after eating	Kali-n.
Back	pain in back ameliorated after stool	Nux-v., ox-ac., puls.
Back	pain in back ameliorated after urinating	Lyc., med.
Back	pain in back ameliorated bending backward	Acon., aeth., am-m., bell., cycl., eupi., fl-ac., hura., lach., petr., puls., rhus-t., sabad., sabin., sil.
Back	pain in back ameliorated bending forward	Chel., meny., nat-a., ph-ac., puls., sang., sec., sep., thuj.
Back	pain in back ameliorated from erructation	Sep.
Back	pain in back ameliorated from exertion	Ruta., sep.
Back	pain in back ameliorated from external warmth	Calc-f., caust., cinnb., nux-v., Rhus-t.
Back	pain in back ameliorated from flatus	Berb., coc-c., ruta.

Body part/Disease	Symptom	Medicines
Back	pain in back ameliorated from leaning back against chair	Eupi., sarr., zing.
Back	pain in back ameliorated from lying on abdomen	Acet-ac., chel., mag-c., nit-ac., sel.
Back	pain in back ameliorated from lying on back	Ambr., bufo., chin., cob., colch., equis., ign., kali-c., lach., Nat-m., nux-v., phos., puls., rhus-t., Ruta., sanic., sep., sil.
Back	pain in back ameliorated from lying on pillow	Carb-v., sep.
Back	pain in back ameliorated from lying on right side	Kali-n., nat-s., ust.
Back	pain in back ameliorated from lying on side	Kali-n., nat-c., nux-v., puls., zinc.
Back	pain in back ameliorated from lying on something hard	Am-m., bell., kali-c., lyc., Nat-m., puls., rhus-t., sep., stann.
Back	pain in back ameliorated from pressure	Aur., camph., carb-ac., cimic., dulc., fl-ac., Kali-c., led., mag-m., nat-m., ph-ac., plb., rhus-t., ruta., Sep., verat., vib.
Back	pain in back ameliorated from rubbing	Aeth., kali-n., lach., lil-t., nat-s., Phos., plb., puls., thuj.
Back	pain in back ameliorated from straightening up the back	Bov., laur.
Back	pain in back ameliorated from throwing shoulder backward	Cycl.
Back	pain in back ameliorated in cold air	Kali-s.
Back	pain in back ameliorated in open air	Acon., nux-v., vib.
Back	pain in back ameliorated on gentle motion	Bell., calc-f., ferr., kali-p., Puls.
Back	pain in back ameliorated on motion	Aesc., aloe., alum., am-c., am-m., bry., calc-f., calc-p., cina., coloc., cupr., dios., Dulc., fl-ac., graph., kali-c., kali-n., kali-p., kali-s., kreos., lach., laur., Lyc., mag-c., mag-m., mang., nat-a., nat-c., nat-s., nux-m., ox-ac., ph-ac., phos., puls., rat., rhod., Rhus-t., samb., sep., sin-n., spig., staph., stront., sulph., ust., vib.
Back	pain in back ameliorated on rising	Lach., nat-c., nat-m., nit-ac.
Back	pain in back ameliorated when turning in bed	Nat-m.
Back	pain in back ameliorated while lying	Agar., ars., asar., bry., cob., kali-c., nat-m., nux-v., phos., psor., ruta., sars., sil.
Back	pain in back ameliorated while sitting	Aeth., bor., caust., mag-c., meny., mur-ac., plb., sars., staph.
Back	pain in back ameliorated while standing	Arg-n., bell., mur-ac.
Back	pain in back ameliorated while walking	Am-c., ant-c., ap-g., Arg-m., arg-n., arn., ars-m., asar., bar-c., bell., bry., calc-f., cob., Dulc., ferr., gamb., kali-n., kali-s., kreos., mag-s., merc., nat-a., nat-m., nux-v., ph-ac., phos., puls., Rhus-t., ruta., sep., staph., stront., tell., thuj., vib., zinc.
Back	pain in back as if menses would come on	Apis., calc-p., calc., cocc., mosch., vib.
Back	pain in back as if struck with a hammer	Sep.
Back	pain in back ascends (move or climb upward) after lying down	Mag-m.
Back	pain in back ascends and descends	Kali-c.
Back	pain in back ascends during every step	Sep.

Body part/Disease	Symptom	Medicines
Back	pain in back ascends during every stool	Phos., podo.
Back	pain in back ascends during labor	Gels., petr.
Back	pain in back ascends on stooping	Arn., sil.
Back	pain in back ascends while sitting	Meny.
Back	pain in back ascends with constriction of anus	Coloc.
Back	pain in back at night	Acon., agar., aloe., am-m., ang., apis., arg-m., arg-n., ars., berb., bry., calc-s., calc., carb-an., carb-s., carb-v., cham., chel., cinnb., dulc., ferr-ac., ferr-i., ferr-p., ferr., hell., helon., hep., ign., kali-i., kali-n., kalm., kreos., lil-t., lyc., mag-c., mag-m., mag-s., mang., Merc-c., merc., naja., nat-a., nat-c., nat-m., nat-p., nat-s., nit-ac., nux-v., ph-ac., phos., phys., plb., podo., rhod., sars., senec., sil., Sulph., Syph., tab.
Back	pain in back before chill	Aesc., aran., ars., bry., carb-v., daph., dios., eup-per., eup-pur., ip., Podo., rhus-t.
Back	pain in back before menses	Acon., am-c., asar., bar-c., berb., bor., brom., calc., carb-an., caust., cinnb., cocc., dig., eupi., gels., hydr., hyos., hyper., Kali-c., kali-n., kreos., lach., lyc., mag-c., mag-m., nit-ac., nux-m., nux-v., ol-an., phos., plat., podo., Puls., ruta., sang., spong., ust., vib., zinc.
Back	pain in back before midnight	Kalm.
Back	pain in back before sneezing	Anag.
Back	pain in back before stool	Bapt., cic., kali-n., nux-v., petr., puls.
Back	pain in back before urinating	Graph., lyc.
Back	pain in back compelling to remain constantly on bed	Phos., puls., Rhus-t.
Back	pain in back compelling to remain constantly on bed but no relief	Lact., Puls.
Back	pain in back compels turning in bed	Phos., Rhus-t.
Back	pain in back descends (To move downward)	Acon., aeth., alum., am-c., chel., cimic., cina., cocc., con., cur., elaps., ferr-s., glon., kali-bi., kali-c., kalm., lil-t., mag-c., mang., merc., nat-m., nat-s., nux-m., nux-v., ox-ac., phys., phyt., pic-ac., podo., psor., rat., sang., sep., thuj., ust., zing.
Back	pain in back descends after dinner	Agar., cob., indg., phel., phos., sep., sulph.
Back	pain in back descends after eating	Agar., ant-t., bry., cham., cina., daph., kali-c.
Back	pain in back descends after emissions (a bodily discharge, especially of semen)	Ant-c., cob., kali-br., ph-ac., sars., staph.
Back	pain in back descends during labour	Nux-v.
Back	pain in back descends while drinking	Chin.
Back	pain in back descends while eating	Chin., coc-c.
Back	pain in back during chill	Ant-t., apis., arn., ars., bell., Bol., calc., caps., carb-s., carb-v., caust., cham., chin-a., Chin-s., chin., elat., eup-per., gamb., hyos., ign., ip., lach., lact-ac., lyc., mosch., myric., nat-m., Nux-v., phos., podo., puls., sang., sep., sulph., verat., zinc.
Back	pain in back during chill extending to occiput and vertex (Top of head)	Puls.

Body part/Disease	Symptom	Medicines
Back	pain in back during fever	Alst., arn., ars., bell., calc., caps., carb-v., caust., chin-s., chin., cocc., eug., eup-per., hyos., ign., kali-ar., kali-c., lach., laur., lyc., nat-m., nat-s., Nux-v., puls., rhus-t., sulph., ziz.
Back	pain in back during labor	Caust., cocc., coff., Gels., Kali-c., nux-v., petr., Puls.
Back	pain in back during perspiration	Carb-v., Merc.
Back	pain in back during sleep	Am-m., ars., kalm., lach., puls., zinc.
Back	pain in back during stool	Apis., ars., carb-an., colch., coloc., cupr., cycl., dulc., ferr-ar., ferr., kali-i., lyc., manc., nicc., nux-v., phos., podo., puls., rheum., squil., stront., sulph., tab., zing.
Back	pain in back during urinating	Ant-c., ip., kali-bi., phos., sulph.
Back	pain in back extending to abdomen	Cham.
Back	pain in back extending to arms	Calc-ar., calc.
Back	pain in back extending to ears	Gels.
Back	pain in back extending to feet	Bor., sep.
Back	pain in back extending to groin	Sabin., sulph.
Back	pain in back extending to head	Calc., chin-s., hell., nat-m., sep., sil.
Back	pain in back extending to head after exertion	Nat-m.
Back	pain in back extending to head on every step	Sep.
Back	pain in back extending to heels	Colch., sep.
Back	pain in back extending to hips	Bol., cimic., lach., lyss., mosch.
Back	pain in back extending to knees	Arn., kali-c.
Back	pain in back extending to lower extremities	Agar., ars., bell., calc-ar., calc., camph., kali-c., lach., lob-c., phos., Rhus-t.
Back	pain in back extending to neck	Sang.
Back	pain in back extending to occiput	Gels., puls.
Back	pain in back extending to occiput (back of head) vertex (top of head) during chill	Puls.
Back	pain in back extending to pelvis	Eupi.
Back	pain in back extending to sacrum	Con., tep.
Back	pain in back extending to shoulder	Chel., chin., kalm., lyc.
Back	pain in back extending to stomach	Cupr., lyc., nicc., nit-ac., puls., rhod., thuj.
Back	pain in back extending to stomach while sitting	Bry., nicc.
Back	pain in back extending to testes	Sulph.
Back	pain in back extending to thighs	Cimic., kali-c., lyc., nux-v., ox-ac.
Back	pain in back extending toward heart	Nat-m.
Back	pain in back from change to cold weather	Calc-p., Dulc., rhod., rhus-t.
Back	pain in back from exertion	Agar., asaf., calc-p., calc., ox-ac., ruta., stry., sulph.
Back	pain in back from lifting	Anag., bor., Calc., Graph., Lyc., nux-v., ph-ac., Rhus-t., sang., sep.
Back	pain in back from lying on abdomen	Arg-n., ust.
Back	pain in back from lying on back	Am-m., ap-g., apis., bell., berb., bry., carb-an., chin., cina., Coloc., cur., eupho., euphr., hyos., ign., kali-n., lyc., mag-s., nat-m., nit-ac., prun-s., psor., puls., sep., staph., tell., zinc.

Body part/Disease	Symptom	Medicines
Back	pain in back from manual labor	Sulph.
Back	pain in back from mental exertion	Cham., con., nat-c.
Back	pain in back from music	Ambr.
Back	pain in back from pressure	Acon., aesc., agar., ang., arn., canth., chel., chin-s., cocc., colch., coloc., crot-t., hep., lach., phos., plat., plb., ruta., sulph., thuj., verb.
Back	pain in back from prolonged stooping	Nat-m.
Back	pain in back from raising arms	Graph.
Back	pain in back from riding from sitting	Aesc., Agar., alum., ant-c., apis., aran., arg-n., ars., Berb., bry., calc-s., calc., cann-i., canth., carb-an., Caust., con., ferr-p., ferr., iris., kali-bi., kali-p., led., lyc., Merc., merl., petr., Phos., ptel., Puls., rhod., Rhus-t., ruta., sep., sil., staph., Sulph., tab., tell., thuj., tus-p., zinc.
Back	pain in back from riding in carriage	Calc., carb-ac., fl-ac., kali-c., lac-c., Nux-m., petr., sep., sulph., ust.
Back	pain in back from sexual excesses	Ars., calc., carb-v., chin., nat-m., nat-p., Nux-v., Ph-ac., phos., puls., sep., Staph., sulph.
Back	pain in back from stooping	Aesc., agar., am-m., berb., bism., chel., eupi., kali-bi., lach., lyc., med., mur-ac., nat-m., ph-ac., phos., Puls., rhus-t., sars., sil., sulph., verat., zinc.
Back	pain in back from stooping prolonged	Nat-m., Puls.
Back	pain in back from straightening up the back	Aeth., agar., bufo., calc., cann-i., carb-ac., chel., kali-bi., kali-c., lach., nat-c., nat-m., nux-v., psor., sep., sulph., thuj.
Back	pain in back from stretching	Calc., mag-c.
Back	pain in back from suppressed menses	Aesc., am-c., apis., bell., cocc., graph., kali-c., nux-m., nux-v., podo., Puls., sang., sep., sil.
Back	pain in back from taking cold	Dulc., mag-p., nit-ac., sars.
Back	pain in back from yawning (to open the mouth wide and take a long deep breath, usually involuntarily, because of tiredness or boredom)	Calc-p., plat.
Back	pain in back has to sit bent	Kali-c., Sulph.
Back	pain in back in afternoon	Abrot., agar., bov., canth., caust., cham., chel., equis., glon., hyos., mag-c., mag-m., nicc., pall., plb., ptel., rumx., ruta., sep., zing.
Back	pain in back in bed	Ang., berb., carb-v., eupho., hep., kali-n., mag-s., nat-m., nit-ac., petr., puls., rat., rhod., ruta., staph.
Back	pain in back in cold air	Agar., bar-c., dulc., merc., nit-ac., nux-v., rhus-t., sabad., sep.
Back	pain in back in damp weather	Calc., Dulc., nux-m., phyt., rhod., Rhus-t., sep.
Back	pain in back in evening	Acon., agar., alumn., ars., calc-p., carb-v., cham., chel., cist., cocc., coloc., cupr-ar., ferr-i., gels., kali-ar., kali-n., kali-s., kalm., lach., led., lil-t., lyc., mag-c., mag-m., naja., nat-a., nat-m., nat-s., nit-ac., nux-v., phys., psor., rhus-t., ruta., sarr., sep., sin-n., sulph., ter., thuj., zing.

Body part/Disease	Symptom	Medicines
Back	pain in back in forenoon	Ars., cham., equis., nat-m., nat-s., ptel.
Back	pain in back in noon	Dios., eupi., rhus-t.
Back	pain in back must sit up to turn over	Kali-p., Nux-v.
Back	pain in back on appearance of menses	Acon., aloe., asar., berb., caust., nit-ac.
Back	pain in back on beginning to move	Bry., Caps., carb-v., caust., Con., Ferr., kali-p., Lyc., phos., Puls., Rhus-t., sep., sil., tab., zinc.
Back	pain in back on going to sleep	Mag-m.
Back	pain in back on retaining urine	Arn., con., nat-s., rhus-t.
Back	pain in back on rising	Am-m., calad., caust., cedr., graph., hep., lyc., nat-m., nit-ac., ran-b., stann., sulph., thuj., verat.
Back	pain in back on swallowing	Caust., kali-c., raph., rhus-t.
Back	pain in back on waking	Abrot., aesc., Aeth., agar., arg-m., berb., calc-p., cham., chel., grat., hep., kali-bi., lac-c., lach., mag-m., mag-s., myric., nat-m., nit-ac., ptel., puls., ran-b., rhod.
Back	pain in back on waking	Abrot., aesc., arg-m., berb., calc-p., chel., hep., lach., mag-m., mag-s., myric., ptel., puls., rhod.
Back	pain in back until sunrise to sunset	Kalm.
Back	pain in back waking him in midnight	Chin-s., nat-c.
Back	pain in back when breathing	Acon., aesc., alum., alumn., am-m., apis., arn., asar., aur., berb., calc., cann-s., carb-an., carb-s., carb-v., cham., chel., cinnb., Coloc., conv., cop., cupr-ar., cupr., dig., dulc., inul., kali-bi., kali-c., kali-n., kali-p., kali-s., kalm., led., lob., merc., mur-ac., nat-a., nat-c., nat-m., nux-v., par., petr., prun-s., psor., ptel., puls., raph., ruta., sabin., sang., sars., seneg., sep., spig., stann., sulph., thuj.
Back	pain in back when coughing	Acon., am-c., arn., arund., Bell., Bry., calc-s., calc., caps., carb-an., chin-s., chin., cocc., cor-r., kali-bi., kali-c., kali-n., kreos., merc., nit-ac., ph-ac., phos., puls., rhus-t., rumx., seneg., sep., stram., sulph., tell.
Back	pain in back when fasting	Kali-n.
Back	pain in back when kneeling	Euphr., sep.
Back	pain in back when sneezing	Arn., arund., sulph.
Back	pain in back when speaking	Cocc.
Back	pain in back when stepping	Acon., carb-ac., carb-an., sep., spong., sulph., ther., thuj.
Back	pain in back when turning	Agar., am-m., bov., bry., dios., hep., kali-bi., merc., nux-v., sanic., sars., sep., sil., thuj., verat.
Back	pain in back when turning in bed	Acon., bry., calad., hep., ign., kali-bi., kali-n., mag-m., merc., nat-c., nux-v., sep., staph., sulph., zinc.
Back	pain in back while leaning sideways	Thuj.
Back	pain in back while lying	Agar., arn., berb., calc., carb-an., chin., coloc., cur., daph., eupho., ferr., hep., ign., kali-i., kali-n., kreos., lyc., mag-m., naja., nat-m., nux-v., puls., rhus-t., spig., staph., tab., tarax., vib.
Back	pain in back while nursing (breast-feeding)	Cham., crot-t., puls., Sil.

Body part/Disease	Symptom	Medicines
Back	pain in back while sewing	Iris., sec.
Back	pain in back while sitting bent	Chel., chin-s., kali-i., laur., nat-c., phos., ran-b., sec., sep., thuj.
Back	pain in back while sitting erect	Kali-c., spong., Sulph.
Back	pain in back while standing	Agar., agn., asar., berb., bry., calc., cann-i., caps., cocc., coff., con., hep., ign., Ind., kali-bi., kali-c., kali-p., kali-s., lil-t., lith., lyc., meny., merc., mur-ac., nit-ac., petr., ph-ac., phos., plan., plb., podo., puls., rumx., ruta., sep., spong., Sulph., thuj., tus-p., Valer., verat., zinc.
Back	pain in back while walking	Aesc., agar., alum., am-c., am-m., arg-n., arn., asaf., bapt., bell., bor., bry., canth., carb-an., caust., cham., chel., cocc., coff., coloc., con., dios., euphr., ferr-p., ferr., grat., hep., hyos., hyper., iris., kali-bi., Kali-c., kali-p., lyc., mag-m., meny., mez., mur-ac., nat-a., nat-c., nux-v., phos., phyt., plat., podo., psor, Ran-b., rhus-t., ruta., sars., sep., spig., spong., stront., sulph., tab., thuj., verat., zinc., zing.
Back	pain in back with convulsions	Acon.
Back	pain in back with desire to urinate	Clem., eupi., lach., nat-s.
Back	pain in back with dyspnoea	Lyc.
Back	pain in back without fever	Arn., ars., calc., caps., cham., cina., ign., nat-m., nit-ac., nux-v., petr., samb., sep., sil., spig., stram., thuj., verat.
Back	pain in back, sitting long almost impossible	Aesc., agar., am-c., bell., berb., calc., phos., Puls., Rhus-t.
Back	pain in back, standing erect almost impossible after sitting	Thuj.
Back	pain in cervical region extending down the back	Aeth., am-c., chel., cimic., cocc., glon., graph., guai., kalm., lil-t., mag-c., nat-m., phyt., podo., psor., rat., sang., sep., stry., thuj., verat.
Back	pain in cervical region extending down the back on going to stool	Verat.
Back	pain in cervical region while lying on back	Graph., spig.
Back	pain in chest ameliorated while lying on back	Phos.
Back	pain in dorsal (back) region while lying	All-c.
Back	pain in dorsal (back) region while riding	Fl-ac., Ind.
Back	pain in dorsal region aggravated on stepping hard	Seneg.
Back	pain in dorsal region during chill	Chin-s., sang.
Back	pain in dorsal region during labor	Petr.
Back	pain in dorsal region extending to arms & legs	Calc.
Back	pain in dorsal region extending to left nipple	Asaf.
Back	pain in dorsal region extending to near edge of spine	Alumn., card-m., chel., nat-c.
Back	pain in dorsal region extending to occiput	Cocc., Ind., kalm., petr.
Back	pain in dorsal region extending to shoulder	Chel.
Back	pain in dorsal region extending to sternum	Kali-bi., laur.
Back	pain in dorsal region extending to stomach	Bry., rhod.

Body part/Disease	Symptom	Medicines
Back	pain in dorsal region extending to stomach on pressure	Bell.
Back	pain in dorsal region from motion of arm	Ail., con., ruta.
Back	pain in dorsal region from motion of right arm	Chel.
Back	pain in dorsal region from stooping	Jug-c.
Back	pain in dorsal region in right scapula	Aesc., ail., all-c., ambr., anac., arn., cahin., Chel., Coloc., con., cund., jug-c., kali-c., lob., lyc., plb., ran-b., sep., sulph., tell., zinc.
Back	pain in dorsal region in right scapula aggravated from bending forward	Lob.
Back	pain in dorsal region in right scapula ameliorated from bending shoulders backward	Conv.
Back	pain in dorsal region in right scapula then left	Kali-p., tell.
Back	pain in dorsal region on bending backwards	Aur.
Back	pain in dorsal region on bending forward	Cimic.
Back	pain in dorsal region on breathing	Aesc., Apis., berb., bry., chel., kali-c., phys., psor., sulph., thuj.
Back	pain in dorsal region on coughing	Calc., caps., kali-bi., merc., sil., stram.
Back	pain in dorsal region on inspiration	Bry., chel., mur-ac.
Back	pain in dorsal region on motion	Agar., bry., cupr-ar., psor., zinc.
Back	pain in dorsal region on motion of head	Agar., sang.
Back	pain in dorsal region on sitting down	Hura., lach.
Back	pain in dorsal region on turning head	Bry., Ind.
Back	pain in dorsal region on while walking	Agar., bell., coloc., nat-c., psor., seneg., sulph.
Back	pain in dorsal region rheumatic	Cimic., dulc., rhus-t., ruta.
Back	pain in dorsal region when moving	Calc., petr.
Back	pain in dorsal region while sitting down	Arg-m., bry., fl-ac., kali-c., mang., ph-ac., phos., tub.
Back	pain in heart ameliorated from lying on back	Cact., psor.
Back	pain in heart at night when lying down on back	Asaf.
Back	pain in heart extending to back	Aloe., ars-i., Cench., crot-t., glon., kali-c., lil-t., naja., spig., Sulph.
Back	pain in heart from lying on back	Asaf., rumx.
Back	pain in hip extending to back	Fago., rhus-t.
Back	pain in ilium extending up the back	Ars., dirc., nat-a., nux-v.
Back	pain in kidney ameliorated while lying on back	Nux-v.
Back	Pain in kidney compells to lie only on back	Colch.
Back	pain in kidneys while lying	Aeth., berb., colch., coloc., nux-v., rhus-t.
Back	pain in kidneys while lying on back	Chel.
Back	pain in kidneys, can lie only on the back	Colch.
Back	pain in mammae extending to back	Phel., plb.
Back	pain in middle of mammae extending to back	Crot-h.
Back	pain in nose extending to dorsum	Agn., canth., chin., hep., kali-bi., kalm., phos.

Body part/Disease	Symptom	Medicines
Back	pain in sacral region while lying on the back	Bapt., bell., ign., lyc., puls., tell.
Back	pain in soles of foot extending to lumbar region	Plb.
Back	pain in spine on lying down on back	Nat-m.
Back	pain in sternum extending back	Con., Kali-bi., stict.
Back	pain in sternum extending to back	Kali-bi., ox-ac., phyt.
Back	pain in thigh with pain in lumbar region	Am-c.
Back	pain in upper limb extending to back	Ars., caust., dios.
Back	pain in uterus ameliorated from pressure on back	Mag-m.
Back	pain in uterus extending to back	Bell., gels., graph.
Back	pain in uterus extending to back and then to groin	Sabin.
Back	palpitation of heart ameliorated while lying on back	Kalm., lil-t.
Back	palpitation of heart while lying on back	Ammc., arg-m., ars., asaf., aur., cact., kali-n., lach.
Back	paralysis (loss of voluntary movement as a result of damage to nerve or muscle function) of muscles of back	Cupr., gels., led.
Back	paralytic pain in back	Cocc., kalm., nat-m., ran-s., sabin., zinc.
Back	paroxysmal (outburst of symptom) pain in back	Asaf., kalm., lyss., nat-c., pall., phos.
Back	patches (small area) on back	Calc., kali-ar., mez.
Back	patches on back	Graph., kali-n., lyc., phos., sil.
Back	periodical pain in back	Ars., chin-s., kali-s.
Back	persistent cough at midnight aggravated from lying on back and ameliorated from lying on side	Nux-v.
Back	perspiration (sweating) on back on waking	Hep.
Back	perspiration at midnight while lying on the back	Cham.
Back	perspiration on back	Lyc., merc., petr., sulph., thuj.
Back	perspiration on back	Acon., Anac., ars., calc-s., calc., camph., casc., caust., Chin-s., Chin., coff., dig., dulc., guai., hep., hyos., ip., kali-bi., lac-c., lach., laur., led., lyc., morph., mur-ac., nat-c., nat-p., nit-ac., Nux-v., par., petr., ph-ac., phos., puls., rhus-t., sabin., Sep., sil., stann., stram., sulph.
Back	perspiration on back after eating	Card-m., par.
Back	perspiration on back after emission	Sil.
Back	perspiration on back during chill	Cann-s.
Back	perspiration on back during effort at stool	Kali-bi.
Back	perspiration on back during menses	Kreos.
Back	perspiration on back during sleep	Tab.
Back	perspiration on back in morning	Chim.
Back	perspiration on back on motion	Chin.
Back	perspiration on back on walking	Caust., lach., lact-ac., nat-c., petr., phos., rhus-t., sep.
Back	pimples in dorsal region	Am-m., berb., cic., cist.
Back	pimples in evening on back	Cocc., fl-ac., ph-ac., rumx.

Body part/Disease	Symptom	Medicines
Back	polyp (a small stalk-shaped growth sticking out from the skin or from a mucous membrane. Polyps are usually benign, but some become malignant) on back	Con.
Back	prickling feeling in back	Acon., aesc., lact., ox-ac., ran-s.
Back	prickling in back	Acon., agar., ant-t., **Apis.**, bar-c., bell., berb., cann-i., cimic., colch., croc., dros., **Ham.**, kali-ar., **Lob.**, **Lyc.**, mag-m., med., mez., mosch., nat-m., nit-ac., nux-v., **Plat.**, ran-s., **Rhus-t.**, sabad., sep., sul-ac., **Sulph.**, sumb., urt-u., zinc.
Back	prickling on back during sleep	Sol-t-ae.
Back	pulsation (to expand and contract with a strong regular beat) pain in back	Am-c., sil.
Back	pulsation in back from suppressed menses	Puls.
Back	pulsation in dorsal region	Calc-p., carb-s., cur., phos.
Back	pulsation in head from lying on back	Sep.
Back	pulsation on back after emotional excitement	Bar-c.
Back	pulsation on back after stool	Alum., caps.
Back	pulsation on back aggravated from coughing	Nit-ac.
Back	pulsation on back alternating with pain in back	Kali-c.
Back	pulsation on back ameliorated during motion	Bar-c.
Back	pulsation on back during motion	Phos.
Back	pulsation on back while sitting	Calc-p., cur., thuj.
Back	pustules on back	Ant-ox., ant-t., cupr-ar., podo.
Back	red rash on back.	Bry., merc., nit-ac., petr., ph-ac., rhus-v., sep., thuj., zinc.
Back	red spots on back	Ant-c., bell., carb-v., cist., cocc., lach., sep., stann., vip.
Back	respiration arrested while lying on back	Sil.
Back	restlessness aggravated on lying on back	Calc-p.
Back	rheumatic pain in back	Acon., ambr., anac., ant-t., ars., asar., aspar., aur., bapt., bar-c., bell., Bry., calc-p., calc., calen., carb-v., cham., chel., Cimic., colch., com., corn., cycl., dros., dulc., ferr., graph., guai., hep., kali-bi., kali-i., lach., lyc., lycps., med., mez., Nux-v., ol-an., petr., phyt., puls., ran-b., Rhod., Rhus-t., ruta., sang., squil., stram., sulph., teucr., ust., valer., verat., zinc.
Back	shaking chill whole day with drawing pains in throat and back	Verat.
Back	shivering extending down the back	Agar., all-c., bry., calc-caust., chel., colch., mag-c., rhus-v.
Back	shivering extending up the back	Canth., dig., puls., rhus-v.
Back	sleeps on back	Acon., aloe., ambr., ant-c., ant-t., apis., arn., ars., aur., bism., **Bry.**, calc., chin., cic., coca., colch., coloc., dig., dros., ferr., hell., hep., ign., kali-p., kreos., lac-c., lyc., mang., med., **Merc-c.**, mez., nat-m., nux-v., op., ox-ac., par, phos., plat., **Puls.**, rhod., **Rhus-t.**, ruta., sabad., sars., sol-n., spig., stann., stram., sulph., verat., viol-o., zinc.
Back	sleeps on back with hand flat over the head	Lac-c.
Back	sleeps on back with hand flat under occiput	Ars., ing., nux-v.
Back	sleeps on back with head low	Dig., nux-v.

Body part/Disease	Symptom	Medicines
Back	smarting (sharp stinging localized pain) with eruption on back	Bry., spig.
Back	spasms in back	Acon., ars., calc-p., crot-c., lach., mygal., nat-m., nat-s., nux-v., oena., phys., stram., syph., tab.
Back	spasms in back on touch	Acon.
Back	spasms in back while nursing	Arn., cham., puls.
Back	spots on back	Calc., cist., lach., lyc., sep., spong., sulph., sumb., zinc.
Back	stiffness (rigid) in back after exertion	Lyc.
Back	stiffness in back after sitting after	Am-m., Ambr., bar-c., bell., caust., cham., con., cupr-ar., Ind., led., phos., Rhus-t., sil., sulph.
Back	stiffness in back after stool	Sep.
Back	stiffness in back after stooping	Bov.
Back	stiffness in back aggravated from standing erect	Bry.
Back	stiffness in back ameliorated from sitting bent	Anac.
Back	stiffness in back ameliorated from walking	Bry., calc-s., cop., Rhus-t., sep., sulph.
Back	stiffness in back ameliorated on moving	Rhus-t., sul-ac.
Back	stiffness in back at night	Lyc.
Back	stiffness in back cramp like	Nit-ac.
Back	stiffness in back during chill	Lyc., nat-s., tub.
Back	stiffness in back from a draft	Rhus-t.
Back	stiffness in back from standing	Stry.
Back	stiffness in back from stooping	Berb., caps., cic., kali-c.
Back	stiffness in back from turning in bed	Sulph.
Back	stiffness in back from walking	Aur., stry.
Back	stiffness in back from writing	Laur.
Back	stiffness in back in evening	Bar-c., dios., lyc., petr.
Back	stiffness in back in morning	Ang., carb-v., ox-ac., phyt., sep., stry., sul-ac., zinc.
Back	stiffness in back in morning ameliorated on rising in bed	Anac.
Back	stiffness in back in morning on rising	Bar-c., calc-s., carb-v., ferr-i., ign., staph., sul-ac.
Back	stiffness in back in morning on waking	Calc., lach., led., sep.
Back	stiffness in back in noon	Valer.
Back	stiffness in back in wet weather	Phyt., Rhus-t.
Back	stiffness in back lying while	Puls.
Back	stiffness in back must walk about some time before he can straighten up	Hydr.
Back	stiffness in back on moving	Acon., aesc., calc., cupr-ar., guai.
Back	stiffness in back on rising	Agar., bry., cham.
Back	stiffness in back on rising from a seat	Agar., am-m., Ambr., anac., bar-c., Bell., berb., bry., carl., Caust., hydr., Ind., led., lyc., petr., puls., Rhus-t., sil., sulph.
Back	stiffness in back painful	Am-m., calc., Caust., helon., manc., nit-ac., puls., Rhus-t.

Body part/Disease	Symptom	Medicines
Back	stiffness in cervical region while lying on back	Spig.
Back	stitching pain in chest extending to back	Alumn., arum-t., bov., chel., chen-a., guai., kali-c., kali-n., lyc., mez., ox-ac., par., sil.
Back	stitching pain in chest extending to back aggravated from lying on left side	Kali-c.
Back	swelling in dorsal region	Am-m., Calc., carb-an., kali-c., lyc., sil., spig., spong.
Back	tension in dorsal region	Aur-m., crot-c., lyc., mag-s., rhus-t., zinc.
Back	tension in dorsal region ameliorated from walking	Mag-s.
Back	tension in dorsal region below scapula from raising arm	Con.
Back	tension in dorsal region between scapula	Colch., ferr., hep., nat-c., nux-v., zinc.
Back	tension in dorsal region between scapula after excitement	Phos.
Back	tension in dorsal region between scapula from lying	Sulph.
Back	tension in dorsal region between scapula from moving	Sulph.
Back	tension in dorsal region in scapula	Alum., bar-c., Carb-an., cic., colch., coloc., con., kali-c., lyc., mag-m., merc-c., merc., mez., mur-ac., nat-c., nux-v., op., rhus-t., sep., sil., sulph., zinc.
Back	tension in dorsal region in scapula from turning the head	Caust., merc.
Back	tension in dorsal region in scapula in evening	Sep.
Back	tension in muscles of back	Aeth., agar., am-m., arg-n., ars., bar-c., berb., bry., coloc., con., hep., ign., lil-t., lyc., med., mez., mosch., nat-c., nat-m., ol-an., olnd., puls., rat., sars., sep., sulph., tarax., teucr., thuj., zinc.
Back	tension in muscles of back aggravated from lying on other side	Sep.
Back	tension in muscles of back ameliorated during motion	Am-m.
Back	tension in muscles of back at night	Nat-c.
Back	tension in muscles of back before dinner	Nicc.
Back	tension in muscles of back during motion	Colch.
Back	tension in muscles of back extending to anus while lying and sitting	Nat-c.
Back	tension in muscles of back extending to chest aggravated from stooping	Chel.
Back	tension in muscles of back extending to neck	Laur.
Back	tension in muscles of back from moving arm	Sulph.
Back	tension in muscles of back in forenoon	Bry.
Back	tension in muscles of back on attempting to straighten up	Bell.
Back	tension in muscles of back on standing	Ign.
Back	tension in muscles of back on turning the body	Hep.
Back	tension in muscles of back while sitting	Am-m., nat-c.
Back	tension in muscles of back while sitting bent	Sulph.

Body part/Disease	Symptom	Medicines
Back	tension in right side of muscles of back	Sep.
Back	tubercles on back	Am-c., lach., lyc., mur-ac., nicc., ph-ac., phos., sec.
Back	tubercles on back	Am-c., am-m., caust., lyc., nicc., squil.
Back	twitching in back on opening the mouth	Stry.
Back	twitching in back while lying on back	Agar.
Back	twitching in dorsal region	Nit-ac., stry.
Back	twitching in dorsal region from manual labour	Nit-ac.
Back	twitching in dorsal region in scapula	Calc-p., calc., lyc., merc., mez., nat-c., phos., rhus-t., sep., squil., thuj.
Back	twitching in right back	Calc.
Back	ulcerative pain in back	Kreos., puls.
Back	ulcer in back	Cist., merc-c.
Back	ulcer in sacrum burn like fire	Ars.
Back	vertigo ameliorated while lying on back	Stram.
Back	vesicles on back	Ars., bov., clem., crot-h., kali-bi., olnd., psor., sep., sulph., tell., tep.
Back	vesicles on back when warm	Cocc., stram.
Back	wandering pain in back	Ang., chel., cimic., dros., kali-s., mag-p., sang., sec., senec., tarent.
Back	warts on back	Nit-ac., sil., thuj.
Back	weakness ameliorated from lying on back	Cast.
Back	weakness extending through back during chill	Thuj.
Back	weakness from pain in stomach & back	Sep.
Back	weakness in back after mental exertion	Calc.
Back	weakness in back after sitting	Sil.
Back	weakness in back after stool	Sumb.
Back	weakness in back after typhoid fever	Sel.
Back	weakness in back after walking	Bapt., petr.
Back	weakness in back aggravated from eating	Nat-m.
Back	weakness in back ameliorated from lying down	Casc., nat-m.
Back	weakness in back ameliorated while walking	Hydr.
Back	weakness in back at night	Petr.
Back	weakness in back from emissions	Sel.
Back	weakness in back from leucorrhoea	Graph.
Back	weakness in back from lying down	Cic., phos.
Back	weakness in back from manual labour	Lach., Nat-m., sil.
Back	weakness in back from riding	Calc-s.
Back	weakness in back from sexual excesses	Agar., calc., nat-m., Nux-v., Ph-ac., phos., Sel.
Back	weakness in back from writing	Lyc.
Back	weakness in back in evening	Nat-p.
Back	weakness in back in forenoon	Calc-s.

Body part/Disease	Symptom	Medicines
Back	weakness in back in morning	Coloc., dios., ox-ac., pall., ther.
Back	weakness in back in morning on rising	Nat-m.
Back	weakness in back on deep breathing	Carb-v.
Back	weakness in back on motion of arms	Clem., par., sil.
Back	weakness in back while sitting	Agar., Calc., cic., graph., lyss., Sulph., Zinc.
Back	weakness in back while walking	Graph., sabad., sep., Sulph.
Back	weakness in back with standing almost impossible	Sul-ac.
Back	weakness in dorsal region between scapula	Agar., sarr.
Back	weakness in dorsal region between scapula ameliorated from leaning on something	Sarr.
Back	weakness in dorsal region in scapula ameliorated from stooping	Alumn.
Back	whistling breath while lying on the back	Aeth.
Bad News	Ailments from bad news	Apis., calc-p., Calc., chin., cinnb., cupr., dros., form., Gels., ign., kali-c., kali-p., lach., lyss., med., nat-m., nat-p., paeon., pall., phos., puls., stram., sulph.
Beard	sycosis (inflammation of hair follicles, especially of the beard marked by pustules and encrustations)	Agar., alum., alumn., anac., ant-c., ant-t., apis., aran., **Arg-m.**, **Arg-n.**, aster., aur-m., aur., bar-c., bry., calc., carb-an., carb-s., carb-v., caust., cham., cinnb., con., dulc., euphr., ferr., fl-ac., graph., hep., iod., kali-c., **Kali-s.**, lach., lyc., mang., **Med.**, merc., mez., **Nat-s.**, **Nit-ac.**, petr., phyt., puls., sabin., sars., sec., sel., **Sep.**, sil., **Staph.**, sulph., **Thuj.**
Beat Rapidly	fluttering (beat rapidly because of a medical disorder or because of nervousness or excitement) in chest after dinner	Sep.
Beat Rapidly	fluttering between shoulders	Cupr.
Beat Rapidly	fluttering commencing in sacrum and gradually rising to occiput	Ol-j.
Beat Rapidly	fluttering in chest after menses	Spig.
Beat Rapidly	fluttering in chest after slight excitement	Aml-n., Lil-t., lith.
Beat Rapidly	fluttering in chest alternating with soreness	Aur-m.
Beat Rapidly	fluttering in chest ameliorated in open air	Nat-m., Nat-s.
Beat Rapidly	fluttering in chest at night	Naja.
Beat Rapidly	fluttering in chest during rest	Lil-t.
Beat Rapidly	fluttering in chest from ascending steps	Bry., Calc.
Beat Rapidly	fluttering in chest in afternoon during headache	Form., sumb.
Beat Rapidly	fluttering in chest in evening	Pic-ac.
Beat Rapidly	fluttering in chest in morning	Naja., stry.
Beat Rapidly	fluttering in chest on raising arms	Dig., sulph.
Beat Rapidly	fluttering in chest on waking	Kali-i., naja.
Beat Rapidly	fluttering in chest wakens her at night	Lil-t.
Beat Rapidly	fluttering in chest while on left side	Daph., dig., gels., nat-m., spig.
Beat Rapidly	fluttering in chest while on right side	Alumn.

Body part/Disease	Symptom	Medicines
Beat Rapidly	fluttering in chest while sitting	Asaf.
Beat Rapidly	fluttering in chest while thinking of it	Arg-n.
Beat Rapidly	fluttering in chest while writing	Naja.
Beat Rapidly	fluttering in thigh	Cench.
Beat Rapidly	fluttering in upper arm	Phyt.
Beat Rapidly	fluttering sensation in region of kidneys	Chim.
Beat Rapidly	fluttering sensation in the region of kidney	Chim.
Bed Wetting	dysuria alternating with bed wetting	Gels.
Bile	urine containig bile (a yellowish green fluid produced in the liver, stored in the gallbladder, and passed through ducts to the small intestine, where it plays an essential role in emulsifying fats)	Acon., card-m., chel., Chion., con., crot-h., cupr-s., kali-i., mag-m., merc., myric., nat-s., nit-ac., osm., phos., sang., sep., sulph., uran., valer.
Bile	vomiting bile (a yellowish green fluid produced in the liver, stored in the gall bladder, and passed through ducts to the small intestine, where it plays an essential role in emulsifying fats) then blood	Agar., carb-v., verat.
Bile	vomiting bile after eating sweets	Iris.
Bile	vomiting bile during fever	Ars., bry., cham., chin., cina., crot-h., cupr., dros., Eup-per., ign., ip., iris., merc., nat-m., nux-v., op., phos., psor., puls., sec., sep., sulph., thuj., verat.
Bile	vomiting bile then food	Bry.
Bile	vomiting bile with colic	Chin., coloc., iod., nux-v.
Bile	vomiting bile with headache	Arg-n., aur., bry., cadm., calc., Chel., crot-h., eup-per., Ip., Iris., lac-d., lept., lob., nat-m., nat-s., nicc., petr., plb., puls., rhus-t., Sang., spig., sulph., verat., zinc.
Bile	vomiting food then bile	Ant-t., bell., bry., colch., dig., nat-m., samb.
Black Head	comedones (a small plug of dark fatty matter blocking a follicle on the skin, especially on the face / Blackhead) on nose	Dros., graph., nit.ac., sabin., sel., sulph., sumb., tub.
Black Head	comedones on chin and upper lip	Sulph.
Black Head	comedones on chin	Dros., tub.
Black Head	comedones on forehead	Sulph.
Black Head	comedones ulcerating	Dig., sel., tub.
Black Head	eruption, pimples with black head in upper limbs	Calc-s.
Bladder	bleeding haemorrhoids in bladder	Ars., Calc., carb-v., ferr., ham., lyc., merc., nit-ac., nux-v.
Bladder	calculi after operation of bladder	Arn., calen., cham., chin., cupr., nux-v., Staph., verat.
Bladder	calculi in bladder	Ant-c., arg-n., Benz-ac., Berb., cact., Calc., Canth., card-m., chin., coc-c., colch., eup-per., lach., lith., Lyc., mez., mill., naja., nat-m., nat-s., nit-ac., nux-m., nux-v., pareir., petr.,phos., puls., raph., ruta., Sars., Sep., sil., tarent., thuj., zinc.
Bladder	chill beginning in and extending from neck of bladder after urinating	Sars.
Bladder	chill in after urination begins in neck of bladder and spreads upwards	Sars.

Body part/Disease	Symptom	Medicines
Bladder	chills spread from the neck of the bladder after urinating	Sars.
Bladder	cold sensation in bladder	Lyss.
Bladder	cold sensation in bladder alternating with heat	Coc-c.
Bladder	constriction in bladder	Alum., berb., cact., caps., caust., chel., cocc., cub., dig., hydrc., lyc., petr., ph-ac., puls., sars., thuj., verat.
Bladder	constriction in bladder after urination	Cub., nat-m.
Bladder	constriction in bladder during urination	Berb., bry., dig., petr., thuj.
Bladder	constriction in neck of bladder	Ant-c., cact., canth., caps., colch., con., elaps., kali-i., mag-p., op., paeon., petr., phos., plb., ruta., sulph.
Bladder	constriction in neck of bladder after urination	Bry., cann-s., cub., sulph.
Bladder	constriction in neck of bladder during urination	Colch., kali-i., petr., polyg-h.
Bladder	cramp (Painful muscle contraction) in bladder	Berb., caps., carb-s., carb-v., coc-c., mag-p., nux-v., ph-ac., plb., prun-s., ruta., sars., sep., zinc.
Bladder	cramp in bladder	Berb., caps., carb-s., carb-v., coc-c., mag-p., nux-v., ph-ac., plb., prun-s., ruta., sars., sep., zinc.
Bladder	cramp in bladder after urination	Caust., nat-m.
Bladder	cramp in bladder during urination	Carb-s.
Bladder	dysuria painful, from spasm of bladder	Colch.
Bladder	dysuria with violent pain in bladder	Calc-p.
Bladder	forcible retention seems to paralyze the bladder	Ars., canth., Caust., gels., hell., hyos., rhus-t., ruta.
Bladder	fungoid growths in bladder	Calc.
Bladder	gangrene in bladder	Canth.
Bladder	gangrene in bladder	Canth.
Bladder	gas passes from bladder	Sars.
Bladder	haemorrhage from bladder	Crot-h., erig., ferr-p., ham., lyc., phos., sec.
Bladder	haemorrhage from urethra with pains in kidneys and bladder	Ip., puls.
Bladder	haemorrhage in bladder	Crot-h., erig., ferr-p., ham., lyc., phos., sec.
Bladder	haemorrhoids, bladder	Acon., ant-c., bor., canth., carb-v., eupho., ham., nux-v., puls., sulph.
Bladder	heat in bladder	All-c., canth., puls., senec.
Bladder	heat in kidneys extending to bladder	Aur.
Bladder	heat in kidneys extending to region of bladder	Aur., Berb., cimic., helon., nat-m., phos., phyt., plb., ter.
Bladder	heat in kidneys extending to region of bladder while sitting	Nat-m.
Bladder	heaviness in bladder	Cann-s., canth., coc-c., dig., kali-i., lyc., nat-m., sep.
Bladder	heaviness in bladder	Cann-s., canth., coc-c., dig., kali-i., lyc., nat-m., sep.
Bladder	hemorrhage from urethra, with pain in bladder & kidney	Ip., puls.
Bladder	inactivity of bladder	Ars., Caust., op., plb.
Bladder	inflammation of bladder , after suppression of menses or hæmorrhoidal flow	Nux-v.

Body part/Disease	Symptom	Medicines
Bladder	inflammation of bladder after scarlatina	Canth.
Bladder	inflammation of bladder from taking cold	Dulc., sulph.
Bladder	inflammation of bladder with pus like discharge after lithotomy	Mill.
Bladder	inflammation of bladder with violent pain and almost clear blood	Nit-ac.
Bladder	inflammation of bladder, after injuries	Arn., staph.
Bladder	insensibility of bladder with violent pain and almost clear blood	Ham.
Bladder	itching in region of bladder with urge to urinate aggravated at night	Sep.
Bladder	muco-pus discharge from bladder from suppressed gonorrhoea	Benz-ac., cub., med., puls., sil., thuj.
Bladder	muco-pus discharge from bladder in old people	Alumn., carb-v., sulph., ter.
Bladder	pain in abdomen extendimg to bladder and testes	Kali-c.
Bladder	pain in bladder after a few drops pass	Berb., calc-p., Canth., caust., fl-ac., lith.
Bladder	pain in bladder after coition	All-c.
Bladder	pain in bladder after lithotomy (surgical removal of stone)	Staph.
Bladder	pain in bladder after urination	Brach., lith., sep.
Bladder	pain in bladder aggravated from drinking	Canth.
Bladder	pain in bladder aggravated from standing	Puls.
Bladder	pain in bladder ameliorated after start of urine	Prun-s.
Bladder	pain in bladder ameliorated from lying on abdomen	Chel.
Bladder	pain in Bladder ameliorated in bed in evening	Alum.
Bladder	pain in bladder before urinating	Berb., fl-ac., lith., manc., nux-v., pall., phyt., prun-s.
Bladder	pain in bladder during menses	Sep.
Bladder	pain in bladder during urging to urinate	Berb., calc-p., eup-pur., hell., nux-v., phyt., puls., rhod., rhus-t., ruta., sul-ac., zinc.
Bladder	pain in bladder during urination	Ant-t., brach., calc-p., calc., carb-v., dig., fl-ac., indg., lil-t., manc., phyt., puls., rhus-a.
Bladder	pain in bladder extending to kidney	Aesc., apis., canth.
Bladder	pain in bladder extending to spermatic cords	Anth., lith.
Bladder	pain in bladder extending to thighs	Puls.
Bladder	pain in bladder extending to uterus	Merl., tarent.
Bladder	pain in bladder from taking cold	Dulc., eup-pur.
Bladder	pain in bladder when beginning to urinate	Acon., apis., ars., cann-s., Canth., caust., Clem., cop., manc., Merc.
Bladder	pain in bladder when coughing	Caps.
Bladder	pain in bladder while sitting	Card-m.
Bladder	pain in bladder with burning after urination	Alum., apis., berb., calc-p., canth., fl-ac., lyc., sep., sil., thuj.
Bladder	pain in bladder with burning aggravated by standing	Eup-pur.

Body part/Disease	Symptom	Medicines
Bladder	pain in bladder with burning ameliorated by walking in open air	Ter.
Bladder	pain in bladder with burning at night	Bell.
Bladder	pain in bladder with burning before urination	Apis., berb., bor., bry., calc., cann-i., canth., caps., chel., clem., colch., fl-ac., lach., nat-c., rheum., rhod., seneg., thuj., zinc.
Bladder	pain in bladder with burning during menses	Sep.
Bladder	pain in bladder with burning during urination	Aloe., canth., caps., cham., eup-pur., kali-bi., lyc., nux-v., phos., prun-s., rheum., ter.
Bladder	pain in bladder with burning while lying	Fl-ac.
Bladder	pain in heart after pain in bladder	Lith.
Bladder	pain in ilium extending to bladder and groin (area between thighs and abdomen)	Bell.
Bladder	pain in kidney extending over bladder	Arg-n., ars., bell., berb., canth., chel., coc-c., kali-i., lyc., nit-ac., oci., petr., phyt., sars., tab.
Bladder	pain in kidneys extending to bladder	Arg-n., ars., bell., berb., canth., chel., coc-c., kali-i., lyc., nit-ac., oci., petr., phyt., sars., tab.
Bladder	pain, cutting in bladder at close of urination	Nat-c., petr., sars., thuj.
Bladder	pain, cutting in bladder before urination	Bry., calc-p., dig., mag-p., manc., ph-ac., phyt., sulph., thuj.
Bladder	pain, cutting in bladder after urination	Calc-p., canth., cub., nat-c., petr., phos., polyg-h.
Bladder	pain, cutting in bladder aggravated from rest	Ter.
Bladder	pain, cutting in bladder aggravated from walking	Mang., thuj.
Bladder	pain, cutting in bladder ameliorated in open air	Ter.
Bladder	pain, cutting in bladder during urination	Calc., canth., eup-pur., kali-c., nat-c., polyg-h., sec., ter., thuj.
Bladder	pain, cutting in bladder while standing	Mang.
Bladder	pain, stitching in kidneys extending to bladder	Arg-n., bell., Berb., coc-c., cupr-ac., Kali-bi., lach., oci.
Bladder	paralysis of bladder after no desire to give birth	Ars., canth., Caust., ferr., hyos., kreos., nux-v., phos., zinc.
Bladder	paralysis of bladder after over distension	Ars., canth., Caust., hell., hyos., nux-v., rhus-t., ruta., stry., sulph.
Bladder	paralysis of bladder from forceful retention	Ars., canth., Caust., gels., hell., hyos., rhus-t., ruta.
Bladder	paralysis of bladder in hysterical subjects	Zinc.
Bladder	paralysis of bladder in old people	Ars., cann-s., cic., con., equis., gels., kali-p., sec., thuj.
Bladder	paralysis of bladder with weakness, fears he will wet the bed in evening	Alum.
Bladder	polyp in bladder	Ant-c., Calc., con., graph., lyc., merc., phos., puls., sil., Teucr., thuj.
Bladder	retention of urine from clots in the bladder	Cact., caust.
Bladder	sensation of contraction in bladder	Ant-c., berb., carb-s., coc-c., hyos., kali-i., lyc., mez., op., petr., ruta., verat.
Bladder	sensation of emptyness bladder	Colch., dig., stram., sumb.
Bladder	sensation of fullness in bladder after urination	Alumn., calc., con., conv., Dig., eup-pur., gnaph., lac-c., lycps., merc., ruta., sars., staph., sulph.

Body part/Disease	Symptom	Medicines
Bladder	sensation of fullness in bladder after urination without desire to urinate	Ars., calad., Caust., fl-ac., hell., op., pall., phos., stann., stram., verat.
Bladder	sensation of stone in bladder	Puls.
Bladder	sensation of worms in bladder	Bell., sep.
Bladder	sensatisons in bladdser as if twisting	Agar., bell.
Bladder	shocks like electric in bladder extending to right thigh	All-c., rhus-t.
Bladder	suppuration from bladder	Canth., sars., ter.
Bladder	swelling in region of the neck of bladder	Puls.
Bladder	swelling in the region of bladder	Puls.
Bladder	tenesmus (an urgent, painful, and unsuccessful attempt to defecate or urinate) of bladder after stool	Canth.
Bladder	tenesmus in bladder after urination	Ferr., squil.
Bladder	tenesmus in bladder with icy cold feet	Elaps.
Bladder	tenesmus in blsadder during menses	Tarent.
Bladder	thickening of walls of bladder	Dulc., pareir.
Bladder	tumours in bladder	Calc.
Bladder	ulcerations in bladder	All-s., canth., eup-pur., merc-c., merc-i-r., ran-b.
Bladder	ulcerations in bladder caused by calculi	All-s.
Bladder	unsatisfactory, as if bladder were not emptied with dribbling	Staph.
Bladder	urging to urinate absent in bladder with distended bladder	Ars., calad., Caust., fl-ac., hell., hyos., op., pall., phos., plb., stann., verat.
Bladder	urging to urinate absent in bladder after menses	Cham., puls.
Bladder	urging to urinate absent in bladder with distended bladder but urine flows freely	Phos.
Bladder	urging to urinate in bladder absent	Ars., bell., calad., Caust., ferr., hell., hyos., lac-c., op., ox-ac., pall., phos., plb., stann., verat.
Bladder	urging to urinate in bladder before menses	Alum., apis., asar., kali-c., Kali-i., nux-v., phos., puls., sars., sulph.
Bladder	urging to urinate in bladder on touching abdomen	Acon.
Bladder	urging to urinate in bladder on waking	Ant-t., caust., dig., eupho., hep., mag-m., murx., sil., staph.
Bladder	urging to urinate in bladder when passing flatus	Puls.
Bladder	urging to urinate in bladder without passing any, the while sitting flows involuntary	Caust.
Bladder	urging to urinate in blasser with menses suppressed	Canth., cham., dig., dros., gels., ign., nat-m., Puls., sulph.
Bladder	urinate five or six times before the bladder is empty	Thuj.
Bladder	urination ineffectual in bladder but as soon as he ceases to strain stool and urine pass involuntarily	Arg-n.
Bladder	urination ineffectual in bladder during standing but while sitting urine flows involuntarily	Caust.

Body part/Disease	Symptom	Medicines
Bladder	urination ineffectual in bladder only a few drops pass until the next stool, when it flows freely	All-s., am-m.
Bladder	urination pain disappears from bladder when menstrual flow starts	Kali-i.
Bladder	urination painful in bladder during perspiration	Ant-t., apis., arn., Bry., canth., caust., dulc., graph., hell., hyos., lyc., Merc., mur-ac., nux-v., ph-ac., phos., puls., rhus-t., squil., staph., sulph., Thuj.
Bleeding	bleeding eczema on face	Alum., ars., dulc., hep., lyc., merc., petr., psor., sep., sulph.
Bleeding	bleeding from eyes	Acon., aloe., am-c., am-caust., arn., bell., Both., calc., camph., carb-v., cham., cor-r., Crot-h., dig., elaps., euphr., kali-chl., Lach., nit-ac., Nux-v., Phos., plb., raph., ruta., sulph.
Bleeding	bleeding from eyes, from blowing nose	Nit-ac.
Bleeding	bleeding from face when scratched	Merc., mez., par., petr., rhus-t., sulph.
Bleeding	bleeding from gums around decayed tooth during menses	Bell.
Bleeding	bleeding from gums around decayed tooth from suppressed menses	Calc.
Bleeding	bleeding from gums in scurvy (vitamin C deficiency which include spongy gums, loosening of the teeth, and bleeding into the skin and mucous membranes)	Ant-t., Ars., carb-an., mur-ac., nat-m., nux-v., sulph.
Bleeding	bleeding from mouth in scarlet fever (Bacterial infection marked by fever, a sore throat, and a red rash, mainly affecting children)	Arum-t.
Bleeding	bleeding from mouth in whooping cough	Cor-r., dros., ip., nux-v.
Bleeding	bleeding from mouth that coagulates (becomes semi solid) easily	Hep., lach., Phos.
Bleeding	bleeding from palate , purpura (bleeding under the skin causes purplish blotches to appear on the skin)	Crot-h., lach., phos., ter.
Bleeding	bleeding from scales after scratching	Lyc.
Bleeding	bleeding from scrotum (the external pouch of skin and muscle containing the testes)	Petr.
Bleeding	bleeding from tongue	Anan., arg-m., ars., Arum-t., Bor., bry., cadm., calc., caps., cham., chlol., clem., cur., guare., kali-bi., kali-chl., lach., lact-ac., lyc., med., merc., nat-m., nat-p., nit-ac., nux-v., phos., podo., sars., sec., sep., spig., ter.
Bleeding	bleeding from ulcer of foot	Ars.
Bleeding	bleeding from ulcer on penis	Cor-r., hep., Merc., nit-ac., staph.
Bleeding	bleeding from varices (swollen or knotted vein) of leg	Ham., puls.
Bleeding	bleeding haemorrhoids in bladder	Ars., Calc., carb-v., ferr., ham., lyc., merc., nit-ac., nux-v.
Bleeding	bleeding of black blood from gums when tooth is extracted	Ars.
Bleeding	bleeding of black blood from mouth	Carb-v., crot-h., lach.
Bleeding	bleeding of clotted blood from mouth	Canth., caust., coch.

Body part/Disease	Symptom	Medicines
Bleeding	Cerebral (the front part of the brain, divided into two symmetrical halves cerebral hemispheres. In humans, it is where activities including reasoning, learning, sensory perception, and emotional responses take place) Hemorrhage	Acon., arn., aur., bar-c., Bell., camph., carb-v., chin., coff., Colch., con., crot-h., cupr., ferr., Gels., hyos., Ip., Lach., laur., lyc., merc., nat-m., nit-ac., nux-m., nux-v., Op., phos., plb., puls., stram.
Bleeding	continuous bleeding from mouth that does not coagulate	Anthr., crot-h.
Bleeding	detatched gums from teeth bleeding easily	Ant-c., Carb-v., phos.
Bleeding	Eruption on head, bleeding after scratching	Alum., ars., bov., calc., cupr-ar., dulc., lach., lyc., merc., nat-a., petr., psor., staph., Sulph.
Bleeding	eruption, bleeding	Calc.
Bleeding	eruption, bleeding after scratching	Cupr-ar.
Bleeding	eruption, bleeding after scratching on upper limbs	Cupr-ar.
Bleeding	eruption, bleeding in foot	Calc.
Bleeding	eruption, bleeding in hands	Alum., lyc., merc., petr.
Bleeding	eruption, elevated bleeding after scratching in upper limbs	Cupr-ar.
Bleeding	eruption, pimples bleeding when scratched in upper limbs	Cob.
Bleeding	eruption, pimples bleeds after scratched in shoulder	Cob., mosch.
Bleeding	eruption, pimples in legs bleeding easily	Agar.
Bleeding	eruption, with petechiæ (a small red or purple spot on the skin caused by minor bleed from tiny blood vessels	Ars., aur-m., berb.
Bleeding	eruptions bleeding	Alum., ant-t., apis., ars., calc., dulc., eupho., hep., kali-ar., kali-c., kali-n., lach., lyc., med., merc-c., **Merc.**, nit-ac., olnd., par., petr., psor., sep., **Sulph.**
Bleeding	eruptions bleeding after scratching	Alum., ars., bov., calc., chin., cocc., cupr-ar., dulc., lach., lyc., nux-v., petr., psor., **Sulph.,** til.
Bleeding	eruptions carbuncle crusty bleeding	Merc., mez.
Bleeding	eruptions carbuncle dry bleeding after scratching	Alum., ars., calc., lyc., petr., sulph.
Bleeding	eruptions herpetic bleeding	Anac., dulc., lyc.
Bleeding	eruptions itching patches bleeding after scratches	**Sulph.**
Bleeding	eruption, pimples bleeding	Cist., par., rhus-t., stront., thuj.
Bleeding	eruption, pustules bleeding	Ant-t.
Bleeding	eruptions, bleeding after scratching in lower limbs	Calc., cupr.
Bleeding	eruptions, bleeding pimples in lower limbs	Agar., thea.
Bleeding	excrescences bleeding	Merc., thuj.
Bleeding	extravasation (to leak, or cause blood or other fluid to leak, from a vessel into surrounding tissue as a result of injury, burns, or inflammation) of blood in lumbar region	Crot-h.
Bleeding	exudation (release through pores or cut) in valves (a membranous structure in a hollow organ or vessel such as the heart or a vein that prevents the return flow of fluid passing through it by folding or closing) of heart	Spong.

Body part/Disease	Symptom	Medicines
Bleeding	fissures on face bleeding	Petr.
Bleeding	growth resembling a wart bleed easily	Calc., cinnb., med., mill., Nit-ac., sulph., thuj.
Bleeding	growth resembling a wart bleeds when touched	Cinnb., Nit-ac., thuj.
Bleeding	growth resembling a wart on penis bleeding	Cinnb., Nit-ac., sulph., thuj.
Bleeding	gums bleeding when scratched	Am-c.
Bleeding	itching in toes scratch until they must bleed	Arg-m.
Bleeding	itching of Scalp, must scratch until bleed	Alum., bov., carb-an., mur-ac., sabad.
Bleeding	large quantity of blood oozes on pressing the gums with fingers	Bapt., graph.
Bleeding	lips bleeding	Aloe., am-c., ars., Arum-t., brom., bry., carb-an., cham., chlor., cob., ign., kali-c., lach., nat-m., ph-ac., plat., stram.
Bleeding	metrorrhagia (excessive bleeding from womb) after abuse of irons	Puls.
Bleeding	metrorrhagia after every stool	Am-m., Ambr., Ind., lyc.
Bleeding	metrorrhagia after exertion	Ambr., aur., bov., Calc., croc., Erig., mill., nit-ac., rhus-t., tril.
Bleeding	metrorrhagia after warm bath	Thuj.
Bleeding	metrorrhagia aggravated at night	Mag-m.
Bleeding	metrorrhagia aggravated by lying on back	Cham.
Bleeding	metrorrhagia aggravated from motion	Arg-n., bell., bry., cact., calc., coff., croc., Erig., helon., Ip., psor., sabin., sec., sulph., tril., ust.
Bleeding	metrorrhagia alternating with dyspnoea	Fl-ac.
Bleeding	metrorrhagia ameliorated from walking	Sabin.
Bleeding	metrorrhagia between the menstrual periods	Ambr., arn., bell., bov., bry., Calc., canth., carb-v., Cham., chin., cimic., cocc., coff., croc., elaps., ferr., hep., Ip., kali-c., lach., lyc., mag-c., mag-s., mang., merc., murx., nit-ac., nux-v., Phos., puls., Rhus-t., Sabin., sec., sep., Sil., stram., sulph., zinc.
Bleeding	metrorrhagia black	Alet., am-c., arn., bell., carb-v., cham., chin., coff., croc., elaps., ferr., helon., ign., kreos., lyc., Plat., puls., sabin., sec., sul-ac., sulph.
Bleeding	metrorrhagia bright red	Acon., aran., arn., bell., calc., cham., chin., cinnam., Erig., ham., hyos., Ip., lac-c., led., lyc., mill., Phos., rhus-t., Sabin., sang., sec., tril., ust., vib.
Bleeding	metrorrhagia coagulated (semi solid)	Alet., apoc., arg-m., arn., Bell., cact., Cham., chin., coc-c., coff., croc., cycl., elaps., ferr., helon., kreos., laur., lyc., merc., murx., nux-v., plat., plb., puls., rhus-t., sabin., sang., sec., stram., tril., ust.
Bleeding	metrorrhagia coagulated expelled with force	Ferr., puls., ust.
Bleeding	metrorrhagia comes suddenly and ceases suddenly	Bell.
Bleeding	metrorrhagia continuous	Apoc., arn., carb-v., cham., erig., hyos., ip., kali-c., kreos., mill., phos., sec., sulph., ust.
Bleeding	metrorrhagia continuous but slow	Carb-v., ham., psor., sec., sulph., ust.
Bleeding	metrorrhagia dark blood	Bell., bry., canth., cham., Chin., croc., crot-h., ferr., ham., helon., kreos., lyc., nux-m., plat., plb., puls., sabin., sec., sep., sul-ac., sulph., tril., ust.

Body part/Disease	Symptom	Medicines
Bleeding	metrorrhagia during and after labor	Acon., alum., apis., arn., bell., bry., cann-s., caul., cham., chin., cinnam., croc., Erig., ferr., Ham., hyos., Ip., kali-c., kreos., lach., lyc., merc., mill., nit-ac., nux-m., nux-v., ph-ac., phos., plat., Sabin., Sec., senec., tril., ust.
Bleeding	metrorrhagia from fibroids (fibrous tissue growth)	Calc-p., calc., hydr., lyc., merc., nit-ac., Phos., sabin., sil., sul-ac., sulph.
Bleeding	metrorrhagia from passing hard stool	Ambr., lyc.
Bleeding	metrorrhagia from polypus (benign growth)	Bell., calc., con., lyc., phos., thuj.
Bleeding	metrorrhagia from retained placenta (organ in uterus of pregnant woman to supply food and oxygen to the fetus through the umbilical cord)	Bell., canth., carb-v., caul., puls., sabin., sec., sep
Bleeding	metrorrhagia gushing	Bell., cham., chin., croc., ham., Ip., mill., Phos., puls., Sabin., sec., tril., ust.
Bleeding	metrorrhagia in little girls	Cina.
Bleeding	metrorrhagia in tall women	Phos.
Bleeding	metrorrhagia in weakly women	Ferr., psor., sulph.
Bleeding	metrorrhagia liquid	Am-c., crot-h., elaps., sec., sul-ac.
Bleeding	metrorrhagia mixed with clots	Bell., cham., chin., croc., ferr., kreos., lyc., puls., sabin., sec., ust.
Bleeding	metrorrhagia mixed with clots	Chin., elaps., ferr., kreos., sabin., sec.
Bleeding	metrorrhagia mixed with fluid	Bry., crot-t., plat., sabin., sec.
Bleeding	metrorrhagia of hot blood	Arn., Bell., bry., lac-c., puls.
Bleeding	metrorrhagia painless	Bov., calc., croc., ham., Kali-fer., mag-c., mill., nux-m., plat., sabin., sec., ust.
Bleeding	metrorrhagia thick blood	Carb-v., nux-m., plat., puls., sulph., tril.
Bleeding	metrorrhagia thin blood	Apoc., bry., carb-v., chin., crot-h., elaps., erig., ferr., kreos., Lach., laur., lyc., phos., plat., puls., Sabin., sec., sul-ac., ust.
Bleeding	metrorrhagia when nursing the child	Sil.
Bleeding	metrorrhagia with clots	Arn., Bell., ip., Sabin., ust.
Bleeding	metrorrhagia with convulsion	Bell., chin., hyos., Sec.
Bleeding	metrorrhagia with fluid	Ham., ust.
Bleeding	nipples bleeding	Ham., lyc., merc., sep., sulph.
Bleeding	pain in teeth ameliorated from bleeding of gums	Bell., caust., sanic., sars., sel.
Bleeding	pimples on chest that bleed easily	Cist.
Bleeding	pimples on tongue bleeding	Graph.
Bleeding	polyp in nose that bleeds easily	Calc-p., calc., phos., thuj.
Bleeding	profuse bleeding from gums on extraction of teeth	Alumn., Arn., ham., kreos., Lach., Phos.
Bleeding	pulsation in head after epistaxis	Bor.
Bleeding	retarded urination, with urging to urinate but can pass no urine until an enormous clot of black blood has passed from the vagina	Coc-c.
Bleeding	skin, crawling must scratch until it bleeds	Agar., alum., arg-m., **Ars.**, bar-c., bov., carb-v., chlol., led., med., psor., puls.

Body part/Disease	Symptom	Medicines
Bleeding	tumour bleeding	Arn., coc-c., kreos., lach., phos., puls., thuj.
Bleeding	ulcer in gums scorbutic (a disease caused by insufficient vitamin C, the symptoms of which include spongy gums, loosening of the teeth, and bleeding into the skin and mucous membranes)	Acet-ac., mur-ac.
Bleeding	ulcer in mouth bleeding	Kreos., merc., sul-ac.
Bleeding	ulcer in tongue bleeding	Merc.
Bleeding	ulcer bleeding	Ant-t., arg-m., arg-n., arn., ars-i., **Ars.**, asaf., bell., calc-s., calc., carb-an., carb-s., carb-v., caust., con., croc., crot-h., dros., graph., ham., **Hep.**, hydr., hyos., iod., kali-ar., kali-c., kali-s., kalm., kreos., **Lach.**, **Lyc.**, **Merc.**, mez., nat-m., **Nit-ac.**, **Ph-ac.**, **Phos.**, puls., ran-b., rhus-t., ruta., sabin., sec., sep., sil., sul-ac., sulph., thuj., zinc.
Bleeding	ulcer bleeding at night	Kali-c.
Bleeding	ulcer bleeding during menses	**Phos.**
Bleeding	ulcer bleeding on edges	Ars., asaf., caust., hep., lach., lyc., merc., ph-ac., phos., puls., sep., sil., sulph., thuj.
Bleeding	ulcer in lower limbs bleeding easily	Carb-v., **Merc.**, ph-ac.
Bleeding	ulcer in skin bleeding when touched	Carb-v., **Hep.**, hydr., lach., mez., nit-ac.
Bleeding	vesicles on tongue bleeding from slightest touch	Mag-c.
Bleeding	warts bleeding	**Caust.**, cinnb., hep., lyc., nat-c., nit-ac., ph-ac., rhus-t., staph., **Thuj.**
Bleeding	warts bleeding from washing	Nit-ac.
Bleeding	wounds bleeding freely	Aran., arn., carb-v., cench., croc., crot-h., ferr., hep., kreos., **Lach.**, merc., mill., nat-m., ph-ac., **Phos.**, puls., rhus-t., sul-ac., sulph., zinc.
Blindness	blindness, after catching cold	Acon.
Blindness	blindness, after headache	Sil.
Blindness	blindness, after injury to eye	Arn.
Blindness	blindness, after lightning stroke	Phos.
Blindness	blindness, after pain in head and eyes	Con.
Blindness	blindness, after sleeping in the sun	Con.
Blindness	blindness, alternates with headaches	Kali-bi.
Blindness	blindness, ameliorated by sleeping	Calc., grat.
Blindness	blindness, ameliorated in open air	Merc., phos.
Blindness	blindness, at sunset	Bell.
Blindness	blindness, by bright objects	Grat., ph-ac.
Blindness	blindness, caused by light	Lyc., mang., thuj.
Blindness	blindness, during delirium (temporary mental disturbance caused by fever, poisoning, or brain injury)	Phos.
Blindness	blindness, during menses	Sep.
Blindness	blindness, during parturition	Aur-m., caust., cocc., cupr.
Blindness	blindness, flickering by day, blind at night	Anac.

Body part/Disease	Symptom	Medicines
Blindness	blindness, in twilight (just after sunset or before dawn)	Lyc., psor.
Blindness	blindness, on looking long at an object	Mang.
Blindness	blindness, paroxysmal (a sudden onset or intensification of a pathological symptom or symptoms, especially when recurrent)	Acon., con., kali-n., mang., nux-v., phos., sil., stram., sulph.
Blindness	blindness, periodic (recurring or reappearing from time to time)	Ant-t., chel., chin., dig., euphr., hyos., merc., nat-m., phos., puls., sep., sil., sulph.
Blindness	blindness, sudden	Aur-m., calc., chin., cupr., mosch., nat-m., phos., psor., sec.
Blindness	blindness, while reading	Agar., arg-n., aur-m., Brom.caust., clem., crot-h., dros., haem., lachn., lyc., nat-c., phos., staph.
Blindness	blindness, with abdominal pain	Crot-t., plb.
Blindness	convulsion at puerperal with blindness	Aur-m., cocc., cupr.
Blindness	headache followed by blindness	Kali-bi.
Blindness	pretended Blindness	Verat.
Blood	Blood Cyst on the scalp	Calc-f., merc., sil.
Blood	blood does not coagulate (make or become semisolid)	Am-c., anthr., apis., ars., both., carb-v., chin., chlol., **Crot-c.**, crot-h., dig., dor., elaps., kali-p., **Lach.**, lat-m., nat-m., **Nit-ac., Phos.**, sec., sul-ac.
Blood	blood does not coagulate after exertion	Mill.
Blood	blood does not coagulate from the orifices (an opening, especially the mouth, anus, vagina, or other opening into a cavity or passage in the body) of the body	Aran., **Both.**, chin., **Crot-h.**, elaps., ip., lach., **Phos.**, sul-ac.
Blood	blood oozing from throat	Acon., arn., ars., bell., canth., carb-v., chin., crot-h., cur., ferr-p., ferr., ham., ip., lach., merc-c., merc-cy., mill., phos., sang., sec., sep.
Blood	blood oozing from tonsils	Crot-h., lach., phos., sec., ter.
Blood	blood oozing from uvula	Lac-c.
Blood	discharge of blood from nose in morning	Am-c., arum-t., calc., kali-c., lach., lyc., petr., sulph.
Blood	discharge of blood from one side on blowing nose	Asc-t.
Blood	discharge of blood on blowing nose	Calad., caust., chel., graph., lach., nit-ac., puls., sulph., thuj., zinc.
Blood	discharge of clear blood from ear	Bry.
Blood	discharge of copious blood from ear	Bar-m.
Blood	discharges of blood from ear	Am-c., arn., arund., asaf., bell., Both., bry., bufo., chin., cic., colch., con., Crot-h., elaps., ery-a., ham., merc., mosch., op., petr., Phos., puls., rhus-t., tell.
Blood	discharges of blood from ear instead of menses	Bry., phos.
Blood	discharges of blood from ear after prolonged suppuration (discharge of pus as a result of an injury or infection)	Chin.
Blood	discharges of blood from ear during cough	Bell.
Blood	discoloration like blood specks in legs	Phos.

Body part/Disease	Symptom	Medicines
Blood	discoloration, blood settles under nails	Apis.
Blood	dry cough with discharge of blood	Zinc.
Blood	dry cough with discharge of blood ends in raising black blood	Elaps.
Blood	epistaxis alternating with spitting of blood	Ferr.
Blood	eruption, blood boils in legs	Mag-c.
Blood	eruption, blood boils in nates	Aur-m.
Blood	eruptions carbuncle discharging blood	Ant-c., calc., crot-h., lach., merc., nux-v.
Blood	eruptions like blood boils	Alum., arn., bell., bry., calc., eupho., hyos., iod., iris., kali-bi., led., lyc., mag-c., mag-m., mur-ac., nat-m., nit-ac., ph-ac., **Phos.**, sec., sep., sil., sul-ac., sulph., thuj.
Blood	eruptions, vesicles in tips of fingers filled with blood	**Ars.**
Blood	excessive flow of blood in brain after a pleasant surprise	Coff.
Blood	excessive flow of blood in brain after lifting	Nat-c.
Blood	excessive flow of blood in brain after menses	Chin., ign., nat-m., sulph., thuj.
Blood	excessive flow of blood in brain aggravated toward evening with terrible pain , would press the head against wall , fears going mad	Stram.
Blood	excessive flow of blood in brain as if blood rushed from heart to head	Nux-m.
Blood	excessive flow of blood in brain at night	Am-c., anac., aster., berb., calc-s., calc., carb-v., cycl., kali-c., mill., Psor., puls., sil., sulph.
Blood	excessive flow of blood in brain at night after anger	Bry., cham., staph.
Blood	excessive flow of blood in brain at night ameliorated in open air	ars., camph., caust., coc-c., grat., hell., mag-m., mosch.
Blood	excessive flow of blood in brain at night during shocks in chest	Tab.
Blood	excessive flow of blood in brain at night on bending head backward	Bell.
Blood	excessive flow of blood in brain at night with anxiety	Acon., aur., cycl.
Blood	excessive flow of blood in brain at night with epistaxis	Ant-c., bell., bry., carb-v., croc., lach., lil-t., meli., nux-v., pic-ac., psor.
Blood	excessive flow of blood in brain before menses	Acon., Apis., bell., bry., cupr., gels., glon., hep., hyper., iod., kali-c., lyc., manc., meli., merc., tril.
Blood	excessive flow of blood in brain compells to sit up	Aloe.
Blood	excessive flow of blood in brain during excitement	Asaf., phos.
Blood	excessive flow of blood in brain during menses	Acon., Apis., bell., bry., cact., calc-p., calc-s., calc., caust., cham., chin., cinnb., con., elaps., ferr-p., gels., glon., iod., mag-c., mag-m., manc., merc., mosch., nat-m., nux-m., nux-v., phos., sang., Sulph., verat-v., verat.
Blood	excessive flow of blood in brain during rage (extreme anger)	Acon., Bell., hyos., lach., nux-v., op., phos., stram., verat.

Body part/Disease	Symptom	Medicines
Blood	excessive flow of blood in brain from 5 p.m., to midnight	Glon.
Blood	excessive flow of blood in brain from fright or grief	Ph-ac.
Blood	excessive flow of blood in brain from suppressed discharges or suddenly ceasing pains	Cimic.
Blood	excessive flow of blood in brain from suppressed lochia (the normal vaginal discharge of cell debris and blood after childbirth) from the vagina	Acon., bell., bry., cimic.
Blood	excessive flow of blood in brain from suppressed menses	Acon., apis., arn., Bell., bry., calc-s., calc., cham., chin., Cimic., coc-c., cocc., Ferr., Gels., Glon., graph., Lach., merc., op., stram., sulph.
Blood	excessive flow of blood in brain in afternoon	Am-c., cham., chin-s., graph., lach., nat-m., paeon., ran-b., sil.
Blood	excessive flow of blood in brain in morning	Calc., cham., chin-s., glon., lach., lact-ac., lyc., mag-c., mag-s., naja., raph., tell.
Blood	excessive flow of blood in brain on raising the head	Lyc.
Blood	excessive flow of blood in brain on rising	Eug., lyc.
Blood	excessive flow of blood in brain on shaking the head	Nit-ac., nux-v.
Blood	excessive flow of blood in brain on taking exercise	Sulph.
Blood	excessive flow of blood in brain on waking	Calc., lyc., ph-ac.
Blood	excessive flow of blood in brain when speaking	Coff., sulph.
Blood	excessive flow of blood in brain when spoken to harshly	Ign.
Blood	excessive flow of blood in brain with redness of face	Acon., Bell., canth., coff., cop., cor-r., glon., graph., meli., merc-c., phos., sil., sol-n.
Blood	excoriating bloody discharge	Ars-i., calc-p., carb-v., fl-ac., hep., lyc., merc., nat-m., puls., rhus-t., Sulph., syph., Tell.
Blood	expectoration containing blood and mucus	Op.
Blood	expectoration with threads of blood mixed with white sputa	Aur-m.
Blood	extravasation (to leak, or cause blood or other fluid to leak, from a vessel into surrounding tissue as a result of injury, burns, or inflammation) of blood in lumbar region	Crot-h.
Blood	faintness at sight of blood	Nux-m.
Blood	haemorrhage of clotted blood from urethra	Cact., caust., chin., coc-c., nux-v.
Blood	haemorrhage of pure blood from urethra	Bry., canth., caps., ham., hell., mez.
Blood	haemorrhagic fever with oozing of dark thin blood from capillaries	Crot-h., sul-ac.
Blood	heaviness of Head as if full of blood	Glon., ign., lil-t.
Blood	hemorrhage of clotted blood from urethra	Cact., caust., chin., coc-c., nux-v.
Blood	hemorrhage of pure blood from urethra	Bry., canth., caps., ham., hell., mez.
Blood	insensibility of bladder with violent pain and almost clear blood	Ham.

Body part/Disease	Symptom	Medicines
Blood	Mass of blood in urine	Plb., ter.
Blood	milk with blood	Bufo., cham., hep., lyc., merc., sep., sulph.
Blood	pain in uterus ameliorated by flow of blood	Arg-n., bell., kali-c., Lach., mosch., sep., sulph., ust., vib.
Blood	pulsation sensation after loss of blood	Chin.
Blood	retention of urine from clots in the bladder	Cact., caust.
Blood	sensation as if blood stagnated (stop flowing)	Acon., bar-c., bell., bry., carb-v., caust., croc., crot-t., dig., gels., hep., ign., lyc., nux-v., olnd., pic-ac., puls., rhod., sabad., seneg., sep., sulph., sumb., zinc.
Blood	sensation of streaming (the rotary flow of protoplasm within some cells and protozoans) of blood	Ox-ac.
Blood	stagnation of blood	Lob.
Blood	Stream of blood from chest to head like a gust of wind with epistaxis (bleeding from nose)	Mill.
Blood	ulcer in gums discharging blood which tastes salty	Alum.
Blood	ulcer in gums exuding blood on pressure	Bov.
Blood	unconsciousness on sight of blood	Nux-m.
Blood	urging to urinate, with but can pass no urine until an enormous clot of black blood has passed from the vagina	Coc-c.
Blood	urticaria vesicular filled with blood	Ail., **Ars.**, aur., bry., camph., canth., carb-ac., fl-ac., graph., kali-p., **Lach.**, nat-c., nat-m., sec., sulph.
Blood	vesicles on ears filled with serum (liquid part of blood)	Rhus-v.
Blood	vomiting bile (a yellowish green fluid produced in the liver, stored in the gall bladder, and passed through ducts to the small intestine, where it plays an essential role in emulsifying fats) then blood	Agar., carb-v., verat.
Blood	vomiting black blood	Card-m., ham.
Blood	vomiting blood after eating	Stram.
Blood	vomiting blood after suppressed haemorrhoidal flow	Acon., carb-v., Nux-v., phos., sulph.
Blood	vomiting blood aggravated on lying	Stann.
Blood	vomiting blood during menses	Sulph.
Blood	vomiting blood during pregnancy	Sep.
Blood	vomiting blood during suppressed menses	Bell., bry., ham.,
Blood	vomiting blood in drunkards	Alumn., ars.
Blood	vomiting blood instead of menses in girls	Ham.
Blood	vomiting blood with cough	Anan.
Blood	vomiting clotted blood	Arn., ars., caust., ham., lyc., merc-c., nux-v., phyt., sec.
Blood	vomiting food then blood	Nux-v.
Blood	weakness from disproportionate loss of blood after menses	Ip.
Blood clot	thrombosis	Ars.

Body part/Disease	Symptom	Medicines
Blood clot	thrombosis (blood clots that may partially or completely block an artery or vein) of lower limbs	Apis.
Blood poisoning	convulsion uremic (form of blood poisoning)	Apoc., crot-h., cupr-ar., cupr., dig., hydr-ac., kali-s., merc-c., mosch., plb., ter.
Blood poisoning	deep sleep during blood poisoning	Agar., anac., ars., bell., lact., op.
Blood vessel	distension of blood vessels	Acon., agar., alum., am-c., arn., ars., bar-c., bar-m., **Bell.**, bry., calc-f., calc., camph., carb-s., carb-v., chel., chin-a., chin-s., **Chin.**, cic., coloc., con., croc., cycl., dig., ferr-ar., ferr-p., **Ferr.**, graph., ham., **Hyos.**, lach., led., lyc., meny., merl., mosch., nat-m., nux-v., olnd., op., ph-ac., phos., plb., podo., **Puls.**, rhod., rhus-t., sars., sec., sep., sil., spig., spong., staph., stront., sulph., **Thuj.**, vip., zinc.
Blood vessel	distension of blood vessels during fever	Agar., bell., camph., chin-s., **Chin.**, **Hyos.**, **Led.**, **Puls.**
Blood vessel	distension of blood vessels in evening	**Puls.**
Blood vessel	feeling of cold in blood vessels	**Acon.**, ant-c., ant-t., **Ars.**, lyc., **Rhus-t.**, verat.
Blood vessel	felon, lymphatic (a network of vessels that transport fluid, fats, proteins, and lymphocytes to the bloodstream) inflamed	All-c., bufo., hep., lach., rhus-t.
Blood vessel	fever with burning heat with distended blood vessels	Aloe., bell., chin-s., **Chin.**, cycl., dig., ferr., hyos., led., **Merl.**, puls., sars.
Blood vessel	haemorrhagic fever with oozing of dark thin blood from capillaries	Crot-h., sul-ac.
Blood vessel	inflammation of blood vessels (an artery, vein, or capillary through which blood flows)	Acon., ant-t., **Arn.**, ars-i., **Ars.**, **Bar-c.**, calc., cham., cupr., ham., kali-c., kreos., lach., lyc., puls., sil., spig., **Sulph.**, thuj., zinc.
Blood vessel	inflammation of pericardium (fibrous membrane that forms a sac surrounding the heart and attached portions of the main blood vessels)	Acon., anac., ant-t., apis., apoc., ars-i., Ars., asc-t., bry., cact., chlor., cimic., colch., dig., iod., kali-ar., kali-c., kali-chl., kali-i., kalm., lach., ox-ac., plat., Psor., Spig., spong., Sulph., verat-v., verat.
Blood vessel	internal chill as if coldness in blood vessels	Acon., ant-c., ant-t., Ars., lyc., Rhus-t., Verat.
Blood vessel	network of blood vessels	Berb., calc., carb-v., caust., clem., crot-h., lyc., nat-m., ox-ac., plat., sabad., thuj.
Blood vessel	pain burning in blood vessels	Agar., **Ars.**, aur., bry., calc., hyos., med., nat-m., nit-ac., op., **Rhus-t.**, sulph., verat.
Blood vessel	sensation of heat in blood vessels	Agar., **Ars.**, aur., bry., calc., hyos., med., nat-m., nit-ac., op., **Rhus-t.**, sulph., verat.
Bloody	bloody discharge from ear after measles	Bov., cact., carb-v., colch., crot-h., lyc., merc., nit-ac., Puls., sulph.
Bloody	bloody discharge from ear threatening caries	Asaf., Aur., calc-f., calc-s., calc., caps., nat-m., Sil., sulph.
Bloody	bloody discharge from urethra	Arg-n., bell., Calc-s., cann-s., Canth., caps., cop., cub., cur., kali-i., lith., lyc., merc-c., merc., mill., mur-ac., nit-ac., psor., puls., thuj., zinc.
Bloody	bloody discharge from urethra in chronic diarrhoea	Eupho.
Bloody	bloody discharge from urethra painful to touch	Caps.
Bloody	bloody milk	Bufo., cham., phyt.
Bloody	bloody perspiration	Arn., calc., cham., chin., clem., **Crot-h.**, cur., **Lach.**, lyc., nux-m., nux-v., petr.

Body part/Disease	Symptom	Medicines
Bloody	bloody perspiration at night	Cur.
Bloody	bloody perspiration staining the linen	Calc., clem., crot-h., cur., **Lach.**, lyc., **Nux-m.**
Bloody	bloody scabs (crust over healing wound) behind ears exuding a glutinous	Rhus-v.
Bloody	bloody, ink-like, albuminous urine from kidney	Colch.
Bloody	crusts on nose, bloody	Am-c., am-m., ambr., calc., kali-bi., nat-a., phos., puls., sep., stront.
Bloody	deep and bleeding cracks on hands	Alum., merc., Nit-ac., Petr., sanic., sars.
Bloody	deep bloody cracks of skin	Merc., **Nit-ac.**, **Petr.**, puls., sars., sulph.
Bloody	discharge from urethra bloody	Canth., Nit-ac., puls.
Bloody	discharge of bloody fluid from umbilicus	Calc-p., calc., nux-m.
Bloody	discharge of bloody mucous from urethra	Canth., Nit-ac., puls.
Bloody	discharge of bloody water from nipple	Lyc., phyt.
Bloody	discharge of bloody wax from ear	Am-m., anac., hep., kali-c., lyc., merc., mosch., nat-m., nit-ac., phos., puls.
Bloody	discharges, bloody from eye	Ars., asaf., carb-s., carb-v., caust., cham., hep., kali-c., kreos., lach., lyc., merc., mez., nat-m., petr., ph-ac., phos., puls., rhus-t., sep., sil., sulph., thuj.
Bloody	eructations bloody	Merc-c., nux-v., phos., raph., sep.
Bloody	eruption, vesicles with bloody serum in lower limbs	Nat-m.
Bloody	eruption, vesicles with bloody serum in sole of foot	Nat-m.
Bloody	expectoration bloody after a fall	Ferr-p., mill.
Bloody	expectoration bloody after drinking	Calc.
Bloody	expectoration bloody after eating	Sep.
Bloody	expectoration bloody after exertion	Ip., mill.
Bloody	expectoration bloody after violent erection	Nat-m.
Bloody	expectoration bloody at night	Arn., ars., ferr., mez., puls., rhus-t., sulph.
Bloody	expectoration bloody at night acrid	Am-c., ars., canth., carb-v., hep., Kali-c., kali-n., rhus-t., Sil., sul-ac., sulph., zinc.
Bloody	expectoration bloody before menses	Zinc.
Bloody	expectoration bloody black at night	Arn., bism., canth., chin., croc., crot-c., dig., dros., Elaps., kali-bi., nit-ac., nux-v., ph-ac., puls., zinc.
Bloody	expectoration bloody during lactation (the production of milk by the mammary glands. the period during which milk is produced by the mammary glands)	Ferr.
Bloody	expectoration bloody during menses	Iod., nat-m., phos., sep., Zinc.
Bloody	expectoration bloody during suppressed menses	Acon., carb-v., dig., led., lyc., Nux-v., phos., puls., sulph.
Bloody	expectoration bloody in afternoon	Alum., clem., lyc., mag-c., mez., mill., nux-v.
Bloody	expectoration bloody in evening	Cub., nat-c., sep.
Bloody	expectoration bloody in evening after lying down	Sep.
Bloody	expectoration bloody in evening when coughing	Nat-c.
Bloody	expectoration bloody in morning during menses	Zinc.

Body part/Disease	Symptom	Medicines
Bloody	expectoration bloody in morning on bed	Nit-ac., Nux-v.
Bloody	expectoration bloody in morning on rising	Aesc., ferr.
Bloody	expectoration bloody in noon	Sil.
Bloody	expectoration bloody on coughing	Bell., sep.
Bloody	expectoration bloody on hawking	Cham., ferr., hyper., kali-n., nit-ac.
Bloody	expectoration bloody when clearing the throat	Am-c.
Bloody	expectoration bloody while lying down in morning	Merc.
Bloody	expectoration bloody while walking	Cham., merc., sul-ac., zinc.
Bloody	expectoration bloody while working	Merc.
Bloody	expectoration blue & white alternately	Arund.
Bloody	expectoration bluish	Arund., brom., kali-bi., nat-a., sulph.
Bloody	ichorous (a watery or slightly bloody discharge from a wound or an ulcer) bloody discharge from ear	Am-c., Ars., calc-p., carb-an., carb-v., Lyc., nit-ac., Psor., sep., sil., tell.
Bloody	leucorrhoea bloody	Acon., agar., aloe., alum., am-m., ant-t., arg-m., arg-n., ars-i., ars., bar-c., bufo., Calc-s., calc., canth., carb-s., carb-v., chin-a., Chin., cinnb., Cocc., coff., con., crot-h., ham., hep., iod., kali-i., kreos., lac-c., lyc., merc-c., merc., murx., Nit-ac., nux-m., petr., ph-ac., phos., phys., podo., sabin., Sep., sil., sul-ac., ter., tril., zinc.
Bloody	leucorrhoea bloody after menses	Ars., caust., chin., pyrog., zinc.
Bloody	lochia bloody	Acon., bry., calc., caul., cham., rhus-t., sil.
Bloody	mucus bloody in throat	Alum., am-br., bad., bism., bor., chel., fl-ac., gels., hep., kali-ar., kali-ma., lyc., mag-c., mag-m., sars., sep., stann., thuj.
Bloody	mucus in larynx blood streaked	Am-c., anan., sol-n.
Bloody	odorless bloody discharge from ear	Lac-c.
Bloody	saliva bloody	Acon., am-c., arg-m., arn., ars., aspar., bad., bell., bry., Bufo., calad., camph., canth., carb-s., carb-v., cic., clem., Crot-c., crot-h., dros., eug., gels., hyos., indg., jatr., kali-i., Mag-c., merc-c., merc., nat-m., Nit-ac., nux-v., op., Phos., rhus-t., sec., staph., stram., sulph., thuj., vip., zinc.
Bloody	saliva bloody before menses	Nat-m.
Bloody	seminal discharge bloody	Cann-s., canth., caust., led., merc., petr., sars., tarent.
Bloody	ulcer with bloody discharge	Ant-t., anthr., arg-m., arn., ars-i., **Ars.**, **Asaf.**, bell., calc-s., canth., carb-an., carb-s., carb-v., caust., com., con., croc., dros., graph., **Hep.**, hyos., iod., kali-ar., kali-c., kali-s., kreos., lach., lyc., **Merc.**, mez., nat-m., nit-ac., petr., ph-ac., phos., puls., pyrog., rhus-t., ruta., sabin., sars., sec., sep., sil., sul-ac., sulph., thuj., zinc.
Blotch	blotches (An irregularly shaped Reddish patch on the skin) on abdomen	Crot-t., merc., nat-c.
Blotch	blotches behind ears	Bry., calc., carb-an., caust., staph.
Blotch	blotches in coccyx	Lach., mez., phos., zinc.
Blotch	blotches of face aggravated at night	Mag-m.
Blotch	blotches of face aggravated before menses	Mag-m.

Body part/Disease	Symptom	Medicines
Blotch	blotches of face aggravated by washing	Am-c., phyt.
Blotch	blotches of face aggravated from warmth of bed	Mag-m.
Blotch	blotches of face itching	Graph.
Blotch	blotches on chest	Nat-c., sars.
Blotch	blotches on chin	Bry., carb-an., eupho., hep., mag-m., olnd.
Blotch	blotches on external throat	Graph., nat-m., sars., sep., spong.
Blotch	blotches on eyelids	Aur., bry., calc., ran-s., staph., thuj.
Blotch	blotches on forehead	Nat-c.
Blotch	blotches on head	Apis., arg-n., Psor. sep.
Blotch	blotches on lips	Arg-m., ars., bar-c., caust., con., hep., kali-i., mag-m., nat-c., sep., sil., sulph.
Blotch	blotches on nose	Bell., iod.
Blotch	blotches on palate	Elaps., fl-ac., syph., zinc.
Blotch	blotches on scrotum	Arn.
Blotch	blotches prepuce (skin covering clitoris)	Sep.
Blotch	eruptions blotches	Anac., ant-c., arn., ars., asaf., bar-c., bell., berb., bry., calc., caps., chel., chlol., cocc., coff., con., croc., crot-h., crot-t., dulc., fl-ac., hell., hep., hyos., ign., kali-c., kreos., lach., led., lyc., mag-c., mang., merc., nat-c., nat-m., nit-ac., nux-v., op., petr., ph-ac., phos., puls., rhus-t., rhus-v., ruta., sabin., sars., sec., sel., sep., sil., spig., squil., staph., stram., sul-ac., sulph., valer., verat., vip.
Blotch	eruptions blotches after scratching	Kali-c., lach., lyc., merc., nat-c., nit-ac., op., rhus-t., spig., verat., zinc.
Blotch	eruptions blotches indurated	Am-m., phos., sars.
Blotch	eruptions blotches inflammed	Hep., mang., merc., phos., sil.
Blotch	eruptions blotches itching & oozing	**Graph.**
Blotch	eruptions blotches red	Arg-n., carb-v., crot-t., fl-ac., merc., mur-ac., op., phos., urt-u.
Blotch	eruptions blotches red & desquamating	Fl-ac.
Blotch	eruptions blotches red & elevated	Fl-ac., rhus-t.
Blotch	eruptions blotches stinging	Petr., sars., stram., zinc.
Blotch	eruptions blotches watey	Graph., mag-c.
Blotch	eruptions blotches yellow	Ant-c., sulph.
Blue Faced	child becomes stiff & blue on face with suffocative cough	Cupr., Ip.
Bodyache	Body aches during dysentery (a disease of the lower intestine caused by infection with bacteria, protozoans or parasites and marked by severe diarrhea, inflammation, and the passage of blood and mucus)	Arn.
Boil	boils (pus-filled abscess on skin) between shoulders	Iod., tarent-c., zinc.
Boil	boils above the eyes	Calc-s., nat-m.
Boil	boils behind ears	Ang., bry., calc., con., nat-c., phyt., sulph., thuj.

Body part/Disease	Symptom	Medicines
Boil	boils in anus	Calc-p., carb-an., caust., petr.
Boil	boils in axila (armpit)	Bor., Hep., lyc., merc., nat-s., petr., ph-ac., phos., sep., sil., sulph., thuj.
Boil	boils in cervical region	Calc., carb-an., coloc., crot-h., cypr., dig., graph., hep., indg., Kali-i., lach., nat-m., nit-ac., petr., phos., psor., rhus-v., sec., Sil., Sulph., thuj., ust.
Boil	boils in coccyx	Caust., coloc., crot-h., graph., kali-bi., Kali-i., lach., mur-ac., ph-ac., phyt., sanic., sul-ac., sulph., tarent-c., thuj., zinc.
Boil	boils in corner of mouth	Am-c., Ant-c.
Boil	boils in front of ears	Bry., carb-v., laur., sulph.
Boil	boils in lumbar region	Hep., psor., rhus-t., thuj.
Boil	boils in margins of ears	Bov., crot-h., Merc., Pic-ac., puls., rhus-t., Sulph.
Boil	boils in meatus	Bov., crot-h., Merc., Pic-ac., puls., rhus-t., Sulph.
Boil	boils in right axila (armpit)	Thuj.
Boil	boils in sacrum	Aeth., thuj.
Boil	boils inside nose	Alum., am-c., carb-an., sep., sil., tub.
Boil	boils near anus	Caust.
Boil	boils on chest	Am-c., chin., hep., Kali-i., lach., mag-c., phos., Psor., Sulph.
Boil	boils on ears	Kali-c., sil., spong., sulph., syph.
Boil	boils on face burning	Alum., am-m., anac., ant-c., apis., ars., calc., caust., chin-s., cic., euphr., graph., kali-c., led., mag-m., merc., nat-m., phos., rat., rhus-t., sars., seneg., sep., staph., sulph.
Boil	boils on face burning when scratched	Nat-s., sars.
Boil	boils on face burning when wet	Euphr.
Boil	boils on face burning, cannot sleep without cold applications	Am-m.
Boil	boils on face painful	Hep.
Boil	boils on forehead	Am-c., led., mag-c., phos., sep.
Boil	boils on gums	Agn., anan., arn., aur., carb-an., carb-v., caust., chel., eupho., jug-r., kali-chl., kali-i., lac-c., lyc., merc., mill., nat-m., nat-p., nat-s., nux-v., petr., ph-ac., phos., plan., plb., Sil., staph.
Boil	boils on lips	Hep., lach., nat-c., petr.
Boil	boils on mammae	Chin., mag-c., phos.
Boil	boils on nose	Acon., alum., am-c., anan., cadm., carb-an., con., hep., mag-m., phos., sars., sil.
Boil	boils on nose burning	Alum., apis., caust., graph., nat-c., nat-m., ol-an., phos.
Boil	boils on occiput	Kali-bi., lyc., nat-c.
Boil	boils on pubes (the part of the abdomen immediately above the external genitalia that is covered with hair from puberty onward)	Apis.
Boil	boils on side of neck	Phos., rhus-t., sec., zinc.

Body part/Disease	Symptom	Medicines
Boil	boils on temples	Mur-ac.
Boil	boils, about the eyes	Sil.
Boil	burning boils in axila	Merc.
Boil	diarrhoea as soon as boils begin to heal	Rhus-v.
Boil	eruption, blood boils in legs	Mag-c.
Boil	eruption, blood boils in nates	Aur-m.
Boil	eruption, boils	All-c., am-c., apoc., ars., aur-m., bell., brom., calc., carb-s., clem., cob., elaps., graph., guare., **Hep.**, hyos., iris., kali-bi., kali-n., lyc., merc., mez., nat-m., nit-ac., nux-v., petr., ph-ac., psor., rat., rhus-t., rhus-v., sec., sep., stram., **Sulph.**, thuj.
Boil	eruption, boils in ankle	Merc.
Boil	eruption, boils in back of hands	Calc.
Boil	eruption, boils in calf	Bell., **Sil.**
Boil	eruption, boils in foot	Anan., calc., led., sars., sil., **Stram.**
Boil	eruption, boils in forearm	Calc., carb-v., cob., iod., lach., lyc., mag-m., nat-s., petr., sil.
Boil	eruption, boils in hands	Calc., coloc., iris., lach., led., lyc., psor.
Boil	eruption, boils in heels	Calc., lach.
Boil	eruption, boils in hips	Alum., am-c., bar-c., graph., hep., jug-r., lyc., nit-ac., ph-ac., rat., sabin.
Boil	eruption, boils in knee	Am-c., calc., nat-m., nux-v.
Boil	eruption, boils in legs	Anan., anthr., ars., calc., cast-eq., mag-c., nit-ac., nux-v., **Petr.**, **Rhus-t.**, sil.
Boil	eruption, boils in nates	Agar., alum., am-c., aur-m., bar-c., bart., cadm., calad., graph., hep., indg., lyc., nit-ac., ph-ac., phos., plb., psor., rat., sabin., sars., sec., sep., sil., sulph., thuj.
Boil	eruption, boils in right thigh	Calc., hell., kali-bi., kali-c., rhus-v.
Boil	eruption, boils in shoulder	Am-c., am-m., bell., hydr., kali-n., nit-ac., ph-ac., sulph.
Boil	eruption, boils in sole of foot	Rat.
Boil	eruption, boils in thighs	Agar., all-s., alum., am-c., apoc., aur-m., bell., calc., carb-s., clem., cocc., hep., hyos., ign., kali-bi., lach., lyc., mag-c., nit-ac., nux-v., petr., ph-ac., phos., plb., rhus-v., sep., **Sil.**, thuj.
Boil	eruption, boils in upper limbs	Aloe., am-c., ars., bar-c., bell., brom., calc., carb-an., carb-v., cob., coloc., elaps., graph., guare., iod., iris., kali-n., lyc., mag-m., mez., **Petr.**, ph-ac., **Rhus-t.**, sil., sulph., syph., zinc.
Boil	eruption, boils in wrists	Iod., sanic.
Boil	eruption, boils on ulnar side of palms	Coloc.
Boil	eruption, large blood boils in shoulder	Calc., jug-r., lyc., zinc.
Boil	eruption, small boils in hands	Iris.
Boil	eruptions boils at injured places	Dulc.
Boil	eruptions boils in the spring	Bell., crot-h., lach.

Body part/Disease	Symptom	Medicines
Boil	eruptions boils maturing slowly	Hep., sil., sulph.
Boil	eruptions boils stinging when touched	Mur-ac., sil.
Boil	eruptions boils with greenish pus	Sec.
Boil	eruptions large boils	Ant-t., apis., bufo., hep., hyos., lach., lyc., merc., nat-c., nit-ac., nux-v., phos., sil., viol-t.
Boil	eruptions like blood boils	Alum., arn., bell., bry., calc., eupho., hyos., iod., iris., kali-bi., led., lyc., mag-c., mag-m., mur-ac., nat-m., nit-ac., ph-ac., **Phos.**, sec., sep., sil., sul-ac., sulph., thuj.
Boil	eruptions like blue boils	Anthr., bufo., crot-h., lach.
Boil	eruptions like boils	Abrot., agar., alum., alumn., am-c., am-m., anac., ant-c., ant-t., anth., apis., **Arn.**, ars-i., ars., aur., bar-c., **Bell.**, brom., bry., bufo., calc-p., calc-s., calc., carb-an., carb-s., carb-v., chin-a., chin., cist., coc-c., cocc., con., crot-h., dulc., elaps., eupho., graph., **Hep.**, hyos., ign., iod., jug-r., kali-i., kali-n., kreos., **Lach.**, laur., led., **Lyc.**, mag-c., mag-m., **Merc.**, mez., mur-ac., nat-a., nat-c., nat-m., nat-p., nit-ac., nux-m., nux-v., **Petr.**, ph-ac., phos., phyt., pic-ac., **Psor.**, puls., **Rhus-t.**, sars., sec., sep., sil., spong., stann., staph., stram., sul-ac., **Sulph.**, tarent., thuj., zinc.
Boil	eruption, periodical boils	**Ars.**, hyos., iod., lyc., merc., nit-ac., phos., phyt., sil., staph., sulph.
Boil	eruption, small boils	**Arn.**, bar-c., dulc., fl-ac., **Kali-i.**, lyc., mag-c., mag-m., nat-m., nux-v., sulph., tarent., viol-t., zinc.
Boil	eruptions, boils in fingers	Calc., lach., sil.
Boil	eruptions, boils in lower limbs	All-c., am-c., apoc., ars., aur-m., bell., carb-s., clem., **Hep.**, hyos., kali-bi., nat-m., nit-ac., nux-v., petr., ph-ac., phos., rhus-t., rhus-v., sec., sep., sil., stram., sulph., thuj.
Boil	eruptions, boils in thumb	Hep., kali-n.
Boil	pain, as from a boil	Hep.
Boil	recurrent boils in axila	Lyc.
Boil	small blood boils on face	Alum., iris., sil.
Boil	small boil near left upper canine (A pointed tooth between the incisors and the first bicuspids two in each jaw), painful to touch	Agn.
Boil	small painful boils in axila	Sep.
Boil	ulcer from boils	Calc-p.
Bone	brittle bones	Calc., symph.
Bone	burning pain in bones of lower limb	Eupho.
Bone	caries (Progressive decay of a tooth or, less commonly, a bone) of bone	**Ang.**, ars., **Asaf.**, aur-m-n., aur-m., aur., bell., bry., calc-f., calc-p., calc-s., calc., caps., carb-ac., chin., cist., clem., con., cupr., dulc., eupho., ferr., **Fl-ac.**, graph., guai., guare., hep., iod., kali-bi., **Kali-i.**, kreos., lach., **Lyc., Merc.**, mez., nat-m., nit-ac., op., petr., ph-ac., phos., puls., rhod., rhus-t., ruta., sabin., sec., sep., **Sil.**, spong., staph., sulph., **Ther.**, thuj.

Body part/Disease	Symptom	Medicines
Bone	caries in bones of head	Arg-m., asaf., Aur., caps., fl-ac., hep., hippoz., nat-m., Nit-ac., ph-ac., Phos., Sil., staph.
Bone	caries of ankle bones , internal malleolus (either of the hammer-shaped bony protuberances at the sides of the ankle joint that project from the lower end of the tibia and fibula)	Sil.
Bone	caries of ankle bones	Asaf., calc., guai., plat-m., puls., sil.
Bone	caries of bone	Ars., Asaf., aur., calc-f., calc-p., calc., con., fl-ac., graph., guai., hep., Lyc., Merc., mez., Nit-ac., ph-ac., phos., puls., ruta., sec., sep., Sil., staph., sulph., ther.
Bone	caries of bone , periosteum	Ant-c., **Asaf.**, aur., bell., chin., cycl., hell., merc., mez., **Ph-ac.**, puls., rhod., rhus-t., ruta., sabin., sil., staph.
Bone	caries of femur (the main bone in the human thigh, the strongest bone in the body)	Calc., Sil., stront.
Bone	caries of fibula (the outer and narrower of the two bones in the human lower leg between the knee and ankle)	Sil.
Bone	caries of hands metacarpal bone (any bone in the human hand between the wrist and digits)	Sil.
Bone	caries of humerus (the long bone of the human upper arm)	Sil.
Bone	caries of tibia (inner and larger of the two bones in the lower leg, extending from the knee to the ankle bone alongside the fibula)	Asaf., aur., calc., guai., hecla., kali-i., lach., ph-ac., phos., Sil.
Bone	chill beginning in and extending from sacrum	Puls.
Bone	coldness in cervical region extending to sacrum on lying down	Thuj.
Bone	coldness in hands during pain in sacrum	Hura.
Bone	coldness in olecranon (elbow bone)	Agar.
Bone	Coldness of Vertex extending to sacrum	Acon.
Bone	constriction in bones	Am-m., anac., aur., chin., cocc., coloc., con., graph., kreos., lyc., merc., nat-m., **Nit-ac.**, nux-v., petr., phos., **Puls.**, rhod., rhus-t., ruta., sabad., sep., sil., stront., **Sulph.**, zinc.
Bone	constrictions in bones of upper limb	Con.
Bone	convulsion from bone in throat	Cic.
Bone	cramp in region of tibia	Am-c.
Bone	cramp in ulnar (the longer of the two bones in the human forearm, situated on the inner side) side of hand	Cocc., puls.
Bone	curvature of cervical bone	Calc., phos., syph.
Bone	curvature of dorsal bone	Bar-c., bufo., calc-s., calc., con., lyc., plb., puls., rhus-t., sil., sulph., syph., thuj.
Bone	discoloration of tibia with spots	Ambr., ant-c., caust., kali-n., lach., mag-c., phos., sil., sul-ac.
Bone	encephalitis of periosteum (the sheath of connective tissue that surrounds all bones except those at joints)	Aur-m., aur., Fl-ac., kali-i., led., mang., merc-c., merc., Mez., nit-ac., Ph-ac., phos., puls., rhod., rhus-t., ruta., sil., staph.

Body part/Disease	Symptom	Medicines
Bone	eruption, in olecranon	Berb.
Bone	eruption, pimples in olecranon	Berb.
Bone	exostoses	Ang., aur-m., aur., bad., calc-f., calc-p., cinnb., dulc., hecla., merc., mez., **Nit-ac.**, ph-ac., phyt., rhus-t., sars., Sil., sulph.
Bone	exostoses (a benign bony growth on the surface of a bone or a tooth root, caused by inflammation or repeated trauma) on sacrum	Rhus-t.
Bone	exostoses in roof of mouth	Asaf.
Bone	exostoses on fingers	Calc-f.
Bone	exostoses on forearm	Dulc.
Bone	exostosis (a benign bony growth on the surface of a bone or a tooth root, caused by inflammation or repeated trauma)	*Arg-m.,* **Aur-m.,** **Aur.,** **Calc-f.,** *calc., crot-c., dulc., fl-ac., hecla., kali-i., merc-c., mez., nit-ac.,* **Phos.,** *puls., rhus-t., ruta.,* **Sil.,** *sulph.*
Bone	Exostosis of nose	Merc., phos.
Bone	exostosis on lower jaw	Ang., Calc-f., hep.
Bone	exostosis on ribs	Merc-c.
Bone	exostosis on right cheek bone	Aur-m.
Bone	feeling of cold in bones	Aran., ars., calc., elaps., lyc., merc., sep., sulph., verat., zinc.
Bone	felon with caries of bone	Asaf., aur., fl-ac., lach., lyc., merc., mez., ph-ac., **Sil.**, sulph.
Bone	felon with caries of bone and deep seated pain aggravated from warmth of bed	Sep.
Bone	felon, bone caries with offensive pus	Fl-ac.
Bone	felon, periosteum (tissue around bone)	Am-c., asaf., calc-p., calc., canth., dios., fl-ac., mez., phos., sep., **Sil.**, sulph.
Bone	fluttering commencing in sacrum and gradually rising to occiput	Ol-j.
Bone	formication in bones of lower limb	Guai.
Bone	formication in sacrum	Bor., crot-t., ph-ac., sars.
Bone	heat in sacrum	Sars., sep., sulph.
Bone	induration (hardness in body tissue) of tendons (tough band connecting muscle to bone) of fingers	Carb-an., Caust.
Bone	inflammation in bone of fingers	Staph.
Bone	inflammation in foot bone	Acon., arn., ars., bor., **Bry.**, calc., calen., carb-an., com., dulc., kali-bi., merc., mygal., phos., puls., rhus-v., sil., **Sulph.**, zinc.
Bone	inflammation in tendo Achillis (tendon that connects the heel bone to the calf muscles)	Sep., zinc.
Bone	inflammation of bone of face	Aur., calc., fl-ac., mez., nit-ac., ph-ac., ruta., sil., staph., still., symph.
Bone	inflammation of bones	Acon., ars-i., ars., asaf., aur-m., aur., bell., bry., calc., chin., clem., coloc., con., cupr., dig., eupho., **Fl-ac.**, guai., hep., iod., kreos., lach., lact-ac., lyc., mag-m., mang., **Merc.**, **Mez.**, nat-c., nit-ac., **Ph-ac.**, phos., plb., psor., **Puls.**, rhus-t., sep., **Sil.**, spig., **Staph.**, sulph., thuj., verat.

Body part/Disease	Symptom	Medicines
Bone	inflammation of periosteum	Ant-c., apis., ars., asaf., aur-m., aur., bell., calc., chin., **Fl-ac.**, kali-i., led., mang., merc-c., merc., **Mez.**, nit-ac., **Ph-ac.**, phyt., psor., Phos., puls., rhus-t., ruta., sil., staph., still., symph.
Bone	inflammation of tendons	Rhod., rhus-t.
Bone	inflammation of the periosteum	Agar., phos., sil.
Bone	injuries in tendons	Anac.
Bone	injuries of bone	Calc-p., calc., **Ruta.**, sul-ac., symph.
Bone	internal chill as if coldness in bones	Berb., elaps., merc., verat.
Bone	itching in olecranon of elbow	Agar., ars-m., mag-m., nit-ac., olnd., phos.
Bone	itching over tibia (inner bone of lower leg)	Aster., bism., cact., calc., chel., cocc., crot-t., grat., hep., kali-c., lach., mang., nit-ac., ph-ac., phos., plb., rumx., sars., sep., stront.
Bone	malignant bone tumour on tibia	Syph.
Bone	moist on sacrum	Graph., led.
Bone	necrosis of bones	**Ars.**, asaf., bell., carb-ac., con., eupho., kreos., *merc-c., merc.*, ph-ac., *phos.*, plb., *sabin.*, sec., sil., sulph., ther., thuj.
Bone	numbness in first finger up radial (radius bone of the forearm) side of arm	Anac., carb-an., phos.
Bone	numbness in head extending to nasal bone	Plat.
Bone	numbness in right illiac fossa (a hollow, pit, or groove in a part of the body such as in a bone) ameliorated by lying on it	Apis.
Bone	numbness in tibia (inner bone of lower leg) of leg	Kalm.
Bone	numbness, in bones of nose	Aml-n., arn.
Bone	ovaries painful extending to shoulder blade (bone in back of shoulder)	
Bone	pain as if bones broken	Aur., bry., cupr., hep., nat-m., puls., ruta., sep., ther., verat., vip.
Bone	pain boring in bones	Agar., aran., asaf., **Aur.**, bar-c., bell., brom., calc., carb-an., clem., dulc., hell., hep., lach., lyc., mang., **Merc.**, mez., nat-c., nat-m., ph-ac., phos., puls., rhod., rhus-t., sabad., sabin., sep., sil., spig., staph., sulph., thuj.
Bone	pain burning in bones	Ars., asaf., aur., bry., carb-v., caust., con., eupho., form., hep., ign., lach., lyc., mang., merc., **Mez.**, nat-c., nit-ac., par., ph-ac., phos., puls., rhus-t., ruta., sabin., sep., sil., staph., sulph., thuj., **Zinc.**
Bone	pain burning in bones at night	Ph-ac.
Bone	pain burning in bones during menses	Carb-v.
Bone	pain digging up bones	Aran., asaf., calc., carb-an., cocc., dulc., mang., rhod., ruta., sep., spig., thuj.
Bone	pain extending to parietal bone (bone forming skull)	Indg., ran-b.
Bone	pain gnawing in bones	Am-m., arg-m., **Bell.**, brom., canth., con., dros., graph., kali-i., lyc., mang., ph-ac., phos., puls., ruta., samb., staph., stront.

Body part/Disease	Symptom	Medicines
Bone	pain gnawing with jerking in bones	**Asaf.**, aur., bell., calc., caust., chin., clem., colch., lyc., merc., nat-m., nux-v., petr., phos., puls., rhod., rhus-t., sep., sil., **Sulph.**, valer.
Bone	pain in attachment of tendons (tough band connecting muscle to bone)	Phyt., rhod., rhus-t.
Bone	pain in bone aggravated from touch	Staph.
Bone	pain in bone as if paralyzed	Nit-ac.
Bone	pain in bone at night	Dros.
Bone	pain in bone in afternoon	Fl-ac.
Bone	pain in bone in afternoon at 3.00 p.m.	Sarr.
Bone	pain in bone lain on	Iod.
Bone	pain in bone of heel	Berb., caps., coloc., crot-h., ign.
Bone	pain in bone of toes	Mez., sep.
Bone	pain in bones at night	Asaf., **Aur.**, caust., *cham.*, cinnb., *fl-ac.*, **Kali-i.**, kalm., *mang.*, *merc-i-f.*, **Merc.**, *mez.*, **Nit-ac.**, *ph-ac.*, *phyt.*, *sars.*, thuj., verat.
Bone	pain in bones of fingers	Alum., apis., ars., crot-h., dios., mez., **Sil.**, verat.
Bone	pain in bones of fingers when grasping	Verat.
Bone	pain in bones of foot	Acon., agar., alum., ars., asaf., aur., bell., bism., carb-v., chin., cocc., cupr., lach., led., merc., mez., nit-ac., plat., ruta., sabin., spig., stann., staph., teucr., verat., zinc.
Bone	pain in bones of leg	**Agar.**, dios., dulc., guai., kali-bi., kali-i., led., lyc., merc., mez., nux-v., phyt., **Syph.**
Bone	pain in bones of leg ameliorated from warmth of bed	Agar., merc., mez.
Bone	pain in bones of lower limb	**Agar.**, aran., carb-v., chin., coloc., con., guai., **Ip.**, kali-bi., kali-c., lyc., mag-m., merc., mez., olnd., petr., rhod., sabin., sulph., valer., zinc.
Bone	pain in bones of lower limb while walking	Mag-m.
Bone	pain in bones of upper limb	Apis., ars., calc-p., iod., kali-bi., **Lyc.**, mag-c., merc., plat., sabad., teucr.
Bone	pain in ear extending to malar bone (cheek bone)	Spig.
Bone	pain in face in left zygoma (cheek bone)	Aur., thuj.
Bone	pain in face in left zygoma aggravated by rest	Mag-c.
Bone	pain in face in left zygoma aggravated at night	Mag-c., mez., plat., sil.
Bone	pain in face in left zygoma ameliorated by pressure	Mez.
Bone	pain in face in left zygoma ameliorated by touch	Thuj.
Bone	pain in face in zygoma	zygoma : Aur., calc-p., caps., caust., chel., cinnb., kali-bi., psor., verb.
Bone	pain in first phalanx (finger bone) of first finger	Osm., plat.
Bone	pain in foot extending to tibia	Nat-m.
Bone	pain in hip extending to sacrum	Ant-c., lyss.
Bone	pain in inner side of bone	Bov., chel., crot-t., led., sil., tarent.
Bone	pain in knee extending to tibia	Indg.

Body part/Disease	Symptom	Medicines
Bone	pain in lumbar region to the pubis	Mag-c., Sabin.
Bone	pain in middle of long bone	Bufo., phyt.
Bone	pain in nose extending to malar bone	Kali-bi.
Bone	pain in olecranon on motion	Hep.
Bone	pain in Periosteum (tissue around bones)	Ant-c., **Asaf.**, aur., bell., bry., camph., cham., chin., colch., coloc., cycl., graph., hell., ign., kalm., led., mang., merc., mez., **Ph-ac.**, phyt., puls., rhod., rhus-t., ruta., sabad., sabin., sil., spig., staph.
Bone	pain in sacral region extending to pubis	Arg-m., helon., laur., Sabin., sulph.
Bone	pain in tendons (tough band connecting muscle to bone)	Anac., Calc., calc-p., chel., chin-s., chin., rhod., rhus-t., sil.
Bone	pain in tendons flexors (muscle bending joint or limb)	Aster.
Bone	pain in tibia ameliorated while standing	**Agar.**, aur-m-n., dulc., tub., verat.
Bone	pain in tibia ameliorated from crossing legs	Aur., bar-c.
Bone	pain in tibia ameliorated on motion	Agar., arg-m., aur-m-n., dulc., psor., rhus-t., verat.
Bone	pain in tibia at night in bed	Aur., carb-an., merc., mez., psor., **Rhus-t.**
Bone	pain in tibia at night	Aur., kali-i., ph-ac., phyt., **Rhus-t.**
Bone	pain in tibia from crossing limbs	**Rhus-t.**
Bone	pain in tibia from damp weather	Dulc., mez., phyt., verat.
Bone	pain in tibia from standing	Aur-m-n., rat.
Bone	pain in tibia in evening	Led.
Bone	pain in tibia in morning	Agar.
Bone	pain in tibia on motion	Berb.
Bone	pain in tibia when extending leg	Aur.
Bone	pain in tibia while sitting	Agar., anac.
Bone	pain in tibia while standing	Bry., carb-an., clem., coc-c., ign., merc., merl., mez., nat-m., nat-s., nux-m., petr., phos., rhod., stry.
Bone	pain in tibia with pain in occiput	Carb-v.
Bone	pain in ulna (bone of human forearm)	Arg-n., calc-s., calc., caust., cham., chin., form., plat., podo., verat-v.
Bone	pain on expansion of tendons	Agar., thuj.
Bone	pain paralytic in bones	**Aur.**, bell., chin., cocc., cycl., dig., led., mez., nat-m., nux-v., petr., puls., rhus-t., sabin., sil., staph., verat., zinc.
Bone	pain paralytic tearing away bones	Bell., bism., chel., chin., cocc., dig.
Bone	pain pinching in bones	Bell., calc., cina., ign., mez., osm., petr., ph-ac., plat., **Verb.**
Bone	pain pressing in bones	Alum., anac., arg-m., ars., asaf., aur., bell., bism., bry., cann-i., canth., carb-s., cham., cocc., colch., coloc., con., cupr., cycl., dros., graph., guai., hell., hep., ign., kali-c., kali-n., merc., mez., nux-m., olnd., phos., plat., puls., rhod., rhus-t., ruta., sabin., sil., spong., stann., staph., thuj., valer., verat., viol-t., zinc.
Bone	pain pressing in glands inward	Aur., *calc.*, cocc., cycl., rheum., *staph.*, zinc.

Body part/Disease	Symptom	Medicines
Bone	pain pressive tearing away bones	**Arg-m.**, arn., asaf., bism., bry., coloc., **Cycl.**, staph., teucr.
Bone	pain stitching in bones	Acon., agar., agn., am-c., anac., ant-c., arg-m., ars., asaf., aur., **Bell.**, **Bry.**, **Calc.**, canth., carb-v., **Caust.**, cedr., chel., chin., cocc., colch., **Con.**, dros., dulc., eupho., graph., **Hell.**, iod., kali-c., kalm., lach., lyc., mag-c., mang., **Merc.**, mez., nit-ac., nux-v., par., petr., ph-ac., phos., **Puls.**, ran-s., ruta., sabin., samb., **Sars.**, **Sep.**, sil., spig., staph., stront., **Sulph.**, thuj., valer., verb., viol-t., zinc.
Bone	pain tearing away bones	Acon., agar., alum., am-m., anac., arg-m., arn., ars., asaf., aur-m., **Aur.**, bar-c., bell., berb., bism., bor., bov., bry., calc-p., cann-s., canth., caps., carb-v., caust., cham., chel., **Chin.**, cina., cocc., coloc., con., crot-t., cupr., cycl., dig., dros., dulc., ferr., graph., hell., hep., ign., iod., **Kali-c.**, kali-n., **Lach.**, laur., lyc., mag-c., mag-m., mang., merc-c., **Merc.**, mez., nat-c., nat-m., nit-ac., nux-v., ph-ac., phos., plb., puls., **Rhod.**, rhus-t., ruta., sabin., samb., sars., sep., **Spig.**, spong., stann., staph., stront., sul-ac., sulph., tab., thuj., valer., verat., verb., zinc.
Bone	pain tearing away bones like cramp	Aur., olnd., valer.
Bone	pain tearing away bones with burning	Sabin.
Bone	pain tearing away bones with jerking	Ang., bry., **Chin.**, cupr., mang.
Bone	pain tearing away periosteum	Bry., mez., ph-ac., rhod.
Bone	pain under scapula (bone forming back of shoulder) after sitting	All-c.
Bone	pain under scapula (bone forming back of shoulder) near spine	Abies-c., aesc., all-c., bad., bry., card-m., Chel., Chen-a., con., conv., cupr., Ind., lac-c., lycps., med., nat-m., nux-v., phos., phys., pic-ac., podo., rhod., ruta., senec.
Bone	pain, constricting bones	Alum.
Bone	pain, cutting in long bones	Calc., osm., sabad.
Bone	pulsation internally in bones	Asaf., calc., carb-v., lyc., merc., nit-ac., phos., rhod., ruta., sabad., sep., sil., sulph., thuj.
Bone	rheumatic pain in bone	Ars-i., ferr., fl-ac.
Bone	sensation of formication in bones	Acon., arn., cham., colch., merc., nat-c., nat-m., nux-v., ph-ac., plat., plb., puls., rhod., rhus-t., sabad., sec., sep., spig., sulph., zinc.
Bone	sensitive tibia (inner bone of lower leg)	Puls.
Bone	sensitiveness to bones	Asaf., aur., bell., bry., calc., carb-an., chel., chin-s., chin., cupr., **Eup-per.**, guai., hyper., lach., lyc., merc-c., merc., mez., nat-c., **Phos.**, puls., rhus-t., sil., stram., sulph., **Tell.**, zinc.
Bone	sensitiveness to Periosteum	Ant-c., aur., bell., bry., chin., ign., **Led.**, merc., mez., ph-ac., puls., rhus-t., ruta., sil., spig., staph.
Bone	slow repair of broken bones	Asaf., **Calc-p.**, **Calc.**, ferr., lyc., merc., mez., nit-ac., ph-ac., phos., puls., ruta., sep., sil., staph., sulph., symph.
Bone	softening of bones	Am-c., **Asaf.**, bell., calc-f., calc-p., **Calc.**, cic., ferr., hep., iod., ip., lyc., **Merc.**, mez., nit-ac., petr., ph-ac., phos., plb., puls., rhod., ruta., sep., **Sil.**, staph., sulph., ther.

Body part/Disease	Symptom	Medicines
Bone	softening of femur (main bone in human thigh)	Sil.
Bone	softening of tibia (inner bone of lower leg)	Guai.
Bone	sore bruised pain in bones	Acon., agar., am-m., **Arg-m.**, asaf., aur., bar-c., bov., calc., cann-s., chin., **Cocc.**, con., cor-r., cupr., graph., **Hep.**, ign., **Ip.**, kali-bi., led., lith., mag-c., mang., mez., nat-m., nux-v., par., petr., ph-ac., phos., puls., **Ruta.**, sabad., sep., sil., spig., valer., verat., zinc.
Bone	stiffness in lower limbs from soreness of tendo achillis (An inelastic cord or band of tough white fibrous connective tissue that attaches a muscle to a bone or other part of heel)	Cimic.
Bone	straining of muscles and tendons from lifting	Alum., ambr., **Arn.**, bar-c., bor., bry., calc-s., **Calc.**, **Carb-an.**, carb-s., carb-v., caust., chin., cocc., coloc., **Con.**, croc., cur., dulc., ferr-p., ferr., **Graph.**, iod., kali-c., lach., lyc., merc., mill., mur-ac., nat-c., nat-m., nit-ac., nux-v., olnd., ph-ac., phos., plat., rhod., **Rhus-t.**, ruta., sec., sep., **Sil.**, spig., stann., staph., sul-ac., sulph., thuj., valer.
Bone	swelling in bone of upper arm	Guare., tep.
Bone	swelling in bones of ankle	Merc., staph.
Bone	swelling in bones of fingers	Carb-an.
Bone	swelling in bones of hand	Aur.
Bone	swelling in bones of upper limbs	Calc., dulc., lyc., mez., sil., sulph.
Bone	swelling in bones	Am-c., **Asaf.**, aur., bell., bry., calc-p., **Calc.**, carb-an., clem., coloc., con., dig., dulc., eupho., ferr., fl-ac., guai., hep., iod., kali-i., kreos., lach., lact-ac., lyc., mang., merc., mez., nat-c., nat-m., nit-ac., petr., **Ph-ac.**, **Phos.**, plb., **Puls.**, rhod., rhus-t., ruta., sabin., sep., **Sil.**, spig., **Staph.**, **Sulph.**, thuj., verat.
Bone	swelling in condyles of elbow	**Calc-p.**, mez.
Bone	swelling in main bone of thigh	Mez., **Sil.**, stront.
Bone	swelling in patella of knee	Coloc., sep
Bone	swelling in Periosteum (tissue around bones)	Ant-c., **Asaf.**, aur., bell., bry., chin., kali-i., mang., merc., mez., nit-ac., **Ph-ac.**, puls., rhod., rhus-t., ruta., sabin., sil., staph.
Bone	swelling in radius (bone in arm or forelimb)	Calc.
Bone	swelling in tendo achillis of leg	Berb., kali-bi., mur-ac., sep., zinc.
Bone	swelling in tendons	Plb.
Bone	swelling in tibia of leg	Aur-m., calc-p., graph., lach., merc., phos., rhus-t., stann., sulph., thuj.
Bone	swelling in tissues around bones of upper limbs	Aur., merc., mez.
Bone	swollen sensation in bones	Ant-c., bell., chel., guai., puls., rhus-t., spig.
Bone	tension in bones	Agar., asaf., **Bell.**, bry., cimic., cocc., con., crot-h., dig., dulc., kali-bi., merc., nit-ac., rhod., ruta., sulph., valer., zinc.
Bone	tumours on metacarpal bones of hand	Ph-ac., tarent.
Bone	twitching (jerk slightly) in tendons (tough band connecting muscle to bone)	Agar., am-c., ambr., ars., asaf., bell., calc., camph., canth., chel., chlor., **Hyos.**, **Iod.**, kali-i., lyc., mez., mur-ac., ph-ac., phos., rhus-t., sec., stry., **Zinc.**

Body part/Disease	Symptom	Medicines
Bone	typhus fever with swelled parotid, and sensitive bones	Mang.
Bone	ulcer in clavicles	Calc-p.
Bone	ulcerative pain in bones	Am-c., am-m., Bar-c., bry., caust., cic., graph., ign., mang., nat-m., puls., rhus-t.
Bone	ulcer in tibia	Asaf., cinnb., cist., graph., lach., mez., nit-ac., ph-ac., **Psor.**, sabin., sang., sulph., syph., vip.
Brain	Anaemia (a blood condition in which there are too few red blood cells or the red blood cells are deficient in hemoglobin, resulting in poor health. Common causes include a lack of dietary iron, heavy blood loss, or the production of too few red blood cells due to disorders such as leukemia) of brain	Alum., ambr., calc-p., calc-s., calc., chin-s., chin., con., dulc., Ferr., fl-ac., hell., kali-c., lyc., mag-c., mosch., mur-ac., nat-c., nat-m., nit-ac., nux-v., petr., Ph-ac., Phos., sang., sel., sep., sil., stry., sulph., zinc.
Brain	aphasia (the partial or total inability to produce and understand speech as a result of brain damage caused by injury or disease)	Both., chen-a., glon., kali-br.
Brain	apoplexy (stroke caused by brain hemorrhage)	**Acon.**, arn., aur., bar-c., **Bell.**, camph., carb-v., chin., **Cocc.**, coff., con., crot-h., cupr., ferr., **Gels.**, hyos., **Ip.**, **Lach.**, laur., lyc., merc., nat-m., nit-ac., nux-m., nux-v., **Op.**, phos., plb., puls., rhus-t., sec., sep., sil., stram.
Brain	boiling sensation in brain	Acon., alum., cann-i., caust., chin., coff., dig., graph., grat., hell., kali-c., kali-s., laur., lyc., mag-m., mang., med., merc., sars., sil., sulph.
Brain	brain feels tired	Colch.
Brain	bubling ,bursting sensation in brain	Form.
Brain	bubling sensation in brain ameliorated by leaning back while sitting	Spig.
Brain	bubling sensation in brain while walking	Nux-v., spig.
Brain	Cancer of breast	Ars.Iod (2nd & 3rd Trituration)
Brain	cancerous affections, encephaloma (protrusion of part of the brain through an opening in the skull)	Acet-ac., ars-i., ars., calc., carb-ac., carb-an., caust., kali-i., kreos., lach., nit-ac., **Phos.**, sil., sulph., thuj.
Brain	cancerous affections, epithelioma	Acet-ac., arg-m., arg-n., **Ars-i.**, ars., aur., bell., brom., calc-p., calc., clem., **Con.**, hydr., kali-s., kreos., **Lyc.**, merc., phos., phyt., ran-b., sep., sil., sulph., thuj.
Brain	Cerebral (the front part of the brain, divided into two symmetrical halves cerebral hemispheres. In humans, it is where activities including reasoning, learning, sensory perception, and emotional responses take place) Hemorrhage	Acon., arn., aur., bar-c., Bell., camph., carb-v., chin., coff., Colch., con., crot-h., cupr., ferr., Gels., hyos., Ip., Lach., laur., lyc., merc., nat-m., nit-ac., nux-m., nux-v., Op., phos., plb., puls., stram.
Brain	cerebral fever	Apis., arn., bapt., bry., canth., cic., gels., **Hyos.**, lach., lyc., nux-m., op., ph-ac., phos., rhus-t., **Stram.**, verat-v., verat.
Brain	cerebro spinal (involving the brain and spinal cord) fever	Acon., aeth., agar., am-c., ant-t., **Apis.**, arg-n., arn., ars., bapt., **Bell.**, bry., cact., camph., canth., cic., cimic., cocc., crot-h., cupr., dig., **Gels.**, glon., hell., hydr-ac., hyos., ign., lyc., nat-m., **Nat-s.**, nux-v., **Op.**, phos., plb., rhus-t., sol-n., tarent., **Verat-v.**, verat., zinc.
Brain	clucking (Voice of hen) sensation in brain	Sulph.

Body part/Disease	Symptom	Medicines
Brain	Concussion of brain	Arn., bell., Cic., hell., hep., hyos., Hyper., kali-p., led., merc., nat-s., ph-ac., rhus-t., sep., sul-ac., zinc.
Brain	congestive fever with threatened brain paralysis with collapse	Carb-v.
Brain	congestive fever with threatened brain paralysis with paralysis of lungs	Ant-t., ars., carb-v., lyc., mosch., phos., sulph.
Brain	congestive fever with threatened brain paralysis	Hell., lach., lyc., **Op.**, ph-ac., phos., tarent., zinc.
Brain	Constriction in brain in morning	Agar., bry., cham., con., gamb., graph., kali-bi., nat-m., nux-m., sulph., sumb., tarax.
Brain	Constriction in brain aggravated from bending forward	Asaf.
Brain	Constriction in brain aggravated from sitting	Fl-ac.
Brain	Constriction in brain aggravated from standing	Mag-c.
Brain	Constriction in brain aggravated from stooping	Berb., coloc., dig., med., thuj.
Brain	Constriction in brain aggravated in open air	Mang., merc., nat-m., valer.
Brain	Constriction in brain aggravated in wet weather	Sulph.
Brain	Constriction in brain ameliorated by heat of sun	Stront.
Brain	Constriction in brain ameliorated from motion	Op., sulph., valer.
Brain	Constriction in brain ameliorated from pressure	Aeth., anac., lach., meny., thuj.
Brain	Constriction in brain ameliorated from uncovering head	Carb-v.
Brain	Constriction in brain ameliorated from vomitting	Stann.
Brain	Constriction in brain ameliorated from walking in open air	Ox-ac.
Brain	Constriction in brain ameliorated from warmth	Stront.
Brain	Constriction in brain ameliorated in morning	Glon.
Brain	Constriction in brain ameliorated in open air	Berb., coloc., kali-i., lach., lyc.
Brain	Constriction in brain ameliorated on lying	Nat-m.
Brain	Constriction in brain ameliorated on rising	Dig., laur., merc.
Brain	Constriction in brain at night	Merc., mez., nux-v.
Brain	Constriction in brain extending to eyes and nose	Nit-ac.
Brain	Constriction in brain from mental exertion	Iris., par., sulph.
Brain	Constriction in brain from sleeping	Graph., merc.
Brain	Constriction in brain in afternoon	Graph., mag-c., naja., nit-ac., phos.
Brain	Constriction in brain in evening	Anac., asaf., hyper., kali-bi., merc., mur-ac., murx., phos., rhus-t., sep., stront., sulph., tab., tarent., valer.
Brain	convulsion epileptic with numbness of brain	Bufo.
Brain	convulsion epileptic with waving sensation in brain	Cimic.
Brain	convulsion from cerebral softening	Caust.
Brain	encephalitis (Inflammation of brain)	Acon., apis., Bell., bry., cadm., camph., canth., cham., cina., con., crot-h., cupr., glon., hell., hyos., lach., merc., nux-v., op., par., phos., phys., plb., puls., rhus-t., stram., sulph., verat-v.

Body part/Disease	Symptom	Medicines
Brain	encephalitis of meninges (protective spine or brain mebranes)	Acon., apis., arg-n., arn., Bell., bry., calc-p., calc., canth., cina., cocc., cupr., gels., glon., Hell., hippoz., hyos., kali-br., lach., merc., nat-m., op., phos., plb., rhus-t., sil., Stram., sulph., Zinc.
Brain	encephalitis of meninges (protective spine or brain mebranes)	Acon., apis., arg-n., arn., Bell., bry., calc-p., calc., canth., cina., cocc., cupr., gels., glon., Hell., hippoz., hyos., kali-br., lach., merc., nat-m., op., phos., plb., rhus-t., sil., Stram., sulph., Zinc.
Brain	encephalitis of periosteum (the sheath of connective tissue that surrounds all bones except those at joints)	Aur-m., aur., Fl-ac., kali-i., led., mang., merc-c., merc., Mez., nit-ac., Ph-ac., phos., puls., rhod., rhus-t., ruta., sil., staph.
Brain	encephalitis with deep sleep or unconsciousness	Bor.
Brain	eruption, bran (husks of cereal grain) like in upper limbs	Bor.
Brain	excessive flow of blood in brain after a pleasant surprise	Coff.
Brain	excessive flow of blood in brain after lifting	Nat-c.
Brain	excessive flow of blood in brain after menses	Chin., ign., nat-m., sulph., thuj.
Brain	excessive flow of blood in brain aggravated toward evening with terrible pain , would press the head against wall , fears going mad	Stram.
Brain	excessive flow of blood in brain as if blood rushed from heart to head	Nux-m.
Brain	excessive flow of blood in brain at night	Am-c., anac., aster., berb., calc-s., calc., carb-v., cycl., kali-c., mill., Psor., puls., sil., sulph.
Brain	excessive flow of blood in brain at night after anger	Bry., cham., staph.
Brain	excessive flow of blood in brain at night ameliorated in open air	ars., camph., caust., coc-c., grat., hell., mag-m., mosch.
Brain	excessive flow of blood in brain at night during shocks in chest	Tab.
Brain	excessive flow of blood in brain at night on bending head backward	Bell.
Brain	excessive flow of blood in brain at night with anxiety	Acon., aur., cycl.
Brain	excessive flow of blood in brain at night with epistaxis	Ant-c., bell., bry., carb-v., croc., lach., lil-t., meli., nux-v., pic-ac., psor.
Brain	excessive flow of blood in brain before menses	Acon., Apis., bell., bry., cupr., gels., glon., hep., hyper., iod., kali-c., lyc., manc., meli., merc., tril.
Brain	excessive flow of blood in brain compells to sit up	Aloe.
Brain	excessive flow of blood in brain during excitement	Asaf., phos.
Brain	excessive flow of blood in brain during menses	Acon., Apis., bell., bry., cact., calc-p., calc-s., calc., caust., cham., chin., cinnb., con., elaps., ferr-p., gels., glon., iod., mag-c., mag-m., manc., merc., mosch., nat-m., nux-m., nux-v., phos., sang., Sulph., verat-v., verat.
Brain	excessive flow of blood in brain during rage (extreme anger)	Acon., Bell., hyos., lach., nux-v., op., phos., stram., verat.

Body part/Disease	Symptom	Medicines
Brain	excessive flow of blood in brain from 5 p.m., to midnight	Glon.
Brain	excessive flow of blood in brain from fright or grief	Ph-ac.
Brain	excessive flow of blood in brain from suppressed discharges or suddenly ceasing pains	Cimic.
Brain	excessive flow of blood in brain from suppressed lochia (the normal vaginal discharge of cell debris and blood after childbirth) from the vagina	Acon., bell., bry., cimic.
Brain	excessive flow of blood in brain from suppressed menses	Acon., apis., arn., Bell., bry., calc-s., calc., cham., chin., Cimic., coc-c., cocc., Ferr., Gels., Glon., graph., Lach., merc., op., stram., sulph.
Brain	excessive flow of blood in brain in afternoon	Am-c., cham., chin-s., graph., lach., nat-m., paeon., ran-b., sil.
Brain	excessive flow of blood in brain in morning	Calc., cham., chin-s., glon., lach., lact-ac., lyc., mag-c., mag-s., naja., raph., tell.
Brain	excessive flow of blood in brain on raising the head	Lyc.
Brain	excessive flow of blood in brain on rising	Eug., lyc.
Brain	excessive flow of blood in brain on shaking the head	Nit-ac., nux-v.
Brain	excessive flow of blood in brain on taking exercise	Sulph.
Brain	excessive flow of blood in brain on waking	Calc., lyc., ph-ac.
Brain	excessive flow of blood in brain when speaking	Coff., sulph.
Brain	excessive flow of blood in brain when spoken to harshly	Ign.
Brain	excessive flow of blood in brain with redness of face	Acon., Bell., canth., coff., cop., cor-r., glon., graph., meli., merc-c., phos., sil., sol-n.
Brain	fever with dry heat at night as if hot vapors rise up to the brain	Ant-t., sarr., sulph.
Brain	Hydrocephalus (increased fluid around brain)	Acon., am-c., Apis., apoc., ars., aur., bell., bry., calc-p., Calc., carb-ac., con., dig., ferr-i., ferr., hell., hyos., indg., iod., kali-i., kali-p., lach., lyc., mag-m., merc., nat-m., op., ph-ac., phos., plat., puls., samb., Sil., stram., sulph., tub., zinc.
Brain	milk disappearing with brain trouble	Agar.
Brain	milk like substance forcibly expelled from breast	Aeth., gamb.
Brain	Mind complaints from anticipation	Arg-n., ars., gels., lyc., med., ph-ac.
Brain	numbness in brain	Apis., bufo., con., kali-br., mag-c., plat.
Brain	pain in cervical region extending to brain	Ferr., kalm., par.
Brain	pain in teeth alternating with stitching pain in left breast	Kali-c.
Brain	pain in uterus extending to breasts	Lyss., murx.
Brain	Painful contraction of the brain that lies below and behind the cerebrum	Absinth.
Brain	paralysis after apoplexy (stroke caused by brain hemorrhage)	Alum., anac., apis., bar-c., cadm., caust., cocc., crot-c., crot-h., cupr., gels., **Lach.**, laur., nux-v., **Op.**, phos., plb., sec., stann., stram., zinc.

Body part/Disease	Symptom	Medicines
Brain	paralysis agitans after apoplexy (stroke caused by Brain haemorrhage)	Anac., arn., bar-c., bell., con., lach., laur., nux-v., **Phos.**, stann., stram., zinc.
Brain	paralysis of left upper limb during meningitis (fatal illness in which a viral or bacterial infection inflames the meninges, causing symptoms such as severe headaches, vomiting, stiff neck, and high fever)	Acon.
Brain	paralysis of lower limb after apoplexy (stroke caused by brain hemorrhage)	**Nux-v.**, phos.
Brain	Pulsation (the rhythmic change in volume that takes place in the heart or an artery) with throbbing pain in middle of brain, every morning, lasts all day	Calc.
Brain	sensation as if cold air passed over brain	Anan., meny., petr., sanic.
Brain	sensation as if cold air passed over brain ameliorated in open air	Laur., sep.
Brain	sensation as if cold air passed over brain spreads from the head	Mosch., valer.
Brain	sensation as if cold cloth around the brain	Glon., sanic.
Brain	sensation as if foreign body in right side of brain	Con.
Brain	sensation as of a ball rising up in brain	Acon., cimic., lach., plat., plb., sep., staph.
Brain	sensation as of a ball rolling on right side of brain	Anan.
Brain	sensation as of a ball rolling in brain	Anan., bufo., hura., lyss.
Brain	sensation in brain as if brain were an ant hill	Agar.
Brain	shocks like electric from concussion (mild brain injury) of brain	Cic.
Brain	tired feeling in brain	Apis., con., iris., lach., nat-m., nux-m., Phos., psor.
Brain	urine inadequate with brain affections	Apis., bell., bry., cupr., squil., stram.
Brain	violent chill with delirium	Arn., ars., bell., bry., cham., **Chin.**, **Nat-m.**, nux-v., puls., sep., stram., sulph., verat.
Breast bone	breathing difficult from pressure on sternum (Breast bone)	All-s., cann-s., ph-ac., phos., rhus-t., squil., thuj.
Breast bone	breathing difficult from pressure on sternum (Breast bone)	All-s., cann-s., ph-ac., phos., rhus-t., squil., thuj.
Breast bone	cancer in sternum (breastbone)	Sulph.
Breast bone	caries of sternum	Con.
Breast bone	constriction in sternum (breastbone)	Acon., cann-s., lob., mur-ac., nux-m., phos., rhus-t., sabin., sulph., zinc.
Breast bone	constriction in sternum on coughing	Phos.
Breast bone	constriction in sternum on motion	Cact., op.
Breast bone	constriction in sternum while eating	Led.
Breast bone	cracking in sternum on bending chest backwards	Am-c.
Breast bone	cracking in sternum on motion	Nat-m., sulph.
Breast bone	formication in sternum	Ran-s.
Breast bone	pain in abdomen extendimg to sternum	Nat-m., rheum.

Body part/Disease	Symptom	Medicines
Breast bone	pain in dorsal region extending to sternum	Kali-bi., laur.
Breast bone	pain in sternum	Bry.
Breast bone	pain in sternum aggravated from stretching	Staph.
Breast bone	pain in sternum from rubbing	Led.
Breast bone	pain in sternum after eating	Chin., con., jug-c.
Breast bone	pain in sternum after smoking	Thuj.
Breast bone	pain in sternum aggravated from pressure	Manc., ph-ac.
Breast bone	pain in sternum ameliorated from sitting erect	Kalm.
Breast bone	pain in sternum as if food had lodged	All-c., led.
Breast bone	pain in sternum at night	Chin.
Breast bone	pain in sternum during inhalation	Bry., caps., chel., laur.
Breast bone	pain in sternum extending back	Con., Kali-bi., stict.
Breast bone	pain in sternum extending to back	Kali-bi., ox-ac., phyt.
Breast bone	pain in sternum from deep respiration	Caust., lyc., nat-m., psor.
Breast bone	pain in sternum from raising arm	Chin.
Breast bone	pain in sternum from respiration	Caps., hep., manc.
Breast bone	pain in sternum from sitting bent	Chin., kalm., rhus-t.
Breast bone	pain in sternum from walking fast	Seneg.
Breast bone	pain in sternum in afternoon	Fl-ac., kali-i.
Breast bone	pain in sternum in spots	Puls., ruta.
Breast bone	pain in sternum on inspiration	Chel., kali-c., manc.
Breast bone	pain in sternum on motion	Bry., led.
Breast bone	pain in sternum on stooping	Kalm., ran-b.
Breast bone	pain in sternum when coughing	Bell., Bry., Caust., chel., chin., cina., cor-r., daph., euphr., hep., Kali-bi., kali-i., kali-n., kreos., osm., ox-ac., ph-ac., phos., phyt., psor., rumx., sang., staph., sulph., thuj.
Breast bone	pain in sternum when drinking	Kali-c., Sep.
Breast bone	pain in sternum when swallowing	All-c., phos.
Breast bone	pain in sternum while ascending	Jug-c.
Breast bone	pain in sternum while talking	Stram.
Breast bone	pain in sternum while walking	Coc-c., jug-c.
Breast bone	pain under left scapula extending to sternum	Chel.
Bronchia	chest symptoms alternating with diarrhoea and bronchitis	Seneg.
Bronchia	cough from sensation of crawling in bronchia (relating to or affecting the tubes bronchi that carry air from the windpipe into the lungs)	Aeth.,Eupi., kreos.
Bronchia	cough from sensation of heat in bronchia	Aeth., eup-per.
Bronchia	inflammation of bronchial tubes (network of airways to and within the lungs) alternates with diarrhoea	Seneg.
Bronchia	inflammation of bronchial tubes in children	Dulc., Ip., Kali-c.
Bronchia	inflammation of bronchial tubes of aged people	Am-c., camph., carb-v., dros., Hippoz., hydr., lyc., nux-v.

Body part/Disease	Symptom	Medicines
Bunion	bunions (an inflammation of the sac bursa around the first joint of the big toe, accompanied by swelling and sideways displacement of the joint) of foot	Am-c., hyper., kali-chl., ph-ac., phos., plb., Sil., zinc.
Bunion	bunions after frost bite (damage to body extremities caused by prolonged exposure to freezing conditions, characterized by numbness, tissue death, and gangrene)	Calc.
Bunion	bunions in soles	Calc.
Bunion	bunions in ulcerated soles	Calc.
Burn	burns	Agar., alum., ant-c., **Ars.**, calc., **Canth.**, carb-ac., carb-v., caust., cycl., eupho., kreos., lach., mag-c., plb., rhus-t., ruta., sec., stram.
Burn	burns of tongues and lips	Ham.
Burn	gangrene from burns or sores	Agar., alum., ant-c., **Anthr.**, apis., **Ars.**, asaf., calc., canth., carb-v., **Caust.**, cycl., eupho., kreos., lach., mag-c., ph-ac., rhus-t., ruta., **Sec.**, stram.
Burning	abscess with burning	**Anthr.**, **Ars.**, pyrog., **Tarent-c.**
Burning	acute angulation of penis with burning in urethra	Calc-p.
Burning	boils on face burning	Alum., am-m., anac., ant-c., apis., ars., calc., caust., chin-s., cic., euphr., graph., kali-c., led., mag-m., merc., nat-m., phos., rat., rhus-t., sars., seneg., sep., staph., sulph.
Burning	boils on face burning when scratched	Nat-s., sars.
Burning	boils on face burning when wet	Euphr.
Burning	boils on face burning, cannot sleep without cold applications	Am-m.
Burning	bubo with burning	Ars-i., ars., bell., carb-an., tarent-c.
Burning	burning	Ail., apis., aster., aur-s., bry., camph., hell., phos., plan., sil., verat.
Burning	burning about anus	Ars., calc.
Burning	burning after itching	Agar., alum., berb., calc., daph., kali-c., mag-c., mez., nux-v., raph.
Burning	burning after itching at night	Nux-v., spong.
Burning	burning after itching between scapula	Rat.
Burning	burning after itching in cervical region	Kali-bi.
Burning	burning after itching in coccyx	Fl-ac.
Burning	burning after itching in evening while undressing	Nux-v.
Burning	burning after itching in lumbar region extending to abdomen and thighs	Nat-m.
Burning	burning after itching in morning while dressing	Nux-v.
Burning	burning after itching while walking in open air	Merc.
Burning	burning after operations	Staph., zinc.
Burning	burning after scratching behind ears	Mag-m.
Burning	burning after scratching ears	Fl-ac.

Body part/Disease	Symptom	Medicines
Burning	burning after scratching in itching	Alum., squil.
Burning	burning after scratching on mammae	Grat.
Burning	burning alternately	Chin.
Burning	burning ameliorated by cold bathing	Apis., aur., nicc., puls., sep., thuj.
Burning	burning ameliorated in open air	Gamb., phyt., Puls.
Burning	burning and redness of left side of cheek	Alum., asaf., lac-c., murx., nat-m., ol-an., ph-ac., spig.
Burning	burning boils in axila	Merc.
Burning	burning during menses	Nicc.
Burning	burning during menses	Cast., mag-c., nicc., nit-ac.
Burning	burning eczema on face	Cic., viol-t.
Burning	burning eruption on head	Ars., bar-c., cic., graph., kali-bi., nit-ac., petr., sars., Sulph.
Burning	burning in coccyx	Am-m., cist., rhus-t.
Burning	burning in coccyx after scratching	Til.
Burning	burning in ear ameliorated by rubbing	Ol-an., phel.
Burning	burning in ear ameliorated by scratching	Caust., mag-c., nat-c.
Burning	burning in ear not ameliorated by rubbing	Zinc.
Burning	burning in ear not ameliorated by scratching	Am-m., arg-m., fl-ac., sars.
Burning	burning in ears aggravated by rubbing	Alum.
Burning	burning in external throat right side	Alum., caust., merc-i-f., vesp.
Burning	burning in kidneys before urination	Rheum., thuj.
Burning	burning in kidneys during urination	Rheum.
Burning	burning in kidneys while lying	Lac-d.
Burning	burning in kidneys with oppressed breathing and faintness	Bufo.
Burning	burning in left kidney	Benz-ac., lachn., zing.
Burning	burning in throat	Caps., manc.
Burning	burning in ureters (either of a pair of ducts that carry urine from the kidneys to the bladder)	Cedr., pin-s., ter.
Burning	burning itching in upper limbs (deltoid region to the hand, including the arm, axilla and shoulder)	Agar., berb., dulc., mez., nux-v., ran-b., spig., stann.
Burning	burning like balls of fire	Ruta.
Burning	burning of external throat left side	Berb., coloc., form., nat-s.
Burning	burning on chest	Alum., bov., cic., mez., rhus-t.
Burning	burning on mammae	Ars., grat., phos., rhus-t.
Burning	burning on one side of cheek and coldnes on other side	Acet-ac., acon., Cham., Ip., kali-c., lach., mosch., nux-v.
Burning	burning one then the other	Chin., nat-c.
Burning	burning pain & crawling in first finger	Agar.
Burning	burning pain after scratching	Kreos.
Burning	burning pain around nails	Con.
Burning	burning pain at night	Kali-c., Aloe., bar-c., calc., Cham., fl-ac., Lach., lyc., mag-m., nat-s., petr., ph-ac., sang., sil., Sulph.

Body part/Disease	Symptom	Medicines
Burning	burning pain beneath shoulder	**Ail.**, lyc., sulph.
Burning	burning pain between fingers	Alum., rhus-v.
Burning	burning pain between index finger and thumb	Alum., berb., iod., rhus-t., sulph.
Burning	burning pain between nates	Arg-m., sep., thuj.
Burning	burning pain between scapula	Acon., alumn., ars-m., berb., bry., cur., glon., graph., helon., Kali-bi., Lyc., mag-m., med., merc., nux-v., ox-ac., ph-ac., Phos., sabad., senec., sil., sulph., thuj., zinc.
Burning	burning pain between scapula after scratching	Mag-c.
Burning	burning pain between scapula ameliorated from rubbing	Phos.
Burning	burning pain between scapula extending down the back	Merc.
Burning	burning pain between scapula extending to nape (back of neck)	Nat-s.
Burning	burning pain between scapula in evening from lying down	Sulph.
Burning	burning pain between scapula in evening from mental exertion	Helon., pic-ac., sil.
Burning	burning pain between scapula in evening in bed	Ferr.
Burning	burning pain between scapula pulsating (throbbing/vibrating)	Phos.
Burning	burning pain between scapula while sitting	Thuj., zinc.
Burning	burning pain during menses	Carb-v.
Burning	burning pain in abdomen after eating	Hydr-ac.
Burning	burning pain in abdomen after ice cream	Ars.
Burning	burning pain in abdomen after stool	Cupr-ar., jug-c., kali-bi., nat-a., sabad.
Burning	burning pain in abdomen ameliorated on lying	Podo.
Burning	burning pain in abdomen before stool	Aloe.
Burning	burning pain in abdomen during stool	Eug., sul-ac.
Burning	burning pain in abdomen while eating	Phos.
Burning	burning pain in acromion (End of shoulder blade)	Mez.
Burning	burning pain in afternoon	Mez.
Burning	burning pain in ankle	Agar., berb., eupho., kreos., laur., manc., nat-c., plat., puls., sulph., zinc.
Burning	burning pain in ankle aggravated from rubbing	Sulph.
Burning	burning pain in ankle extending over the soles to the toes	Kreos.
Burning	burning pain in ankle in evening	Sulph.
Burning	burning pain in ankle while walking	Agar.
Burning	burning pain in back after coition	Mag-m.
Burning	burning pain in back after emission	Merc., phos.
Burning	burning pain in back after grief	Naja.
Burning	burning pain in back after scratching	Mag-c.

Body part/Disease	Symptom	Medicines
Burning	burning pain in back ameliorated after scratching	Rhus-v.
Burning	burning pain in back ameliorated from motion	Mag-m., pic-ac., rat.
Burning	burning pain in back ameliorated from walking in open air	Kali-n.
Burning	burning pain in back at night	Helon., ph-ac.
Burning	burning pain in back before menses	Kreos.
Burning	burning pain in back from mental exertion	Pic-ac., sil.
Burning	burning pain in back from walking in open air	Arn., kali-c., sil.
Burning	burning pain in back from walking in open air	Arn., kali-c., sil.
Burning	burning pain in back in forenoon	Kali-bi.
Burning	burning pain in back in morning	Mag-m., zinc.
Burning	burning pain in back in morning after coition aggravated by rest ameliorated by motion	Mag-m.
Burning	burning pain in back in morning on rising ameliorated by motion	Rat.
Burning	burning pain in back in noon	Rhus-t.
Burning	burning pain in back in spots	Nit-ac., ph-ac., Phos., zinc.
Burning	burning pain in back of finger	Brom., cocc., ran-s., sil.
Burning	burning pain in back of hand	Agar., apis., aur-m., berb., bry., calc., carl., cop., dulc., fl-ac., laur., nat-s., nux-v., rhus-v., sulph.
Burning	burning pain in back when getting warm in bed	Sil.
Burning	burning pain in back while lying	Lyc.
Burning	burning pain in back while lying on back	Ars.
Burning	burning pain in back while sitting	Ars., asar., bor., Zinc.
Burning	burning pain in ball of finger	Sulph., Zinc.
Burning	burning pain in ball of thumb	Laur., lith., nux-v.
Burning	burning pain in bones of lower limb	Eupho.
Burning	burning pain in calf	Agar., alum., am-c., aur., dig., eupi., mez., plb., ran-s., rhus-t., sars., sulph., tarent.
Burning	burning pain in calf from walking in open air	Mez.
Burning	burning pain in cervical region after scratching	Mag-c.
Burning	burning pain in cervical region aggravated from moving head	Nat-s., plb.
Burning	burning pain in cervical region ameliorated from sleep	Calc.
Burning	burning pain in cervical region extending down back	Med.
Burning	burning pain in cervical region extending to clavicle (the long curved bone that connects the upper part of the breastbone with the shoulder blade at the top of each shoulder in humans)	Nat-s.
Burning	burning pain in cervical region extending to occiput (back of head)	Calc.
Burning	burning pain in cervical region in afternoon	Fago.

Body part/Disease	Symptom	Medicines
Burning	burning pain in cervical region in evening	Mag-c.
Burning	burning pain in cervical region in morning	Am-c.
Burning	burning pain in cervical region in morning	Am-c.
Burning	burning pain in cervical region in spots	Kali-br.
Burning	burning pain in cervical region stinging	Glon.
Burning	burning pain in cervical region when touched	Nat-m.
Burning	burning pain in cervical region while swallowing	Petr.
Burning	burning pain in coccyx	Apis., canth., cist., colch., laur., mur-ac., phos., staph.
Burning	burning pain in coccyx during menses	Carb-v., mur-ac.
Burning	burning pain in coccyx extending up the spine	Mur-ac.
Burning	burning pain in coccyx in evening	Apis.
Burning	burning pain in coccyx when touched	Apis.
Burning	burning pain in coccyx while sitting	Apis., cist.
Burning	burning pain in dorsal region from needle work or writing	Ran-b., sep.
Burning	burning pain in dorsal region	Caps., dios., mang., zinc.
Burning	burning pain in elbow	Agar., alum., arg-m., arund., asaf., bell., berb., calc-p., carb-an., carb-v., coc-c., colch., coloc., kali-n., merc., mur-ac., ph-ac., phos., plat., sep., sulph., ter.
Burning	burning pain in elbow at night	Sep.
Burning	burning pain in elbow in evening	Arg-m., carb-an.
Burning	burning pain in elbow in forenoon	Sulph.
Burning	burning pain in evening in bed	Carb-v.
Burning	burning pain in finger in evening	Alum.
Burning	burning pain in finger in forenoon	Fago.
Burning	burning pain in first finger	Acon., agar., alum., arund., berb., card-m., chel., ferr-ma., hura., kali-c., olnd., sil.
Burning	burning pain in foot after walking	Kali-c.
Burning	burning pain in foot aggravated from touch	Bor.
Burning	burning pain in foot at night	Ars-m., coloc., lac-c., nat-c., sep., sil., **Sulph.**
Burning	burning pain in foot at night in bed	Nat-p., **Sulph.**
Burning	burning pain in foot at night in bed during menses	Nat-p.
Burning	burning pain in foot at night in bed during menses	Nat-p.
Burning	burning pain in foot between the toes	Nat-c.
Burning	burning pain in foot from climacteric	Sang.
Burning	burning pain in foot from warmth of bed	Agar., calc., merc., stront., **Sulph.**
Burning	burning pain in foot in bed in evening	Agar.
Burning	burning pain in foot in bed in morning	Hep.
Burning	burning pain in foot in evening	Calc., nat-s., sang., sulph.
Burning	burning pain in foot in evening in bed	Calc., hep., merc., stront., **Sulph.**
Burning	burning pain in foot in morning in bed	Hep., nat-s.
Burning	burning pain in foot in noon	Am-c., hura.

Body part/Disease	Symptom	Medicines
Burning	burning pain in foot while walking	Carb-an., nat-c., nat-m., phyt.
Burning	burning pain in foot with perspiration	Sil.
Burning	burning pain in forearm ameliorated from rubbing	Ol-an.
Burning	burning pain in forearm (part of the human arm between the elbow and the wrist) at night on lying on it	Graph.
Burning	burning pain in forearm after scratching	Bor., caust., clem., laur., sulph.
Burning	burning pain in forearm aggravated from pressure	Bell.
Burning	burning pain in forearm at night	Graph., zinc.
Burning	burning pain in forearm during motion	Thuj.
Burning	burning pain in forearm near the wrist	Agar., bov., caust., kali-bi., rhus-v., zinc.
Burning	burning pain in forearm with stinging in spots	Ran-s.
Burning	burning pain in fourth finger	Spig., stann., tarax.
Burning	burning pain in hand after eating	Sulph.
Burning	burning pain in hand aggravated from washing in cold water	Caps.
Burning	burning pain in hand at night	Lac-c., pall.
Burning	burning pain in hand during chill	Spong.
Burning	burning pain in hand during fever	Hura.
Burning	burning pain in hand during menses	Carb-v., sec.
Burning	burning pain in hand in afternoon	Cham., fago., phos.
Burning	burning pain in hand in afternoon	Nat-s.
Burning	burning pain in hand in eczema	Merc.
Burning	burning pain in hand in evening	Cedr., phos., **Puls., Sulph.**
Burning	burning pain in hand in forenoon	Fago., nat-s.
Burning	burning pain in hand in forenoon while the other is cold	Fago.
Burning	burning pain in hand in morning	Petr., sulph.
Burning	burning pain in hand in noon	Am-c., mag-c.
Burning	burning pain in hand with one hot and pale, the other cold and red	Mosch.
Burning	burning pain in heel at night in bed	Kali-n.
Burning	burning pain in heel extending to tongue	Vip.
Burning	burning pain in heel in morning	Eupi.
Burning	burning pain in heel in morning in bed	Fago., graph.
Burning	burning pain in hip at night	Bell., eupho., mag-m.
Burning	burning pain in hip before menses	Kali-c.
Burning	burning pain in hip during menses	Med.
Burning	burning pain in hip during rest	Kali-n.
Burning	burning pain in hip extending to heel	Arund.
Burning	burning pain in hip in afternoon	Mag-m.
Burning	burning pain in hip in evening	Mag-m., nicc.

Body part/Disease	Symptom	Medicines
Burning	burning pain in hip in evening after lying down	Mag-m.
Burning	burning pain in hip in evening after scratching	Mag-m., nicc.
Burning	burning pain in hip in noon	Nicc.
Burning	burning pain in hip in noon after scratching	Nicc.
Burning	burning pain in hollow of knee	Am-c., ars-h., bar-c., berb., cast-eq., chel., grat., indg., iod., lith., petr., sul-ac., sulph., thuj.
Burning	burning pain in hollow of knee ameliorated from walking	Grat.
Burning	burning pain in hollow of knee at night in bed	Bell., chin., sep.
Burning	burning pain in hollow of knee extending down back of leg	Bar-c.
Burning	burning pain in hollow of knee while sitting	Bar-c., grat.
Burning	burning pain in inner side of thigh	Agar., bry., cocc., lachn., lyc., mez., sars., sulph.
Burning	burning pain in inner side of thigh after rubbing	Samb.
Burning	burning pain in inner side of thigh during menses	Sars.
Burning	burning pain in inner side of thigh in evening	Agar., bry.
Burning	burning pain in inner side of thigh near female genitalia	Bor., kreos., laur., sulph.
Burning	burning pain in inner side of thigh near male genitalia	Bar-c., crot-t., ferr-ma.
Burning	burning pain in inner side of thigh on touch	Lyc.
Burning	burning pain in inner side of thigh while walking	Agar., lyc.
Burning	burning pain in joints	Abrot., ant-t., carb-v., guare., kali-c., mang., nat-c., nat-n., nit-ac., plat., thuj., zinc.
Burning	burning pain in joints of finger	Apis., bufo., cann-i., carb-v., caust., vinc.
Burning	burning pain in joints of fingers	Nat-c.
Burning	burning pain in joints of lower limb	Bar-c., nat-c., phos., stront.
Burning	burning pain in joints of thumb	Spig.
Burning	burning pain in joints of toes	Berb.
Burning	burning pain in joints of upper limbs	Carb-v., graph., nat-c., stront.
Burning	burning pain in knee ameliorated while walking	Phos.
Burning	burning pain in knee from ascending steps	Sulph.
Burning	burning pain in knee in afternoon	Lyc.
Burning	burning pain in knee in morning	Phos.
Burning	burning pain in knee while walking	Stram.
Burning	burning pain in knee with stinging	Bell.
Burning	burning pain in larynx after talking	Ferr., kali-bi.
Burning	burning pain in last lumbar vertebra (a bone of the spinal column, typically consisting of a thick body, a bony arch enclosing a hole for the spinal cord, and stubby projections that connect with adjacent bones)	Acon., aesc., cham., pic-ac.
Burning	burning pain in left scapula	Ambr., bar-c., card-m., com., euphr., fl-ac., nat-m., sil., teucr., zinc.

Body part/Disease	Symptom	Medicines
Burning	burning pain in left scapula at night	Bar-c.
Burning	burning pain in left upper limbs	Cocc.
Burning	burning pain in leg after dinner	Agar.
Burning	burning pain in leg after exercise	Sulph.
Burning	burning pain in leg aggravated from stretching	Berb.
Burning	burning pain in leg aggravated from touch	Bov., con.
Burning	burning pain in leg as from sparks	Anac.
Burning	burning pain in leg at night	Sep.
Burning	burning pain in leg from scratching	Corn., ir-foe., seneg., sulph.
Burning	burning pain in leg from warm bed	Sep.
Burning	burning pain in leg in afternoon while sitting	Sulph.
Burning	burning pain in leg in evening	Agar., nat-s., sang., seneg., sulph.
Burning	burning pain in leg in morning	Agar., nat-s., sulph.
Burning	burning pain in leg when rising	Sulph.
Burning	burning pain in liver	Acon., agar., aloe., am-c., anan., bry., carb-s., carb-v., crot-c., gamb., kali-c., Lept., med., nit-ac., plb., stann., ther.
Burning	burning pain in liver after stool	Lept., stann.
Burning	burning pain in lower limb at night	Fago.
Burning	burning pain in lower limb at night in bed	Kali-c.
Burning	burning pain in lower limb at noon	Agar.
Burning	burning pain in lower limb when undressing	Mez.
Burning	burning pain in lumbar region ameliorated from walking	Bar-c.
Burning	burning pain in lumbar region during pregnancy	Rhus-t.
Burning	burning pain in lumbar region during sleep	Zinc.
Burning	burning pain in lumbar region extending across abdomen	Bar-c.
Burning	burning pain in lumbar region extending to right side & shoulder	Clem.
Burning	burning pain in lumbar region extending up the spine to between scapula	Ars., phos., sep., sil., thuj.
Burning	burning pain in lumbar region from sitting	Asar.
Burning	burning pain in lumbar region in afternoon	Mag-m.
Burning	burning pain in lumbar region in evening	Mag-m.
Burning	burning pain in lumbar region in evening after lying down	Sulph.
Burning	burning pain in lumbar region in morning	Zinc.
Burning	burning pain in lumbar region in spot	Bar-c., ph-ac., zinc.
Burning	burning pain in lumbar region on rising from sitting	Arg-m., bar-c., berb.
Burning	burning pain in lumbar region sudden as from hot needle	Aeth.
Burning	burning pain in lumbar region when breathing deeply	Sep.

Body part/Disease	Symptom	Medicines
Burning	burning pain in morning	Phos.
Burning	burning pain in nail of second finger	Kali-c.
Burning	burning pain in nails	Alum., ant-c., calc., caust., **Graph.**, hep., merc., nat-m., nux-v., puls., sep., sulph.
Burning	burning pain in nates (buttock)	Bar-c., bry., calc-p., coloc., lyc., mag-m., mang., **Merc.**, mez., sep., stront., sulph.
Burning	burning pain in nates in evening after lying down	Sulph.
Burning	burning pain in nates while sitting	Mang.
Burning	burning pain in nose aggravated during menses	Carb-an.
Burning	burning pain in nose during coryza	Aesc., all-c., aloe., am-c., Ars., calad., caust., gels., mez., senec., seneg., sulph.
Burning	burning pain in olecranon	Chel., ph-ac.
Burning	burning pain in palm & soles at night	Lach.
Burning	burning pain in palm after rubbing	**Sulph.**
Burning	burning pain in palm after warm bath	Nat-c.
Burning	burning pain in palm at midnight	Rhus-t.
Burning	burning pain in palm at night	**Lach.**
Burning	burning pain in palm during menses	Carb-v., petr.
Burning	burning pain in palm in evening	**Lach.**, rumx., upa.
Burning	burning pain in palm with stinging	Bor.
Burning	burning pain in palms & soles at night	Lach.
Burning	burning pain in pancreas (a large elongated glandular organ lying near the stomach. It secretes juices into the small intestine and the hormones insulin, glucagon, and somatostatin into the bloodstream)	Iris.
Burning	burning pain in right calf	Agar.
Burning	burning pain in right leg	Agar.
Burning	burning pain in right scapula	Bar-c., cann-s., carb-v., caust., iod., lachn., laur., lyc., plb., seneg., sulph., verat., zinc.
Burning	burning pain in right shoulder	Am-m., carb-v.
Burning	burning pain in right upper limbs	Plb.
Burning	burning pain in roots of nails	Asaf.
Burning	burning pain in sacral region after stool	Coloc.
Burning	burning pain in sacral region aggravated from warmth of bed	Coloc.
Burning	burning pain in sacral region during menses	Carb-v., ferr.
Burning	burning pain in sacral region while sitting	Bor.
Burning	burning pain in sacral region	Bor., carb-v., colch., coloc., ferr., helon., lachn., mur-ac., murx., ph-ac., phos., podo., rhus-t., sabin., sep., sil., sulph., tarent., thuj.
Burning	burning pain in scapula	Alum., Bar-c., carb-s., carb-v., caust., cund., iod., kali-c., lachn., laur., lyc., mang., Merc., mez., mur-ac., nat-c., nat-m., nux-v., rob., seneg., sep., sil., stann., sul-ac., sulph., zinc.

Body part/Disease	Symptom	Medicines
Burning	burning pain in scapula ameliorated from walking	Bar-c.
Burning	burning pain in scapula while sewing	Ran-b.
Burning	burning pain in scapula while writing	Ran-b.
Burning	burning pain in sciatic parts of lower limb	Ars., bufo., gels., lach., lyc., phos., rhus-t., ruta.
Burning	burning pain in second finger	Apis., coloc., kali-c., mez., sul-ac.
Burning	burning pain in shoulder after scratching	Kali-c.
Burning	burning pain in shoulder at night	Puls.
Burning	burning pain in shoulder extending over the arm	Puls., sulph.
Burning	burning pain in shoulder extending to hip	Mag-m.
Burning	burning pain in shoulder in evening	Alumn., dios., sep., sulph.
Burning	burning pain in shoulder in evening after lying down	Sulph.
Burning	burning pain in shoulder in evening while walking	Rhus-t.
Burning	burning pain in shoulder while sitting	Merc.
Burning	burning pain in sole in afternoon	Gels., ol-an.
Burning	burning pain in sole in evening	Berb., **Lach.**, lyc., mag-m., merc., nat-c., phos., zinc.
Burning	burning pain in sole in evening after scratching	Am-c.
Burning	burning pain in sole in morning	Ph-ac., phyt., zinc.
Burning	burning pain in sole in morning in bed	Hep.
Burning	burning pain in soles after eating	Sil.
Burning	burning pain in soles after long sitting	**Sulph.**
Burning	burning pain in soles after standing	Carb-v., merc., sul-i.
Burning	burning pain in soles ameliorated in bed	Nat-c.
Burning	burning pain in soles ameliorated while walking	Ol-an.
Burning	burning pain in soles cold to touch	Sulph.
Burning	burning pain in soles during menses	Carb-v., petr.
Burning	burning pain in soles from walking in open air	Hep.
Burning	burning pain in soles in bed	Canth., **Cham.**, hep., ph-ac., plb., sang., **Sulph.**
Burning	burning pain in soles in summer	Vesp.
Burning	burning pain in soles while sitting	Anac., carb-v., lyc., mur-ac.
Burning	burning pain in soles while walking	Carb-v., coc-c., graph., kali-c., lyc., nat-c., **Sulph.**
Burning	burning pain in spine	Acon., agar., Ars., asaf., bell., cham., gels., glon., helon., kalm., Lach., lachn., lyc., mag-m., med., nat-c., nat-p., ph-ac., Phos., pic-ac., plb., puls., Sec., sep., thuj., verat., zinc.
Burning	burning pain in spine	Ars-m., graph., lach., pic-ac., sep., sil.
Burning	burning pain in spine above small of back	Zinc.
Burning	burning pain in spine ameliorated from rubbing	Phos.
Burning	burning pain in spine as if a hot iron were thrust through lower vertebræ	Alum.
Burning	burning pain in spine at night	Ph-ac.
Burning	burning pain in spine from mental exertion	Pic-ac., sil.

Body part/Disease	Symptom	Medicines
Burning	burning pain in spine in small place	Agar.
Burning	burning pain in spine in spots	Agar., phos.
Burning	burning pain in spine shooting	Acon.
Burning	burning pain in spine stitching	Mag-m., zinc.
Burning	burning pain in spine stitching ameliorated by motion	Mag-m.
Burning	burning pain in spine while lying	Lyc.
Burning	burning pain in spine while sitting	Zinc.
Burning	burning pain in spleen	Anan., bell., carb-an., coc-c., ign., sec.
Burning	burning pain in spots	Plan.
Burning	burning pain in spots of upper limbs	Am-c., bry., merc., ph-ac.
Burning	burning pain in thigh after rubbing	Sulph.
Burning	burning pain in thigh after scratching	Grat., plan.
Burning	burning pain in thigh aggravated from touch	Phos.
Burning	burning pain in thigh ameliorated after scratching	Alum.
Burning	burning pain in thigh at night in bed	Carb-v., eupho.
Burning	burning pain in thigh extending to ankles	Apis., arund.
Burning	burning pain in thigh while sitting	Asaf., grat.
Burning	burning pain in thigh while standing	Ph-ac.
Burning	burning pain in thigh while walking	Coloc., ph-ac.
Burning	burning pain in third finger	Osm., tarax.
Burning	burning pain in thumb	Agar., arum-t., arund., berb., chel., gran., graph., hep., lach., laur., mag-arct., mag-aust., merc., nux-v., ol-an., olnd., sars., staph., vesp., zinc.
Burning	burning pain in thumb at night	Sars.
Burning	burning pain in thumb in afternoon	Agar.
Burning	burning pain in tip of fourth finger	Apis., aur-m-n., fl-ac., kali-c., sul-ac.
Burning	burning pain in tip of thumb	Con., croc., gymn., lach., mur-ac., olnd., sil., sulph., teucr.
Burning	burning pain in tips of finger	Am-m., anthr., apis., bell., caust., con., croc., crot-c., gins., mag-m., mur-ac., nat-s., sabad., sars., sil., sulph., tab.
Burning	burning pain in tips of toes	Mur-ac., sars.
Burning	burning pain in toes after wetting feet	Nit-ac.
Burning	burning pain in toes aggravated in warm bed	Nux-v.
Burning	burning pain in toes at day time	Ind.
Burning	burning pain in toes at night	Plat.
Burning	burning pain in toes on walking	Phos.
Burning	burning pain in toes with cold feet	Apis.
Burning	burning pain in trachea when speaking	Dros.
Burning	burning pain in trachea with cough	Caust., ferr., gels., mag-s., phyt., Spong.
Burning	burning pain in upper arm after scratching	Mosch.

Body part/Disease	Symptom	Medicines
Burning	burning pain in upper arm at night in bed	Arg-n.
Burning	burning pain in upper arm in deltoid	Nux-v.
Burning	burning pain in upper arm in spots	Berb., graph., sulph.
Burning	burning pain in upper limbs after scratching	Kreos., led., merc., til.
Burning	burning pain in upper limbs after washing	Bov.
Burning	burning pain in upper limbs aggravated from covering	Rhus-v.
Burning	burning pain in upper limbs aggravated from touch	Crot-t.
Burning	burning pain in upper limbs aggravated from uncovering	Crot-t.
Burning	burning pain in upper limbs ameliorated after scratching	Jug-c.
Burning	burning pain in upper limbs at night	Chin., til.
Burning	burning pain in upper limbs at night in bed	Chin.
Burning	burning pain in upper limbs extending over body	Apis.
Burning	burning pain in upper limbs extending to fingers	Mag-m.
Burning	burning pain in upper limbs extending to hand	Fl-ac.
Burning	burning pain in upper limbs from rubbing	Crot-t.
Burning	burning pain in upper limbs in evening	Puls.
Burning	burning pain in upper limbs in forenoon	Cast.
Burning	burning pain in upper limbs in morning	Agar.
Burning	burning pain in upper limbs on motion	Crot-t.
Burning	burning pain in urethra after stool	Nat-c.
Burning	burning pain in urethra when stream is interrupted	Clem.
Burning	burning pain in urethra after coition	Berb., canth., nat-p., sep., sul-ac., Sulph.
Burning	burning pain in urethra after emission	Carb-an., carb-v., caust., cob., dig., merc., sep., sulph., thuj.
Burning	burning pain in urethra after erection	Anag., cahin., calc-p., canth., carb-s., ferr-i., mag-m., mosch., nat-m., nit-ac.
Burning	burning pain in urethra after rising	Thuj.
Burning	burning pain in urethra ameliorated during urination	Berb., bry., cocc.
Burning	burning pain in urethra at all times	Calad., canth.
Burning	burning pain in urethra at close of urination	Cann-s., kali-n., mez., Nat-c., ph-ac.
Burning	burning pain in urethra before urination	Alum., apis., aspar., berb., Bor., bry., calc., Cann-i., Canth., chel., coc-c., colch., cop., dig., ery-a., fl-ac., merc-c., merc., nat-c., nit-ac., nux-v., ph-ac., phos., prun-s., puls., rhod., seneg., sulph., zinc.
Burning	burning pain in urethra ceases during coition	Anag.
Burning	burning pain in urethra during coition	Agar., ant-c., calc., canth., kreos., merc., sulph., thuj.
Burning	burning pain in urethra during emission	Ant-c., bor., clem., sars., sep., Sulph., thuj.
Burning	burning pain in urethra during exercise	Alum.
Burning	burning pain in urethra during menses	Nat-m.

Body part/Disease	Symptom	Medicines
Burning	burning pain in urethra during stool	Coloc.
Burning	burning pain in urethra during urination	Anag., Caust., con., fl-ac., ign., seneg., teucr., thuj.
Burning	burning pain in urethra last drop cause violent burning	Arg-n., carb-v., clem., colch., coloc., lyc., merc., mez., nux-m., sel., tell.
Burning	burning pain in urethra on touching	Berb., bor., merc.
Burning	burning pain in urethra on waking after emission	Carb-an.
Burning	burning pain in urethra urinating while	Ant-c., ant-t., Canth., con., nit-ac., phos., prun-s., sabad., sulph.
Burning	burning pain in urethra when beginning to urinate	Apis., ars., cann-s., clem., Merc., nat-a., prun-s., teucr.
Burning	burning pain in urethra when effort is made to pass urine	Calad., prun-s.
Burning	burning pain in urethra when not urinating	Asaf., berb., bov., bry., calad., cedr., clem., graph., merc-c., Merc., nat-c., nit-ac., sabad., staph., sulph., teucr., thuj.
Burning	burning pain in urethra when semen is discharged	Agar., ant-c., arg-n., berb., bor., calc., canth., clem., kreos., merc., nat-m., nit-ac., sars., sep., sul-ac., Sulph., thuj.
Burning	burning pain in urethra while sitting	Card-m., par.
Burning	burning pain in urethra while walking	Stry.
Burning	burning pain in wrist after scratching	Calc-p., plb.
Burning	burning pain in wrist aggravated from rubbing	Berb.
Burning	burning pain in wrist extending to index finger	Arund.
Burning	burning pain in wrist extending to index finger & thumb	Agar., asar.
Burning	burning pain in wrist extending to little finger	**Sulph.**
Burning	burning pain in wrist in afternoon	Sulph.
Burning	burning pain in wrist in evening	Stront.
Burning	burning pain near last rib	Kali-bi., lyss.
Burning	burning pain on top of shoulder	Carb-v.
Burning	burning pain under right scapula	Bry., cann-s., lob., pall., staph., tab.
Burning	burning pain with itching in hip	Lith.
Burning	burning periodic	Asaf.
Burning	burning perspiration	Merc., mez., **Nat-c.**, verat.
Burning	burning pimples in cervical region	Am-c.
Burning	burning pimples in lumbar region	Lyc.
Burning	burning prepuce	Caust., merc.
Burning	burning swelling of foot	Canth.
Burning	burning throat pit	Calc-p., chel., elaps., lach.
Burning	burning vesicles (a very small blister filled with clear fluid serum) on chest	Alum.
Burning	burning vesicles on penis	Caust., merc.
Burning	burning, back of the eyes	Form.
Burning	chancres burning	Ars-m.

Body part/Disease	Symptom	Medicines
Burning	cicatrices burn	Ars., carb-an., graph., lach.
Burning	coldness in foot in noon while the other one burns	Hura.
Burning	coldness in foot with burning soles	Cupr.
Burning	coldness in foot with burning soles during chill	Ant-c., aur., ferr., Meny., phos., sep., Verat., zinc.
Burning	coldness in leg with burning in thighs	Tab.
Burning	coldness in upper arm with burning	Graph.
Burning	Coldness of right side of head but feels burning hot	Bar-c., calc.
Burning	condylomata on skin burning	Apis., cinnb., nit-ac., ph-ac., sabin., thuj.
Burning	corns burning	Agar., alum., am-c., ant-c., arg-m., bar-c., bry., calc-s., calc., carb-v., caust., graph., hep., Ign., lith., lyc., meph., nat-m., nux-v., petr., ph-ac., phos., ran-b., ran-s., rhus-t., Sep., sil., sulph., thuj.
Burning	cough with burning in chest	Am-c., caust., coc-c., eupho., euphr., led., mag-m., ph-ac.
Burning	cracks of skin with burning	Petr., sars., zinc.
Burning	cracks on hands burning	Petr., sars., zinc.
Burning	discoloration with red spots in thigh with burning	Ph-ac.
Burning	discoloration, redness in spots with burning	Berb., sulph., tab.
Burning	eructations burning	Caust., coff., crot-t., ferr., iod., lyc.
Burning	eruption, burning after scratching in upper limbs	Staph., til.
Burning	eruption, burning in upper limbs	Con., merc., nat-c., **Rhus-t.**, spig.
Burning	eruption, burning after scratching in hands	Mez., **Staph.**
Burning	eruption, burning after scratching in thighs	Til.
Burning	eruption, burning after scratching	Staph., til.
Burning	eruption, burning in foot	Bov., mez.
Burning	eruption, burning in hands	Bufo., rhus-t.
Burning	eruption, burning in hollow of knee	Merc.
Burning	eruption, burning in knee	Nux-v.
Burning	eruption, burning in legs	Lact-ac., rhus-t.
Burning	eruption, burning in pimples when scratched in thighs	Staph., til.
Burning	eruption, burning in thighs	Fago., til.
Burning	eruption, burning on touch in hands	Canth., **Cic.**
Burning	eruption, burning pimples in hands	Bov., rhus-t.
Burning	eruption, burning pimples in thighs	Mang.
Burning	eruption, burning vesicles between the fingers	Canth.
Burning	eruption, burning vesicles in back of hands	Mez.
Burning	eruption, burning vesicles in forearm	Sil.
Burning	eruption, burning vesicles in hands	Canth., rhus-v.
Burning	eruption, burning vesicles in lower limbs	Verat.
Burning	eruption, burning vesicles in thighs	Verat.
Burning	erupion, burning vesicles in wrists	Am-m., bufo., mez.

Body part/Disease	Symptom	Medicines
Burning	eruption, burning	**Ars.**, bov., fago., lact-ac., **Merc.**, nux-v., **Rhus-t.**, til.
Burning	eruption, itching burning in foot	Bov., mez.
Burning	eruption, itching burning rash in thighs during menses	Rhus-v.
Burning	eruption, pemphigus (an autoimmune disease characterized by large blisters on the skin and mucous membranes, often accompanied by itching or burning sensations) in upper limbs	Sep., ter.
Burning	eruption, pemphigus in back of hands	Sep.
Burning	eruption, pemphigus in wrists	Sep.
Burning	eruption, pimples between index finger and thumb burning on touch	Canth.
Burning	eruption, pimples burning after scratching in upper limbs	Canth., carb-an.
Burning	eruption, pimples burning in elbow	Kali-n.
Burning	eruption, pimples burning in forearm	Am-c., calad., mang., nat-s.
Burning	eruption, pimples burning in shoulder	Mag-m.
Burning	eruption, pimples burning in upper limbs	Am-c., bov., mag-m., nat-s., rhus-t.
Burning	eruption, pimples in wrists with burning after scratching	Carb-an.
Burning	eruption, pustules burns in thighs	Mez.
Burning	eruption, rash in wrists burning after scratching	Calad.
Burning	eruption, vesicles in wrists burning when scratched	Am-m.
Burning	eruption, with burning in wrists	Merc.
Burning	eruptions (rash or blemish) burning at night	Ars., caust., merc., **Rhus-t.**, staph., til.
Burning	eruptions burning	Agar., alum., am-c., am-m., ambr., anac., ant-c., ant-t., **Apis.**, arg-m., **Ars.**, aur., bar-c., bell., berb., bov., bry., bufo., calad., calc-s., calc., cann-s., canth., caps., **Carb-ac.**, carb-an., carb-s., carb-v., **Caust.**, chin-a., chin., **Cic.**, clem., cocc., coff., colch., com., con., crot-t., cub., dig., dulc., eupho., **Graph.**, guai., hell., hep., ign., kali-ar., kali-bi., kali-c., kali-i., kali-n., kali-s., kreos., lach., laur., led., lyc., mang., **Merc.**, mez., nat-a., nat-c., nat-m., nat-p., nit-ac., nux-v., olnd., par., petr., ph-ac., phos., plat., plb., psor., puls., ran-b., **Rhus-t.**, sabad., sars., seneg., sep., sil., spig., spong., squil., stann., staph., stram., stront., sulph., teucr., thuj., urt-u., verat., viol-o., viol-t., zinc.
Burning	eruptions burning aggravated from touch	Cann-s., canth., merc.
Burning	eruptions burning ameliorated after scratching	Kali-n.
Burning	eruptions burning in open air	Led.
Burning	eruptions burning pocks	**Ars.**, lach., merc.
Burning	eruptions burning when washing	Merc.
Burning	eruptions burning when washing in cold water	Clem., thuj.
Burning	eruptions carbuncle burning	Anthr., apis., ars., coloc., crot-c., crot-h., hep., **Tarent-c.**

Body part/Disease	Symptom	Medicines
Burning	eruptions carbuncle crusty burning	Am-c., ant-c., calc., cic., puls., sars.
Burning	eruptions herpetic burning	Agar., alum., am-c., ambr., anac., **Ars.**, aur., bar-c., bell., bov., bry., calad., calc., caps., carb-an., carb-v., **Caust.**, cic., clem., cocc., con., dulc., hell., hep., kali-c., kali-n., kreos., lach., led., lyc., mang., **Merc.**, mez., nat-c., nat-m., nux-v., olnd., par., petr., ph-ac., phos., plb., psor., puls., ran-b., **Rhus-t.**, sabad., sars., sep., sil., spig., spong., squil., staph., stram., sulph., teucr., thuj., verat., viol-t., zinc.
Burning	eruption, pimples burning	Agar., **Ars.**, bov., canth., caust., graph., kali-c., mag-m., merc., nat-s., ph-ac., rhus-t., squil., staph., stront., sulph., til.
Burning	eruption, pustules burning	Am-c., jug-r., petr.
Burning	eruption, tubercles burning	Am-c., am-m., calc., carb-an., cocc., dulc., kali-i., mag-m., mag-s., mang., merc., mur-ac., nicc., nit-ac., phos., staph.
Burning	eruptions, burning after scratching in lower limbs	Til.
Burning	eruptions, burning in fingers	Ran-b.
Burning	eruptions, burning in lower limbs	Bov., fago., lact-ac., merc., nux-v., til.
Burning	eruptions, burning pimples when scratched in lower limbs	Staph.
Burning	felon, burning panaritium	**Anthr.**
Burning	felon, malignant (likely to spread or cause death) with burning	Anthr., ars., **Tarent-c.**
Burning	fever alternating with chilliness, dry burning heat	Bell., sang.
Burning	fever at night with dry burning heat	**Acon.**, anac., arn., **Ars.**, bar-c., **Bell.**, **Bry.**, calc., carb-v., caust., cedr., chel., chin-s., cina., coc-c., coff., colch., coloc., con., dulc., graph., hep., kali-n., lach., lyc., nit-ac., nux-m., nux-v., **Phos.**, puls., ran-s., rhod., **Rhus-t.**, rhus-v., spig., thuj., tub.
Burning	fever at night with dry burning heat and anxiety	Acon., apis., **Ars.**, bar-c., bry., rhus-t.
Burning	fever at night with dry burning heat and sleeplessness	Bar-c., cham., graph., hyos., phos.
Burning	fever at night with dry burning heat without thirst	Apis., **Ars.**
Burning	fever with burning heat after midnight	**Ars.**, ign., lyc., merc., nat-m., phos., sulph., thuj.
Burning	fever with burning heat at night	**Acon.**, agar., apis., **Ars.**, arund., bapt., **Bell.**, berb., bry., **Cact.**, cann-s., canth., carb-s., carb-v., cham., cina., con., hep., ign., lyc., merc., nat-m., nit-ac., nux-v., op., petr., **Phos.**, **Puls.**, rhus-t., staph., stram., sulph., thuj., verat.
Burning	fever with burning heat at night in bed with intolerable burning heat	**Puls.**
Burning	fever with burning heat before midnight	Agar., ars., **Bry.**, cham., laur., puls., sep., verat.
Burning	fever with burning heat in afternoon	**Apis.**, ars., **Bell.**, berb., bry., hep., hyos., ign., lyc., nat-m., nit-ac., nux-v., **Phos.**, puls., rhus-t., stram., sulph.

Body part/Disease	Symptom	Medicines
Burning	fever with burning heat in afternoon with transient (short in duration) chill	Cur.
Burning	fever with burning heat in evening	Acon., agar., apis., ars., **Bell.**, berb., bry., carb-v., cham., cina., hell., hep., hyos., ign., ip., **Lyc.**, merc-c., mosch., nat-m., nit-ac., nux-v., **Phos., Puls., Rhus-t.**, staph., sulph., thuj., verat.
Burning	fever with burning heat in forenoon	Bry., lyc., **Nat-m.**, nux-v., phos., rhus-t., sulph., thuj., verat.
Burning	fever with burning heat in morning	Ars., bry., cham., ign., nat-m., nux-v., rhus-t., sulph., thuj.
Burning	fever with burning heat with distended blood vessels	Aloe., bell., chin-s., **Chin.**, cycl., dig., ferr., hyos., led., **Merl.**, puls., sars.
Burning	fever with dry burning heat and desire to be covered	Manc.
Burning	fever with dry burning heat during sleep	Gins., **Samb.**, thuj.
Burning	fever with dry burning heat except head and face, which are covered with sweat	Stram.
Burning	fever with dry burning heat except head and face, which are covered with sweat which he does not feel	Canth.
Burning	fever with dry burning heat extending from head and face with thirst for cold drinks	Acon.
Burning	fever with dry burning heat in parts lain on	Lyss., manc.
Burning	fever with dry burning heat increased by walking in open air	Chin.
Burning	fever with dry burning heat lasting all day	Chin., thuj.
Burning	fever with dry burning heat mostly internal, blood seems to burn in the veins	**Ars.**, bry., med., **Rhus-t.**
Burning	fever with dry burning heat outside & cold inside	Ars.
Burning	fever with dry burning heat spreading from the hands over the whole body	**Chel.**
Burning	fever with dry burning heat with and without body turning hot	**Bell.**
Burning	fever with dry burning heat with pricking over the whole body	**Chin.**, gels.
Burning	fever with dry burning heat with stinging sensation	Apis., merc-c.
Burning	fever with dry burning heat with sweat even when bathed in with red face	Op.
Burning	fever with dry burning heat with thirst for cold drinks	Acon., **Phos.**
Burning	fever with dry burning heat with unquenchable thirst	**Ars.**, bell., colch., hep., **Phos.**
Burning	fever with dry heat in evening with distended veins and burning hands that seek out cool places	**Puls.**
Burning	fever with internal burning heat	Ars., bell., brom., caps., hyos., mez., mosch., **Sec.**
Burning	fever with internal burning heat at 9.00 a.m.	Brom.

Body part/Disease	Symptom	Medicines
Burning	foot burning	Agar., ars., aster., calc., cham., cocc., fl-ac., graph., kali-ar., kali-c., lyc., **Med.**, nat-s., **Ph-ac.**, phyt., plan., **Puls.**, sang., sanic., **Sec.**, sep., stann., **Sulph.**, zinc.
Burning	foot burning uncovers them	Agar., cham., mag-c., **Med., Puls.**, sang., sanic., **Sulph.**
Burning	growth resembling a wart on penis burning	Apis., cinnb., Nit-ac., ph-ac., psor., sabin., thuj.
Burning	haemorrhage with burning in urethra	Ambr., chin., coch., graph., kali-c., kali-i., merc., nux-v., puls., seneg., sulph., ter.
Burning	hemorrhage from urethra with burning	Ambr., chin., coch., graph., kali-c., kali-i., merc., nux-v., puls., seneg., sulph., ter.
Burning	inflammation of urethra with burning, shooting pain and increased gonorrhœa	Arg-n., cann-s.
Burning	insensibility in hand to burning	Plb.
Burning	interrupted sleep after midnight with burning in veins	Verat.
Burning	itching behind ear followed by burning	Nat-m.
Burning	itching in ankle with burning	Berb., lith.
Burning	itching in back of foot with burning	Berb.
Burning	itching in back of hand with burning	Stann.
Burning	itching in bend of knee with burning after scratching	Rat.
Burning	itching in buttock with burning	Am-c.
Burning	itching in calf with burning	Berb., mez.
Burning	itching in first toe with burning	Nat-c.
Burning	itching in foot with burning	Berb., stram.
Burning	itching in forearm with burning	Agar., calad., kali-bi.
Burning	itching in hand with burning	**Agar.**, apis., arg-m., kali-bi.
Burning	itching in hip with burning after scratching	Mag-c.
Burning	itching in lower limbs with burning	Agar., alum., anac., apis., berb., calc., dulc., hep., kali-n., led., lith., mez., mur-ac., nat-c., nux-v., paeon., rhus-t., sars.
Burning	itching in palm at midnight with burning	Agar., aur-m., ran-b., spig.
Burning	itching in palm at midnight with burning after rubbing	**Sulph.**
Burning	itching in sole of foot with burning	Berb., kali-n.
Burning	itching in thigh with burning	Agar., alum., anac., apis., bar-c., berb., calc., dulc., led., nux-v., rhus-t., sars.
Burning	itching in thigh with burning in spots	Rhus-t.
Burning	itching in thumb with burning	Aur-m.
Burning	itching in toes with burning	Berb., hep., Ind., mur-ac., nat-c., paeon.
Burning	itching in upper arm with burning	Berb., dulc., nux-v.
Burning	itching of Forehead with burning	Kali-bi.
Burning	itching, burning after scratching	Lach., nat-p., phos., rumx., sabad., sabin., **Sulph.**
Burning	leucorrhoea burning	Alum., am-c., ars-i., ars., bar-c., Bor., Calc-s., Calc., canth., carb-an., carb-s., carb-v., cast., con., ferr-i., fl-ac., iod., kali-ar., kali-c., kali-p., kali-s., Kreos., mag-s., meph., nit-ac., phos., Puls., Sep., sul-ac., Sulph., tarent., thuj.

Body part/Disease	Symptom	Medicines
Burning	new cracks of skin with burning	Sars.
Burning	pain burning in blood vessels	Agar., **Ars.**, aur., bry., calc., hyos., med., nat-m., nit-ac., op., **Rhus-t.**, sulph., verat.
Burning	pain burning in bones	Ars., asaf., aur., bry., carb-v., caust., con., eupho., form., hep., ign., lach., lyc., mang., merc., **Mez.**, nat-c., nit-ac., par., ph-ac., phos., puls., rhus-t., ruta., sabin., sep., sil., staph., sulph., thuj., **Zinc.**
Burning	pain burning in bones at night	Ph-ac.
Burning	pain burning in bones during menses	Carb-v.
Burning	pain burning in glands	Alum., ant-c., arn., **Ars.**, bell., brom., bry., calc., cann-s., carb-v., caust., cic., clem., cocc., con., graph., hep., ign., kali-c., laur., merc., mez., nat-m., nux-v., phos., phyt., plat., **Puls.**, rhus-t., sep., sil., staph., sul-ac., sulph., teucr., zinc.
Burning	pain burning in kidney with oppressed breathing and faintness	Bufo.
Burning	pain burning in left upper part of body	Kreos.
Burning	pain burning in parts grasped with the hands	Bry., **Caust.**
Burning	pain in bladder with burning after urination	Alum., apis., berb., calc-p., canth., fl-ac., lyc., sep., sil., thuj.
Burning	pain in bladder with burning aggravated by standing	Eup-pur.
Burning	pain in bladder with burning ameliorated by walking in open air	Ter.
Burning	pain in bladder with burning at night	Bell.
Burning	pain in bladder with burning before urination	Apis., berb., bor., bry., calc., cann-i., canth., caps., chel., clem., colch., fl-ac., lach., nat-c., rheum., rhod., seneg., thuj., zinc.
Burning	pain in bladder with burning during menses	Sep.
Burning	pain in bladder with burning during urination	Aloe., canth., caps., cham., eup-pur., kali-bi., lyc., nux-v., phos., prun-s., rheum., ter.
Burning	pain in bladder with burning while lying	Fl-ac.
Burning	pain stitching & burning like cold needles	**Agar.**
Burning	pain stitching (Sensation while closing a wound with one or more stitches) & burning	**Ars.**, aur., mez., ol-an., spig.
Burning	pain stitching with burning in muscles	Acon., alum., am-m., anac., arg-m., arn., **Asaf.**, aur., bar-c., bry., calc., caust., cic., cina., **Cocc.**, colch., dig., eupho., ign., laur., lyc., mag-c., mang., merc., **Mez.**, mur-ac., **Nux-v.**, olnd., par., phyt., plat., plb., rhod., **Rhus-t.**, sabad., sabin., samb., sep., spig., stann., **Staph.**, **Sul-ac.**, tarax., **Thuj.**, viol-t., zinc.
Burning	pain stitching with burning in muscles like hot needles	**Ars.**, ol-an.
Burning	pain tearing away bones with burning	Sabin.
Burning	pain tearing with burning in muscles	Bell., carb-v., caust., kali-c., led., lyc., nit-ac., ruta., sabin., tarax., zinc.
Burning	pain, burning at bottom throat	Ars.

Body part/Disease	Symptom	Medicines
Burning	pain, burning in larynx during coryza	Am-m., seneg.
Burning	pain, burning in larynx during cough	Ars., bell., bufo., carb-v., caust., cham., chel., coc-c., dros., gels., iod., mag-m., phos., pyrog., rumx., seneg.
Burning	pain, burning in larynx extending to abdomen	Ambr.
Burning	pain, burning in larynx extending to epiglottis (flap of cartilage situated at the base of the tongue that covers the opening to the air passages when swallowing, preventing food or liquids from entering the windpipe trachea)	Wye.
Burning	pain, burning in larynx extending to nostrils	Kali-bi.
Burning	pain, burning in larynx on deep inspiration	Rumx.
Burning	pain, burning in trachea as if nails in larynx	Spong.
Burning	pain, burning in trachea	Am-m., ant-c., ars., bar-c., canth., carb-v., caust., cham., cina., cycl., ferr-ar., gels., graph., hydr-ac., iod., lach., lact., lob., lyc., mag-m., merc-c., merc., mez., myric., par., phos.,puls., rumx., seneg., sep., spong., staph., sulph., ter., zinc.
Burning	pain, burning in trachea during cough	Ant-c., carb-v., caust., cina., iod., lach., mag-m., pyrog., Spong., sulph., zinc.
Burning	pain, burning in trachea on coughing	All-c., staph., sulph.
Burning	pain, burning in trachea on swallowing	Merc-cy.
Burning	painful burning swelling of lower limbs	Ant-c., ars., mur-ac., petr., ph-ac., puls.
Burning	perspiration in foot with burning	Calc., lyc., mur-ac., petr., sep., sulph., thuj.
Burning	pimples burning before menses	Aur-m., verat.
Burning	pimples burning during menses	All-s., caust., hep., lyc., petr.
Burning	pimples on chest with burning	Agar., bov., staph.
Burning	pimples on face burning	Aphis., cic.
Burning	pustules on tongue with burning and stinging	Am-c.
Burning	rash on face burning	Teucr.
Burning	sciatic pain in lower limb with burning	Ars., bufo., coloc., gels., lach., lyc., phos., rhus-t., ruta.
Burning	side of external throat burning after dinner	Grat.
Burning	skin burning after coition	Agar.
Burning	skin burning after scratching	Agar., am-c., am-m., ambr., anac., ant-c., arn., ars., bar-c., bell., bov., bry., calad., calc., cann-s., canth., caps., carb-an., carb-s., carb-v., **Caust.**, chel., cic., cocc., coff., con., crot-t., cycl., dros., dulc., eupho., graph., hep., kali-ar., kali-c., kali-p., kali-s., kreos., lac-c., **Lach.**, laur., led., lyc., mag-c., mag-m., mang., **Merc.**, mez., mosch., nat-c., nat-m., nat-s., nit-ac., nux-v., **Olnd.**, par., petr., ph-ac., phos., puls., ran-b., rhod., **Rhus-t.**, sabad., sabin., samb., sars., sel., seneg., **Sep., Sil.**, spig., spong., squil., staph., stront., **Sulph.**, thuj., til., verat., viol-t., zinc.
Burning	skin burning after sleep	Urt-u.
Burning	skin burning after working in cold water	Thuj.
Burning	skin burning as from flames	Viol-o.
Burning	skin burning as from mental excitement	Bry.

Body part/Disease	Symptom	Medicines
Burning	skin burning as from sparks	Agar., arg-m., calc-p., calc., nat-m., **Sec.**, sel.
Burning	skin burning as from stings	Calc-p., cocc., **Urt-u.**
Burning	skin burning at night	Ars., carb-v., cinnb., clem., con., dol., merc., nux-v., olnd., rhus-t.
Burning	skin burning from perspiration	Merc., **Mez.**, **Nat-c.**, verat.
Burning	skin burning in spots	Agar., am-c., am-m., apis., ars., bell., canth., carb-v., caust., chel., croc., cupr., ferr., fl-ac., iod., kali-ar., kali-c., lach., lyc., mag-c., mag-m., merc., mez., nat-s., **Ph-ac.**, plat., rhus-t., sel., sul-ac., **Sulph.**, tab., thuj., viol-o., zinc.
Burning	skin burning on parts lain on	Lyss., manc., sulph.
Burning	skin burning on touch	Canth., ferr., sabin.
Burning	skin dry & burning with inability to persspire	Acon., alum., am-c., ambr., anac., apis., apoc., arg-m., arn., ars-i., **Ars.**, **Bell.**, bism., bry., calc., cann-s., cham., chin., coff., **Colch.**, con., cupr., dulc., eup-pur., **Graph.**, hyos., iod., ip., kali-ar., **Kali-c.**, kali-s., laur., led., lyc., mag-c., merc-c., merc., nat-m., nit-ac., **Nux-m.**, nux-v., olnd., op., ph-ac., phos., plat., **Plb.**, psor., puls., rhus-t., sabad., samb., sec., seneg., sep., **Sil.**, spong., **Squil.**, staph., sulph., teucr., thuj., verb., viol-o.
Burning	skin dry & burning with inability to persspire when exercising	Arg-m., calc., nat-m., **Plb.**
Burning	skin, burning after coition	Agar.
Burning	skin, burning ameliorated in cold air	Kali-bi.
Burning	skin, burning at night	Bov., lachn., mez., til.
Burning	skin, burning at night as from nettles	Calc-p., **Chlol.**, cocc., **Urt-u.**
Burning	skin, burning during chill	Hep., petr.
Burning	skin, burning in cold air	Apis., cadm., kali-ar., lact-ac., nit-ac., rumx., sep., spong., staph., tell., tub.
Burning	skin, indurations burning	Hep.
Burning	skin, swelling & burning	Acon., ant-c., arn., **Ars.**, bell., **Bry.**, calc., carb-an., carb-v., caust., chin., cocc., colch., coloc., crot-h., dulc., eupho., hell., hep., hyos., iod., kali-ar., kali-c., lach., led., **Lyc.**, mang., merc., mez., nat-a., nat-c., nux-v., op., ph-ac., **Phos.**, puls., rhus-t., samb., sec., sep., sil., spig., spong., squil., stann., **Sulph.**
Burning	sleeplessness from burning in vein	Ars.
Burning	swelling in fingers with burning	Olnd.
Burning	swelling in joints of fingers with burning	Bufo.
Burning	tears, burning	Apis., arn., ars-i., ars., aur., bell., cadm., calc., canth., chin-a., Chin., dios., eug., Euphr., kreos., lyc., merc., nat-s., nit-ac., nux-v., phyt., plb., psor., Rhus-t., sang., sil., spig., staph., stict., stront., Sulph., verb., zinc.
Burning	toes burning	Bor.
Burning	tubercles stinging & burning	Calc., carb-ac., merc., phos.
Burning	tumour burning	Calc., carb-an., thuj.
Burning	ulcer in face burning	Nux-v.

Body part/Disease	Symptom	Medicines
Burning	ulcer in mouth burning	Alum., ars., caps., carb-v., caust., chin., cic., hydr., kali-ar., kali-i., kreos., merc., nat-c., nat-m., ph-ac., sep., sin-n.
Burning	ulcer burning	Ars., hep.
Burning	ulcer in buttocks with burning	Vinc.
Burning	ulcer in fauces with burning	Caps.
Burning	ulcer in lower limbs burning with touch	Merc.
Burning	ulcer in nose with burning	Ars., sil.
Burning	ulcer in skin with burning	Ambr., **Anthr., Ars.,** asaf., aur., bar-c., bar-m., bell., bov., bry., bufo., calc-s., calc., canth., carb-ac., carb-an., **Carb-s., Carb-v., Caust.,** cham., chin-a., chin., cinnb., clem., con., dros., ferr-ar., graph., hep., hydr., ign., kali-ar., kali-c., kali-p., kali-s., kreos., lach., **Lyc.,** mang., **Merc.,** mez., mur-ac., nat-a., nat-c., nat-m., nat-p., nit-ac., nux-v., petr., ph-ac., plb., **Puls.,** ran-b., **Rhus-t.,** sars., sec., sel., sep., **Sil.,** squil., staph., stront., **Sulph.,** syph., thuj., zinc.
Burning	ulcer in skin with burning in margins	**Ars.,** asaf., carb-an., caust., clem., hep., lach., **Lyc., Merc.,** mur-ac., petr., ph-ac., phos., puls., ran-b., sep., **Sil.,** staph., sulph., thuj.
Burning	ulcer in skin with burning when touched	Ars., bell., canth., carb-v., lach., lyc., merc., mez., puls., rhus-t., sil., sulph.
Burning	ulcer with burning around	Ars., asaf., bell., caust., cham., hep., lach., lyc., merc., mez., mur-ac., nat-c., nux-v., petr., phos., **Puls.,** rhus-t., sep., sil., staph.
Burning	ulcer with burning at night	Anthr., carb-v., hep., lach., merc., rhus-t., staph.
Burning	ulcer with burning during menses	Carb-v.
Burning	ulcer with burning in leg	**Anthr., Ars.,** carb-v., lyc., merc., nit-ac., puls., **Sil.,** syph.
Burning	ulcer with burning in lower limbs	**Anthr., Ars.,** carb-ac., **Carb-s., Carb-v.,** caust., **Lyc.,** mag-c., **Merc., Puls., Sil.,** sulph., zinc.
Burning	ulcer with burning in tips of fingers	**Ars.,** sep.
Burning	urine burning before menses	Apis., canth., verat., zinc.
Burning	urine burning during menses	Nux-v., zinc.
Burning	varicose veins burning	Apis., **Ars.,** calc.
Burning	vesicles on face burning	Agar., anac., aur., caust., cic., nat-m., ran-b.
Burning	vesicles on gums burning	Bell., mag-c., mez.
Burning	vesicles on tongue burning like fire on right side	Phel.
Burning	wandering burning pain	Plat.
Burning	warts burning	Am-c., ars., hep., lyc., petr., phos., rhus-t., sep., sulph.
Bursa	bursa (a fluid-filled body sac that reduces friction around joints or between other parts that rub against one another) on wrist	Ruta., stann.
Bursa	bursa (a fluid-filled body sac that reduces friction around joints or between other parts that rub against one another)	Arn., calc-p., cann-s., Nat-m., Sil., stann., Stict.
Bursa	inflammation in bursa (fluid-filled body sac that reduces friction around joints or between other parts that rub against one another)	Ruta.

Body part/Disease	Symptom	Medicines
Buttock	abscess in nates (Buttock)	Carb-o., sulph., thuj.
Buttock	bubbling sensation in nates	Ant-c., zinc.
Buttock	bubbling sensation in nates while standing	Ant-c.
Buttock	burning pain between nates	Arg-m., sep., thuj.
Buttock	burning pain in nates (buttock)	Bar-c., bry., calc-p., coloc., lyc., mag-m., mang., **Merc.**, mez., sep., stront., sulph.
Buttock	burning pain in nates in evening after lying down	Sulph.
Buttock	burning pain in nates while sitting	Mang.
Buttock	carbuncles on nates	Agar., thuj.
Buttock	chill beginning in and extending from buttocks	Puls.
Buttock	coldness in gluteal region	Agar., calc.
Buttock	coldness in nates	Agar., daph., hydr.
Buttock	coldness in nates at night in bed	Cench.
Buttock	coldness in nates during menses	Mang.
Buttock	constrictions in nates	Plat., thuj.
Buttock	contraction of muscles & tendons of nates	Rhus-t.
Buttock	convulsion of nates	Bar-c., calc., nux-v., sep.
Buttock	cramp in buttock muscles	Agar., bell., gels., hyos., hyper.
Buttock	cramp in nates	Bell., bry., cann-s., caust., graph., rhus-t., sep.
Buttock	cramp in nates at night in bed	Sep.
Buttock	cramp in nates while standing	Rhus-t.
Buttock	cramp in nates while stooping	Cann-s.
Buttock	discoloration with redness in nates	Cann-s., hyos.
Buttock	discoloration with redness in spots in nates	Cann-s., mag-c.
Buttock	emaciation of buttocks (either of the two fleshy mounds above the legs and below the hollow of the back)	Bar-m., lach., nat-m., sacc.
Buttock	eruption in nates	Ant-c., bor., canth., caust., graph., mez., nat-c., nat-m., nux-v., sel., thuj., til.
Buttock	eruption, between nates	Olnd.
Buttock	eruption, blood boils in nates	Aur-m.
Buttock	eruption, blotches in nates	Ant-c., bry., sars.
Buttock	eruption, boils in nates	Agar., alum., am-c., aur-m., bar-c., bart., cadm., calad., graph., hep., indg., lyc., nit-ac., ph-ac., phos., plb., psor., rat., sabin., sars., sec., sep., sil., sulph., thuj.
Buttock	eruption, corroding vesicles in nates	Bor.
Buttock	eruption, excoriation in nates	Rhus-t., thuj.
Buttock	eruption, herped in nates	Bor., caust., kreos., nat-c., nicc.
Buttock	eruption, in upper parts between nates	Hep.
Buttock	eruption, itching in nates	Calc-p., caust., graph., thuj., til.
Buttock	eruption, itching pimples in nates	Kali-n., lyc., til.
Buttock	eruption, knots in nates	Ther.

Body part/Disease	Symptom	Medicines
Buttock	eruption, leprous spots annular (shaped like ring) in nates	Graph.
Buttock	eruption, moisture between nates	Arum-t., thuj.
Buttock	eruption, painful in nates	Graph.
Buttock	eruption, painful pimples in nates	Ham., sulph.
Buttock	eruption, pimples between nates	Sulph.
Buttock	eruption, pimples in nates	Ant-c., ars-h., bar-c., berb., calc., canth., chel., cob., graph., ham., hura., kali-n., lyc., mag-c., mang., meph., merc., nat-p., nux-v., petr., plan., rhus-t., sel., sulph., thuj., til.
Buttock	eruption, pustules between nates	Phos.
Buttock	eruption, pustules in nates	Ant-c., calc., grat., hyos., jug-c., ph-ac.
Buttock	eruption, scabs in nates	Chel., graph., psor.
Buttock	eruption, scurfy in nates	Calc-p.
Buttock	eruption, tubercles in nates	Hep., mang., phos.
Buttock	eruption, urticaria in nates	Hydr., lyc.
Buttock	eruption, vesicles in nates	Bor., cann-s., carb-an., crot-t., iris., olnd., ph-ac., rhus-t.
Buttock	excoriation between nates	Arg-m., arum-t., bufo., carb-s., **Graph.,** nat-m., nit-ac., puls., sep., sulph.
Buttock	formication in nates	Ars.
Buttock	induration of nates	Ph-ac., thuj.
Buttock	infiltration of nates	Vip.
Buttock	itching between buttock	Alum., bar-c., con.
Buttock	itching between buttock	Alum., bar-c., con.
Buttock	itching in buttock	Am-c., ant-t., asc-t., bar-c., calc-p., calc., carb-ac., caust., cham., con., dulc., gran., kali-c., lyc., mag-c., mag-m., mez., olnd., petr., prun-s., sel., sil., staph., stront., **Sulph.,** ther., thuj., zinc.
Buttock	itching in buttock after dinner	Laur.
Buttock	itching in buttock aggravated from scratching	Petr.
Buttock	itching in buttock ameliorated from cold water	Petr.
Buttock	itching in buttock ameliorated from scratching	Kali-i., olnd., thuj.
Buttock	itching in buttock at night	Petr.
Buttock	itching in buttock at night in bed	Merc-i-f.
Buttock	itching in buttock in bed	Rumx.
Buttock	itching in buttock in evening	Sars.
Buttock	itching in buttock in evening in bed	Lyc.
Buttock	itching in buttock in evening while undressing	Mag-c.
Buttock	itching in buttock in morning on rising	Nat-c.
Buttock	itching in buttock in open air	Rumx.
Buttock	itching in buttock with burning	Am-c.
Buttock	itching in gluteal (muscle that form the buttock or and move the thigh) region of hip	Coloc., fl-ac., mur-ac., ph-ac., tarax.

Body part/Disease	Symptom	Medicines
Buttock	numbness in nates of lower limb	Calc-p., dig., plb., raph., spong., sulph.
Buttock	numbness in nates of lower limb on rising after sitting	Calc-p.
Buttock	numbness in nates of lower limb while sitting	Alum., calc-p., dig., guai., sulph.
Buttock	pain in gluteal (buttock muscle) region	Eup-per., euphr., hura., kalm., laur., lepi., med., nit-ac., puls., rhus-t., sol-t-ae., spig., tab.
Buttock	pain in gluteal region after sitting	Laur., puls.
Buttock	pain in gluteal region from walking	Spig., tab.
Buttock	pain in ilium extending to the glutei (buttock) muscles and thighs	Kali-c.
Buttock	pain in lumbar region to the nates (buttock)	Kali-c., thuj.
Buttock	pain in nates of lower limb	Agar., bry., calc-p., calc., caust., cina., cist., coca., coloc., cupr., eup-per., eupho., iod., kali-bi., kali-c., kalm., merc., mez., mill., nit-ac., phos., plb., puls., sep., staph., **Sulph.**, tarent.
Buttock	perspiration in nates	Thuj.
Buttock	sensitive nates	Ars.
Buttock	shocks in buttocks	Cocc.
Buttock	shuddering buttocks	Croc.
Buttock	shuddering buttocks while sitting	Croc.
Buttock	swelling in the buttocks	Coloc., crot-t., dulc., ph-ac., sulph.
Buttock	tingling in gluteal muscles	Calc-p.
Buttock	twitching in buttocks	**Agar.**, ant-c., calc., kali-c., mag-m., nat-c., ph-ac., phos., prun-s., sep., spong., stann.
Buttock	twitching in buttocks in evening	Ant-c.
Buttock	twitching in buttocks while sitting	Ant-c., calc., nat-c.
Buttock	ulcer in buttocks	Bor., sabin., sulph., vinc.
Buttock	ulcer in buttocks with burning	Vinc.
Buttock	ulcer in upper part of buttocks	Sabin.
Buttock	warts on buttocks	Con.

Body part/Disease	Symptom	Medicines
Calculi	calculi (a stone or concretion, especially one in the kidney, gallbladder, or urinary bladder)	Ant-c., arg-n., Benz-ac., Berb., cact., Calc., Canth., card-m., chin., coc-c., colch., eup-per., lach., lith., Lyc., mez., mill., naja., nat-m., nat-s., nit-ac., nux-m., nux-v., pareir., petr., phos., puls., raph., ruta., Sars., Sep., sil., tarent., thuj., zinc.
Calculi	calculi after operation of bladder	Arn., calen., cham., chin., cupr., nux-v., Staph., verat.
Calculi	calculi in bladder	Ant-c., arg-n., Benz-ac., Berb., cact., Calc., Canth., card-m., chin., coc-c., colch., eup-per., lach., lith., Lyc., mez., mill., naja., nat-m., nat-s., nit-ac., nux-m., nux-v., pareir., petr.,phos., puls., raph., ruta., Sars., Sep., sil., tarent., thuj., zinc.
Calculi	calculi, after operation	Arn., calen., cham., chin., cupr., nux-v., Staph., verat.
Calf	abscess in calf (the fleshy part at the back of the leg below the knee)	Chin.
Calf	bubbling sensation in calf	Crot-h., rheum., spig.
Calf	burning pain in calf	Agar., alum., am-c., aur., dig., eupi., mez., plb., ran-s., rhus-t., sars., sulph., tarent.
Calf	burning pain in calf from walking in open air	Mez.
Calf	burning pain in right calf	Agar.
Calf	chill beginning in and extending from calves	Lach., lyc., ox-ac.
Calf	coldness in calf	Ars., berb., bufo., chel., hyper., lach., mang., rumx.
Calf	coldness in calf ameliorated while rising from sitting	Mang.
Calf	coldness in calf in evening	Mang.
Calf	coldness in calf in forenoon	Berb.
Calf	coldness in foot extending to calves	Aloe., crot-t.
Calf	compression of calf	Jatr., led., sol-n.
Calf	contraction of muscles & tendons of calf of leg	Agar., agn., arg-n., ars., bov., calc-p., caps., caust., jatr., led., med., nat-c., nat-m., puls., sil.
Calf	contraction of muscles & tendons of calf of leg while walking	Agar., lyc.
Calf	contraction of muscles & tendons of calf of leg with cramp like pain	Ferr.
Calf	convulsion of calf	Berb., cupr., ferr-m.
Calf	convulsive twitching of calf	Op.
Calf	cramp in ankle extending to calf	Cupr.
Calf	cramp in calf after coition	Coloc.
Calf	cramp in calf after mortification (the death and decaying of a part of a living body, e.g. because the blood supply to it has been cut off)	Coloc.

Body part/Disease	Symptom	Medicines
Calf	cramp in calf after stool	Ox-ac., trom.
Calf	cramp in calf after walking	Carb-an., plat., **Rhus-t.**
Calf	cramp in calf ameliorated on motion	Arg-m., bry., ferr., rhus-t.
Calf	cramp in calf at day time	Graph., petr.
Calf	cramp in calf at night	Ambr., anac., arg-n., ars., berb., bry., Calc., carb-an., carb-v., caust., coca., cocc., dig., eupi., ferr-m., ferr., graph., kali-c., Lyc., lyss., mag-c., mag-m., med., nit-ac., nux-m., nux-v., petr., plb., rhus-v., sars., sep., stann., Sulph., zinc.
Calf	cramp in calf at night from bending foot	Chin.
Calf	cramp in calf before menses	Phos.
Calf	cramp in calf before sleep	Nux-m.
Calf	cramp in calf during coition	Cupr., graph.
Calf	cramp in calf during labor	Nux-v.
Calf	cramp in calf during menses	Cupr., phos., verat.
Calf	cramp in calf during pregnancy	Sep.
Calf	cramp in calf during sleep	Ant-t., graph., inul., kali-c., nat-m., tep.
Calf	cramp in calf from ascending	Berb.
Calf	cramp in calf from lifting the foot	Agar.
Calf	cramp in calf in afternoon	Ant-t., elaps.
Calf	cramp in calf in bed	Ars., bov., Calc., Carb-s., caust., eupi., ferr-m., ferr., graph., hep., ign., kali-c., lachn., lact-ac., mag-c., nux-v., phys., Rhus-t., sep., sil., Sulph.
Calf	cramp in calf in bed on flexing thigh	Nux-v.
Calf	cramp in calf in cholera	Ant-t., camph., colch., **Cupr.**, jatr., kali-p., mag-p., **Sulph.**, **Verat.**
Calf	cramp in calf in evening	Kali-n., mag-c., nux-v., sel., sulph.
Calf	cramp in calf in evening in bed	Ars., mag-c., puls.
Calf	cramp in calf in evening on going to sleep	Berb., nux-m.
Calf	cramp in calf in forenoon	Nat-m., sulph.
Calf	cramp in calf in morning	Bry., carb-an., lach., nit-ac.
Calf	cramp in calf in morning in bed	Bov., caust., graph., hep., ign., lach., lact-ac., nit-ac., sil., sulph.
Calf	cramp in calf in morning on rising	Ferr., lact-ac.
Calf	cramp in calf in morning on waking	Lob.
Calf	cramp in calf on attempting to coition	Cupr.
Calf	cramp in calf on bending knee	Cocc., hep., ign.
Calf	cramp in calf on crossing feet	Alum.
Calf	cramp in calf on descending	Coca.
Calf	cramp in calf on drawing up knee	Coff.
Calf	cramp in calf on drawing up leg	Kali-c., nit-ac.
Calf	cramp in calf on flexing leg	Cocc., coff., kali-c., nux-v.
Calf	cramp in calf on motion	Bapt., bufo., calc., coca., hyos., ign., lyc., nux-m.

Body part/Disease	Symptom	Medicines
Calf	cramp in calf on pulling boot	Calc.
Calf	cramp in calf on rising from a bed	Ferr., mag-c.
Calf	cramp in calf on rising from a seat	Alum., anac.
Calf	cramp in calf on standing long	Euphr.
Calf	cramp in calf on standing	Euphr., ferr., nat-m.
Calf	cramp in calf on stepping	Sulph.
Calf	cramp in calf on waking	Graph., lob., staph., verat-v.
Calf	cramp in calf on walking	Agar., am-c., **Anac.**, arg-m., arg-n., ars., berb., **Calc-p.**, cann-s., coca., dulc., ign., lact., lyc., mag-m., nat-m., nit-ac., puls., sul-ac., **Sulph.**
Calf	cramp in calf when stretching foot after waking	Aspar.,Chin., nit-ac., thuj.
Calf	cramp in calf when stretching foot in bed after waking	**Calc.**, carl., cham., lyss., nat-c., pin-s., sulph.
Calf	cramp in calf when stretching leg	Bar-c., bufo., **Calc.**, carl., lyc., nux-v., sep., sulph.
Calf	cramp in calf when thinking about it	Spong., staph.
Calf	cramp in calf when turning foot while sitting	Nat-m.
Calf	cramp in calf when turning over in bed	Mag-c.
Calf	cramp in calf while dancing	Sulph.
Calf	cramp in calf while lying	Bry., led., mag-c., sel.
Calf	cramp in calf while sitting bent	Lyc.
Calf	cramp in calf while sitting	Ign., lyc., olnd., plat., **Rhus-t.**
Calf	cramp in calf while walking	Phos.
Calf	cramp in right calf	Agar., kali-c., lyss., trom.
Calf	cramp like twitching of calf	Jatr.
Calf	discoloration on calf with blotches	Petr.
Calf	discoloration on calf with blue spots	Kali-p.
Calf	discoloration with red spots on calf	Con., graph., kali-br., lach.
Calf	discoloration with spots on calf	Con., graph., sars.
Calf	emaciation of calf	Sel.
Calf	eruption, blotches in calf	Aur., carb-v., lach., merc., petr., phos., thuj.
Calf	eruption, boils in calf	Bell., **Sil.**
Calf	eruption, desquamation in calf	Mag-c.
Calf	eruption, eczema in calf	Graph.
Calf	eruption, elevated spots in calf	Mag-c.
Calf	eruption, herpes in calf	Cycl., lyc., sars.
Calf	eruption, in calf	Apis., bell., caust., kali-ar., mag-c., petr., phyt., sars., sep., sil., thuj.
Calf	eruption, itching in calf	Sil.
Calf	eruption, lumps in calf	Nit-ac.
Calf	eruption, pimples in calf	Agar., arg-n., asc-t., bov., bry., elaps., hura., kali-bi., lach., nat-c., ph-ac., puls., rumx., sabin., sars., sep., staph., zinc.
Calf	eruption, pimples in calf becoming ulcer	Ph-ac.

Body part/Disease	Symptom	Medicines
Calf	eruption, pustules in calf becoming ulcer	Kali-bi., kali-br.
Calf	eruption, rash in calf	Calc.
Calf	eruption, red in calf	Mag-c.
Calf	eruption, red spots in calf	Con., lyc., phyt.
Calf	eruption, scabs in calf	Kali-br.
Calf	eruption, tubercles in calf	Petr.
Calf	eruption, urticaria in calf	Carb-v.
Calf	eruption, vesicles in calf	Caust., sars., sep.
Calf	eruption, white nodes in calf	Thuj.
Calf	flashes of pain in calf	Xan.
Calf	formication in calf	Agar., alum., ant-c., bar-c., cast., caust., cham., coloc., ip., lach., nux-v., onos., plb., rhus-v., sang., sol-n., spig., sul-ac., sulph., zinc.
Calf	formication in calf after walking in open air	Nux-v.
Calf	formication in calf in evening	Alum.
Calf	formication in calf while sitting	Bar-c.
Calf	formication in calf while standing	Verat.
Calf	formication in calf while walking	Sul-ac.
Calf	heaviness in calf	Agar., aloe., arg-n., ars-i., berb., cham., euphr., lyss., rhus-t., sep., sulph.
Calf	itching in calf	Aloe., alum., berb., cact., calc., carb-ac., carb-s., **Caust.**, chel., cinnb., cocc., crot-c., cycl., euphr., graph., hep., hura., ip., kali-bi., laur., lyc., mag-c., mag-m., mang., mez., nat-c., nat-m., nit-ac., ol-an., paeon., phos., phyt., rumx., sabad., sars., sul-i., sulph., tarax., ther., thuj., verat-v., verat., zinc.
Calf	itching in calf ameliorated from rubbing	Paeon.
Calf	itching in calf ameliorated from scratching	Laur., mag-c., mag-
Calf	itching in calf at night	Rumx., zinc.
Calf	itching in calf in evening	Cycl., daph., sars.
Calf	itching in calf in evening on lying down	Tarax.
Calf	itching in calf in morning	Rumx., sars.
Calf	itching in calf in spots	Graph., sars.
Calf	itching in calf while standing	Verat.
Calf	itching in calf while undressing	Cact.
Calf	itching in calf while walking	Cocc.
Calf	itching in calf with burning	Berb., mez.
Calf	jerking in calf	Graph., **Op.**, tarax.
Calf	lameness in calf	Ars-i., pic-ac.
Calf	lumps in calf	Merc., nit-ac.
Calf	numbness in calf of leg	Acon., ars., berb., bry., cham., coloc., dulc., graph., lach., nux-v., phos., sil., verat-v.
Calf	numbness in calf of leg in afternoon	Dulc.

Body part/Disease	Symptom	Medicines
Calf	numbness in calf of leg in evening	Dulc.
Calf	pain in calf after bathing	Pip-m.
Calf	pain in calf after walking	Am-m., cinnb., rhus-t.
Calf	pain in calf ameliorated from drawing feet	Cham.
Calf	pain in calf ameliorated from warmth of bed	Nux-v.
Calf	pain in calf ameliorated on motion	Agar., am-c., ars-i., cupr., rhus-t.
Calf	pain in calf at night	Anac., arg-n., cham., gels., lyc., nux-v., pic-ac., sabad., sulph.
Calf	pain in calf during chill	Ars., thuj.
Calf	pain in calf during menses	Berb.
Calf	pain in calf extending down tibia	Led.
Calf	pain in calf from ascending steps	Arg-n., rhus-t., sulph.
Calf	pain in calf from descending steps	Arg-m., puls-n.
Calf	pain in calf from touch	Calc.
Calf	pain in calf from walking	Alum., anac., ars., arund., **Calc.**, caps., carb-an., gymn., ign., iris., jatr., lyc., mur-ac., nux-v., onos., puls., spig., sulph., verat-v., zinc.
Calf	pain in calf in afternoon	Rhus-t.
Calf	pain in calf in evening	Alum., calc., nux-v., puls., staph., verat.
Calf	pain in calf in evening in bed	Staph.
Calf	pain in calf in evening while sitting with knees bent	Coca.
Calf	pain in calf in morning	Calc-p.
Calf	pain in calf in morning on going down stairs	Rhus-t.
Calf	pain in calf in morning on waking	Gels.
Calf	pain in calf on bending foot	Calc.
Calf	pain in calf on coughing	Nux-v.
Calf	pain in calf on first rising	Nat-p.
Calf	pain in calf on motion of feet	Cham.
Calf	pain in calf while sitting	Agar., puls., sul-ac., sulph.
Calf	pain in foot extending to calves	Dros.
Calf	pain in kidney extending to calves	Berb.
Calf	pain in kidneys extending to calves	Berb.
Calf	pain in lumbar region down the legs to calves	Berb., ph-ac., tep.
Calf	sensation as if calf bandaged	Card-m., nat-p.
Calf	sensation of vibration in calf	Phel.
Calf	sensitive calf	Nat-m., plb., sil.
Calf	stiffness in calf	Arg-n.
Calf	swelling of foot extending to calf	Am-c., puls.
Calf	swelling in calf of leg	Berb., bry., calc., carb-v., chin., dulc., graph., hyos., led., mez., puls., sil., sulph.
Calf	tingling in calf	Bar-c., berb., cham., lach., onos.
Calf	trembling in calf	Meny., nat-m., sulph.

Body part/Disease	Symptom	Medicines
Calf	tumours on calf	Kali-br., sulph.
Calf	twitching in calf from stretching out foot	Laur.
Calf	twitching in calf from touch	Tarax.
Calf	twitching in calf in forenoon while sitting	Nat-c.
Calf	twitching in calf in morning	Eupi.
Calf	twitching in calf in morning in bed	Laur., puls., zinc.
Calf	ulcerative pain in calf	Agar.
Calf	varices of calf	Clem., plb.
Calf	weakness in calf after walking	Calc-s.
Calf	weakness in calf ameliorated while sitting	Nicc.
Calf	weakness in calf ameliorated while walking	Plb.
Calf	weakness in calf at night	Sulph.
Calf	weakness in calf during chill	Thuj.
Calf	weakness in calf in afternoon	Cast., valer.
Calf	weakness in calf in evening	Dulc., eupi.
Calf	weakness in calf on motion	Cast.
Calf	weakness in calf when kneeling	Ars-i.
Calf	weakness in calf when rising from a seat	Zinc.
Calf	weakness in calf while sitting	Stront.
Calf	weakness in calf while walking	Aloe., croc., gran., nicc., osm.
Callosity	callosities (a local thickening of the outer layer of the skin caused by repeated friction or pressure) of hand	Phos.
Callosity	horny callosities (thickening of skin) on hands	Am-c., Graph., kali-ar., rhus-v., sil., Sulph.
Callosity	horny callosities on soles	Ant-c., ars., calc., plb., sil., sulph.
Callosity	horny callosities on toes	Ant-c., graph.
Callosity	horny callosities with deep cracks	Cist., graph.
Callosity	horny callositieson soles with tenderness	Alum., lyc., med., nat-s.
Can Not	cannot be quieted	Cina.
Can Not	cannot bear a draft of air on nape	Hep., merc., sil.
Can Not	cannot bear a draft of air on spine	Sumb.
Can Not	cannot bear to have fingers touch each other	Lac-c., lach., sec.
Can Not	cannot lie dow & sits bent forward during cough	Iod.
Can Not	cannot look at Blood and Knife	Alumina
Can Not	cannot pronounce name	Chin-s.
Can Not	cannot rest , when things are not in proper place	Anac., ars.
Can Not	cannot tell direction of sound	Carb-an.
Can Not	cannot walk in chorea, must run or jump	Bufo., kali-br., nat-m.
Cancer	cancer (a malignant tumor or growth caused when cells multiply uncontrollably, destroying healthy tissue. The different forms are sarcomas, carcinomas, leukemias, and lymphomas)	Acet-ac., ars-i., Ars., Aur-m-n., bar-c., bell., Bism., cadm., Calc., caps., Carb-ac., Carb-an., carb-v., Cinamon. (3,6 or 30)., Con., crot-h., Cund., hydr., iris., kreos., lach., Lyc., merc-c., mez., nux-v., Phos., plat., sep., sil., staph., sulph., thuj.

Body part/Disease	Symptom	Medicines
Cancer	cancer in epithelioma (a tumor composed of epithelial tissue) in mammae	Arg-n., ars-i., ars., brom., Bufo., calc-p., calc., clem., Con., hydr., kreos., lach., merc-i-f., merc., phos., phyt., sep., sil., sulph., thuj.
Cancer	cancer in old cicatrices of mammae	Graph.
Cancer	cancer in sternum (breastbone)	Sulph.
Cancer	cancer of axilla	Aster.
Cancer	Cancer of breast	Ars.Iod (2nd & 3rd Trituration)
Cancer	cancer of face	aur., carb-an., con., kali-ar., kali-c., kali-i., lach., nit-ac., phos., sil., sulph., zinc.
Cancer	cancer of larynx	Ars., nit-ac., phos., sang., thuj.
Cancer	cancer of lips	Ant-chl., Ars., aur-m., aur., camph., carb-an., caust., cic., cist., clem., Con., cund., kali-chl., kali-s., kreos., lach., lyc., phos., phyt., sep., sil., sulph.
Cancer	cancer of Mammae	Aster.
Cancer	cancer of mammae with nightly pains	Aster.
Cancer	cancer of nose	Alumn., ars., aur-m., Aur., calc., carb-ac., carb-an., cund., kreos., merc., phyt., sep., sulph.
Cancer	cancer of ovaries	Ars., con., graph., kreos., lach., psor.
Cancer	cancer of palate	Aur., hydr.
Cancer	cancer of rectum	Alum., nit-ac., ruta., sep.
Cancer	cancer of scrotum	Carb-an., ph-ac.
Cancer	cancer of testes	Spong.
Cancer	cancer of throat	Carb-an., led., tarent.
Cancer	cancer of tongue	Alumn., apis., ars., aur-m., aur., benz-ac., calc., carb-an., caust., con., crot-h., cund., hydr., kali-chl., kali-cy., kali-i., lach., mur-ac., nit-ac., phos., phyt., sep., sil., sulph., thuj.
Cancer	cancer of uterus	Alum., alumn., anan., apis., arg-m., arg-n., Ars-i., Ars., aur-m-n., aur., brom., bufo., calc., carb-an., carb-s., carb-v., chin., cic., clem., Con., crot-h., cund., elaps., Graph., Hydr., iod., kali-ar., kaol., Kreos., Lach., lap-a., Lyc., mag-m., merc-i-f., merc., Murx., nat-c., nat-m., nit-ac., Phos., phyt., plat., rhus-t., sabin., sang., sec., Sep., Sil., staph., sulph., tarent., Thuj., zinc.
Cancer	cancer, advanced stage	Carb-an., sil.
Cancer	Cancer, epithelioma (Tumour)	Cund., lach.
Cancer	Cancer, epithelioma of cornea (the transparent convex membrane that covers the pupil and iris of the eye)	Hep.
Cancer	cancer,epithelioma of lachrymal glands (relating to tears)	Carb-an.
Cancer	Cancer,epithelioma of lids	Hydr., lach., phyt., thuj.
Cancer	canceros ulcer in glands	Arn., Ars., aur., bell., Bufo., calc., carb-an., carb-v., caust., clem., Con., cupr., dulc., hep., kali-c., kreos., lyc., merc-i-f., merc., nit-ac., ph-ac., phos., rhus-t., sep., sil., squil., sul-ac., Sulph., zinc.

Body part/Disease	Symptom	Medicines
Cancer	cancerous affections, encephaloma (protrusion of part of the brain through an opening in the skull)	Acet-ac., ars-i., ars., calc., carb-ac., carb-an., caust., kali-i., kreos., lach., nit-ac., **Phos.**, sil., sulph., thuj.
Cancer	cancerous affections, epithelioma	Acet-ac., arg-m., arg-n., **Ars-i.**, ars., aur., bell., brom., calc-p., calc., clem., **Con.**, hydr., kali-s., kreos., **Lyc.**, merc., phos., phyt., ran-b., sep., sil., sulph., thuj.
Calf	coldness in left foot	Aeth., hydrc., pip-m., sumb., tub.
Cancer	cancerous affections, fungus hæmatodes (immature blood cell, especially a red blood cell)	Ant-t., **Ars.**, bell., calc., **Carb-an.**, carb-v., clem., kreos., **Lach.**, lyc., merc., nat-m., nit-ac., **Phos.**, puls., sep., **Sil.**, staph., sulph., **Thuj.**
Cancer	cancerous affections, glands	Aur-m., **Carb-an.**, **Con.**
Cancer	cancerous affections, lupus	Agar., alum., alumn., ant-c., arg-n., ars-i., **Ars.**, aur-m., bar-c., calc., carb-ac., carb-s., carb-v., caust., cist., graph., hep., hydrc., kali-ar., kali-bi., kali-c., kali-chl., kali-s., kreos., lach., **Lyc.**, nit-ac., phyt., psor., sep., sil., spong., staph., sulph., **Thuj.**
Cancer	cancerous affections, lupus in rings	Sep.
Cancer	cancerous affections, melanotic (having a dark complexion and dark hair)	Arg-n., card-m., lach., ph-ac.
Cancer	cancerous affections, noma (severe gangrenous inflammation of the mouth or genitals, usually occurring in children who are malnourished or otherwise debilitated)	Alum., alumn., ars., calc., carb-v., con., elat., kali-p., merc., sil., sulph.
Cancer	cancerous affections, scirrhus (a cancerous tumor carcinoma that is hard and fibrous)	Alumn., arg-m., ars., aster., calc-s., **Carb-an.**, carb-s., carb-v., **Con.**, graph., hydr., lap-a., phos., phyt., sep., **Sil.**, staph., sulph.
Cancer	convulsion after metastasis (spread of Cancer)	Cupr.
Cancer	cough from malignant tumour/cancer with the sound of croup	Cupr.
Cancer	eruption, tubercles malignant	Ars.
Cancer	leukemia (fatal cancer in which white blood cells displace normal blood, leading to infection, shortage of red blood cells anemia, bleeding, and other disorders. Certain types of childhood leukemias respond well to treatment, which includes drugs chemotherapy and radiotherapy)	Acet-ac., ars., calc-p., calc., carb-s., carb-v., chin., crot-h., ip., kali-p., **Nat-a.**, nat-m., nat-p., **Nat-s.**, nux-v., pic-ac., sulph., thuj.
Cancer	malignant (used to describe a disease or condition that is liable to cause death or serious disablement unless effectively treated) tumours (mass of tissue) on neck	Calc-p.
Cancer	malignant bone tumour on tibia	Syph.
Cancer	malignant eruption on head	Brom., phos.
Cancer	malignant ulcer in nose	Carb-an., kali-bi.
Cancer	malignant ulcer of upper limbs	Lach.
Cancer	metastasis (malignant tumor / Cancer) of male gentialia	**Abrot.**, carb-v., colch., cupr., lac-c., puls., sang., sulph.
Cancer	metastasis (spread of cancer) to testes (either of the paired male reproductive glands, roundish in shape, that produce sperm and male sex hormones, and hang in a small sac scrotum)	Ars., carb-v., jab., nat-m., Puls., rhus-t.

Body part/Disease	Symptom	Medicines
Cancer	metastasis (the spread of a cancer from the original tumor to other parts of the body by means of tiny clumps of cells transported by the blood or lymph) of face	Agar.
Cancer	metastasis of face	Abrot., carb-v., puls.
Cancer	metastasis to mammae (milk-secreting organ)	Puls.
Cancer	pain in cancer of prostate gland	Crot-h.
Cancer	pain in prostate gland in cancer	Crot-h.
Cancer	tumour, malignant in mouth	Calc.
Cancer	tumours sarcoma	Bar-c., calc-f.
Cancer	tumours steatoma (a malignant tumor containing solid fat) reappearing every 4 weeks	Calc.
Cancer	tumours steatoma suppurating	Calc., carb-v.
Cancer	ulcer cancerous of lips	Ars., aur-m., carb-an., clem., Con., kali-bi., lyc., phos., phyt.
Cancer	ulcer in skin with cancerous growth	Ant-c., apis., ars., **Hep.**, kreos., merc., **Nit-ac.**, phos., sabin., sulph., thuj.
Cancer	ulcer malignant	Ars., lach., phos.
Cancer	ulcer cancerous	Ambr., ant-c., anthr., apis., ars-i., **Ars.**, aur., bell., **Bufo.**, calc-s., calc., carb-ac., carb-an., carb-s., carb-v., caust., chel., clem., con., crot-c., cund., dulc., graph., **Hep.**, hippoz., hydr., kali-ar., kali-c., kali-i., kreos., lach., **Lyc.**, lyss., mang., merc., mur-ac., nit-ac., petr., ph-ac., phos., phyt., rhus-t., rumx., sars., sep., **Sil.**, spong., squil., staph., **Sulph.**, thuj.
Carbuncle	carbuncle (inflamed swelling / a multiple-headed boil) in cervical region	Anthr., caust., crot-h., hep., Lach., rhus-t., Sil., sulph.
Carbuncle	carbuncle in coccyx	Anthr., ars., crot-h., lach., sil.
Carbuncle	carbuncle in dorsal region	Hep., lach., tarent.
Carbuncle	carbuncle on head	Anthr., ars., hep., lach., sil., sulph.
Carbuncle	carbuncles	Anthr., arn., Ars., hep., Lach., Sil., Sulph., tarent-c.
Carbuncle	carbuncles on chin	Lyc.
Carbuncle	carbuncles on eye	Agar., Arg-n., cann-i., kali-c., zinc.
Carbuncle	carbuncles on forearm	Hep.
Carbuncle	carbuncles on nates	Agar., thuj.
Carbuncle	carbuncles on thigh	Agar., arn., asim., hep.
Carbuncle	eruptions (rash or blemish) carbuncle stinging	**Apis.**, carb-an., nit-ac.
Carbuncle	eruptions carbuncle	Agar., ant-t., anthr., apis., arn., **Ars.**, **Bell.**, bufo., caps., carb-an., coloc., crot-c., crot-h., echi., hep., hyos., lach., mur-ac., nit-ac., phyt., pic-ac., rhus-t., sec., **Sil.**, sulph., tarent-c.
Carbuncle	eruptions carbuncle after abuse of mercury	**Kali-i.**
Carbuncle	eruptions carbuncle after scratching	Alum., am-c., am-m., ant-c., ars., bar-c., bell., bov., bry., calc., caps., carb-an., carb-s., carb-v., cic., con., dulc., graph., hep., kali-ar., kali-c., kali-s., kreos., led., **Lyc.**, merc., mez., nat-m., petr., phos., puls., ran-b., **Rhus-t.**, sabad., sabin., sars., sep., sil., staph., **Sulph.**, thuj., verat., viol-t., zinc.

Body part/Disease	Symptom	Medicines
Carbuncle	eruptions carbuncle burning	Anthr., apis., ars., coloc., crot-c., crot-h., hep., **Tarent-c.**
Carbuncle	eruptions carbuncle clustered	Agar., calc., ph-ac., ran-b., rhus-t., staph., verat.
Carbuncle	eruptions carbuncle confluent	Agar., ant-t., caps., chlol., cic., hyos., ph-ac., phos., rhus-v., valer.
Carbuncle	eruptions carbuncle coppery	Alum., ars-i., ars., aur., calc., cann-s., **Carb-an.**, carb-v., cor-r., kali-i., kreos., led., lyc., merc., mez., nit-ac., phos., psor., rhus-t., ruta., syph., verat.
Carbuncle	eruptions carbuncle corrosive (gradually destructive)	Ars., calc., caps., carb-s., clem., graph., merc-i-r., merc., nat-m., ran-s., rhus-t., **Sulph.**, thuj.
Carbuncle	eruptions carbuncle crusty black	Ars., bell., chin., vip.
Carbuncle	eruptions carbuncle crusty bleeding	Merc., mez.
Carbuncle	eruptions carbuncle crusty brown	Am-c., ant-c., berb.
Carbuncle	eruptions carbuncle crusty burning	Am-c., ant-c., calc., cic., puls., sars.
Carbuncle	eruptions carbuncle crusty dry	Ars-i., ars., **Aur-m.**, **Aur.**, bar-c., calc., chin-s., graph., lach., led., merc., ran-b., sulph., thuj., viol-t.
Carbuncle	eruptions carbuncle crusty over whole body	Ars., **Dulc.**, psor.
Carbuncle	eruptions carbuncle desquamating	Acet-ac., agar., **Am-c.**, am-m., ant-t., apis., ars-i., ars., arum-t., aur., bar-c., **Bell.**, bor., bov., calc-s., calc., canth., caps., carb-an., caust., cham., clem., coloc., con., crot-h., crot-t., cupr., dig., dulc., elaps., eupho., ferr-p., ferr., graph., hell., iod., kali-ar., kali-c., **Kali-s.**, kreos., lach., laur., led., mag-c., manc., merc., **Mez.**, mosch., nat-a., nat-c., nat-m., nat-p., **Olnd.**, op., par., ph-ac., phos., plat., plb., **Psor.**, puls., ran-b., ran-s., rhus-t., rhus-v., sabad., sec., sel., **Sep.**, sil., spig., staph., sul-ac., sulph., tarax., teucr., thuj., urt-u., verat.
Carbuncle	eruptions carbuncle destroying hair	Ars., lyc., merc., nat-m., rhus-t.
Carbuncle	eruptions carbuncle dirty	Merc., psor., sulph., syph.
Carbuncle	eruptions carbuncle disappearing from cold air	Calc.
Carbuncle	eruptions carbuncle discharging after scratching	Alum., ars., bar-c., bell., bov., bry., calc., carb-an., carb-v., caust., cic., con., dulc., **Graph.**, hell., hep., kali-c., kreos., **Lach.**, led., **Lyc.**, merc., mez., nat-c., nat-m., nit-ac., olnd., petr., **Rhus-t.**, ruta., sabin., sars., sel., sep., sil., squil., staph., sul-ac., sulph., tarax., thuj., viol-t.
Carbuncle	eruptions carbuncle discharging blood	Ant-c., calc., crot-h., lach., merc., nux-v.
Carbuncle	eruptions carbuncle discharging glutinous	Calc., carb-s., **Graph.**, nat-m., sulph.
Carbuncle	eruptions carbuncle discharging greenish	Ant-c., kali-chl., rhus-t.
Carbuncle	eruptions carbuncle discharging ichorous	Ant-t., clem., ran-s., *rhus-t.*
Carbuncle	eruptions carbuncle discharging moist	Alum., anac., anag., ant-c., ars-i., ars., bar-c., bell., bov., bry., bufo., cact., cadm., calc-s., calc., canth., caps., carb-an., **Carb-s.**, **Carb-v.**, caust., cham., cic., cist., dem., con., crot-h., crot-t., cupr., **Dulc.**, **Graph.**, hell., hep., hydr., iod., jug-c., kali-ar., kali-br., kali-c., kali-p., kali-s., kreos., lach., led., **Lyc.**, manc., merc., **Mez.**, mur-ac., nat-a., nat-c., **Nat-m.**, nat-p., nat-s., nit-ac., olnd., petr., ph-ac., phos., phyt., psor., ran-b., **Rhus-t.**, rhus-v., ruta., sabin., sars., sel., **Sep.**, **Sil.**, **Sol-n.**, squil., staph., still., sul-ac., sul-i., sulph., tarax., tell., thuj., vinc., viol-t., zinc.

Body part/Disease	Symptom	Medicines
Carbuncle	eruptions carbuncle discharging pus	Clem., graph., hep., lyc., nat-m., nit-ac., sulph.
Carbuncle	eruptions carbuncle discharging thin	Cupr., dulc., hell., **Nat-m.**, rhus-t., rhus-v., sol-n.
Carbuncle	eruptions carbuncle discharging white	Bor., **Calc.**, carb-v., caust., dulc., graph., lyc., merc., nat-m., phos., **Puls.**, sep., **Sil.**
Carbuncle	eruptions carbuncle discharging yellow	Alum., anac., **Ant-c.**, ars., bar-c., calc., canth., carb-an., **Carb-s.**, **Carb-v.**, caust., clem., cupr., dulc., graph., hep., iod., kali-c., kali-s., lach., lyc., merc., nat-m., nat-p., **Nat-s.**, **Nit-ac.**, **Phos.**, **Puls.**, rhus-t., **Sep.**, **Sil.**, sol-n., **Sulph.**, thuj., viol-t.
Carbuncle	eruptions carbuncle dry	Alum., anac., anag., **Ars-i.**, **Ars.**, **Aur-m.**, **Aur.**, **Bar-c.**, bor., bry., bufo., cact., calad., **Calc-s.**, **Calc.**, carb-s., carb-v., caust., clem., cocc., corn., cupr., dulc., fl-ac., graph., hep., hydr-ac., hyos., kali-ar., kali-c., kali-chl., kali-i., kali-s., kreos., **Led.**, lyc., mag-c., merc., **Mez.**, nat-c., nat-m., nat-p., par., petr., ph-ac., **Phos.**, psor., rhus-t., sars., sel., **Sep.**, **Sil.**, stann., staph., sulph., teucr., thuj., valer., **Verat.**, viol-t., zinc.
Carbuncle	eruptions carbuncle dry bleeding after scratching	Alum., ars., calc., lyc., petr., sulph.
Carbuncle	eruptions carbuncle fetid	Graph., lyc., merc., plb., psor., staph., **Sulph.**
Carbuncle	eruptions carbuncle from cold air	Apis., caust., dulc., kali-c., mang., nit-ac., **Rhus-t.**, rumx., sep.
Carbuncle	eruptions carbuncle gray	Ars., merc., sulph.
Carbuncle	eruptions carbuncle greenish	Ant-c., calc., petr., sulph.
Carbuncle	eruptions carbuncle hard	**Ran-b.**
Carbuncle	eruptions carbuncle honey coloured	Carb-v.
Carbuncle	eruptions carbuncle horny	Ant-c., graph., **Ran-b.**
Carbuncle	eruptions carbuncle in covered parts	Led., thuj.
Carbuncle	eruptions carbuncle in warm weather	Bov.
Carbuncle	eruptions carbuncle inflammed	Calc., lyc.
Carbuncle	eruptions carbuncle like chicken pox	Acon., **Ant-c.**, ant-t., ars., asaf., bell., canth., carb-v., caust., coff., con., cycl., hyos., ip., led., merc., nat-c., nat-m., **Puls.**, rhus-t., sep., sil., **Sulph.**, thuj.
Carbuncle	eruptions carbuncle moist	Alum., anac., anthr., **Ars.**, bar-c., **Calc.**, **Carb-s.**, cic., clem., **Graph.**, hell., hep., kali-s., **Lyc.**, **Merc.**, **Mez.**, olnd., phos., plb., ran-b., **Rhus-t.**, ruta., sep., sil., **Staph.**, **Sulph.**
Carbuncle	eruptions carbuncle oozing greenish bloody	Ant-c.
Carbuncle	eruptions carbuncle patchy	Hydr., kali-c., merc., **Nit-ac.**, sabin., sil., thuj., zinc.
Carbuncle	eruptions carbuncle purple with small vesicles around	Crot-c., **Lach.**
Carbuncle	eruptions carbuncle renewed daily	Crot-t.
Carbuncle	eruptions carbuncle serpiginous	Clem., psor., sulph.
Carbuncle	eruptions carbuncle smarting	Puls.
Carbuncle	eruptions carbuncle suppurating	Ars., plb., sil., sulph.
Carbuncle	eruptions carbuncle white	Alum., calc., mez., **Nat-m.**, tell., thuj.
Carbuncle	eruptions carbuncle with coppery spots	Merc., mez., nit-ac., ust.

Body part/Disease	Symptom	Medicines
Carbuncle	eruptions carbuncle yellow	Ant-c., aur-m., aur., bar-m., calc-s., calc., carb-v., cic., cupr., dulc., hyper., iod., kali-bi., kali-s., kreos., merc., mez., nat-p., petr., ph-ac., spong., staph., sulph., viol-t.
Carbuncle	eruptions carbuncle yellow white	Mez.
Caressing	trembling while caressing	Caps.
Caries	bloody discharge from ear threatening caries	Asaf., Aur., calc-f., calc-s., calc., caps., nat-m., Sil., sulph.
Caries	caries (Progressive decay of a tooth or, less commonly, a bone) of bone	**Ang.**, ars., **Asaf.**, aur-m-n., aur-m., aur., bell., bry., calc-f., calc-p., calc-s., calc., caps., carb-ac., chin., cist., clem., con., cupr., dulc., eupho., ferr., **Fl-ac.**, graph., guai., guare., hep., iod., kali-bi., **Kali-i.**, kreos., lach., **Lyc.**, **Merc.**, mez., nat-m., nit-ac., op., petr., ph-ac., phos., puls., rhod., rhus-t., ruta., sabin., sec., sep., **Sil.**, spong., staph., sulph., **Ther.**, thuj.
Caries	caries in bones of head	Arg-m., asaf., Aur., caps., fl-ac., hep., hippoz., nat-m., Nit-ac., ph-ac., Phos., Sil., staph.
Caries	caries of ankle bones , internal malleolus (either of the hammer-shaped bony protuberances at the sides of the ankle joint that project from the lower end of the tibia and fibula)	Sil.
Caries	caries of ankle bones	Asaf., calc., guai., plat-m., puls., sil.
Caries	caries of bone	Ars., Asaf., aur., calc-f., calc-p., calc., con., fl-ac., graph., guai., hep., Lyc., Merc., mez., Nit-ac., ph-ac., phos., puls., ruta., sec., sep., Sil., staph., sulph., ther.
Caries	caries of bone , periosteum	Ant-c., **Asaf.**, aur., bell., chin., cycl., hell., merc., mez., **Ph-ac.**, puls., rhod., rhus-t., ruta., sabin., sil., staph.
Caries	caries of clavicles	Sil.
Caries	caries of elbow	Sil.
Caries	caries of femur (the main bone in the human thigh, the strongest bone in the body)	Calc., Sil., stront.
Caries	caries of fibula (the outer and narrower of the two bones in the human lower leg between the knee and ankle)	Sil.
Caries	caries of fingers	Sil.
Caries	caries of foot	Asaf., calc., hecla., merc., Sil.
Caries	caries of gums	Calc.
Caries	caries of heel (the back part of a person's foot immediately below the ankle)	Calc., plat-m., sil.
Caries	caries of humerus (the long bone of the human upper arm)	Sil.
Caries	caries of joints	Nit-ac.
Caries	caries of knee	Sil.
Caries	caries of left toe	Sil.
Caries	caries of lower jaw	Asaf., aur-m-n., aur-m., aur., cist., con., fl-ac., kali-i., merc., mez., nit-ac., phos., phyt., sil., staph.
Caries	caries of lower limbs	Aur-m-n., aur-m., aur., calc., mez., nit-ac., sep., Sil.

Body part/Disease	Symptom	Medicines
Caries	caries of lumbar vertebrae	Sil.
Caries	caries of metacarpal bone of hands (any bone in the human hand between the wrist and digits)	Sil.
Caries	caries of nose	Asaf., aur-m-n., aur-m., Aur., cadm., calc., fl-ac., hecla., hep., hippoz., kali-i., merc-i-r., phos., phyt., Sil., still.
Caries	caries of palate	Aur., guare., hippoz., merc., nit-ac.
Caries	caries of shoulder joint	Sil.
Caries	caries of sternum	Con.
Caries	caries of tibia (inner and larger of the two bones in the lower leg, extending from the knee to the ankle bone alongside the fibula)	Asaf., aur., calc., guai., hecla., kali-i., lach., ph-ac., phos., Sil.
Caries	caries of upper limbs	Sil.
Caries	caries of wrist	Sil.
Caries	felon with caries of bone	Asaf., aur., fl-ac., lach., lyc., merc., mez., ph-ac., **Sil.**, sulph.
Caries	felon with caries of bone and deep seated pain aggravated from warmth of bed	Sep.
Caries	felon, bone caries with offensive pus	Fl-ac.
Cartilage	affections of cartilages (the tough elastic tissue that is found in the nose, throat, and ear and in other parts of the body and forms most of the skeleton in infancy, changing to bone during growth) of heart	Acon., am-c., ars-i., ars., Aur-m., Aur., bad., brom., Cact., calc., caust., cench., coll., crot-h., cupr., ferr., gels., hydr., hyos., iod., kalm., Lach., laur., lil-t., Lith., Lob., lycps., mosch., Naja., nat-m., op., phos., psor., Puls., seneg., Spig., Spong.
Cartilage	cracking in knee as if cartilage slipped	Petr.
Cartilage	inflammation of cartilages	**Arg-m.**, nat-m.
Cartilage	pain in nose extending to junction of cartilage	Kali-bi.
Cartilage	sensitiveness to cartilages	**Arg-m.**
Cartilage	sore bruised pain in cartilages	**Arg-m.**, rhod., rhus-t.
Cartilage	swelling in cartilages	**Arg-m.**
Catalepsy	deep sleep in afternoon after catalepsy (unconsciousness during which muscles become rigid and remain in any position in which they are placed)	Grat.
Cautious	cautious	Caust., graph., ip., mag-arct.
Cautious	cautious anxiously	Caust.
Chatter	chattering (make high-pitched sounds from teeth grinding due to fear or cold)	Bar-c., calc., cocc., ip., kali-p., phos.
Cheek	biting of cheek when talking or chewing	Carb-an., caust., Ign., Nit-ac.
Cheek	burning and redness of left side of cheek	Alum., asaf., lac-c., murx., nat-m., ol-an., ph-ac., spig.
Cheek	burning on one side of cheek and coldnes on other side	Acet-ac., acon., Cham., Ip., kali-c., lach., mosch., nux-v.
Cheek	covulsions in masseters (cheek muscle)	Ambr., ang., cocc., cupr., mang., nux-v.
Cheek	cystic tumor on cheek	Graph.
Cheek	discolouration of cheeks	Cham.
Cheek	exostosis on right cheek bone	Aur-m.

Body part/Disease	Symptom	Medicines
Cheek	headache extending around the cheek	Hep., hyper., indg., rhus-t.
Cheek	headache extending down the zygoma	Hyper.
Cheek	induration inside of cheek	Caust.
Cheek	inflammation with sore spots inside cheek	Aloe.
Cheek	itching of cheeks	Agar., agn., alum., anan., ang., ant-c., asaf., bell., berb., hyper., kali-p., mag-m., nat-m., puls., rhus-t., ruta., spong., stront., sulph., thuj., viol-t.
Cheek	one cheek cold and red, the other hot and pale	Mosch.
Cheek	pain in ear extending to malar bone (cheek bone)	Spig.
Cheek	pain in face in left zygoma (cheek bone)	Aur., thuj.
Cheek	pain in face in left zygoma aggravated by rest	Mag-c.
Cheek	pain in face in left zygoma aggravated at night	Mag-c., mez., plat., sil.
Cheek	pain in face in left zygoma ameliorated by pressure	Mez.
Cheek	pain in face in left zygoma ameliorated by touch	Thuj.
Cheek	pain in face in zygoma	zygoma : Aur., calc-p., caps., caust., chel., cinnb., kali-bi., psor., verb.
Cheek	pain in nose extending to malar bone	Kali-bi.
Cheek	pain in teeth ameliorated from rubbing cheek	Merc., phos.
Cheek	pain in teeth with swelling of cheek	Arn., ars., Bell., Bry., calc., caps., Lach., lyc., Merc., nat-m., nux-v., petr., ph-ac., phos., puls., staph., sulph.
Cheek	pimples in inner cheeks and lips	Berb.
Cheek	redness of right nostrils extending to cheek	Anthr.
Cheek	remitent fever with redness of one cheek, paleness of the other	Acon., **Cham.**
Cheek	swelling in face with shining cheeks	Apis., arn., aur., spig.
Cheek	tingling (stinging or prickling) on cheeks and lips	Agn., arn., ars., berb., dros.
Cheek	ulcer in cheek	Ant-t., calc., iod., nat-m., phos.
Cheerful	cheerful after coition	Nat-m.
Cheerful	cheerful after convulsions (uncontrollable shaking)	Sulph.
Cheerful	Cheerful after stool	Bor., nat-c., Nat-s., ox-ac.
Cheerful	cheerful after supper	Cist.
Cheerful	cheerful after urination	Eug., hyos.
Cheerful	cheerful afternoon	Anac., ang., arg-m., aur-m., calc-s., calc., mag-c., nat-s., ox-ac., phos., plb., sars., thuj.
Cheerful	cheerful alternating with aversion to work	Spong.
Cheerful	cheerful alternating with physical sufferings	Plat.
Cheerful	cheerful alternating with sadness	Acon., agar., asar., canth., carb-an., caust., chin., cimic., clem., croc., ferr., fl-ac., gels., hell., ign., iod., kali-chl., lyc., med., nat-c., nat-m., nit-ac., nux-m., phos., plat., psor., senec., sep., spig., tarent., zinc., ziz.
Cheerful	cheerful alternating with violence	Aur., croc., stram.
Cheerful	cheerful Ameliorated in room	Tarent.
Cheerful	cheerful at night	Alum., bell., caust., croc., cupr., hyos., kreos., lyc., op., ph-ac., sep., sil., stram., sulph., verat.

Body part/Disease	Symptom	Medicines
Cheerful	cheerful before menses	Acon., fl-ac., hyos.
Cheerful	cheerful daytime	Anac., arg-m., aur., caust., mag-m., mur-ac., sars.
Cheerful	cheerful during chill	Cann-s., nux-m., phos., puls., rhus-t., verat.
Cheerful	cheerful during Delirium	Acon., bell., cact., con., op., sulph., verat.
Cheerful	cheerful during heat	Acon., op.
Cheerful	cheerful during menses	Fl-ac., stram.
Cheerful	cheerful during perspiration	Apis., ars., bell., clem.
Cheerful	cheerful evening	Agar., aloe., alum., aster., bell., bism., bufo., calc., carb-ac., cast., chin-s., chin., cist., clem., cupr., cycl., ferr., graph., lach., lachn., lyss., mag-c., med., merc-i-f., merc-i-r., nat-c., nat-m., nux-m., ol-an., phel., plat., sulph., sumb., teucr., valer., verb., viol-t., zinc.
Cheerful	cheerful followed by irritability	Clem., hyos., nat-s., ol-an., op., seneg., tarax.
Cheerful	cheerful followed by prostration	Clem., spong.
Cheerful	cheerful followed by sleepiness	Bell., calc.
Cheerful	cheerful forenoon	Aeth., bor., caust., clem., com., graph., nat-m., nat-s., phos., plb., zinc.
Cheerful	cheerful in bed	Hep.
Cheerful	cheerful in company	Bov.
Cheerful	cheerful in morning	Bor., calc-s., carb-s., caust., cinnb., con., fl-ac., graph., hep., hura., lach., nat-s., plat., psor., spig., sulph.
Cheerful	cheerful in open air	Merc-i-f., plat., plb., tarent., teucr.
Cheerful	cheerful on rising	Hydr.
Cheerful	cheerful on thinking of death	Aur.
Cheerful	cheerful on waking	Aloe., clem., hydr., nux-m., tarent.
Cheerful	cheerful on walking in open air	Alum., ang., cinnb., fl-ac., plb., tarent.
Cheerful	cheerful when constipated	Calc., psor.
Cheerful	cheerful when thunders and lightnings	Sep.
Cheerful	cheerful with all pain	Spig.
Cheesy	cheesy deposits	Helon.
Cheesy	cheesy discharge from urethra	Hep.
Chest	acne on chest	Bar-c.
Chest	anxiety from pressure on the chest	Sulph.
Chest	bladder, constant urging to urinate with pain in liver, chest & kidneys	Ferr.
Chest	blood blisters on chest	Ars.
Chest	blotches on chest	Nat-c., sars.
Chest	boils on chest	Am-c., chin., hep., Kali-i., lach., mag-c., phos., Psor., Sulph.
Chest	boring pain in right scapula to front of chest	Acon.
Chest	breathing difficult from anxiety in chest in morning	Puls.
Chest	burning on chest	Alum., bov., cic., mez., rhus-t.

Body part/Disease	Symptom	Medicines
Chest	burning vesicles (a very small blister filled with clear fluid serum) on chest	Alum.
Chest	catarrh of nose extends to chest	Bry.
Chest	chest fever	Am-c., ant-t., **Bry.**, carb-v., chel., chin., hyos., kali-bi., lyc., nit-ac., **Phos.**, rhus-t., sulph.
Chest	chest symptoms aggravated from clothing	Ail., aur-m., benz-ac., bov., calc., Caust., chel., con., kali-bi., Lach., lact., lycps., merc., tarent., zinc.
Chest	chest symptoms alternating with diarrhoea and bronchitis	Seneg.
Chest	chest symptoms alternating with eye symptoms	Ars.
Chest	chest symptoms alternating with rectal symptoms	Calc-p., Sil., verat.
Chest	chest symptoms alternating with skin symptoms	Crot-h.
Chest	chill beginning in and extending from chest	**Apis.**, ars., carb-an., cic., cina., kreos., lith., merl., nux-v., rhus-t., sep., spig.
Chest	chill beginning in and extending from right side of chest	Merl.
Chest	chill beginning in chest with violent congestion and suffocation in warm room	Apis.
Chest	chillines in chest	Alum., ars., bry., nat-c., par., ran-b.
Chest	chillines in chest after stool	Plat.
Chest	chillines in left side of chest	Nat-c., nat-m.
Chest	chilliness with well covered but chest chilly	Ran-b.
Chest	clawing sensation in chest	Samb., stront.
Chest	clucking (Voice of hen) sound in chest	Cina., kali-c., nat-m.
Chest	congestion (condition of having an excessive amount of blood or fluid accumulate in an organ or body part) in chest after exertion	Spong.
Chest	congestion in chest after exposure to cold air	Cimic., phos.
Chest	congestion in chest after menses	Ign.
Chest	congestion in chest after motion	Spong.
Chest	congestion in chest after uterine haemorrhage	Aur-m., chin., phos.
Chest	congestion in chest after writing	Am-c.
Chest	congestion in chest at climaxis	Arg-n., Lach.
Chest	congestion in chest at night	Ferr., puls.
Chest	congestion in chest before menses	Kali-c.
Chest	congestion in chest during menses	Glon.
Chest	congestion in chest during pregnancy	Glon., nat-m., sep.
Chest	congestion in chest during sleep	Mill., puls.
Chest	congestion in chest in afternoon	Seneg.
Chest	congestion in chest in morning	Elaps., pall.
Chest	congestion in chest on walking	Lach.
Chest	congestion in chest upon delayed menses	Graph., nux-m., puls.
Chest	congestion in chest while walking rapidly	Nux-m.

Body part/Disease	Symptom	Medicines
Chest	congestion in chest with weakness & nausea	Spong.
Chest	constriction as from band in lower part of chest	Agar., chlor., thuj.
Chest	constriction in chest from inclination to cough	Sep.
Chest	constriction in chest after breakfast	Agar., sulph.
Chest	constriction in chest after coition	Staph.
Chest	constriction in chest after dinner	Carb-s., hep., phel.
Chest	constriction in chest after drinking	Cupr.
Chest	constriction in chest after eating	Arn., carb-an., cupr., hep., phel., puls.
Chest	constriction in chest after suppressed foot sweat	Sil.
Chest	constriction in chest after talking	Hep.
Chest	constriction in chest after vomiting	Verat-v.
Chest	constriction in chest after waking	Dig., psor.
Chest	constriction in chest aggravated after supper	Mez.
Chest	constriction in chest aggravated from covering of bed	Ferr.
Chest	constriction in chest aggravated from motion	Agar., ang., ars., ferr., led., lyc., nux-v., spong., verat.
Chest	constriction in chest aggravated from touch	Arn., cupr.
Chest	constriction in chest aggravated lying on left	Myric.
Chest	constriction in chest aggravated lying on right	Lycps.
Chest	constriction in chest aggravated lying quiet	Caps.
Chest	constriction in chest alternating with pain in abdomen	Calc.
Chest	constriction in chest alternating with sudden expansion	Sars.
Chest	constriction in chest ameliorated after eating	Sulph.
Chest	constriction in chest ameliorated during deep respiration	Sulph.
Chest	constriction in chest ameliorated from bending backwards	Caust.
Chest	constriction in chest ameliorated from drawing shoulders back	Calc.
Chest	constriction in chest ameliorated from expectoration	Calc., manc.
Chest	constriction in chest ameliorated from motion	Seneg.
Chest	constriction in chest ameliorated from perspiration	Sulph.
Chest	constriction in chest ameliorated from straightening up	Mez.
Chest	constriction in chest ameliorated from warmth of bed	Phos.
Chest	constriction in chest ameliorated from weeping	Anac.
Chest	constriction in chest ameliorated while lying	Calc-p.
Chest	constriction in chest ameliorated while lying head high	Ferr.
Chest	constriction in chest ameliorated while sitting	Nux-v.

Body part/Disease	Symptom	Medicines
Chest	constriction in chest ameliorated while sitting bent	Lach.
Chest	constriction in chest ameliorated while standing	Mez.
Chest	constriction in chest ameliorated while walking	Ferr.
Chest	constriction in chest ameliorated while walking in open air	Alum., chel., dros., puls.
Chest	constriction in chest as from band	Acon., aml-n., arg-n., ars., bry., Cact., chlor., led., lob., lyc., op., Phos., pic-ac., sil.
Chest	constriction in chest asthmatic	Ang., coff., led., mez., naja., nux-v., sulph.
Chest	constriction in chest at day time	Mez., phos.
Chest	constriction in chest at night	Alum., aral., bry., coloc., ferr., kali-n., lach., mez., myric., puls., seneg., sep., sil., stram., tab.
Chest	constriction in chest at night in bed	Ferr., nux-v.
Chest	constriction in chest before menses	Phos.
Chest	constriction in chest before vomiting	Cupr.
Chest	constriction in chest convulsive	Asaf., Bell., Cupr.
Chest	constriction in chest during chill	Ars., cimx., kali-c., Nux-v., phos.
Chest	constriction in chest during cough	Calc., cham., cimx., con., cupr., form., hell., lyc., mag-p., merc., myrt., Phos., puls., stram., sulph.
Chest	constriction in chest during deep respiration	Agar., aspar., caust., cham., cic., coc-c., dulc., euon., ferr., ham., kali-bi., kali-n., lact., lyc., mag-m., mosch., nat-c., nux-v., puls., sang., seneg., stry., sulph., tab., tarax., thuj.
Chest	constriction in chest during expiring	Bor., caust., chel., kali-c.
Chest	constriction in chest during inspiration	Agar., aspar., cham., chel., con., dros., mez., raph., sabad., seneg., sulph.
Chest	constriction in chest during menses	Sep.
Chest	constriction in chest during spasmodic cough	Mosch.
Chest	constriction in chest during stool	Coloc.
Chest	constriction in chest during whooping cough (an infectious bacterial disease that causes violent coughing mainly affects children)	Caust., mur-ac., spong.
Chest	constriction in chest from anger	Cupr.
Chest	constriction in chest from ascending	Ang., Ars., Calc., led., mag-c., nux-v.
Chest	constriction in chest from becoming cold	Mosch., phos.
Chest	constriction in chest from bending backwards	Nit-ac.
Chest	constriction in chest from bending forward	Dig.
Chest	constriction in chest from bringing arms together in front	Sulph.
Chest	constriction in chest from cold air	Bry., phos., sabad.
Chest	constriction in chest from cold bathing	Nux-m.
Chest	constriction in chest from exertions	Ars., calc., ferr., nat-m., nux-v., spong., verat.
Chest	constriction in chest from flatulance	Nux-v., rheum., sil.
Chest	constriction in chest from manual labuor	Calc.
Chest	constriction in chest from stooping	Alum., laur., merc., mez., seneg.

Body part/Disease	Symptom	Medicines
Chest	constriction in chest from straightening up	Sars.
Chest	constriction in chest from stretching	Nat-m.
Chest	constriction in chest in afternoon	Bapt., eupi., lac-c., mag-c., nat-m., petr., sulph.
Chest	constriction in chest in evening	Ars., bry., calc-p., carb-s., carb-v., hyper., puls., raph., rhus-t., stann., sulph., verb., zinc.
Chest	constriction in chest in evening in bed	Ars., bell., berb.
Chest	constriction in chest in hydrothorax (fluid in pleural cavity)	Apis., apoc., colch., lact., merc., psor., spig., stann.
Chest	constriction in chest in morning	Arg-n., calc., carb-v., cycl., lyc., nat-m., phos., puls., sars., sep.
Chest	constriction in chest in morning during fasting	Sulph.
Chest	constriction in chest in morning on waking	Sep.
Chest	constriction in chest in noon	Agar.
Chest	constriction in chest on swallowing	Kali-c.
Chest	constriction in chest on waking	Alum., dig., graph., Lach., lact., seneg., sep.
Chest	constriction in chest one sided	Cocc., zinc.
Chest	constriction in chest painful	Sulph., verat.
Chest	constriction in chest preventing talking	Cact.
Chest	constriction in chest spasmodic	Am-c., Asaf., aur., calc., carb-s., carb-v., caust., cupr., glon., hep., Ign., ip., kali-c., kali-p., lact., led., nat-m., op., phos., sars., sec., sep., spong., sulph., verat.
Chest	constriction in chest when falling asleep	Bry., graph., lach.
Chest	constriction in chest while cough	Carb-v., clem., dros., ip., mosch., samb., stram., sulph.
Chest	constriction in chest while lying	Aral., lach., nat-m., nux-v.
Chest	constriction in chest while rapid walking	Puls.
Chest	constriction in chest while sitting	Agar., ars., mez., nit-ac.
Chest	constriction in chest while standing	Verat.
Chest	constriction in chest while walking	Am-c., anac., ang., Ars., dig., ferr., jug-c., kali-c., led., lyc., nux-v., puls., sulph., verat.
Chest	constriction in chest while walking in open air	Am-c., calc., lith.
Chest	constriction in heart ameliorated by bending chest forward	Lact-ac., lil-t.
Chest	constriction in lower part of chest aggravated from lying on right side	Lycps.
Chest	constriction in right side of chest	Cocc., zinc.
Chest	constriction in stomach extendig to chest	Alum.
Chest	constriction in upper part of chest	Cham., phos., rhus-t.
Chest	coppery patches in chest	Stram.
Chest	coryza, extending to chest	All-c., carb-v., euphr., ip., merc., nux-v.
Chest	cough aggravated from motion of chest	Anac., bar-c., Chin., cocc., dros., lach., mang., merc., mur-ac., nat-m., Nux-v., phos., sil., Stann.
Chest	cough aggravated from mucous in upper chest	Anac., bar-c., Chin., cocc., dros., lach., mang., merc., mur-ac., nat-m., Nux-v., phos., sil., Stann.

Body part/Disease	Symptom	Medicines
Chest	cough from cold wind on chest	Phos., rumx.
Chest	cough from cramps in chest	Bell.
Chest	cough from dryness in chest	Bell., benz-ac., kali-chl., lach., laur., merc., puls.
Chest	cough from fullness of chest	Chin-a., sulph.
Chest	cough from fullness of chest in morning	Chin-a., sulph.
Chest	cough from pressure in chest	Iod., op.
Chest	cough from sensation of crawling in chest	Cahin., caust., con., kreos., nux-m., rhus-t., squil.
Chest	cough from sensation of heat in chest	Carb-v.
Chest	cough from stitching in chest	Acon., bry., nit-ac., nux-v.
Chest	cough from tingling in chest	Sep., squil.
Chest	cough with burning in chest	Am-c., caust., coc-c., eupho., euphr., led., mag-m., ph-ac.
Chest	cough with mucous in chest	Ant-t., arg-m., ars., arum-t., asar., bar-c., calc., caust., cham., cina., euphr., graph., guare., iod., ip., Kali-bi., kali-n., kreos., med., nat-m., plb., Puls., sep., spong., Stann., sulph.
Chest	cough with oppression (trouble) in epigastrium	Kali-bi.
Chest	cracking in sternum in region of heart	Nat-c.
Chest	cracking in sternum on bending chest backwards	Am-c.
Chest	cracking in sternum on motion	Nat-m., sulph.
Chest	cramps in chest after eating	Nat-m.
Chest	cramps in chest after exertion	Plb.
Chest	cramps in chest aggravated from motion	Ferr., sulph.
Chest	cramps in chest ameliorated on lying down	Sulph.
Chest	cramps in chest at night	Nat-a.
Chest	cramps in chest during menses	Cocc.
Chest	cramps in chest in evening in warm room	Sulph.
Chest	cramps in chest in evening while riding	Phos.
Chest	cramps in chest in open air	Iod.
Chest	cramps in chest in warm room	Sulph.
Chest	cramps in chest on coughing	Kali-c., laur.
Chest	cramps in chest on walking	Ferr.
Chest	cramps in chest with eructations	Dig.
Chest	crusts on chest	Anac., ars., fl-ac., hep., mez., nat-s.
Chest	cyanosis in chest	Ant-t., bor., carb-an., dig., ip., Lach., Laur.
Chest	desquamation on chest	Led., mez., sulph.
Chest	diarrhoea after pain in chest	Sang.
Chest	difficulty in speech from weakness of chest	Stann.
Chest	dropsy of chest can lie only on affected side	Ars.
Chest	dropsy of chest can lie only on right side with head low	Spig.
Chest	dropsy of chest with asthma	Psor.

Body part/Disease	Symptom	Medicines
Chest	dropsy of chest with asthma	Psor.
Chest	ecchymosis in chest	Lach., phos., sul-ac.
Chest	eczema on chest	Anac., calc-s., calc., carb-v., cycl., Graph., hep., kali-s., petr., Psor., Sulph.
Chest	emaciation of chest	Kali-i.
Chest	empyema (accumulation of pus) in chest	Apis., ars-i., Ars., Calc-s., calc., carb-s., carb-v., chin-a., chin., dig., ferr., hep., iod., kali-c., Kali-s., lach., lyc., Merc., nat-a., nit-ac., phos., sep., Sil., Sulph.
Chest	eruptions herpetic alternating with chest affections and dysenteric stools	Rhus-t.
Chest	eruptions on skin alternating with tightness of chest	Calad., kalm., rhus-t.
Chest	eruptions on skin of chest in every spring	Nat-s.
Chest	eruption, rash from tightness of chest alternating with asthma	Calad.
Chest	extremities flexed over chest	Morph., olnd., tab.
Chest	faintness from constriction of chest	Acon.
Chest	fluttering (a condition marked by rapid, but regular heartbeat) in chest after dinner	Sep.
Chest	fluttering in chest after menses	Spig.
Chest	fluttering in chest after slight excitement	Aml-n., Lil-t., lith.
Chest	fluttering in chest alternating with soreness	Aur-m.
Chest	fluttering in chest ameliorated in open air	Nat-m., Nat-s.
Chest	fluttering in chest at night	Naja.
Chest	fluttering in chest during rest	Lil-t.
Chest	fluttering in chest from ascending steps	Bry., Calc.
Chest	fluttering in chest in afternoon during headache	Form., sumb.
Chest	fluttering in chest in evening	Pic-ac.
Chest	fluttering in chest in morning	Naja., stry.
Chest	fluttering in chest on raising arms	Dig., sulph.
Chest	fluttering in chest on waking	Kali-i., naja.
Chest	fluttering in chest wakens her at night	Lil-t.
Chest	fluttering in chest while on left side	Daph., dig., gels., nat-m., spig.
Chest	fluttering in chest while on right side	Alumn.
Chest	fluttering in chest while sitting	Asaf.
Chest	fluttering in chest while thinking of it	Arg-n.
Chest	fluttering in chest while writing	Naja.
Chest	formication in chest from warm food	Mez.
Chest	formication in chest in warm room	Mez.
Chest	formication in chest on entering house	Phos.
Chest	freckles (a harmless small brownish patch on skin) in chest	Nit-ac.
Chest	fullness in chest after coffee	Canth.

Body part/Disease	Symptom	Medicines
Chest	fullness in chest after eating	Ant-c., caps., lyc.
Chest	fullness in chest after eating in evening	Alumn.
Chest	fullness in chest ameliorated after expectoration	Ail.
Chest	fullness in chest before menses	Brom., Sulph.
Chest	fullness in chest during exertion	Nat-a.
Chest	fullness in chest if desire to urinate is delayed	Lil-t.
Chest	fullness in chest in afternoon	Alumn., coca.
Chest	fullness in chest in bed in evening	Nat-s., sulph.
Chest	fullness in chest in evening	Carb-v., eupi., lact., Puls., sulph.
Chest	fullness in chest in morning	Con., lyc., sulph.
Chest	fullness in chest in morning after smoking	Cycl.
Chest	fullness in chest in open air	Lyc.
Chest	fullness in chest on deep inspiration	Kali-n., nat-a., sulph.
Chest	fullness in chest on waking	Con., ph-ac.
Chest	fullness in chest when ascending	Bar-c.
Chest	fullness in chest while sitting	Caps.
Chest	fullness in chest while walking in forenoon	Acon.
Chest	fullness in chest while writing in forenoon	Fl-ac.
Chest	haemorrhage (the loss of blood from a ruptured blood vessel, either internally or externally) black from chest	Kreos.
Chest	haemorrhage brown from chest	Bry., rhus-t.
Chest	haemorrhage dark from chest	Arn., coll., ham., mag-c., puls.
Chest	haemorrhage from chest after exertion	Acon., arn., ferr., ip., mill., puls., rhus-t., urt-u.
Chest	haemorrhage from chest after suppression of menses	Acon., ars., bell., bry., con., dig., ferr., graph., ham., mill., phos., Puls., sang., senec., sep., sulph., ust.
Chest	haemorrhage from chest after whiskey	Merc., puls.
Chest	haemorrhage from chest after wine	Acon.
Chest	haemorrhage from chest alternating with rheumatism (stiffness in joints or muscles)	Led.
Chest	haemorrhage from chest ameliorated from walking slowly	Ferr.
Chest	haemorrhage from chest as a result of pneumonia (an inflammation of one or both lungs, usually caused by infection from a bacterium or virus)	Calc-s., sul-ac.
Chest	haemorrhage from chest before menses	Dig.
Chest	haemorrhage from chest from anger	Nux-v.
Chest	haemorrhage from chest in drunkards	Ars., hyos., Nux-v., op.
Chest	haemorrhage from chest in lying in women	Acon., arn., chin., hyos., ip., puls., sulph., tril.
Chest	haemorrhage from chest in nursing mothers	Chin.
Chest	haemorrhage frothy foamy from chest	Acon., arn., dros., ferr., ip., led., mill., op., ph-ac., phos., sec., sil.
Chest	headache alternating with pain in chest	Lachn.

Body part/Disease	Symptom	Medicines
Chest	headache extending around the chest	Con., nat-m.
Chest	herpes on chest	Ars., graph., hep., lyc., mag-c., petr., staph., syph.
Chest	holds chest with hands during cough	Arn., bor., Bry., cimic., Dros., eup-per., kreos., merc., nat-m., nat-s., phos., sep.
Chest	impeded, obstructed breath from constriction of chest	Bell., brom., Cact., caps., chel., cic., cupr-ac.
Chest	impeded, obstructed breath with pain in chest	Brom., bry., caps., colch., croc., merc., plb., ran-s., ruta., spong., sulph., valer., verb.
Chest	impeded, obstructed breath with pain in diaphragm	Ip., spig.
Chest	impeded, obstructed breath with spasms of chest	Hyos., stram.
Chest	impeded, obstructed breath with stitches of chest	Aloe., arg-m., arn., berb., bry., chin-s., kreos., mez., rhod., stann., sul-ac., thuj., verb.
Chest	inflammation of diaphragm (curved muscular membrane that separates the abdomen from the area around the lungs)	Bry., cact., dulc., hep., lyc., nux-m., nux-v., ran-b., stram., verat.
Chest	interrupted sleep from oppression in chest	Seneg.
Chest	itching and tingling in chest	Con.
Chest	itching in chest at night	Lith.
Chest	itching in chest biting	Laur., spong.
Chest	itching in chest biting aggravated by cold	Nicc.
Chest	itching in chest biting aggravated from scratching	Con.
Chest	itching in chest biting ameliorated from scratching	Nicc.
Chest	itching in chest in afternoon	Nicc.
Chest	itching in chest in evening	Cact., chin., mez., stront., sulph.
Chest	itching in chest in evening on becoming warm in bed	Puls., rhus-v.
Chest	itching in chest in evening while walking	Fl-ac.
Chest	itching in chest in morning	Brom.
Chest	itching in chest in morning in bed	Rhus-t.
Chest	itching in chest in spots	Aster., nit-ac.
Chest	itching in chest when warm	Bov., cocc.
Chest	itching in external throat extended to chest	Fl-ac.
Chest	itching on chest	Cann-s., graph., led., rhus-t., stram., urt-u.
Chest	jerking in chest	Agar., anac., arg-m., calc-p., cina., con., lyc., spong., squil., valer.
Chest	jerking in chest when breathing	Lyc.
Chest	jerking in chest when moving the arm	Anac.
Chest	loose cough from tickling deep in chest	Graph.
Chest	miliary on chest	Hydrc., mez.
Chest	motion of upper limbs forward over chest during cramp	Atro.
Chest	motion of upper limbs forward over chest during cramp thrown violently	Ip.
Chest	must hold chest with both hands while whooping cough	Arn., bor., Bry., cimic., Dros., eup-per., kreos., merc., nat-m., nat-s., phos., sep.

Body part/Disease	Symptom	Medicines
Chest	nodules on chest	Bar-c., carb-an., hippoz., hydr., mang., merc-c., nat-s.
Chest	numbness in chest	Chel., cupr-ar., glon., merc., nux-m., rhus-t., urt-u.
Chest	numbness in fingers from chest affection	Carb-an.
Chest	numbness in left side of chest	Cupr-ar., cur., plb.
Chest	numbness in right side of chest	Chel.
Chest	ovaries painful extending to chest	Apis., lach.
Chest	pain in abdomen extendimg into chest	Aloe., alum., dulc., grat., hyos., kali-c., lach., mag-c., merl., nat-m., par., phos., plb., raph.
Chest	pain in chest from excitements	Stann., stram.
Chest	pain in chest from exertion	Alum., ang., caust., ferr., laur., plb., ran-b.
Chest	pain in chest after dinner	Bry., canth., carb-s., cimic., lob., mez., nat-p., rat., sulph., zinc.
Chest	pain in chest after drinking cold water	Carb-v., nit-ac., psor., staph., thuj.
Chest	pain in chest after eating	Alum., anag., arg-n., aspar., brom., caust., chin., cimic., kali-c., laur., mez., nat-c., nux-v., phos., sulph., sumb., thuj., verat., zinc.
Chest	pain in chest after every breath	Nat-m.
Chest	pain in chest after hawking	Asaf.
Chest	pain in chest after herpes zoster	Mez., ran-b.
Chest	pain in chest after hiccoughing (an abrupt involuntary contraction of the diaphragm that causes an intake of breath and closes the vocal cords, resulting in a convulsive gasp with the gulping sound)	Am-m., stront.
Chest	pain in chest after inflammation of lungs	Am-c., ars., lach., Lyc., Phos., Sulph.
Chest	pain in chest after midnight	Rhus-t.
Chest	pain in chest after sneezing	Bor., cina., crot-h., merc., thuj.
Chest	pain in chest after stool	Agar.
Chest	pain in chest after stooping	Nat-s.
Chest	pain in chest after wine	Bor.
Chest	pain in chest aggravated by arms near chest	Psor.
Chest	pain in chest aggravated from bending right	Rhod.
Chest	pain in chest aggravated from bending sideways	Acon.
Chest	pain in chest aggravated from blowing nose	Chel.
Chest	pain in chest aggravated from lying on painful side	Bell., nux-v., ran-b., rumx.
Chest	pain in chest aggravated from motion	Abrot., arn., bad., bapt., Bell., Bry., Calc., caps., carb-s., card-m., chel., chin., cimic., equis., gamb., graph., hep., hyos., kali-c., kali-p., kalm., lact-ac., laur., lyc., manc., meny., merc., naja., nat-m., nit-ac., nux-v., phos., psor., ran-b., sabad., sars., sec., Spig., squil., stront., sulph., viol-t.
Chest	pain in chest aggravated from pressure	Ant-c., meny., merc-i-f., nat-p., ran-b., seneg., sul-ac., tarax.
Chest	pain in chest aggravated from singing	Am-c.
Chest	pain in chest aggravated in warm room	Mag-s., sil.

Body part/Disease	Symptom	Medicines
Chest	pain in chest alternating with pain in abdomen	Aesc., ran-b.
Chest	pain in chest alternating with pain in stomach	Caust.
Chest	pain in chest ameliorated after eating	Chel., rhod.
Chest	pain in chest ameliorated after rising in bed	Kali-c.
Chest	pain in chest ameliorated by arms near chest	Lact-ac.
Chest	pain in chest ameliorated during inspiration	Merc.
Chest	pain in chest ameliorated from bending forward	Asc-t., chel., chin-s., Puls.
Chest	pain in chest ameliorated from eructations	Bar-c., kali-c., lyc.
Chest	pain in chest ameliorated from expectoration (to cough up and spit out phlegm, thus clearing the bronchial passages)	Chel., euon., mag-s.
Chest	pain in chest ameliorated from heat	Phos.
Chest	pain in chest ameliorated from lieing on painful sides	Ambr., Bry., calad., nux-v., stann.
Chest	pain in chest ameliorated from lieing on sides	Alum.
Chest	pain in chest ameliorated from lying on back	Ambr., cact.
Chest	pain in chest ameliorated from lying on painful side	Ambr., bry., kali-c.
Chest	pain in chest ameliorated from motion	Lob., phos., rhus-t., seneg.
Chest	pain in chest ameliorated from pressure	Arn., bor., Bry., cimic., Dros., eup-per., kreos., merc., nat-m., nat-s., phos., ran-b., sep.
Chest	pain in chest ameliorated from pressure on sides	Bor., bry., cimic., phos.
Chest	pain in chest ameliorated from rubbing	Calc., phos.
Chest	pain in chest ameliorated from sitting	Alum., am-m., asaf.
Chest	pain in chest ameliorated from standing	Chin., graph.
Chest	pain in chest ameliorated from warmth	Ars., caust., Phos.
Chest	pain in chest ameliorated in open air	Nat-m.
Chest	pain in chest ameliorated in open air	Nat-m.
Chest	pain in chest ameliorated on motion	Aur-m-n.
Chest	pain in chest ameliorated on stretching the arm	Berb.
Chest	pain in chest ameliorated while lying	Alum., ox-ac.
Chest	pain in chest ameliorated while lying on abdomen	Bry.
Chest	pain in chest ameliorated while lying on back	Phos.
Chest	pain in chest ameliorated while sitting bent	Chel., ran-b.
Chest	pain in chest ameliorated while walking	Chin., dros., mez., nat-m., ph-ac., seneg.
Chest	pain in chest as if splinter (a small thin sharp piece of wood, metal, stone, glass)	Arg-n.
Chest	pain in chest at 4.00 a.m.	Asc-t.
Chest	pain in chest at night	Alum., am-c., ant-t., apis., arg-n., Ars., caust., chel., con., graph., lyc., mag-s., merc-c., nit-ac., nux-v., ran-b., ran-s., rhus-t., sabad., seneg., sil., sin-n.
Chest	pain in chest at night	Am-c., chel., con., graph., iod., myris., rumx.
Chest	pain in chest at night on falling asleep	Nux-m.

Body part/Disease	Symptom	Medicines
Chest	pain in chest at night on going into open air	Am-m.
Chest	pain in chest before chill	Ars., plan.
Chest	pain in chest before going to sleep	Carb-v., sulph.
Chest	pain in chest before menses	Puls.
Chest	pain in chest before stool	Calc-s.
Chest	pain in chest can lie only on back	Acon., bry., phos.
Chest	pain in chest during chill (a moderate but often unpleasant degree of coldness	Ars., bell., Bry., chin-s., Kali-c., lach., puls., rhus-t., sabad., seneg.
Chest	pain in chest during chilliness	Eupi., sep.
Chest	pain in chest during cough	Apis., arn., ars., bell., Bry., calc-s., calc., caps., caust., chel., coff., con., kali-n., lact., lyc., Merc., nat-s., phos., psor., puls., rhus-t., sabad., seneg., sep., Squil., stram., Sulph., tarent., verat., zinc.
Chest	pain in chest during deep respiration	Acon., ant-c., arg-m., arn., aur., bar-c., bor., Bry., bufo., calc-p., calc., canth., caps., carb-an., carb-v., cham., chel., chin-s., chin., cycl., ferr-p., ferr., fl-ac., form., graph., grat., Kali-c., kali-n., lyc., meny., mez., nit-ac., oena., ph-ac., phos., phyt., plat., rhus-t., rumx., seneg., sil., spong., stann., sulph., sumb., thuj., verat.
Chest	pain in chest during expiration	Ambr., cina., raph., spig., staph., zinc.
Chest	pain in chest during hawking (to clear the throat noisily of phlegm)	Plb., spig.
Chest	pain in chest during heat	Ant-c., ars., canth., caps., carb-v., cina., guare., kali-c., kalm., nux-v.
Chest	pain in chest during inspiration	Acon., aesc., arn., ars., aspar., aur., benz-ac., bor., bov., brom., Bry., calc-s., canth., caps., carb-s., caust., cham., Chel., cocc., colch., con., grat., kali-c., kali-n., led., lyc., mez., nat-a., nat-s., nicc., oena., op., phyt., plb., ran-b., Rumx., sang., sep., sil., spig., Squil., sumb., tarax., viol-t.
Chest	pain in chest during menses	Cocc., graph., phos., puls.
Chest	pain in chest during palpitation	Sep.
Chest	pain in chest during palpitation (to beat in an irregular or unusually rapid way, either because of a medical condition or because of exertion, fear, or anxiety)	Sep., spig., spong.
Chest	pain in chest during respiration (the act of breathing air in and out)	Aesc., Bry., chel., puls.
Chest	pain in chest during riding in a wagon	Dig.
Chest	pain in chest during riding on horse back	Nat-c.
Chest	pain in chest during sleep	Cupr.
Chest	pain in chest from anxiety	Phos.
Chest	pain in chest from ascending	Acon., bor., cact., crot-h., graph., kali-bi., ran-b., rat., staph., stram.
Chest	pain in chest from bending backward	Rhod.
Chest	pain in chest from bending forward	Aloe., alum., alumn., arg-m., brom., nat-m.

Body part/Disease	Symptom	Medicines
Chest	pain in chest from carrying a load	Alum.
Chest	pain in chest from change in weather	Ran-b.
Chest	pain in chest from cold air	Ph-ac.
Chest	pain in chest from eructations	Cocc., phos., staph.
Chest	pain in chest from fasting	Iod.
Chest	pain in chest from laughing	Acon., laur., mez., nicc., psor.
Chest	pain in chest from lieing on affected sides	Ant-t., bell., calc., sabad.
Chest	pain in chest from lieing on painful sides	Bell., bry., nux-v., ran-b., rumx.
Chest	pain in chest from lieing on sides	Canth., hydr., ran-b.
Chest	pain in chest from lifting	Alum., Arn., bar-c., brom., phos., psor., sulph.
Chest	pain in chest from motion of arms	Carb-an., card-m., caust., nux-m., seneg., sulph.
Chest	pain in chest from motion of head	Guai.
Chest	pain in chest from pressure of clothing	Benz-ac., ran-b.
Chest	pain in chest from pressure on sides	Brom., meny., merc-i-f., sul-ac., tarax.
Chest	pain in chest from returning winter every year	Arg-m., kalm.
Chest	pain in chest from rising from a seat	Kali-c., nat-c.
Chest	pain in chest from sitting bent	Am-m., dig.
Chest	pain in chest from smoking	Seneg.
Chest	pain in chest from sneezing	Acon., bor., Bry., caust., chel., coc-c., crot-t., dros., lact., merc., rhus-t., seneg., thuj.
Chest	pain in chest from standing	Aur-m., bov., calc., nat-m., nat-s., ran-b., spig., stann., zinc.
Chest	pain in chest from stooping	Nicc.
Chest	pain in chest from wine	Bor.
Chest	pain in chest from yawning	Bell., bor., hep., nat-s., phel., sang.
Chest	pain in chest if desire to urinate be delayed	Lil-t.
Chest	pain in chest in afternoon	Am-m., bad., bar-c., canth., chel., coloc., eupi., fago., gamb., iod., kali-bi., kali-n., led., lyc., nicc., op., sang., sulph., tarent.
Chest	pain in chest in afternoon	Alum., bar-c., canth., chel., coloc., form., kali-bi., led., lyc., nicc.
Chest	pain in chest in damp weather	Cupr., kali-c., Nat-s., ran-b., sil.
Chest	pain in chest in evening	Acon., alum., ambr., ant-t., bad., bar-c., cahin., calad., calc., chel., coloc., dig., dios., euphr., eupho.,gamb., hyper., kali-bi., Kali-c., kali-i., kali-n., lyc., mag-s., mez., mur-ac., nat-m., nicc., nux-m., olnd., phos., ran-b., ran-s., rumx., seneg., sulph., tab., thuj., verb., zinc.
Chest	pain in chest in evening in bed	Benz-ac., cahin., kali-c., nat-c., nit-ac., ran-b., rhus-t., sep.
Chest	pain in chest in forenoon	Agar., am-m., caust., cham., coloc., puls., ran-b.
Chest	pain in chest in morning	Acon., am-m., bov., bry., caust., chel., chin., chin-s., con., elaps., fago., ferr-p., fl-ac., hep., lil-t., lyc., mang., merc-c., merc., nat-s., nit-ac., nux-v., ox-ac., phos., puls., ran-b., rhus-t., sang., sep., squil., sulph., sumb., thuj.

Body part/Disease	Symptom	Medicines
Chest	pain in chest in morning in bed	Colch., lact., mag-s., phel., rumx., seneg., sil.
Chest	pain in chest in noon	Dig., naja., rumx.
Chest	pain in chest in open air	Am-m.
Chest	pain in chest on expiration	Chin., crot-t., spig., staph., tarax., viol-o., zinc.
Chest	pain in chest on getting warm in bed	Rhus-v.
Chest	pain in chest on motion	Aster., bad., brom., Bry., calc., Chel., gamb., graph., hell., hyper., lyc., phos., psor., ran-b., sabad., sars., sulph., viol-t., zinc.
Chest	pain in chest on motion	Aster., bad., brom., Bry., calc., Chel., gamb., graph., hell., hyper., lyc., phos., psor., ran-b., sabad., sars., sulph., viol-t., zinc.
Chest	pain in chest on rising	Puls.
Chest	pain in chest on rising in bed	Am-c.
Chest	pain in chest on stooping	Am-c., ars., card-m., chel., fago., lyc., merc., merl., mez., nat-s., nit-ac., ran-b., rhod., seneg.
Chest	pain in chest on straightening up	Acon., aloe., nicc.
Chest	pain in chest on stretching the arm	Ran-b.
Chest	pain in chest on swallowing	All-c., alum., calc-p.
Chest	pain in chest on waking	Arg-n., Graph., kali-bi., merc-i-r., phos., seneg., thuj.
Chest	pain in chest paroxysmal (a sudden onset or intensification of a pathological symptom or symptoms, especially when recurrent)	Caul., nit-ac., ox-ac., plb., sep., stront., stry.
Chest	pain in chest rheumatic	Abrot., ambr., ant-t., arg-n., arn., berb., Bry., cact., cadm., carb-v., caust., chin., cimic., colch., con., corn., guai., hydr., kali-i., Kalm., lach., Lact-ac., lyc., nux-v., phos., plb., Ran-b., rhod., Rhus-t., rumx., Spig., tarent.
Chest	pain in chest undulating (move sinuously like waves)	Dig., dulc., spig.
Chest	pain in chest when stooping	Am-c., lyc., nit-ac., sep.
Chest	pain in chest when touched	Dros., phos., ran-b.
Chest	pain in chest when turning	Ran-b.
Chest	pain in chest when turning in bed	Caust., thuj.
Chest	pain in chest while ascending steps	Kali-bi., staph.
Chest	pain in chest while bending backward	Rhod.
Chest	pain in chest while bending forward	Aloe., alum., alumn.
Chest	pain in chest while bending right	Cocc.
Chest	pain in chest while blowing nose	Sumb.
Chest	pain in chest while clearing throat	Spig.
Chest	pain in chest while eating	Kali-bi., led., ol-an.
Chest	pain in chest while lying	Alumn., asaf., bry., calc., caps., caust., con., kali-n., psor., puls., ran-b., rumx., seneg.
Chest	pain in chest while lying in bed	Calc., con.
Chest	pain in chest while lying on left side	Am-c., eup-per., Phos.
Chest	pain in chest while lying on right side	Lyc., lycps., phyt.

Body part/Disease	Symptom	Medicines
Chest	pain in chest while riding on carriage	Alum., dig.
Chest	pain in chest while riding on horse back	Nat-c., ol-j.
Chest	pain in chest while sitting	Am-m., bry., chin., dig., nat-s., nit-ac., paeon., ph-ac., plan., seneg., spig., staph.
Chest	pain in chest while sitting bent	Am-c., anac.
Chest	pain in chest while standing	Calc., nat-s., stann., zinc.
Chest	pain in chest while talking	Am-c., Bor., cann-s., Kali-c., kali-n., nat-m., prun-s., rhus-t., tab.
Chest	pain in chest while talking	Bor., kali-n., rhus-t., tab.
Chest	pain in chest while turning right	Rumx.
Chest	pain in chest while walking	Agar., am-c., bell., brom., bry., bufo., cact., calc., camph., card-m., cham., chel., cimic., cinnb., cocc., colch., coloc., dig., hep., kali-i., lact., merc., merl., nat-m., olnd., ox-ac., Ran-b., rhus-t., sars., spig., stann., stront., sul-ac., sulph., tarax., tarent., viol-t., zinc.
Chest	pain in chest while walking in open air	Caust., lyc., ran-b., sulph., zinc.
Chest	pain in chest while walking slowly	Bor.
Chest	pain in chest while writing	Mag-s., ran-b.
Chest	pain in chest while yawning	Nat-s.
Chest	pain in external throat extending to pectoral (Chest) muscles	Ars.
Chest	pain in kidneys extending to chest	Benz-ac.
Chest	pain in left side of chest extending to groin	Fl-ac.
Chest	pain in left side of chest extending to right shoulder	Carb-v., graph.
Chest	pain in left side of chest extending to shoulder	Verat.
Chest	pain in left side of chest extending to throat	Sulph.
Chest	pain in left upper limb with angina pectoris (chest pain)	Cimic., dig., lat-m.
Chest	pain in lower chest ameliorated from lying	Chel.
Chest	pain in lower chest ameliorated from lying on back	Ambr.
Chest	pain in lower chest ameliorated from walking	Chin.
Chest	pain in lower chest ameliorated from walking extending transversely (lying or extending crosswise or at right angles to something)	Bism.
Chest	pain in lower chest from deep inspiration	Carb-s., chel., naja.
Chest	pain in lower chest while lying on left side	Phos.
Chest	pain in lower chest while sitting	Chin., seneg.
Chest	pain in lower chest while walking	Bism., sep.
Chest	pain in lower left side of chest	Cact., carb-s., carb-v., colch., kali-p., lith., Ox-ac., Phos., rhod., tarent.
Chest	pain in lower left side of chest ameliorated from eating	Rhod.
Chest	pain in lower right side of chest	Ambr., chel., kali-c., merc-c., naja.
Chest	pain in lumbar region to the pectoral muscles (chest muscles) and arms after riding	Brach.

Body part/Disease	Symptom	Medicines
Chest	pain in pectoral muscles	Bry., echi., merc., rhus-t.
Chest	pain in region of diaphragm	Echi., nux-m.
Chest	pain in region of diaphragm in forenoon	Nux-m.
Chest	pain in shoulder extending to chest	Sars.
Chest	pain in thigh extending to chest	Puls.
Chest	pain in upper limb extending to chest	Vip.
Chest	pain in uterus extending to chest	Lach., murx.
Chest	pain in uvula extending to chest	Agar., sang.
Chest	pain of face extending to chest	Sil.
Chest	pain under left scapula extending to chest	Bar-c., kali-c., sars., sep.
Chest	palpitation of heart on bending chest forward	Kalm., Spig.
Chest	periodic Constriction of chest	Phos.
Chest	perspiration in chest after coition	Agar.
Chest	perspiration in chest aggravated from cold	Agar., camph., canth., cocc., hep., lyc., merc., petr., sep., stann.
Chest	perspiration in chest during chilliness	Sep.
Chest	perspiration in chest during menses	Bell., kreos.
Chest	perspiration in chest offensive	Arn., graph., hep., Lyc., phos., Sel., sep.
Chest	perspiration in chest oily	Arg-m.
Chest	petechia on chest	Ars., cop., stram.
Chest	petechia on chest , purple	Ars.
Chest	phthisis after injury to the chest	Ruta.
Chest	pimples hard under the skin of chest	Alum.
Chest	pimples on chest , elevated	Valer.
Chest	pimples on chest that bleed easily	Cist.
Chest	pimples on chest with burning	Agar., bov., staph.
Chest	pimples on chest with red areola	Bov.
Chest	pimples on chest, flattening	Rhus-t.
Chest	pimples on chest, hard	Bov., valer.
Chest	pimples on chest, indolent (disease or condition that is slow to develop or be healed, and causes no pain)	Cund.
Chest	pimples on chest, itching	Cann-s., dulc., gins., mag-m., nat-c., tab.
Chest	pimples on chest, red	Am-c., apis., arund., bov., cocc., iod., mez., ph-ac., plb., stram., zinc.
Chest	pimples on chest, red in evening	Ph-ac.
Chest	pimples on chest, white	Valer.
Chest	pimples pointed with whitish semi-transparent vesicles on chest	Bry.
Chest	pustules on chest	Agar., ant-t., ars., arund., asar., aur., bar-c., calc., chel., chlor., cocc., euon., fl-ac., graph., hep., hydr., hydrc., kali-bi., kali-s., mag-m., merc-c., petr., psor., rhus-t., sil., stront.

Body part/Disease	Symptom	Medicines
Chest	rash on chest	Am-c., ant-t., bry., calad., calc-s., calc., Chel., cupr., ferr., ip., lach., Led., merc., mez., plb., sil., staph., sulph., syph., ter.
Chest	rash red on chest aggravated by warmth	Stram.
Chest	rash red on chest	Am-c., calc., camph., Chel., corn., staph., stram., sulph.
Chest	rash with itching on chest	Calad., caust., staph.
Chest	reddish patches on the skin of chest	Apis., chlol., cinnb.
Chest	redness in chest	Aster., aur., bar-c., bell., chin-s., graph., iod., kali-ar., lac-c., rhus-t., rhus-v., sulph., tarax., vesp.
Chest	respiration arreasted during constriction of chest	Hell., sep.
Chest	rheumatic pain in extremities alternating with chest affection	Led.
Chest	rubeola (a red rash on the skin, seen in diseases such as measles, scarlet fever, and syphilis) on chest after abuse of mercury	Kali-i.
Chest	sensation as if drops of boiling water were falling into chest	Acon.
Chest	sensation of bar of iron across the centre of chest	
Chest	sensation of bar of iron around chest	Arg-n.
Chest	sensation of emptyness in chest after cough	Ill., kali-c., nat-s., sep., stann., zinc.
Chest	sensation of emptyness in chest after eating	Nat-p.
Chest	sensation of emptyness in chest after expectoration	Calad., stann., zinc.
Chest	sensation of emptyness in chest at night	Sep.
Chest	sensation of emptyness in chest during cough	Sep., stann., sulph.
Chest	sensation of emptyness in chest on beginning to sing	Stann.
Chest	sensation of plug (close up something) in chest	Anac., aur.
Chest	spots on chest, black	Vip.
Chest	spots on chest, brown	Cadm., carb-v., lyc., mez., petr., phos., Sep., thuj.
Chest	spots on chest, brown on mammae with itching	Cadm., carb-v., lyc., phos., sep.
Chest	spots on chest, brown with itching	Hydr., lyc., sulph.
Chest	spots on chest, dark	Phos.
Chest	spots on chest, yellow	Ars., phos.
Chest	spots on chest, yellow become dark	Mez.
Chest	spots on chest, yellow with itching in evening	Sulph.
Chest	stitching pain in chest ameliorated from pressure of hand	Aur-m., puls.
Chest	stitching pain in chest ameliorated from scratching	Plat.
Chest	stitching pain in chest extending to arms	Brom., nat-m.
Chest	stitching pain in chest extending to back	Alumn., arum-t., bov., chel., chen-a., guai., kali-c., kali-n., lyc., mez., ox-ac., par., sil.
Chest	stitching pain in chest extending to back aggravated from lying on left side	Kali-c.
Chest	stitching pain in chest extending to back ameliorated from lying on right side	Kali-c.

Body part/Disease	Symptom	Medicines
Chest	stitching pain in chest extending to elbow	Sil.
Chest	stitching pain in chest extending to hypochondrium	Berb.
Chest	stitching pain in chest extending to sacral region	Thuj.
Chest	stitching pain in chest extending to scapula	Arum-t., chel., chen-a., lact., nat-m., seneg., Sulph.
Chest	stitching pain in chest extending to shoulder	Indg., kali-c., nat-m., sang.
Chest	stitching pain in chest extending to sternum	Laur.
Chest	stitching pain in chest extending to submaxillary gland (gland of lower jaw)	Calc.
Chest	stitching pain in chest while reading aloud	Calc., nat-m.
Chest	stitching pain in chest with fainting	Arn.
Chest	stitching pain in chest with numbness and lameness of left arm	Rhus-t.
Chest	stitching sensation in chest after anger	Arg-n., caust.
Chest	stitching sensation in chest after hawking	Asaf.
Chest	stitching sensation in chest aggravated from bending sideways	Acon.
Chest	stitching sensation in chest aggravated from sneezing	Acon., bor., bry., chel., Dros., Merc., rhus-t.
Chest	stitching sensation in chest ameliorated from bending forward	Chel., chin.
Chest	stitching sensation in chest ameliorated from rubbing	Calc., phos.
Chest	stitching sensation in chest at night	Alum., am-c., apis., ip., lyc., merc-c., nit-ac., phos., ran-s., rhus-t., sabad., seneg.
Chest	stitching sensation in chest at night in bed	Phos.
Chest	stitching sensation in chest at night on waking	Seneg.
Chest	stitching sensation in chest compelling to bend	Sars.
Chest	stitching sensation in chest compelling to bend backeard or forward	Agar.
Chest	stitching sensation in chest during fever	Acon., Bry., kali-c., nux-v.
Chest	stitching sensation in chest from cold drinks	Staph., thuj.
Chest	stitching sensation in chest from hiccoughing	Am-m.
Chest	stitching sensation in chest from yawning	Aur., bell., bor., mag-c., nat-s., phel.
Chest	stitching sensation in chest in afternoon	Coloc., iod., sulph.
Chest	stitching sensation in chest in evening	Calad., kali-bi., kali-i., kali-n., mag-c., ran-s., rumx., verb.
Chest	stitching sensation in chest in evening in bed	Benz-ac., nat-c.
Chest	stitching sensation in chest in forenoon	Caust.
Chest	stitching sensation in chest in morning	Chin., hep., kali-bi., mang., merc., rhus-t., squil.
Chest	stitching sensation in chest in morning on rising	Ran-b.
Chest	stitching sensation in chest in noon	Agar.
Chest	stitching sensation in chest on ascending steps	Bor., rat., stram.
Chest	Stream of blood from chest to head like a gust of wind with epistaxis (bleeding from nose)	Mill.

Body part/Disease	Symptom	Medicines
Chest	sudden outburst of pain in chest	Ox-ac., phos.
Chest	swelling in chest	Calc., dulc., iod., kali-m., merc., nat-c., sep., sil., sulph.
Chest	swelling in hand extending to chest muscles	Crot-h.
Chest	tension in muscles of back extending to chest aggravated from stooping	Chel.
Chest	tubercles on chest	Am-c., caust., mang., nicc.
Chest	tubercles on chest	Hydrc., thuj.
Chest	urticaria on chest	Calad., hydrc., sars., sulph., urt-u.
Chest	vesicles on chest	Alum., arund., calc-s., calc., camph., carb-s., caust., graph., kali-i., led., merc., rhus-t., sep., stram., sulph.
Chest	weakness in chest after exertion	Aloe., Spong.
Chest	weakness in chest after expectoration	Stann.
Chest	weakness in chest aggravated from reading	Sulph.
Chest	weakness in chest aggravated from sitting long	Dig., ph-ac.
Chest	weakness in chest aggravated from wine	Bor.
Chest	weakness in chest ameliorated from bending forward	Nux-v.
Chest	weakness in chest ameliorated from lying	Alum.
Chest	weakness in chest ameliorated from walking	Ph-ac.
Chest	weakness in chest from cough	Graph., nit-ac., ph-ac., psor., ruta., sep., Stann.
Chest	weakness in chest from cough before menses	Graph.
Chest	weakness in chest from deep respiration	Carb-v., plat.
Chest	weakness in chest from lying on side	Sulph.
Chest	weakness in chest from reading aloud	Cocc., sulph.
Chest	weakness in chest from walking	Lyss., rhus-t.
Chest	weakness in chest from walking in open air	Rhus-t.
Chest	weakness in chest from walking rapid	Kali-c.
Chest	weakness in chest from walking rapid in open air	Nat-m.
Chest	weakness in chest in evening	Ran-s.
Chest	weakness in chest in evening while lying	Sulph.
Chest	weakness in chest in morning on waking lasting until 3.00 p.m.	Merc-i-r.
Chest	weakness in chest on beginning to sing	Stann.
Chest	weakness in chest on waking	Carb-v.
Chest	weakness in chest when singing	Carb-v., sulph.
Chest	weakness in chest when talking	Calc., ph-ac., rhus-t., Stann., sul-ac., sulph.
Chest	weakness in chest when talking loud	Calc., gels., laur., Sulph.
Chest	weakness in chest while eating	Carb-an.
Chest	yawning with oppression of chest	Stann.
Chest	yellow , scaly , itching spots on chest	Kali-c.
Chest	yellow , scaly , itching spots on chest	Kali-c.

Body part/Disease	Symptom	Medicines
Chest Sound	murmur (soft blowing or fluttering sound, usually heard via a stethoscope, that originates from the heart, lungs, or arteries and may indicate disease or structural concerns) blood flow.	Agar., aml-n., apis., ars-i., ars., aspar., aur-m., aur., bar-c., Cact., calc., carb-ac., chel., chin-a., cocc., colch., Coll., crot-h., cupr-s., Dig., ferr-ar., ferr-i., Ferr., glon., hep., hydr-ac., hydr., iber., iod., ip., kali-ar., kali-br., kali-c., Kalm., lach., lith., lob., lyc., lycps., merc., Naja., nat-a., nat-c., nat-m., nit-ac., phos., plb., psor., puls., Rhus-t., Spig., Spong., stann., stram., sumb., tab., tarent., tub.
Chicken Pox	cough after chicken pox (a highly infectious viral disease, especially affecting children, characterized by a rash of small itching blisters on the skin and mild fever)	Ant-c.
Chicken Pox	eruption, like chicken pox in upper limbs	Led.
Chicken Pox	eruption, like varicella (chicken pox) in lower limbs	Ant-t.
Chicken Pox	eruption, like varicella in legs	Ant-t.
Chicken Pox	eruption, varicella like	Ant-t.
Chicken Pox	eruptions carbuncle like chicken pox	Acon., **Ant-c.**, ant-t., ars., asaf., bell., canth., carb-v., caust., coff., con., cycl., hyos., ip., led., merc., nat-c., nat-m., **Puls.**, rhus-t., sep., sil., **Sulph.**, thuj.
Chilblain	chilblains (red itchy swelling on the fingers, toes, or ears caused by exposure to cold and damp)	Agar.
Chilblain	chilblains inflamed	Ars., cham., lyc., nit-ac., nux-v., Puls., staph., sulph.
Chilblain	chilblains on feet cracked	Merc., nux-v., petr.
Chilblain	chilblains on feet suppurating	Lach., sil., sulph.
Chilblain	chilblains on feet swollen	Merc.
Chilblain	chilblains on feet with inflammation	Lach., merc., nit-ac., Petr.
Chilblain	chilblains on feet with purple	Lach., merc., puls., sulph.
Chilblain	chilblains on fingers	Berb., carb-an., lyc., nit-ac., nux-v., petr., puls., sul-ac., sulph.
Chilblain	chilblains on fingers with itching	Sulph.
Chilblain	chilblains on fingers, painful	Sul-ac.
Chilblain	chilblains on hands With Itching	Puls., zinc.
Chilblain	chilblains on hands, In mild weather	Stann.
Chilblain	chilblains on hands, with swelling	Zinc.
Chilblain	chilblains on toes	Agar., alum., aur., bor., carb-an., croc., kali-c., nit-ac., nux-v., Petr., phos., Puls., rhod.
Chilblain	chilblains painful	Arn., ars., aur., hep., nit-ac., petr., ph-ac., phos., puls., sep.
Chilblain	chilblains pulsating	Nux-v.
Chilblain	chilblains with heel swollen and red	Petr.
Children	anxiety in children	Bor., calc-p., calc., gels., kali-c.
Children	aphthae of mouth in children	Bor., casc., kali-chl., Merc., mur-ac., nux-m., nux-v., plan., sacc., Sul-ac., sulph.
Children	asthmatic in children	Acon., ambr., Cham., Ip., kali-br., kali-i., mosch., Nat-s., nux-v., psor., Puls., Samb., stram., sulph.
Children	asthmatic in children after vaccination	Thuj.

Body part/Disease	Symptom	Medicines
Children	breathing difficult in children	Ambr., calc-p., calc., lyc., Nat-s., puls.
Children	cancerous affections, noma (severe gangrenous inflammation of the mouth or genitals, usually occurring in children who are malnourished or otherwise debilitated)	Alum., alumn., ars., calc., carb-v., con., elat., kali-p., merc., sil., sulph.
Children	child becomes stiff & blue on face with suffocative cough	Cupr., Ip.
Children	child boring fingers in ears	Arund., cina., psor., sil.
Children	child coughs at sight of strangers	Ambr., ars., bar-c., phos.
Children	child Holds person who is near	Stram.
Children	child leans head to left side all time	Nux-m.
Children	child leans head to right side all time	Am-c., ferr.
Children	child leans head, all time	Cina.
Children	child refuses mother's milk	Bor., Calc-p., calc., cina., lach., merc., sil.
Children	child wakes but cannot get out of bed soon enough	Kreos.
Children	children grasp the genitals and cry out during painful urging	Acon., merc.
Children	children put finger in mouth	Calc., cham., Ip.
Children	children with red face, flabby muscles, who sweat easily and take cold readily in consequence	Calc.
Children	chorea in children who has grown too fast	Phos.
Children	chronic dry cough in scrofulous (diseased, or shabby in appearance due to tuberculosis of the lymph glands, especially of the neck) children	Bar-m.
Children	chronic obstruction in nose of children	Bry., Calc., con., fl-ac., sars., sel., sil., sulph.
Children	constriction in chest during whooping cough (an infectious bacterial disease that causes violent coughing mainly affects children)	Caust., mur-ac., spong.
Children	convulsion in children	Acon., aeth., agar., ambr., apis., **Art-v.**, **Bell.**, bry., calc., camph., caust., cham., cic., **Cina.**, cocc., coff., crot-c., cupr., dol., gels., **Hell.**, hep., hydr-ac., hyos., ign., ip., kali-c., lach., laur., lyc., mag-p., nux-v., **Op.**, plat., sec., sil., **Stram.**, sulph., **Verat.**, **Zinc.**
Children	convulsion in children from approach of strangers	Op.
Children	cough following scarlatina (bacterial infection marked by fever, a sore throat, and a red rash, mainly affecting children)	Ant-c., con., hyos.
Children	cough from exposure to snowfall in children	Sep.
Children	cough in child which must be raised that gets blue in face cannot exhale	Meph.
Children	cyanosis in infants	Arn., ars., bor., cact., camph., carb-v., chin., **Dig.**, **Lach.**, **Laur.**, naja., op., phos., psor., rhus-t., sec., sulph.
Children	deep sleep in children	Cupr.
Children	discoloration of skin in new born children	Acon., bov., chin., nat-s., sep.

Body part/Disease	Symptom	Medicines
Children	distension of abdomen in children	Bar-c., Calc., Caust., cina., cupr., sil., staph., Sulph.
Children	dysuria child cries at the close of urination	Sars.
Children	dysuria painful, child cries at close of urination	Sars.
Children	dysuria painful, child cries before urine starts	Bor., lach., lyc., nux-v., Sars.
Children	enlarged abdomen of children	Bar-c., Calc., cupr., mag-m., psor., sanic., sars., Sil., sulph.
Children	enlarged abdomen of children with marasmus (a gradual wasting away of the body, generally associated with severe malnutrition or inadequate absorption of food and occurring mainly in young children)	Calc., sanic., sars.
Children	enlarged abdomen of fat children	Am-m., calc.
Children	enlarged liver in children	Calc-ar., nux-m.
Children	eruption, rash in children	Acon., bry., cham., ip., sulph.
Children	haemorrhoids in children	Mur-ac.
Children	hardness of abdomen in children	Calc., sil.
Children	hernia inguinal in right side of abdomen in children	Aur., lyc.
Children	hernia inguinal in children	Aur., lyc., nit-ac., nux-v.
Children	hernia inguinal in left side of abdomen in children	Nux-v.
Children	Hydrocephalitic (head of the baby is greatly enlarged and the forehead is seen to bulge)	Calc Phos 6X to 30 X
Children	infant scream before the urine passes	Bor., lach., lyc., nux-v., sars.
Children	inflammation of lungs in infants	Acon., ant-t., bry., ferr-p., Ip., kali-c., lob., lyc., merc., nux-v., op., phos.
Children	inflammation of bronchial tubes in children	Dulc., Ip., Kali-c.
Children	Inflammation of eye in infants	Acon., alumn., Apis., arg-m., Arg-n., arn., Ars., arund., bell., bor., bry., Calc., cham., dulc., euphr., hep., ign., lyc., merc-c., merc., Nit-ac., nux-v., Puls., rhus-t., sulph., Thuj., zinc.
Children	inflammation of throat of children	Cham.
Children	involuntary urination in weak children	Chin.
Children	irritability in children	Abrot., ant-c., ant-t., ars., benz-ac., bor., calc-p., Cham., Cina., graph., iod., lyc., Mag-c., puls., sanic., sep., sil., zinc.
Children	itching in nose, child starts out of sleep and rubs constantly	Lyc.
Children	learning to walk late	Agar., bar-c., bell., **Calc-p.**, **Calc.**, **Caust.**, **Nat-m.**, nux-v., sanic., sil., sulph.
Children	marasmus (gradual wasting away of the body) of children	Abrot., alum., ant-c., arg-n., **Ars-i.**, **Ars.**, bar-c., **Calc-p.**, **Calc.**, carb-v., caust., chin., cina., hydr., **Iod.**, kali-c., kreos., lyc., mag-c., **Nat-m.**, nux-m., nux-v., ol-j., op., petr., phos., plb., psor., puls., sars., sep., **Sil.**, sulph.
Children	nursing children	Acon., agn., ars., bell., **Bor.**, bry., calc-p., **Calc.**, carb-an., carb-v., cham., chel., chin., cina., con., crot-t., dulc., ferr., graph., ign., iod., ip., kali-c., lach., lyc., mag-c., merc., nat-c., nat-m., **Nat-p.**, nux-v., ph-ac., phel., phos., phyt., **Puls.**, rheum., rhus-t., samb., sec., sel., **Sep.**, sil., spig., squil., stann., staph., stram., sulph., zinc.

Body part/Disease	Symptom	Medicines
Children	obstinate (difficult to control) children, yet cry when kindly spoken to	Sil.
Children	obstruction in nose in children	Am-c., ars., asc-t.
Children	obstruction in nose while nursing infants (a very young child that can neither walk nor talk)	Aur., kali-bi., Lyc., Nux-v., samb.
Children	open fontanelles (a soft, membrane-covered space between the bones at the front and the back of a young baby's skull)	Apis., Calc-p., Calc., ip., merc., sep., Sil., sulph., syph.
Children	premature decay and hollowness of teeth in children	Calc-f., calc-p., calc., coff., fl-ac., Kreos., Staph.
Children	prolapsus of anus in children	Ferr., hydr., nux-v., Podo.
Children	remitent fever in infants	**Acon.**, ars., **Bell.**, bry., **Cham.**, **Gels.**, ip., nux-v., sulph.
Children	respiration arressted suddenly in children	Cham.
Children	restless children	Ant-t., bor., cham., jal., rheum.
Children	retention of urine every time child catches cold	Acon., cop., dulc., puls., sulph.
Children	retention of urine in children	Acon., Apis., art-v., bell., benz-ac., calc., caust., cop., dulc., eup-pur., ferr-p., gels., ip., op.
Children	retention of urine in new born infants	Acon., apis., ars., benz-ac., camph., canth., caust., erig., hyos., lyc., puls.
Children	skin, becomes sore in a child	Ant-c., bar-c., bell., calc., **Cham.**, chin., ign., kreos., lyc., merc., puls., ruta., sep., sil., squil., **Sulph.**
Children	sleeplessness child must be carried	Cham.
Children	sleeplessness child must be rocked (away to and fro)	Cina.
Children	snuffles in new-born infants	Dulc., Lyc., Nux-v., puls., Samb.
Children	suffocation in new born infant	Acon., Ant-t., arn., bell., Camph., chin., laur., op.
Children	sunken fontanelles	Apis., calc.
Children	trembling after nursing infant	Olnd.
Children	Tuberculous Children	Beta Vul. 2X
Children	urination painful, child cries	Bor., lach., Lyc., nux-v., Sars.
Children	urination painful, child grasps the genital and cry out	Acon., merc.
Children	urination painful, child jumps up & down if cannot be gratified (satisfied)	Petros.
Children	vomiting in teething children	Bism., calc., hyos.
Children	weakness in ankle in children learning to walk	**Carb-an.**, nat-p.
Children	weakness in children	Bar-c., bell., calc., lach., lyc., nux-v., sil., sulph.
Children	weakness in lower limbs in child learning to walk late	**Calc.**
Children	weakness in lumbar region in child does not learn to walk	All-s.
Chill	Aching in back before chill	Carb-v., daph., dios., Eup-per., ip., Podo., rhus-t.
Chill	Aching in lumbar region during chill	Gamb., myric.
Chill	annual chill	Ars., **Carb-v.**, **Lach.**, nat-m., psor., rhus-r., **Rhus-v.**, sulph., thuj., tub., urt-u.

Body part/Disease	Symptom	Medicines
Chill	anxiety after chill	Chel., kali-c.
Chill	anxiety before chill	Ars-h., ars., Chin.
Chill	anxiety caused by chill	Acon., ars., gels., tub.
Chill	biting skin during chill	Gamb.
Chill	breathing difficult during chill	Apis., ars., bry., cimx., gels., gins., guare., kali-c., mez., nat-m., nux-m., nux-v., puls., seneg., thuj., zinc.
Chill	burning pain in hand during chill	Spong.
Chill	cheerful during chill	Cann-s., nux-m., phos., puls., rhus-t., verat.
Chill	chill (a moderate but often unpleasant degree of coldness) never at night	Chin.
Chill	chill after anger	Acon., ars., **Bry.**, cham., **Nux-v.**, teucr.
Chill	chill after eating	Agar., alum., am-c., am-m., anac., arg-n., **Ars.**, **Asar.**, **Bell.**, bor., bry., calc., camph., **Carb-an.**, carb-s., carb-v., caust., cham., chin., coc-c., coloc., con., croc., cycl., dig., graph., ign., ip., kali-ar., **Kali-c.**, kali-p., lach., lyc., nat-c., nat-m., nat-p., nit-ac., nux-v., petr., ph-ac., phos., puls., **Ran-b.**, rhus-t., sel., sep., sil., staph., sulph., **Tarax.**, teucr., ther., verat., zinc.
Chill	chill after epilepsy	Calc., **Cupr.**, sulph.
Chill	chill after excitement	Calc., cic., **Gels.**, ign., teucr.
Chill	chill after exertion	Arn., ars., bar-c., eup-per., kali-s., merc., nux-v., rhus-t., sil., sulph.
Chill	chill after exposure during rains	Aran., bell., calc., cedr., cur., dulc., ferr., **Nat-s.**, **Rhus-t.**, zinc.
Chill	chill after exposure from residing at seashore	Nat-m., nat-s.
Chill	chill after exposure from sleeping in damp rooms	Aran., ars., calc., carb-v., chin-a., lach., nat-s., rhus-t.
Chill	chill after exposure from standing in water	Arn., calc., led., rhus-t.
Chill	chill after exposure from too frequent cold bath	Ant-c., calc., rhus-t., tarent.
Chill	chill after exposure to a draft	Acon., bar-c., calc., canth., ferr., hep., merc., tarent.
Chill	chill after exposure to area submerged in water	Ang., cedr., chin-s., chin., eucal., nat-m., **Nat-s.**, nux-v.
Chill	chill after exposure to malarial influences	**Arn.**, carb-ac., **Cedr.**, chin-a., chin-s., chin., eucal., eup-per., ferr., ip., nat-m., nat-s., nux-v., **Psor.**, sulph.
Chill	chill after exposure to soil freshly turned up	Nat-m.
Chill	chill after exposure to the heat of sun	Bell., cact., glon., lach., nat-c.
Chill	chill after exposure to tropical (the area between or near the tropic of Cancer and the tropic of Capricorn) countries	Ang., bry., **Cedr.**, chin., nat-m., **Nat-s.**, podo., ter.
Chill	chill after exposure when heated	Acon., carb-v., sil.
Chill	chill after exposure when lying on path of river	Calc., nat-m., nat-s., nux-v.
Chill	chill after exposure	Acon., ang., ant-c., aran., arn., ars., bar-c., bol., bry., cact., **Calc.**, canth., carb-v., **Cedr.**, chin-s., chin., dros., dulc., eucal., eup-per., hep., kali-c., lach., led., nat-m., nat-s., **Rhus-t.**, sep., spig., tarent., zinc.
Chill	chill after menses	Jug-r., kali-c., nat-m., nux-v., phos., puls.
Chill	chill after mental exertion	Aur., colch., nux-v.

Body part/Disease	Symptom	Medicines
Chill	chill after midnight	**Ars., Calad.,** coff., dros., hep., mag-s., merc., op., petr., sil., thuj.
Chill	chill after motion	Agar., **Ars.,** cadm., kali-c., nux-v., phos., **Puls.,** rat., **Rhus-t.,** sep., stann., valer., zinc.
Chill	chill after perspiration	Ant-c., ars., bry., calad., **Caps.,** carb-v., **Caust.,** cham., dig., eup-per., kali-c., lach., **Lyc.,** mag-s., mez., nat-m., op., petr., ph-ac., phos., puls., rhus-t., sabad., sarr., sep., sulph., thuj., verat.
Chill	chill after sleep	Acon., agar., **Alum., Am-m.,** ambr., arn., ars., bry., cadm., calc., caust., con., crot-t., cycl., lyc., merc., nit-ac., nux-v., phos., puls., rhus-t., sabad., samb., sars., sep., sil., staph., sulph., tarent., thuj., verat., zinc.
Chill	chill after sleep alternating with attacks of colfdness	Nux-m.
Chill	chill after stool	Ambr., bufo., canth., dios., grat., lyc., mag-p., merc-c., mez., ox-ac., paeon., petr., plat., stront.
Chill	chill after vexation	Acon., ars., bry., gels., merc., nux-v., rhus-t., tarent.
Chill	chill after walking in the open air	Am-c., anac., ars., bry., cann-s., carb-v., kali-c., laur., nit-ac., nux-v., puls., rhus-t., sep., spong., staph., zinc.
Chill	chill aggravated during drinking	Alum., ant-t., arn., **Ars., Asar.,** bry., cadm., **Calc.,** cann-s., **Caps.,** chel., chin-a., **Chin.,** cimx., cocc., con., croc., elaps., **Eup-per.,** hep., kali-ar., lob., lyc., mez., nat-m., nit-ac., **Nux-v.,** puls., rhus-t., sep., sil., sulph., tarax., tarent., thuj., **Verat.**
Chill	chill aggravated from rising from bed	Bar-c., bism., bor., **Calc.,** canth., cham., ferr-i., mag-c., **Merc.,** mez., **Nux-v.,** phos., rhus-t., sil.
Chill	chill aggravated from swallowing	Merc-c.
Chill	chill aggravated from touch	**Acon.,** ang., apis., bell., cham., **Chin.,** colch., hep., hyos., lyc., **Nux-v.,** phos., puls., sep., spig., staph., sulph.
Chill	chill aggravated from warm drinks	Alum., cham.
Chill	chill aggravated from warm things	Alum., bell., bry., **Puls.**
Chill	chill aggravated in warm room	Acon., **Apis.,** arg-n., bry., cinnb., **Ip.,** merc., nat-m., puls., **Sec.,** sep., staph.
Chill	chill aggravated when thinking of it	Chin-a.
Chill	chill alternating with sweat	Ant-c., ars., calc., eupho., led., lyc., nux-v., phos., sabad., sulph., thuj., verat.
Chill	chill ameliorated after eating	Acon., **Ambr.,** ars., bov., cann-s., chel., cop., cur., ferr., ign., **Iod.,** kali-c., laur., mez., nat-s., petr., phos., rhus-t., sabad., squil., stront.
Chill	chill ameliorated after exercise in open air	Alum., **Caps.,** mag-c., mag-m., **Puls.,** spong., staph., sul-ac.
Chill	chill ameliorated after motion	Acon., apis., arn., asar., bell., caps., cycl., dros., kreos., mag-m., merc., mez., nit-ac., nux-v., podo., **Puls.,** rhus-t., sep., sil., spig., staph., sul-ac., tarent.
Chill	chill ameliorated after sleep	Arn., ars., bry., calad., calc., caps., chin., colch., cupr., ferr., kreos., nux-v., **Phos.,** rhus-t., samb., sep.

Body part/Disease	Symptom	Medicines
Chill	chill ameliorated during drinking	Bry., carb-an., **Caust.**, **Cupr.**, graph., ip., mosch., nux-v., olnd., phos., rhus-t., sil., spig., tarax.
Chill	chill ameliorated from external warmth	Aesc., arg-m., arn., **Ars.**, bar-c., **Bell.**, canth., **Caps.**, carb-an., caust., chel., chin-a., chin., cic., cimx., cocc., colch., con., cor-r., eup-per., ferr., gels., hell., hep., hyos., **Ign.**, **Kali-c.**, kali-i., lach., lachn., laur., **Meny.**, merl., mez., mosch., nat-c., **Nux-m.**, **Nux-v.**, plat., podo., **Rhus-t.**, **Sabad.**, samb., sep., sil., squil., stram., stront., sulph., tarent., ther.
Chill	chill ameliorated from rising from bed	Am-c., ambr., ant-t., arg-m., ars., aur., bell., dros., eupho., ferr., ign., **Iod.**, led., lyc., mag-c., merc-c., merc., nat-c., plat., puls., rhod., rhus-t., sel., sep., stront., sulph., verat.
Chill	chill ameliorated from sun shine	Anac., con.
Chill	chill ameliorated from uncovering and undressing	Apis., **Camph.**, ip., med., puls., **Sec.**, sep.
Chill	chill ameliorated from warm drinks	Bry., eupi.
Chill	chill ameliorated from wrapping up followed by severe fever and sweat	Sil.
Chill	chill ameliorated in bed	Am-c., bry., canth., **Caust.**, cimx., cocc., con., hell., **Kali-c.**, kali-i., kali-n., lachn., mag-c., **Mag-m.**, mag-s., mez., mosch., nat-c., nit-ac., nux-v., podo., puls., **Pyrog.**, rhus-t., sars., squil., stram., sulph.
Chill	chill ameliorated in open air	Acon., alum., ang., ant-c., **Apis.**, arg-m., **Asar.**, **Bry.**, **Caps.**, cocc., graph., **Ip.**, mag-c., mag-m., mez., nat-m., phos., **Puls.**, sabin., staph., **Sul-ac.**
Chill	chill ameliorated in warm room	Aesc., agar., am-c., **Ars.**, bar-c., bell., brom., camph., canth., carb-an., carb-v., caust., **Chel.**, chin-a., chin., cic., con., gels., hell., hep., **Ign.**, **Kali-ar.**, kali-bi., **Kali-c.**, kreos., lach., laur., mag-c., mang., **Meny.**, merc-c., merc., mez., nat-a., **Nux-m.**, nux-v., petr., plat., ran-b., rat., rhod., rhus-t., **Sabad.**, sel., sep., sil., spig., sul-ac., sulph., tarent., ther., valer., zinc.
Chill	chill ameliorated on bed but not by heat of stove	Kali-i., kreos., podo., tarent.
Chill	chill ameliorated on bed but not from external covering	Lachn.
Chill	chill ameliorated on rising	Rhus-t.
Chill	chill ameliorated on sitting	Ign., nux-v.
Chill	chill ameliorated while lying	Arn., asar., bry., canth., colch., kali-n., nat-m., nux-v., sil., zinc.
Chill	chill appearing every other day	Aesc., alum., anac., ant-c., ant-t., apis., **Aran.**, arn., ars-i., **Ars.**, bar-c., bar-m., bell., bol., brom., **Bry.**, calc., canth., **Caps.**, carb-an., carb-v., cedr., cham., chin-a., chin-s., chin., cic., cimx., cina., cor-r., dros., dulc., elat., **Eup-per.**, **Eup-pur.**, ferr-ar., ferr., gamb., gels., hyos., ign., iod., **Ip.**, kali-ar., lach., lyc., mez., mill., nat-m., nux-m., **Nux-v.**, petr., plan., podo., **Puls.**, rhus-t., sabad., sarr., sep., staph., sulph., thuj., verat.
Chill	chill as if cold wind were blowing between the shoulder blades	Caust.

Body part/Disease	Symptom	Medicines
Chill	chill as if cold wind were blowing upon the body	Asar., camph., caust., chin., cimx., croc., cupr., hep., laur., mosch., rhus-t., samb.
Chill	chill as if cold wind were blowing upon the body when walking	Chin.
Chill	chill as if cold wind were blowing upon the body while writing	Agar.
Chill	chill as if ice-water were rising and falling through a cylindrical opening in left lung	Elaps.
Chill	chill as if water running down the back	Agar., alumn., ars.
Chill	chill as if water were poured over him	Anac., ant-t., ars., bar-c., chin., cimx., led., mag-c., **Merc.**, mez., rhus-t., stram.
Chill	chill as if wind blowing upon soles while body sweating	Acon.
Chill	chill as often as he wakes	**Am-m.**, arn.
Chill	chill at day time	Alum., ant-c., ars., arund., asar., bapt., camph., carb-an., **Chin.**, dros., gels., graph., kali-ar., kali-c., kali-p., lyc., mag-s., merc., mosch., nat-c., nat-m., nat-s., nit-ac., plan., sabin., sars., sil., tarent.
Chill	chill at day time with fever at night	Alum.
Chill	chill at day time with sweat at night	Ars.
Chill	chill at midnight	Ars., cact., canth., **Caust.**, chin-a., chin., grat., mez., mur-ac., nat-m., raph., sep., sulph.
Chill	chill at night after nausea	Phyt.
Chill	chill at night before falling asleep	Carb-v., lyc., nux-v., phos.
Chill	chill at night during sweat	Eup-per.
Chill	chill at night in a warm room	Rat.
Chill	chill at night in bed	Canch., canth., **Carb-an.**, dros., euphr., ferr-i., ferr-p., mag-c., mag-s., meny., sars., sulph.
Chill	chill at night on putting hand out of bed	Canth., hep., sil.
Chill	chill at night on rising	Ant-t.
Chill	chill at night on waking	Aloe., carb-an., chel., graph., sars., sil.
Chill	chill at night with hot head	Colch.
Chill	chill automnal	**Aesc.**, ars., bapt., **Bry.**, chin., **Colch.**, **Nat-m.**, nux-v., rhus-t., **Sep.**, verat.
Chill	chill before menses	Am-c., berb., calc., kali-c., kreos., **Lyc.**, nux-v., **Puls.**, sep., **Sil.**, sulph., thuj., verat.
Chill	chill before midnight	Alum., am-c., arg-m., arund., cact., carb-an., caust., mur-ac., nit-ac., phos., **Puls.**, sabad., sulph., verat.
Chill	chill before stool	Aloe., ant-c., ars., bapt., bar-c., benz-ac., calad., chin-s., dig., ip., mag-m., merc., mez., nat-c., phos., puls., verat.
Chill	chill beginning from soles	Dig.
Chill	chill beginning in and extending from abdomen	**Apis.**, bell., calad., calc., camph., cann-s., coloc., cur., **Ign.**, merc., par., teucr., verat.
Chill	chill beginning in and extending from ankles	Chin., lach., puls.

Body part/Disease	Symptom	Medicines
Chill	chill beginning in and extending from arm and hand	Carb-v.
Chill	chill beginning in and extending from arms	**Bell.**, dig., **Hell.**, ign., mez., plat.
Chill	chill beginning in and extending from both arms and thighs	Psor.
Chill	chill beginning in and extending from both arms at once	Bell., hell., mez.
Chill	chill beginning in and extending from buttocks	Puls.
Chill	chill beginning in and extending from calves	Lach., lyc., ox-ac.
Chill	chill beginning in and extending from chest	**Apis.**, ars., carb-an., cic., cina., kreos., lith., merl., nux-v., rhus-t., sep., spig.
Chill	chill beginning in and extending from face	Acon., arn., bar-c., berb., bor., calc., carb-ac., caust., cham., ign., kreos., laur., merc., petr., phos., puls., rhod., ruta., staph., stram.
Chill	chill beginning in and extending from feet	Apis., arn., bar-c., bor., calc-s., calc., chel., cimx., dig., **Gels.**, hyos., kali-bi., lyc., mag-c., **Nat-m.**, nux-m., nux-v., puls., rhus-t., sabad., sarr., sep., sulph.
Chill	chill beginning in and extending from fingers	Bry., coff., dig., **Nat-m.**, nux-v., sep., sulph.
Chill	chill beginning in and extending from hands	Bry., chel., dig., eup-per., **Gels.**, ip., nux-v., puls., rhus-t., sabad., sep., sulph.
Chill	chill beginning in and extending from hands and feet	Apis., bry., carb-v., chel., dig., ferr., gels., **Nat-m.**, nux-m., op., sabin., samb., sulph.
Chill	chill beginning in and extending from head	Bar-c., mosch., nat-m., stann., valer.
Chill	chill beginning in and extending from knees	Apis., benz-ac., puls., thuj.
Chill	chill beginning in and extending from left arm and lower limbs	Nux-m.
Chill	chill beginning in and extending from left hand	Carb-v., nux-m.
Chill	chill beginning in and extending from left side of body	Carb-v., caust.
Chill	chill beginning in and extending from left wrist	Nux-m.
Chill	chill beginning in and extending from legs	Cedr., chin., kali-bi., nux-m., ox-ac., puls., rhus-t., sep., thuj.
Chill	chill beginning in and extending from lips	**Bry.**
Chill	chill beginning in and extending from neck	Puls., staph., valer.
Chill	chill beginning in and extending from neck of bladder after urinating	Sars.
Chill	chill beginning in and extending from nose	Nat-c., sabad., sulph., tarax., tub., zinc.
Chill	chill beginning in and extending from nose	Nat-c., sabad., sulph., tarax., tub., zinc.
Chill	chill beginning in and extending from palms and soles	Dig.
Chill	chill beginning in and extending from right arm and right side	Merl.
Chill	chill beginning in and extending from right foot	Chel., lyc., sabin.
Chill	chill beginning in and extending from right hand	Merl.
Chill	chill beginning in and extending from right side of body	Bry., nat-m., rhus-t.

Body part/Disease	Symptom	Medicines
Chill	chill beginning in and extending from right side of chest	Merl.
Chill	chill beginning in and extending from sacrum	Puls.
Chill	chill beginning in and extending from scalp (skin on top of head)	Mosch.
Chill	chill beginning in and extending from thighs	Cedr., cham., rhus-t., ther., **Thuj.**
Chill	chill beginning in and extending from throat	Sep.
Chill	chill beginning in and extending from tips of fingers	**Bry.**, nat-m., puls.
Chill	chill beginning in and extending from tips of fingers and toes	**Bry.**, cycl., dig., meny., nat-m., **Sep.**, stann., sulph.
Chill	chill beginning in and extending from toes	Bry., coff., **Nat-m.**, sep., sulph.
Chill	chill beginning in and extending from toes	Bry., coff., **Nat-m.**, sep., sulph.
Chill	chill beginning in and extending from umbilicus	Puls.
Chill	chill beginning in and extending from vertex	Arum-t.
Chill	chill beginning in chest with violent congestion and suffocation in warm room	Apis.
Chill	chill beginning in hands and extending to palms and soles	Dig.
Chill	chill causes cough	Cimx., psor.
Chill	chill developing slowly after stool	Ambr., grat.
Chill	chill developing slowly after urinating	Eug., plat., sars., sep.
Chill	chill developing slowly at night	Hep., merc-c., puls., tub.
Chill	chill developing slowly at night alternating with heat	Anthr.
Chill	chill developing slowly before stool	Mez.
Chill	chill developing slowly during stool	Nat-m.
Chill	chill developing slowly from 4.00 to 6.00 p.m.	Alum., arg-n.
Chill	chill developing slowly in a warm room	Aloe., puls., ran-b.
Chill	chill developing slowly in afternoon	Alum., arg-n., calc., calen., carb-an., caust., psor.
Chill	chill developing slowly in afternoon after dinner	Thuj.
Chill	chill developing slowly in afternoon after rest	Bry.
Chill	chill developing slowly in cold air	Anac., bufo.
Chill	chill developing slowly in evening	Am-m., arg-n., ars-h., ars., bell., calc., chlor., gins., kali-i., lyc., nat-m., psor., puls., rhus-t., sul-ac., thuj., tub., zing.
Chill	chill developing slowly in forenoon	Chlor.
Chill	chill developing slowly in forenoon on going in a warm room	Aloe.
Chill	chill developing slowly in morning	Cina., lyc., spig., viol-t.
Chill	chill developing slowly in morning on rising from bed with cold developing slowly on abdomen	Meny.
Chill	chill developing slowly on motion	Acon., sin-a.
Chill	chill developing slowly when rising from sitting	Coff.
Chill	chill developing slowly while standing	Coloc., ham.
Chill	chill during cold damp weather	Am-c., aran., calc., dulc., lyc., mang., merc., **Nux-m.**, rhus-t., sulph., verat.

Body part/Disease	Symptom	Medicines
Chill	chill during descending	Acon., **Agar.**, am-m., aml-n., apis., ars-h., ars., arum-t., bar-c., bell., bor., brom., calad., canth., carb-ac., caust., cedr., chel., cic., cocc., coff., colch., croc., eup-per., eup-pur., kreos., lach., lil-t., lob., mag-c., mez., **Mosch.**, phos., psor., sabad., staph., **Stram.**, sul-ac., sulph., thuj., valer., **Verat.**, zinc.
Chill	chill during diarrhoea	Aloe., ambr., apis., kali-n., sulph.
Chill	chill during disordered stomach	Ant-c., **Ip.**, puls.
Chill	chill during menses	Aloe., am-c., bell., berb., bry., bufo., calc., carb-an., cast., caul., cham., coff., cycl., eupi., graph., ip., kali-i., kreos., lach., led., lyc., mag-c., nat-m., nat-p., nat-s., nux-v., phos., **Puls.**, sec., **Sep.**, **Sil.**, **Sulph.**, thuj., verat., vib., zinc.
Chill	chill during menses when uncovered	Mag-c.
Chill	chill during menses while walking	Mag-c.
Chill	chill during motion	Acon., agar., aloe., alum., ant-c., ant-t., **Apis.**, arn., ars-i., ars., asaf., asar., bell., brom., **Bry.**, camph., cann-s., canth., **Caps.**, casc., caust., cedr., cham., chin., **Coff.**, colch., con., crot-t., cur., cycl., eup-per., gels., hell., hep., iod., kali-ar., kali-c., kali-n., **Merc-c.**, merc., mez., nat-m., nit-ac., **Nux-v.**, petr., plan., plb., podo., psor., **Rhus-t.**, rumx., sang., **Sep.**, **Sil.**, spig., **Squil.**, staph., sul-ac., sulph., thuj.
Chill	chill during sleep	Aeth., am-c., ars., bell., **Bor.**, bov., bry., cadm., calc., carb-an., carb-s., carb-v., caust., cham., chin., grat., hep., hyos., ign., indg., lyc., mur-ac., nat-m., op., ph-ac., phos., puls., sabad., samb., sep., sulph., zinc.
Chill	chill during stool	Aloe., alum., ars., bell., bry., cact., calad., calc., caps., cast., coloc., con., ferr-m., grat., Ind., ip., jatr., lyc., mag-m., merc., nat-c., phos., plat., podo., puls., rheum., rhus-t., sec., sil., spig., stann., sulph., trom., verat., vib.
Chill	chill felt most severely in pit of stomach with violent congestion of head, cold body, with thirst and body feels bruised	**Arn.**
Chill	chill from abuse of alcohol	Led., nux-v.
Chill	chill from abuse of arsenic	Ip.
Chill	chill from bathing in cold water	Aran., cedr.
Chill	chill from becoming wet	Acon., aran., bar-c., bell., bry., calc., cedr., dulc., nat-s., **Rhus-t.**, sep., tarent.
Chill	chill from becoming wet when over heated	Acon., calc., clem., colch., **Rhus-t.**, sep., sil.
Chill	chill from being overheated	Acon., ant-c., ant-t., bell., bry., camph., **Carb-v.**, dig., kali-c., nat-m., nat-s., nux-v., op., phos., **Puls.**, rhus-t., sep., **Sil.**, thuj., zinc.
Chill	chill from coughing	Ars., bry., calc., carb-v., con., cupr., hyos., mez., nat-c., nux-v., phos., **Puls.**, rhus-t., sabad., sep., sulph., verat.
Chill	chill from fright	Acon., **Gels.**, ign., lyc., merc., nux-v., op., plat., puls., sil., verat.
Chill	chill from getting wet	Acon., aran., bar-c., bell., bry., calc., cedr., dulc., nat-s., **Rhus-t.**, sep., sil.

Body part/Disease	Symptom	Medicines
Chill	chill from grief (sorrow)	Gels., ign.
Chill	chill from putting hand out of bed	**Bar-c.**, canth., **Hep.**, phos., **Rhus-t.**, sil.
Chill	chill from sad news	Calc., cic., ign., teucr.
Chill	chill from the least draught of cold air	Bar-c., bell., bry., **Calc.**, canth., **Caps.**, carb-an., cham., **Chin.**, dulc., hep., kali-c., mag-c., merc., **Nux-v.**, pyrus., rhod., sel., sil., sulph., zinc.
Chill	chill from turning over in bed	Acon., bry., caps., hep., lyc., nat-m., **Nux-v.**, **Puls.**, sil., staph., stram., sulph.
Chill	chill from uncovering and undressing	Acon., **Agar.**, am-c., am-m., arg-m., arg-n., **Arn.**, ars-h., ars., asar., aur., bell., bor., calc., canth., caps., carb-an., card-m., **Cham.**, chin-a., **Chin.**, clem., cocc., colch., con., **Cycl.**, dig., dros., eup-per., ferr., **Hep.**, kali-n., lach., mag-c., merc., merl., mez., mosch., nat-m., nit-ac., nux-m., **Nux-v.**, phos., plat., puls., rhod., **Rhus-t.**, samb., sep., **Sil.**, spong., squil., **Stram.**, stront., tarent., thuj.
Chill	chill from walking in the open air	Acon., anac., ant-t., **Ars.**, bell., bor., bry., carb-an., carb-v., cham., **Chel.**, chin-a., **Chin.**, cocc., colch., con., dig., **Eupho.**, hep., mag-m., mang., merc-c., merc., nux-m., **Nux-v.**, ph-ac., sel., sil., spig., sul-ac., sulph., tarax.
Chill	chill from working in clay	**Calc.**
Chill	chill from working in water	**Calc.**, rhus-t.
Chill	chill hastens and increases the chill and causes nausea	Eup-per.
Chill	chill hastens and increases the chill and causes vomiting	**Ars.**, cadm., nux-v.
Chill	chill heavy in morning of one day and light chill in afternoon of other day	Eup-per.
Chill	chill heavy in morning of one day and light in afternoon of next day	Eup-per.
Chill	chill in affected parts	Ars., caust., cocc., dulc., graph., lach., led., merc., nux-v., petr., plat., plb., rhod., rhus-t., sil., thuj.
Chill	chill in after urination	Arn., calc., eug., hep., med., nat-m., **Plat.**, puls., rhod., sars., sep., sulph., thuj.
Chill	chill in after urination begins in neck of bladder and spreads upwards	Sars.
Chill	chill in afternoon after diarrhoea	Ox-ac.
Chill	chill in afternoon after dinner	**Anac.**, bor., carb-an., caust., coc-c., colch., cycl., mag-m., merc., nit-ac., nux-v., puls., spig., sulph., thuj.
Chill	chill in afternoon after sleep	Acon., bry., con., cycl., merc., sabad.
Chill	chill in afternoon after stool	Dios.
Chill	chill in afternoon after waking	Graph.
Chill	chill in afternoon at 3.00 p.m. lasting until bed time	Puls.
Chill	chill in afternoon by a warm stove	Bapt., ferr-i., lyc.
Chill	chill in afternoon during menses	Nat-c., nat-m., nat-s.
Chill	chill in afternoon during sleep	Phos.

Body part/Disease	Symptom	Medicines
Chill	chill in afternoon even in a warm room	Mag-m., rhus-t.
Chill	chill in afternoon following heat	Nux-v., **Puls.**, stram.
Chill	chill in afternoon following heat and sweat	Nux-v.
Chill	chill in afternoon in a hot room	Sil.
Chill	chill in afternoon lasting 4 hours	Nux-v.
Chill	chill in afternoon lasting until morning	Canth., kali-i., sars.
Chill	chill in afternoon lasting untill falling asleep in evening	Graph.
Chill	chill in afternoon on first day of mense	Nat-m.
Chill	chill in afternoon on waking	Canth.
Chill	chill in afternoon with cold perspiration	Gels., sarr.
Chill	chill in afternoon with perspiration	Dig., nat-m.
Chill	chill in afternoon with violent chill with thirst and red face	**Ferr.**
Chill	chill in and extending from abdomen to fingers and toes	Calad.
Chill	chill in autumn (season after summer and before winter) & spring (season between winter & summer)	Apis., ars., **Lach.**, psor., sep.
Chill	chill in before urination	Arn., bor., bry., coloc., hyper., med., **Nit-ac.**, nux-v., puls., rhus-t., sulph., thuj.
Chill	chill in during urination	Bell., eug., gels., lyc., merc., nit-ac., nux-v., phos., **Plat.**, puls., senec., sep., stram., sulph., thuj., verat.
Chill	chill in evening after drinking	Nat-m.
Chill	chill in evening after drinking tea	Ox-ac.
Chill	chill in evening after eating	Calc., kali-c., nux-v.
Chill	chill in evening after lying down	Acon., am-m., aur., bov., bry., camph., caps., cham., grat., hell., lac-c., lyc., merc., nat-c., nat-m., nicc., nit-ac., nux-v., par., ph-ac., phos., podo., **Puls.**, sabad., sars.
Chill	chill in evening ameliorated in bed	Chin-s., mag-c., mag-m., nat-s., rat.
Chill	chill in evening at sunset	Ars., carb-ac., ign., puls., thuj.
Chill	chill in evening continuing all night	Bov., cina., gamb., hyos., ip., lyc., nux-v., puls., rhus-t., sarr.
Chill	chill in evening continuing until midnight	Calad., merc., phos., tub.
Chill	chill in evening during external warmth	Mur-ac.
Chill	chill in evening during motion	Apis., brom., bry., calad., colch., nux-v.
Chill	chill in evening during stool	Alum., sulph.
Chill	chill in evening followed by convulsion and heat lasting all night	Cina.
Chill	chill in evening followed by sweat	Carb-an., cedr., sabad.
Chill	chill in evening from external cold	Nux-m.
Chill	chill in evening in a warm room	Arg-n., chlor., laur., nat-m., puls.

Body part/Disease	Symptom	Medicines
Chill	chill in evening in bed	Agar., **Alum.**, am-c., ars., aur., bry., calc-ar., calc., carb-an., cast., chel., chin-s., chin., coc-c., colch., dros., ferr., guare., kali-n., lyc., mag-c., mag-s., merc., mur-ac., nat-a., nat-c., nat-m., nat-p., nit-ac., nux-v., op., petr., phos., raph., rhus-t., sang., sil., sulph., tarent., thuj., tub.
Chill	chill in evening mingled with heat, then heat no sweat	Kali-s.
Chill	chill in evening not relieved by external warmth	Calc., canth., chin., cina., laur., **Nux-v.**, rhus-t.
Chill	chill in evening on falling asleep	Calc., graph., sil.
Chill	chill in evening on rising	Bor., canth.
Chill	chill in evening on walking	Nat-c., nux-m.
Chill	chill in evening while eating	Bov., con.
Chill	chill in evening while undressing	Acon., calc., cocc., fago., mag-c., merc., nat-a., nit-ac., op., plat., rhus-t., spig., tarent., tub.
Chill	chill in evening while walking	Petr.
Chill	chill in evening with burning in abdomen	Nat-c., phos.
Chill	chill in evening with colic	Led.
Chill	chill in evening with flushes of heat	Petr., thuj.
Chill	chill in evening with pains	Cycl., ign., **Puls.**
Chill	chill in evening without subsequent heat	Calc., lyc., sabad., sulph.
Chill	chill in fever alternating with thirst, then sweat	Sabad.
Chill	chill in fever followed by heat with sweat of the face	Alum.
Chill	chill in fever followed by heat without sweat	Graph., nat-m.
Chill	chill in fever followed by heat, then sour sweat	Lyc.
Chill	chill in fever followed by thirst then sweat	Kali-c.
Chill	chill in fever followed by thirst then sweat then heat without thirst	Hep., kali-n., nat-m.
Chill	chill in fever followed with internal chill, then heat and sweat	Phos.
Chill	chill in fever followed with thirst	Rhus-t.
Chill	chill in fever followed without thirst	Am-m., nit-ac.
Chill	chill in hot weather of summer	Ang., bapt., bell., bry., chin.
Chill	chill in morning after breakfast	Calc-s., carb-an., eupi., gels., verat.
Chill	chill in morning after nightly emissions	Merc.
Chill	chill in morning after perspiration	Mag-s., op.
Chill	chill in morning after rising	Acon., aloe., bor., calc-p., **Calc.**, canth., hep., mag-m., mang., meny., merc., nat-c., nat-s., nux-v., spig., **Verat.**
Chill	chill in morning by a warm stove	Ferr-i., lyc., mag-c.
Chill	chill in morning continuing through the forenoon	Arn., ars., eup-per., nat-m., petr., plb.
Chill	chill in morning continuing through the forenoon until evening	Bapt., hell., mag-c., nat-c., plb.
Chill	chill in morning during breakfast	Carb-an., eupi., gels., graph., verat.

Body part/Disease	Symptom	Medicines
Chill	chill in morning during menses after faintness	**Nux-v.**
Chill	chill in morning during sleep	Caust., nat-m.
Chill	chill in morning if uncovered	Clem., **Nux-v.**
Chill	chill in morning in bed	Ang., apis., arn., bov., carb-s., caust., chin-a., chin-s., chin., con., graph., kali-c., kali-n., led., lyc., mag-s., **Merc.**, mur-ac., **Nat-m.**, nit-ac., **Nux-v.**, rhod., sars., staph., sulph., **Verat.**
Chill	chill in morning on waking	Ant-t., arn., ars., bry., canth., chel., cimic., con., lyc., mag-s., merc., nat-c., nat-s., nit-ac., rhus-t., sep., sulph., tarent., thuj., trom., zinc.
Chill	chill in noon after bathing	Sulph.
Chill	chill in noon after dinner	Grat., mag-s.
Chill	chill in noon after sleep	Bry.
Chill	chill in noon followed by heat	Colch.
Chill	chill in spring	Ant-t., ars., canth., carb-v., cham., gels., **Lach.**, nux-m., **Psor.**, sep., sulph.
Chill	chill in stormy weather	Bry., cham., chin., nux-m., nux-v., phos., puls., rhod., rhus-t., **Zinc.**
Chill	chill in summer	Caps., casc., cedr., lach., nat-m., **Psor.**
Chill	chill in the open air	**Agar.**, alum., am-c., **Anac.**, ant-t., **Ars.**, **Asar.**, **Bapt.**, bar-c., bell., bol., bor., bov., brom., bry., bufo., calad., calc-p., **Calc.**, calen., camph., cann-s., canth., caps., carb-ac., carb-an., carb-v., cham., chel., chin-a., **Chin.**, cocc., **Coff.**, colch., con., **Cycl.**, dulc., eupho., guai., **Hep.**, **Ign.**, kali-ar., kali-c., kali-chl., kali-n., kali-p., kreos., laur., mag-m., mag-s., mang., merc-c., **Merc.**, mosch., nat-m., nit-ac., **Nux-m.**, **Nux-v.**, **Petr.**, ph-ac., phos., **Plat.**, **Plb.**, puls., ran-b., rhod., rhus-t., sars., seneg., **Sep.**, sil., spig., stram., stront., sul-ac., sulph., tab., tarax., thuj., viol-t., zinc., zing.
Chill	chill in upper part of body	Ip.
Chill	chill in warm room on coming in from open air	Arg-n.
Chill	chill in warm room, desire to be near stove	Gels., mosch., rhus-t.
Chill	chill in warm room, desire to be near stove but gets sick near stove	Laur.
Chill	chill in warm room, desire to be near stove but it increases the chill	Chin.
Chill	chill irregular	**Ars.**, eup-per., ign., ip., kali-ar., meny., mill., **Nux-v.**, **Psor.**, **Puls.**, samb., **Sep.**
Chill	chill is felt as if cold water pouring over outside of thorax (part between head and abdomen)	Verat.
Chill	chill left sided	Bar-c., **Carb-v.**, **Caust.**, **Dros.**, elaps., ferr., lach., **Lyc.**, nat-c., rhus-t., ruta., sil., spig., stann., sulph., **Thuj.**
Chill	chill left sided before epilepsy	Sil.
Chill	chill like clock	Aran., cact., cedr.
Chill	chill makes headache and all other symptoms unbearable	**Cimx.**

Body part/Disease	Symptom	Medicines
Chill	chill not ameliorated in warm room nor by warm stove	Acon., alum., **Anac.**, ant-c., **Apis.**, aran., arg-n., ars-i., ars., asar., bapt., bell., **Bov.**, **Bry.**, cact., calc., canth., carb-ac., chin., cic., cina., cinnb., clem., **Cocc.**, colch., dios., dros., dulc., euphr., ferr-i., guai., hell., hep., iod., **Ip.**, kali-i., kreos., lach., laur., lyc., mag-m., merc., **Mez.**, nat-m., nux-m., **Nux-v.**, ph-ac., phos., podo., **Puls.**, ruta., sabin., sars., sep., sil., spong., staph., stry., sul-ac., sulph., teucr., thuj., til., **Verat.**
Chill	chill not marked	Acon., am-m., ambr., bell., camph., canth., carb-an., carb-v., caust., chel., cic., coloc., mag-c., **Psor.**, **Sep.**
Chill	Chill on closing the eyes	Mag-m.
Chill	chill on going into the cold air	Aesc., **Agar.**, ars., bry., calc., camph., **Caps.**, caust., cham., **Coff.**, **Cycl.**, dig., hell., hep., kali-ar., kali-c., **Mez.**, mosch., nat-a., nat-c., nat-p., nux-m., **Nux-v.**, petr., phos., rhod., rhus-t., sabad., sep., sil., spig., verat., zinc.
Chill	chill on going into the cold air from a warm room	Puls.
Chill	chill on rising	Acon., arn., ars., bell., bry., cham., **Merc-c.**, merc., mur-ac., nux-v., phos., puls., rhus-t., squil., sulph., verat.
Chill	chill on side not lain on	Ferr-ma.
Chill	chill on side which he lies	Arn., mur-ac.
Chill	chill on single parts	**Ambr.**, ars., asar., bar-c., bell., bry., calad., calc., caust., cham., hep., **Ign.**, led., lyc., **Mez.**, mosch., nux-v., **Puls.**, rhus-t., **Sep.**, sil., thuj., verat.
Chill	chill on waking	**Alum.**, ambr, **Am.**, ars., bry., calc., card-m., caust., hep., lyc., merc., nit-ac., nux-v., phos., puls., rhus-t., sabad., samb., sars., sep., sil., staph., sulph., tarent., thuj., verat., zinc.
Chill	chill one sided	Alum., ambr., anac., ant-t., arn., bar-c., bell., **Bry.**, **Carb-v.**, **Caust.**, cham., chel., chin., cocc., croc., dig., dros., elat., ferr., ign., kali-c., kali-p., lach., **Lyc.**, nat-c., nat-m., nat-p., **Nux-v.**, par., ph-ac., phos., plat., **Puls.**, ran-b., **Rhus-t.**, ruta., sabad., sabin., sars., sep., **Sil.**, spig., stann., stram., sul-ac., sulph., thuj., verat., verb.
Chill	chill pernicious (causeing serious harm)	Apis., **Arn.**, ars., bell., cact., camph., caps., chin-s., cur., elat., **Gels.**, hyos., lyc., nat-s., **Nux-v.**, op., **Psor.**, puls., stram., sul-ac., sulph., tarent., verat-v., **Verat.**
Chill	chill right sided	Arn., **Bry.**, caust., **Chel.**, eupi., lyc., nat-m., nux-v., par., phos., puls., ran-b., **Rhus-t.**, sabin.
Chill	chill when overheated	Acon., calc., clem., colch., rhus-t., sep., sil.
Chill	chill while eating	Apis., bov., carb-an., carb-v., cocc., con., eupho., kali-c., lyc., nit-ac., ran-s., raph., rhus-t., sep., sil., staph.
Chill	chill while lying	Am-m., cham., cimx., nux-v., phel., podo.
Chill	chill while walking	Arn., asaf., cham., chin.
Chill	chill with coldness of right side and heat of left	Rhus-t.
Chill	chill with numbness	Puls.
Chill	chill with pain	Ang., aran., ars., asaf., aur., bar-c., **Bov.**, bry., caps., cocc., **Coloc.**, cycl., **Dulc.**, eupho., graph., hep., ign., kali-bi., kali-c., **Kali-n.**, lach., led., lyc., **Mez.**, nat-c., nat-m., petr., plb., **Puls.**, ran-b., rhus-t., **Sep.**, sil., squil., sulph.

Body part/Disease	Symptom	Medicines
Chill	chill with perspiration	Alum., ars., calc., cedr., **Cham.**, cinnb., cupr., dig., eup-per., eupho., ferr., gels., kali-ar., led., lyc., nat-m., nux-v., **Puls.**, pyrog., rhus-t., sabad., sang., sars., sulph., thuj., verat.
Chill	chill with trembling & shivering	Acon., agar., agn., **Anac.**, **Ant-t.**, apis., arn., ars., asaf., bell., berb., bor., bov., brom., bry., calc., cann-s., canth., caps., carb-an., cham., chin-s., chin., cic., cimic., cina., cocc., con., croc., eup-per., ferr-ar., ferr., kali-n., led., merc-i-f., merc., mygal., nat-c., nat-m., nux-v., olnd., op., par., petr., ph-ac., phos., **Plat.**, psor., puls., rhus-t., sabad., **Sil.**, stram., sulph., tarent., teucr., ther., valer., zinc.
Chill	chill with trembling & shivering at night	Bor.
Chill	chill with trembling & shivering in afternoon	Asaf., carb-an.
Chill	chill with trembling & shivering in evening	Nat-m., plat., teucr.
Chill	chill with trembling & shivering in morning	Anac.
Chill	chill with trembling & shivering in noon	Gels.
Chill	chill without subsequent heat	Acon., aran., bov., calc., camph., chin., hep., led., lyc., mez., mur-ac., nit-ac., ph-ac., ran-b., sabad., sep., staph., sulph.
Chill	chill, but warmth unbearable	**Apis.**, camph., **Ip.**, **Puls.**, **Sec.**, **Sep.**, staph.
Chill	chill, desire for sun	Anac., con.
Chill	chill, desire warmth which does not relieve	Acon., alum., **Aran.**, bell., bov., calc., camph., chin., cic., cina., cocc., colch., con., dros., ferr., hep., kali-i., **Lach.**, lyc., meny., merc., nat-m., **Nux-v.**, phos., podo., pyrog., sil., tarent., verat.
Chill	chillines in chest	Alum., ars., bry., nat-c., par., ran-b.
Chill	chillines in chest after stool	Plat.
Chill	chillines in chest in evening	Ars.
Chill	chillines in chest on walking in open air	Chin., ran-b.
Chill	chillines in left side of chest	Nat-c., nat-m.
Chill	chillines in mammae in shivering	Cocc., guai., petr.
Chill	chilliness after coition	Nat-m.
Chill	chilliness after eating	Ars., asar., calc., carb-an., caust., kali-c., nux-v., rhus-t., sil., sulph., tarax., teucr., zinc.
Chill	chilliness after labor pain	Kali-c., kali-i.
Chill	chilliness after stool	Bufo., grat., mag-m., plat.
Chill	chilliness after urination	Arn., **Plat.**, puls., sep., sulph., thuj.
Chill	chilliness after walking	Gins.
Chill	chilliness ameliorated after urination	Med.
Chill	chilliness as if cold air were blowing on uncovered parts	Mosch.
Chill	chilliness at night	Acon., agar., aloe., am-c., bov., caps., card-m., caust., croc., kali-i.
Chill	chilliness at night after lying down and as often she wakes without thirst	**Am-m.**

Body part/Disease	Symptom	Medicines
Chill	chilliness at night at 9.30 p.m. followed by shaking chill and has to go to bed	Sabad.
Chill	chilliness at night before menses	Aloe.
Chill	chilliness at night during menses	Lach.
Chill	chilliness at night during sleep	Am-c., grat.
Chill	chilliness at night during undressing	Acon., merc-c., op.
Chill	chilliness before menses	Aloe., am-c., calc., caul., kali-c., kreos., **Lyc.**, mag-c., nat-m., nux-v., **Puls.**, sep., **Sil.**, verat.
Chill	chilliness before stool	Ars., bapt., bar-c., benz-ac., calad., dig., ip., mang., merc., mez., nat-c., phos., puls., verat.
Chill	chilliness before urination	Med., nit-ac.
Chill	chilliness during apyrexia (during lack of fever	Anac., ars., bry., caps., cocc., daph., dig., hep., led., nat-m., puls., ran-s., sabad., sil., verat.
Chill	chilliness during headache	Sil.
Chill	chilliness during menses	Am-c., bell., berb., bry., bufo., calc., carb-an., carb-s., cast., caul., cocc., cycl., graph., ip., kali-i., kreos., mag-c., nat-m., nat-p., nux-v., phos., **Puls.**, sec., **Sep.**, **Sil.**, **Sulph.**, tab., zinc., zing.
Chill	chilliness during stool	Aesc., ars., bell., calc-s., mag-m., mez., rheum., sil., stann., **Verat.**
Chill	chilliness during urination	Lyc., nit-ac., **Plat.**, sep., stram., thuj.
Chill	chilliness during vomiting	Dulc.
Chill	chilliness followed by urging to urinate	Senec.
Chill	chilliness from abuse of coffee	Cham., nux-v.
Chill	chilliness from bad news	Sulph.
Chill	chilliness from exciting news	Gels., sulph.
Chill	chilliness from part touched	Spig.
Chill	chilliness from washing	Bry., zinc.
Chill	chilliness in afternoon	Acon., am-c., arg-m., bar-c., carb-an., caust., chin-s., cina., con., croc., cycl., dulc., graph., kali-chl., kali-n., lyc., mag-m., meny., nit-ac., petr., phos., ran-b., stram.
Chill	chilliness in afternoon , not relieved by heat of stove but relieved by covering up warmly on bed	Podo.
Chill	chilliness in afternoon after dinner	Anac., ars., carb-an.
Chill	chilliness in afternoon after rest	Anac., bry., merc.
Chill	chilliness in afternoon during menses	Nat-m.
Chill	chilliness in afternoon without subsequent heat	Nit-ac., ph-ac.
Chill	chilliness in ball of right big toe	Ars-h.
Chill	chilliness in evening after eating	Croc., kali-c.
Chill	chilliness in evening aggravated from warm stove	Merc.
Chill	chilliness in evening ameliorated on lying on bed	Kali-i., kali-n., mag-m., mag-s.
Chill	chilliness in evening as often as she wakes	**Am-m.**
Chill	chilliness in evening on falling asleep	Lyc., phos.

Body part/Disease	Symptom	Medicines
Chill	chilliness in evening on lying on bed	Am-m., aur., bov., bry., colch., lyc., merc-c., merc., mur-ac., podo., zinc.
Chill	chilliness in evening while walking	Puls.
Chill	chilliness in evening with cold legs lasting all night	Aur.
Chill	chilliness in evening with flashes of heat in the face	Nit-ac., petr.
Chill	chilliness in evening with headache	Acon., bry.
Chill	chilliness in evening with nausea & cold limbs	Apis.
Chill	chilliness in evening with sleepiness	Lycps., nat-m., op.
Chill	chilliness in feet	Agar., ant-c., bry., cedr., dros., nit-ac., petr., phos., rhus-t., sulph., thuj.
Chill	chilliness in feet after motion	Calc.
Chill	chilliness in feet in summer	Ant-c.
Chill	chilliness in first toe	Nit-ac.
Chill	chilliness in forenoon	Aeth., agar., ambr., arg-n., asar., bar-c., chin-s., gamb., guai., kali-c., laur., led., mag-c., mag-m., mur-ac., **Nat-m.**
Chill	chilliness in forenoon before dinner ameliorated by eating	Ambr.
Chill	chilliness in hip	Ham.
Chill	chilliness in knee	Card-m., coloc., ign.
Chill	chilliness in legs	Ars., cinnb., hep., mosch., par., rhod., samb., sep., spong.
Chill	chilliness in legs in sciatica	Nux-v.
Chill	chilliness in lower limbs	Cocc., par., sep.
Chill	chilliness in morning	Am-c., anac., ang., arg-m., arn., asaf., bov., carb-an., chin-a., con., eup-per., eupho., ferr., hep., mag-s., mang., mur-ac., nat-m., nit-ac., rhod.
Chill	chilliness in morning after rising	Acon., arg-n., mang., mur-ac., nat-c., nux-v.
Chill	chilliness in morning and lasting all day	Ferr., mag-c., mang., mez., nat-m., sabin., **Sil.**
Chill	chilliness in morning and lasting all forenoon	Arn.
Chill	chilliness in morning on waking	Ang., arn., chel., mag-s., rhod., zinc.
Chill	chilliness in noon	Apis., lact-ac., lob.
Chill	chilliness in noon after sleep	Bry.
Chill	chilliness in posterior surface of upper limb	Raph.
Chill	chilliness in right upper limb extending to back and legs	Mez.
Chill	chilliness in right upper limbs	Phys., plat.
Chill	chilliness in right upper limbs in open air	Lyss.
Chill	chilliness in shoulder	Lept.
Chill	chilliness in thighs	Acon., arn., ars-i., psor., spong.
Chill	chilliness in toes	Agar., asar., bor., carb-an., carb-v., cast-eq., croc., cycl., op., Petr., phos., puls., sulph., thuj., Zinc.
Chill	chilliness in upper arm	Chel.

Body part/Disease	Symptom	Medicines
Chill	chilliness in upper limb after stool	Plat.
Chill	chilliness in upper limb in evening after lying down	Nux-v.
Chill	chilliness in upper limbs	Astac., bar-c., bell., berb., calc., carb-ac., caust., cham., cinnb., euphr., ign., mez., petr., plat., puls., thuj., zinc.
Chill	chilliness lasting all night	Graph.
Chill	chilliness more in warm room than in open air	Bry., grat., puls.
Chill	chilliness on urging to urinate	Hyper., med.
Chill	chilliness on waking	Card-m., staph.
Chill	chilliness when drinking	Ars.
Chill	chilliness when going from open air in warm room	Am-c., ars., bar-c., bry.
Chill	chilliness when in warm room	Carb-ac., cinnb., grat., iod., lact., puls.
Chill	chilliness while eating	Carb-an., eupho., ran-s.
Chill	chilliness while walking in the open air	Acon., cham., chin., dig., eupho., led., merc-c., plb.
Chill	chilliness with pain	Ars., caust., puls., sep.
Chill	chilliness with perspiration	Acon., ail., am-c., aml-n., ant-c., arg-n., ars., bry., calc., caps., chin., dig., **Eup-per.,** eup-pur., eupho., led., nat-m., **Nux-v.,** petr., phos., psor., puls., pyrog., sabad., sang., sulph., thuj., **Tub.**
Chill	chilliness with perspiration as soon as gets warm in bed	Arg-n.
Chill	chilliness with slightest movement of the bed clothes	Acon., **Arn.,** calc., **Nux-v.,** rhus-t., stram., sulph.
Chill	chilliness with well covered but chest chilly	Ran-b.
Chill	chilliness without subsequent heat	Agn., lyc.
Chill	chills spread from the neck of the bladder after urinating	Sars.
Chill	clenching at beginning of chill	Cimx.
Chill	coldness in foot with burning soles during chill	Ant-c., aur., ferr., Meny., phos., sep., Verat., zinc.
Chill	coldness in hands during chill	Aur., cact., camph., canth., carb-v., cedr., chel., colch., con., hep., ip., lyc., meny., Mez., nat-m., Nux-v., op., petr., Phos., plb., samb., Sec., stram., Verat.
Chill	coldness in knee at night during chill	Apis, Carb-v., ign., Phos., sil.
Chill	coldness in left leg during chill	Carb-v., caust., thuj.
Chill	coldness in right leg during chill	Bry., chel., elaps., sabad., sep.
Chill	coldness in thigh at night during chill	Thuj.
Chill	coldness in tips of finger during chill	Ran-b.
chill	coldness in upper limbs during chill	Bell., dig., hell., mez.
Chill	constant chill during menses	Cast., cycl., kreos., rhus-t.
Chill	constriction in chest during chill	Ars., cimx., kali-c., Nux-v., phos.
Chill	contraction of muscles & tendons during chill	Cimx.
Chill	contraction of muscles & tendons of fingers before chill	Cimx.
Chill	contraction of muscles & tendons of hamstrings during chill	Cimx.

Body part/Disease	Symptom	Medicines
Chill	contraction of muscles & tendons of hollow of knee during chill	Cimx.
Chill	convulsion during chill	Ars., Lach., merc., nux-v.
Chill	cramp during chill	Cupr., sil.
Chill	cramp in foot during chill	Cupr., elat., nux-v.
Chill	cramp in leg during chill	Cupr., elat., nux-v.
Chill	deep sleep during chill	Bell., hep., laur., nat-m., **Op.**
Chill	discoloration of skin with different colours during chill	Ars., crot-h., nux-v., rhus-t.
Chill	discoloration with blueness on hand during chill	Camph., nux-v., spong., stram., **Verat.**
Chill	discoloration with purple hands during chilliness	Thuj.
Chill	discoloration, blueness of nails during chill	Apis., arn., **Ars.**, asaf., carb-s., carb-v., chel., chin-s., chin., cocc., con., dros., eup-pur., ip., kali-ar., mez., **Nat-m.**, **Nux-v.**, petr., ph-ac., **Rhus-t.**, sulph., thuj., verat.
Chill	distesion, during chill	Cocc.
Chill	dry cough after dry chill	Nux-m., samb.
Chill	dry cough before dry chill	Mag-c., Rhus-t., samb., tub.
Chill	dry cough during dry chill	Ferr., rhus-t.
Chill	dysuria during chill	Canth., cham., lyc., merc., nux-v., ph-ac., puls., sulph., thuj.
Chill	external chill	**Acon.**, aeth., agar., alum., am-c., **Am-m.**, ant-t., apis., aran., arn., ars-i., **Ars.**, bar-c., bar-m., bell., bry., calc., **Camph.**, canth., caps., caust., cham., chel., chin., cimic., cimx., cina., colch., con., cupr-ar., dig., dulc., euphr., ferr-m., gamb., gels., hyos., **Ign.**, iod., ip., kali-ar., kali-bi., kali-c., kali-chl., kali-p., lach., laur., mag-c., meny., merc-c., merc., mez., mosch., mur-ac., naja., nat-m., nat-s., **Nit-ac.**, nux-v., **Olnd.**, petr., phos., plb., rhus-t., sabad., sec., sil., sul-ac., sulph., til., verat-v., **Verat.**, verb., **Zinc.**
Chill	external chill at night	Nit-ac., phos.
Chill	external chill at night after waking	Bov., bry.
Chill	external chill at night during sleep	Crot-h.
Chill	external chill during desire for stool	Ant-c.
Chill	external chill during stupor (dazed state)	Hep.
Chill	external chill in afternoon	Chel., puls.
Chill	external chill in afternoon during sweat	Gels.
Chill	external chill in evening	Am-c., calc., dulc., gamb., nux-m., ran-b., rhus-t.
Chill	external chill in evening in bed	Nat-m.
Chill	external chill in evening lasting until 4.00 a.m.	Gamb.
Chill	external chill in morning	Acon., aeth.
Chill	external chill in spots	*Ambr., ars., bell., bry., **Caust.**, cham., hep., **Ign.**, led., lyc., merc., **Mez.**, mosch., nux-v., par., petr., **Puls.**, rhus-t., **Sep.**, sil., spig., thuj.*

Body part/Disease	Symptom	Medicines
Chill	external chill on uncovering	Arg-m.
Chill	external coldness in back after eating	Coc-c., lyc.
Chill	faintness during chill	Ars., asar., **Sep.**
Chill	feels better before chill	Psor.
Chill	fever alternating with chill during menses	Am-c., thuj.
Chill	fever alternating with chill after eating	Oct
Chill	fever alternating with chill at night	**Acon.**, ang., bar-c., hura., ip., mag-s., merc., phos., sabad., sep., sulph.
Chill	fever alternating with chill at night with perspiration	Ip.
Chill	fever alternating with chill in afternoon	Calc., chin-s., chin., kali-n., lob., myric., rhus-t., sep., sulph.
Chill	fever alternating with chill in evening	All-c., all-s., alum., am-c., ant-s., bar-c., cocc., kali-c., kali-n., lyc., merc., ph-ac.
Chill	fever alternating with chill in evening in bed	Am-c.
Chill	fever alternating with chill in forenoon	Chin., colch., elaps., thuj.
Chill	fever alternating with chill in open air	Chin.
Chill	fever alternating with chill on motion	Ant-t.
Chill	fever alternating with chill then heat	Verat.
Chill	fever alternating with chill then heat then finally sweat	Bry., kali-c., spig.
Chill	fever alternating with chill then sweat then cold sweat	Caps., verat.
Chill	fever alternating with chill with fright	Lyc.
Chill	fever alternating with chill, followed by sweat	Kali-c., meny., verat.
Chill	fever alternating with chilliness, dry burning heat	Bell., sang.
Chill	fever at night with chilli during day and heat at night	Dros.
Chill	fever at night with chilliness	Acon., agar., apis., ars., bapt., carb-s., carb-v., caust., cham., coca., coff., colch., cur., elaps., graph., kali-bi., rhus-t., sil., **Sulph.**, thuj., tub.
Chill	fever followed chill then cold sweat	Ars., verat.
Chill	fever followed chill then cold sweat then heat	**Bell.**
Chill	fever followed chill then cold sweat then sweat then heat	Bell.
Chill	fever followed chill then cold sweat then sweat without heat or thirst	Am-m., bry., caust., staph.
Chill	fever followed heat then chill then heat	Am-m., stram.
Chill	fever followed heat then chill then sweat	Rhus-t.
Chill	fever in afternoon alternating with chill	**Calc.**, kali-n.
Chill	fever in afternoon followed by chilliness	Kali-n.
Chill	fever in afternoon with chilliness	Anac., **Apis.**, ars., caust., coff., colch., cur., hyos., kali-c., podo., rhus-t., sil., sulph.
Chill	fever in evening after chill	Acon., apis., ars., berb., graph., guai., petr., sulph.

Body part/Disease	Symptom	Medicines
Chill	fever in evening lasting all night followed by shuddering	Cocc.
Chill	fever in evening with chilliness	Acon., anac., apis., arn., ars., bapt., bor., carb-v., caust., cham., coff., elaps., ferr-i., hep., kali-c., kali-i., nat-m., sabin., sil., sulph., thuj.
Chill	fever in forenoon alternating with chill	Calc., cham., thuj.
Chill	fever in forenoon with chilliness	Ars., bapt., **Cham.**, kali-c., sil., sulph., thuj.
Chill	fever in morning in bed at 5.00 a.m. followed by shaking chill	Apis.
Chill	fever in morning on waking	Acon-c., aeth., camph., chel., eup-per., lac-c., petr., sep., sulph.
Chill	fever in morning with chilliness	**Apis.**, arn., **Ars.**, caust., cham., coff., kali-bi., kali-c., kali-i., sulph., thuj.
Chill	fever with burning heat alternating with chill	Laur.
Chill	fever with burning heat alternating with chilliness	**Bell.**
Chill	fever with burning heat in afternoon with transient (short in duration) chill	Cur.
Chill	fever with chill	**Acon.**, ambr., anac., ant-c., ars-i., **Ars.**, asar., **Bell.**, benz-ac., bry., bufo., **Calc.**, caps., carb-v., **Cham.**, chel., chin-s., chin., cocc., coff., coloc., dig., dros., ferr-ar., ferr., graph., **Hell.**, **Ign.**, iod., ip., kali-ar., kreos., led., lyc., merc., mez., nat-c., nat-m., nat-s., nicc., **Nit-ac.**, **Nux-v.**, olnd., petr., phos., plb., podo., puls., pyrog., ran-b., **Rhus-t.**, sabad., sabin., samb., sang., sep., sil., spig., staph., stram., **Sulph.**, tarent., thuj., verat., zinc.
Chill	fever with chill with and shaking	Sec.
Chill	fever with chill without subsequent perspiration	Graph.
Chill	fever with chilliness	Acon., agar., anac., **Apis.**, arn., ars., bapt., bar-m., bell., bor., **Calc.**, carb-v., caust., cham., **Coff.**, colch., cur., dros., elaps., hep., kali-ar., **Kali-bi.**, kali-c., kali-i., kali-s., lach., lachn., led., merc., nat-m., phos., podo., **Puls.**, pyrog., sabin., sec., sep., sil., spig., squil., sulph., tarent., **Thuj.**, tub., **Verat.**, zinc.
Chill	fever with chilliness alternating with heat not perceptible to the touch	Merc.
Chill	fever with chilliness and pain from uncovering	Squil.
Chill	fever with chilliness from putting the hands out of bed	Arn., bar-c., bor., hep., **Nux-v.**, pyrog., stram., tarent., **Tub.**
Chill	fever with chilliness from uncovering	Acon., agar., apis., **Arn.**, bar-c., bell., calc., carb-an., cham., chin-s., **Chin.**, **Nux-v.**, psor., pyrog., **Rhus-t.**, sarr., sep., squil., tarent., **Tub.**
Chill	fever with chilliness from uncovering in any stage of symptoms	Arn., ars., aur., carb-an., chin., gels., graph., hell., hep., **Nux-v.**, pyrog., **Rhus-t.**, **Samb.**, squil., stram., tarent.
Chill	fever with constant shuddering with one cheek hot and red	Coff.
Chill	fever with dry heat in afternoon with chilliness	Arg-n.

Body part/Disease	Symptom	Medicines
Chill	fever with dry heat in evening between 7.00 to 9.00 p.m. followed by chill until 10 p.m.	Elaps.
Chill	fever with dry heat in evening in bed with chilliness in back	Coff.
Chill	fever with external heat in afternoon with chillliness	Ars.
Chill	fever with external heat with chilliness	Acon., agn., alum., anac., arn., **Ars.**, asar., atro., bell., berb., bry., calc-ar., **Calc.**, cann-i., cocc., coff., coloc., dig., dros., gamb., hell., hep., **Ign.**, kali-n., lac-c., lach., laur., lyc., meny., merc., mur-ac., nat-m., **Nux-v.**, par., phos., plb., **Pyrog.**, ran-b., raph., rat., rheum., **Sep.**, sil., squil., sulph., tab., **Thuj.**, verat.
Chill	fever with internal heat at night must uncover, which causes chilliness	**Mag-c.**
Chill	fever with internal heat with external chill	**Acon.**, arn., ars-i., **Ars.**, bell., bry., calc., **Camph.**, caps., cham., chel., ferr-ar., ferr-i., ferr., ign., iod., ip., kali-ar., kali-c., mez., **Mosch.**, nit-ac., ph-ac., phos., puls., rhus-t., sabad., sang., sec., sil., squil., sul-ac., sulph., **Verat.**, zinc.
Chill	fever with internal heat with external chill with coldness of single parts	Chin., ign., nux-v., rhus-t.
Chill	fever with long lasting heat followed by chill	Apis.
Chill	fever with shivering	Acon., anac., ant-t., apis., **Arn.**, bell., bov., bry., calc., carb-s., carb-v., **Caust.**, cham., chin-s., chin., cina., cocc., coff., cur., cycl., dros., elaps., eup-per., **Gels.**, graph., **Hell.**, hep., ign., lach., mag-m., mag-p., meny., merc., **Nux-v.**, petr., ph-ac., podo., psor., puls., rhus-t., sabad., sep., **Sulph.**, tarent., verat., zinc.
Chill	fever with shivering alternating with heat	Acon., ars., bell., bov., bry., calc., caust., chin., cocc., cycl., dros., elaps., hep., ip., kali-bi., lach., lob., merc., mosch., nux-v., ph-ac., plat., sabad.
Chill	fever with shivering and perspiration with heat	**Nux-v.**, podo., rhus-t., sulph.
Chill	fever with shivering from drinking	Bell., **Caps.**, eup-per., **Nux-v.**
Chill	fever with shivering from motion	Apis., arn., **Nux-v.**, podo., stram.
Chill	fever with shivering from uncovering	Apis., **Arn.**, bar-c., calc., chin-s., chin., lach., **Nux-v.**, psor., rhus-t., stram., tarent., **Tub.**
Chill	fever with shuddering (shiver violently) alternating with heat	Bov.
Chill	fever with shuddering (shiver violently) with the heat	Acon., bell., caps., **Cham.**, hell., ign., kali-i., nat-m., nux-v., rheum., rhus-t., zinc.
Chill	fever without chill	Acet-ac., acon., aesc., alum., ambr., anac., ang., ant-c., **Apis.**, arn., **Ars.**, bapt., **Bell.**, benz-ac., bov., **Bry.**, cact., calc., carb-s., carb-v., caust., **Cham.**, chin-a., chin., cina., clem., coff., con., cur., elaps., eup-per., ferr-ar., ferr-p., ferr., **Gels.**, graph., hep., ip., kali-ar., kali-bi., kali-c., lach., lyc., lyss., mang., merl., nat-m., nicc., nux-m., nux-v., petr., podo., puls., **Rhus-t.**, spig., stann., stram., sulph., thuj.
Chill	fever without chill after midnight	**Ars.**, bor., ferr., kali-c., lyc., nat-m., sulph., tax., thuj.
Chill	fever without chill at 5.30 p.m. with pricking in tongue	Cedr.

Body part/Disease	Symptom	Medicines
Chill	fever without chill at midnight	**Ars.**, nux-v., stram., sulph.
Chill	fever without chill at night	Acon., ang., ant-t., apis., **Ars., Bapt., Bell., Bry.,** calc., carb-v., caust., cham., cina., coff., ferr-ar., ferr., gels., hep., ip., kali-bi., lachn., lyc., nat-m., nicc., nux-v., petr., phos., podo., puls., **Rhus-t.,** stram., sulph., thuj.
Chill	fever without chill before midnight	Acon., ant-c., ars., **Bry.,** carb-v., cham., elaps., lyc., mag-m., mag-s., nat-m., petr., puls., sabad.
Chill	fever without chill in afternoon	Aesc., anac., ang., apis., **Ars., Bell.,** bry., calc., caust., chin-a., chin., clem., coff., con., cur., eup-per., ferr-ar., ferr., gels., graph., ip., kali-ar., kali-bi., kali-c., lyc., nat-m., nux-v., puls., rhus-t., sang., sil., sulph.
Chill	fever without chill in afternoon lasting all night	Ars., hep., puls., stann.
Chill	fever without chill in evening	Acon., aesc., alum., ambr., anac., ang., ant-t., apis., arn., ars., bapt., **Bell.,** bor., **Bry.,** calc., carb-v., caust., cham., chin-a., chin., cina., coff., coloc., eup-per., ferr-ar., ferr-p., ferr., hep., ip., kali-ar., kali-bi., kali-c., lach., lyc., nat-m., nicc., nux-m., nux-v., petr., plat., podo., **Puls., Rhus-t.,** stann., sulph., thuj.
Chill	fever without chill in evening at same hour, daily fever, with short breath	Cina.
Chill	fever without chill in evening lasting all night	Cham., lyc., nux-v., rhus-t.
Chill	fever without chill in forenoon	Ars., bapt., cact., calc., cham., Gels., lyc., nat-m., nux-m., nux-v., rhus-t., spig., sulph., thuj.
Chill	fever without chill in morning	Arn., ars., bry., calc., caust., eup-per., hep., kali-bi., kali-c., nat-m., petr., podo., rhus-t., sulph., thuj.
Chill	fever without chill in noon	Ars., spig., stram., sulph.
Chill	fever without chill with very ill humored	Con.
Chill	flushes of heat alternating with chill	Acon., ars., asar., calc., chin-s., corn., iod., kali-bi., med., sep., spig.
Chill	flushes of heat followd by chill	**Caust.,** sang.
Chill	flushes of heat with chilliness	Agar., apis., ars., carb-v., colch., corn., eup-per., kali-bi., lach., lob., merc., plat., puls., sep., sulph., ter., thuj.
Chill	foot hot during chill	Cann-s., rat., spong.
Chill	formication at night during chill	Gamb.
Chill	formication during chill	Gamb.
Chill	formication in foot during chill	Canth.
Chill	formication in hand during chill	Canth.
Chill	frequent attacks of chilliness after intermediate sleep	**Nux-m.**
Chill	frequent chill from 1.00 to 7.00 a.m.	Sil.
Chill	frequent urination, during chill	Ars., canth., hyper., lec., meph., Merc., petros., ph-ac., phos., sulph.
Chill	goose flesh with sudden chill with hair standing on end	Bar-c., dulc.
Chill	grinding of teeth during chill	Ant-c., apis., ars., calc., cham., lyc., phos., stram.
Chill	hand hot in evening during shivering	Sulph.

Body part/Disease	Symptom	Medicines
Chill	hand hot during chill	Apis., chin., cina., nat-c., nux-v., ph-ac., phos., puls., spong.
Chill	hand hot in evening during chilliness	Asaf.
Chill	hands hot during shivering	Ign.
Chill	head heat after chilliness	Sang., Sil.
Chill	headache with chilliness	Sil.
Chill	heat during chilliness over back	Gins.
Chill	heat in back alternating with cold with shivering	Cham.
Chill	heaviness in extremities before chill	Ther.
Chill	heaviness in extremities during chill	Coc-c.
Chill	heaviness in foot during chilliness	Hell.
Chill	heaviness in leg before chill	Cimx.
Chill	hot breath during chill	Anac., camph., cham., Rhus-t.
Chill	intermission of chill during menses	Eupi.
Chill	internal chill in afternoon	Ars., cocc., guai., phos., psor.
Chill	internal chill in afternoon following heat	Guai.
Chill	internal chill in afternoon without subsequent heat	Ang.
Chill	internal chill in evening	Atro., caust., cocc., eupi., gamb., guai., lyc., nit-ac., par., petr., phos., plb., psor.
Chill	internal chill in evening on falling sleep	Phos.
Chill	internal chill in evening worse lying down	Hell.
Chill	internal chill in noon	Kali-c., psor.
Chill	internal chill aggravated by external heat	Ip.
Chill	internal chill as if coldness in blood vessels	Acon., ant-c., ant-t., Ars., lyc., Rhus-t., Verat.
Chill	internal chill as if coldness in bones	Berb., elaps., merc., verat.
Chill	internal chill at midnight	Caust.
Chill	internal chill at night	Ambr., dros., nux-v., petr., sil.
Chill	internal chill at night in open air	Anac.
Chill	internal chill during first sleep	Dig.
Chill	internal chill in a warm room	Anac., cist., kreos., puls.
Chill	internal chill in forenoon	Merc., sulph.
Chill	internal chill in morning	Arg-n., con., lyc., merc., sulph.
Chill	internal chill in morning during breakfast	Ther.
Chill	internal chill in morning in bed	Lyc., merc.
Chill	internal chill on waking	Arn.
Chill	internal chill with trembling & shivering	Par.
Chill	internal chill with trembling & shivering in evening	Par.
Chill	internal chill with trembling & shivering in forenoon	Lyc., par.
Chill	involuntary urination before chill	Gels.
Chill	involuntary urination during chill	Caust., dulc., puls., rhus-t., sulph.
Chill	itching in thigh from becoming chilly	Dios.

Body part/Disease	Symptom	Medicines
Chill	lachrymation during chill	Elat.
Chill	lameness in lower limbs during chill	Ign., lyc., rhus-t., tub.
Chill	lower limbs hot after chilliness	Nit-ac.
Chill	menses suppressed from chill	Bell., dulc., nux-m., puls., sep., sulph.
Chill	motion brings on chilliness during fever	Ant-t., apis., arn., chin-s., merc., **Nux-v.**, podo., **Rhus-t.**, stram.
Chill	nausea during chill	Arg-n., ars., bell., bov., bry., calc., cham., chel., cina., cob., cocc., con., Eup-per., hyper., ign., ip., kali-ar., kali-c., kali-s., kreos., lach., lyc., nat-m., nit-ac., petr., puls., raph., rhus-t., rumx., sabad., sang., sec., sep., sul-ac., verat., zinc.
Chill	nausea with chilliness	Alum., bov., con., kreos.
Chill	numbness during chill	Rhus-t.
Chill	numbness in fingers during chill	Cedr., cimx., ferr., **Sep.**, stann., thuj.
Chill	numbness in foot with chill	Cedr., cimx., ferr., lyc., nux-m., **Puls.**, sep., stann., stram.
Chill	numbness in left hand during chill	Apis., cimx., ferr., guare., lyc., nux-m., nux-v., ph-ac., **Puls.**, sec., **Sep.**, stann.
Chill	numbness in leg during chill	Eup-pur., nux-v.
Chill	numbness in lower limb during chill	Con.
Chill	pain between scapula during chill	Sang.
Chill	pain in arm after chill	Ars-h.
Chill	pain in back before chill	Aesc., aran., ars., bry., carb-v., daph., dios., eup-per., eup-pur., ip., Podo., rhus-t.
Chill	pain in back during chill	Ant-t., apis., arn., ars., bell., Bol., calc., caps., carb-s., carb-v., caust., cham., chin-a., Chin-s., chin., elat., eup-per., gamb., hyos., ign., ip., lach., lact-ac., lyc., mosch., myric., nat-m., Nux-v., phos., podo., puls., sang., sep., sulph., verat., zinc.
Chill	pain in back during chill extending to occiput and vertex (Top of head)	Puls.
Chill	pain in back extending to occiput (back of head) vertex (top of head) during chill	Puls.
Chill	pain in calf during chill	Ars., thuj.
Chill	pain in cervical region during chill	Ail., ars-h.
Chill	pain in chest before chill	Ars., plan.
Chill	pain in chest during chill (a moderate but often unpleasant degree of coldness	Ars., bell., Bry., chin-s., Kali-c., lach., puls., rhus-t., sabad., seneg.
Chill	pain in chest during chilliness	Eupi., sep.
Chill	pain in dorsal region during chill	Chin-s., sang.
Chill	pain in ear during chill	Acon., apis., calc., gamb., graph., nux-v., puls., sulph.
Chill	pain in elbow during chill	Ang., **Podo.**
Chill	pain in extremities alternating with chill and heat	Brom.

Body part/Disease	Symptom	Medicines
Chill	pain in extremities during chill	Ang., aran., arn., **Ars.**, asaf., aur., bar-c., **Bov.**, bry., calc-s., calc., caps., carb-s., caust., chin-s., cimx., cina., cocc., **Coloc.**, cycl., **Dulc.**, **Eup-per.**, eup-pur., eupho., ferr., form., gels., graph., hell., hep., ign., **Ip.**, kali-ar., kali-c., **Kali-n.**, kali-s., lach., led., **Lyc.**, **Mez.**, mur-ac., nat-a., nat-c., nat-m., **Nux-v.**, op., petr., ph-ac., plb., psor., **Puls.**, **Pyrog.**, ran-b., **Rhus-t.**, sabad., **Sep.**, sil., squil., stram., sulph., **Tub.**, xan.
Chill	pain in fingers during chill	Nux-v.
Chill	pain in foot during chill	Cupr.
Chill	pain in hand during chill	Nux-v.
Chill	pain in heart during chill	Calc.
Chill	pain in hip during chill	Arn., calc., lyc., nux-v., rhus-t., sep.
Chill	pain in joints during chill	**Cimx.**, ferr., hell.
Chill	pain in kidneys during chill	Ars., canth., kali-c., lyc., nux-v., puls., zinc.
Chill	pain in knee during chill	Agar., ars-h., chin., cimx., cocc., nat-m., nat-s., nux-v., podo., puls., rhus-t., sep., sulph.
Chill	pain in leg before chill	Eup-per., eup-pur., puls.
Chill	pain in leg during chill	Ars., cimx., lyc., nat-m., puls., **Pyrog.**, sep., spong., tub.
Chill	pain in lower limb before chill	Nux-v.
Chill	pain in lower limb during chill	Arn., **Ars.**, bry., caps., **Chin.**, ferr., led., lyc., mez., nat-m., **Nux-v.**, phos., puls., **Pyrog.**, rhus-t., sep., sulph., thuj.
Chill	pain in lumbar region before chill	Aesc., eup-pur., Podo.
Chill	pain in lumbar region during chill	Ars., calc., nux-v., ph-ac., phos., puls., rhus-t., sep., sil.
Chill	pain in sacral region during chill	Ars., gamb., hyos., Nux-v., psor., verat.
Chill	pain in teeth during chill	Agar., carb-v., graph., hell., kali-c., Rhus-t., sep., staph.
Chill	pain in teeth with chilliness	Daph., eupho., hell., lach., puls., rhod., rhus-t.
Chill	pain in thigh during chill	Ars., **Bor.**, chin., cimx., dulc., nat-m., puls., **Pyrog.**
Chill	pain in upper limb before chill	Eup-per., phel.
Chill	pain in upper limb during chill	Bry., chin., lyc., nux-v., ph-ac., phos., puls., rhus-t.
Chill	pain of face during chill	Acon., caust., chin., lach., mez., nux-v., rhus-t., spig.
Chill	pain under left scapula (bone forming back of shoulder) during chill	Chin., rhus-t., Sep.
Chill	palpitation of heart before chill	Chin.
Chill	palpitation of heart during chill	Gels., lil-t., merc., ph-ac., phos., sep., sulph.
Chill	palpitation of heart from becoming chilled	Acon.
Chill	periodicity of chill regular & distinct	Aesc., ang., apis., **Aran.**, bov., **Cact.**, caps., **Cedr.**, **Chin-s.**, cina., ferr., gels., hell., lyc., nat-s., podo., pyrog., sabad., spig., stann., staph., tarent., thuj.
Chill	perspiration brings on chilliness	Eup-per., eup-pur., hep., **Nux-v.**, psor., tub.
Chill	perspiration in chest during chilliness	Sep.
Chill	perspiration in foot during chill	Cann-s.

Body part/Disease	Symptom	Medicines
Chill	perspiration in hand during chill	Eup-per., ip., puls.
Chill	perspiration on back during chill	Cann-s.
Chill	perspiration with scanty sweat after a severe chill	Eup-per.
Chill	predominating (be in majority) chill at night	Apis., gamb., merc., phos.
Chill	predominating chill at night long lasting chill with little heat, and no thirst	Lyc., puls.
Chill	predominating chill at night long lasting chill without heat, sweat or thirst	**Aran.**, bov.
Chill	predominating chill in afternoon	Apis., arn., **Ars.**, **Lyc.**, plb., **Puls.**, rhus-t., thuj.
Chill	predominating chill in evening	Alum., arn., cina., cycl., hep., kali-s., mur-ac., ph-ac., phos., **Puls.**, **Rhus-t.**, sulph.
Chill	predominating chill in morning	Bry., **Eup-per.**, hep., **Nat-m.**, **Nux-v.**, podo., sep., **Verat.**
Chill	predominating chill in noon	Ant-c., elat., **Sulph.**
Chill	predominating chill without heat or thirst	Mur-ac., sep., staph., sulph.
Chill	predominating paroxysm consists only of chill	*Aran., bov., camph., canth., hep., led., lyc., mez., mur-ac., ran-b., sabad.*
Chill	pulsation in head during chill	Cann-i., eup-per.
Chill	pulsation in lumbar region during chill	Nux-v.
Chill	Pulsation with chilliness	Sil.
Chill	quartan (recurring every fourth day) of chill	Acon., anac., ant-c., apis., arn., **Ars-i.**, **Ars.**, bapt., bell., brom., bry., bufo., carb-v., chin-a., chin-s., chin., **Cimx.**, cina., clem., coff., cor-r., elat., **Hyos.**, ign., **Iod.**, ip., kali-ar., lach., **Lyc.**, meny., mill., nat-m., nux-m., nux-v., plan., podo., **Puls.**, rhus-t., **Sabad.**, sep., sulph., thuj., **Verat.**
Chill	quotidian (recurring daily) chill	Acon., aesc., agar., alum., anac., ang., ant-c., ant-t., apis., **Aran.**, arn., **Ars.**, arund., asaf., bapt., bar-c., bell., bol., bry., **Cact.**, calc., camph., caps., carb-v., cedr., cham., chel., chin-a., chin-s., chin., cic., cina., con., cur., cycl., dros., elaps., elat., eup-per., eup-pur., ferr-ar., ferr., gamb., gels., graph., hep., ign., **Ip.**, kali-ar., kali-bi., kali-c., kali-s., lach., led., lob., lyc., mag-c., meny., **Nat-m.**, nat-s., nit-ac., **Nux-v.**, op., petr., phos., plan., podo., **Puls.**, pyrog., rhus-t., sabad., samb., sarr., sep., spig., stann., staph., stram., sulph., tarent., thuj., verat.
Chill	restless sleep after chill	Spong.
Chill	restless sleep before chill	Anthr., arn., chin.
Chill	semi annual chill	Lach., sep.
Chill	Sensation of death during chill	Cann-i.
Chill	sensation of paralysis of leg during chill	Ars., ign., stram.
Chill	shaking chill from a draft of air	Acon., bar-c., bry., caps., **Chin.**, mosch., phys., verat.
Chill	shaking chill after stool	Carb-an., plat.
Chill	shaking chill after vomiting	Thuj., zinc.
Chill	shaking chill at 11.00 a.m. until 4.00 p.m.	Sep.

Body part/Disease	Symptom	Medicines
Chill	shaking chill at night	Acon., calc., dros., gamb., kali-c., kali-i., merc., nat-m., nat-s., petr., phos., rhus-t., sars., sulph.
Chill	shaking chill at night before going to bed	Cocc., laur., nat-m., samb.
Chill	shaking chill at night in open air	**Ars.**, calc-p., calc., caust., cham., chel., chin., coff., lach., mag-m., nux-v., plat., rhus-t., tab.
Chill	shaking chill at night on lying down	Acon.
Chill	shaking chill before stool	Carb-an., caust., chin-s., mag-m., merc., mez.
Chill	shaking chill during & after swallowing	Merc-c.
Chill	shaking chill during motion	Alum., ant-t., caps., cedr., eup-per., sang., sil., sulph., thuj.
Chill	shaking chill during pain	Ars.
Chill	shaking chill during stool	Bell., mag-m., nit-ac., stann.
Chill	shaking chill from fright	Merc.
Chill	shaking chill in afternoon	Ang., **Ars.**, canth., cast., cham., chel., chin-s., chin., cocc., coff., con., croc., **Ferr.**, ip., petr., ph-ac., **Phos.**, psor., rhus-t., sabad., staph., sulph.
Chill	shaking chill in afternoon lasting until next morning	Kali-i.
Chill	shaking chill in afternoon on slightest contact with open air	Nux-v.
Chill	shaking chill in evening after undressing	Spong.
Chill	shaking chill in evening ameliorated in bed	Mag-m., mag-s.
Chill	shaking chill in evening in bed	Am-c., chel., chin., mag-c., merc., mez., nat-m., rhus-t., sabad., sil., tab., thuj.
Chill	shaking chill in evening in open air	Mang.
Chill	shaking chill in evening in the house	Mang.
Chill	shaking chill in evening on going to sleep	Am-c., phos., staph.
Chill	shaking chill in evening while undressing	Agar., mag-c.
Chill	shaking chill in evening while walking in open air	**Ars., chin.**
Chill	shaking chill in evening without subsequent heat	Led.
Chill	shaking chill in morning	Ant-c., ars., caps., carb-v., chin., cocc., coff., cor-r., hell., mang., merc., nat-a., nat-c., nat-m., nux-m., podo., rat., sarr., spong., verat.
Chill	shaking chill in morning in bed	Chin., coff., mag-s., nat-s.
Chill	shaking chill in morning on rising	Acon., kreos., mag-s., nux-v.
Chill	shaking chill in morning while walking	Sep.
Chill	shaking chill in morning without subsequent heat	Cocc.
Chill	shaking chill in noon	Ant-c., sep.
Chill	shaking chill in noon after dinner	Mag-m.
Chill	shaking chill in noon during dinner	Grat.
Chill	shaking chill in the open air not ameliorated by covering	Rhus-t.
Chill	shaking chill long lasting not relieved by any thing	**Aran.**, nux-v.
Chill	shaking chill long lasting with little heat and no thirst	Puls.

Body part/Disease	Symptom	Medicines
Chill	shaking chill long lasting without heat or sweat	**Aran.**, bov., canth., lyc.
Chill	shaking chill long lasting without subsequent heat	**Aran.**, bov., camph., hep., led., lyc., mez., verat.
Chill	shaking chill maniacal (so uncontrolled as to appear to be affected by mania) delirium (a state marked by extreme restlessness, confusion, and sometimes hallucinations, caused by fever, poisoning, or brain injury)	Cimx., tarent.
Chill	shaking chill on drinking	Alum., arn., ars., calc-s., calc., cann-s., **Caps.**, chel., chin., elaps., lyc., **Nux-v.**
Chill	shaking chill on entering the house from open air	Aeth., arg-n., caust., chin.
Chill	shaking chill on going into warm room	Colch., rhus-t.
Chill	shaking chill on inspiring	**Brom.**
Chill	shaking chill on putting hand out of bed	**Hep.**, phos., **Rhus-t.**
Chill	shaking chill on yawning	Arn., cina.
Chill	shaking chill while eating	Caps., graph., lyc., mag-m.
Chill	shaking chill while walking in open air	Chel.
Chill	shaking chill whole day with drawing pains in throat and back	Verat.
Chill	shaking chill with deep sleep & snoring (to breathe noisily while asleep because of vibrations of the soft palate)	Op.
Chill	shaking chill with flying heat	Bov.
Chill	shaking chill with heat	**Arn.**, ars., bell., bry., cann-i., cham., chel., chin., cocc., hell., hep., hyos., ign., lach., merc., mosch., puls., rhus-t., sep., tab.
Chill	shaking chill with heat of face	Thuj.
Chill	shaking chill with heat of head	**Arn.**, **Bell.**, bry., cact., mang.
Chill	shaking chill with perspiration	Alum., cedr., cupr., eup-per., **Nux-v.**, rhus-r., rhus-t., verat.
Chill	shaking chill with pulsating pain in occiput	Bor.
Chill	shaking chill with skin cold and blue	Camph., carb-v., chin., nux-m., nux-v., rhus-t., sec.
Chill	shaking chill without subsequent heat	**Aran.**, bov., camph., canth., cocc., graph., hep., kali-c., kali-n., led., lyc., mez., mur-ac., **Staph.**, sulph., verat.
Chill	shaking chill without subsequent heat or sweat	**Aran.**, bov., canth., cast.
Chill	shaking chill without subsequent heat or thirst	**Sep.**, staph., sulph.
Chill	shaking chill without subsequent heat	Kali-n., nat-c.
Chill	shaking chill, wants to be held so he may not shake so hard	Gels., lach.
Chill	shivering at night	Carb-v.
Chill	shivering at night in bed	Raph.
Chill	shivering during stool	Coloc., trom.
Chill	shivering extending down the back	Agar., all-c., bry., calc-caust., chel., colch., mag-c., rhus-v.
Chill	shivering extending up the back	Canth., dig., puls., rhus-v.

Body part/Disease	Symptom	Medicines
Chill	shivering in afternoon	Mag-c.
Chill	shivering in evening	Apis., bry., canth., caps., cham., cocc., mag-m., mag-s., verat.
Chill	shivering in evening in bed	Sang.
Chill	shivering in forenoon	Graph., mag-c.
Chill	shivering in lumbar region	Coff-t., jatr., lyc., petr.
Chill	shivering in lumbar region after stool	Puls.
Chill	shivering in lumbar region in warm room	Petr.
Chill	shivering in morning	Apis., cham., meny., staph.
Chill	shivering in morning after rising	Staph.
Chill	shivering in morning in bed	Kali-c.
Chill	shivering in warm room	Petr.
Chill	shivering near warm stove	Nicc.
Chill	shivering of legs	Graph., kali-c., meny.
Chill	shivering on lying down	Nat-c.
Chill	shivering with perspiration	Aml-n., ant-t., arg-n., cedr., coff., eup-per., hell., led., lyc., merc., **Nux-v.**, puls., pyrog., raph., rhus-t., sep., sulph., tab., verat.
Chill	short attacks of chilliness	Ferr.
Chill	skin, burning during chill	Hep., petr.
Chill	sleepiness after chilliness	Nux-v.
Chill	sleepiness before chill	Ars., nicc., puls., sabad., ther.
Chill	sleepiness between chill	Nux-m.
Chill	sleepiness during chill	Aeth., ambr., ant-c., ant-t., cimx., hell., iris., kali-bi., kali-i., mez., nat-m., nux-m., nux-v., **Op.**, phos., tarax.
Chill	sleepiness in noon during chilliness	Ferr-i.
Chill	sleeplessness with anxiety and heat, must cover which causes chilliness	Mag-c.
Chill	sleeplessness with chill	Bry., lyc., mur-ac.
Chill	sore bruised pain during chill	Tarent.
Chill	stiffness before chill	Chin-s., psor., rhus-t.
Chill	stiffness during chill	Chin-s., eup-per., nat-s., op., rhus-t.
Chill	stiffness in back during chill	Lyc., nat-s., tub.
Chill	stiffness in fingers during chill	Eup-per., ferr., rhus-t.
Chill	stiffness in hand during chilliness	Kali-chl.
Chill	stiffness in joints during chill	Bry., calc., **Caust.**, led., lyc., nux-v., op., petr., rhus-t., sep., sulph., thuj.
Chill	stiffness in lower limbs before chill	Petr., phos., psor., rhus-t.
Chill	stiffness in lower limbs during chill	Nat-s., tub.
Chill	stiffness in right upper limbs during chill	Eup-per.
Chill	stretching before chill	Aesc., ant-t., arn., ars., bry., eup-per., ign., ip., nat-m., nux-v., plan., rhus-t.

Body part/Disease	Symptom	Medicines
Chill	stretching during chill	Alum., ars., bry., caps., coff., daph., elat., eup-per., ip., kreos., laur., mur-ac., nat-s., nit-ac., nux-v., petr., rhus-t., ruta., tab., teucr.
Chill	stretching in evening during chill	Tab.
Chill	sudden weakness during chilliness	Sep.
Chill	sweat & chilliness as soon as he gets warm in bed	Arg-n.
Chill	sweating during chill	Acon., bry., calc., chin., cina., dig., led., nat-s.
Chill	trembling during chill	Anac., ang., ars., bry., chin-s., chin., cina., **Cocc.**, con., eup-per., ferr., gels., merc., par., petr., plat., sabad., sul-ac., zinc.
Chill	trembling in foot during chill	Canth.
Chill	trembling in hand during chill	Canth., chin.
Chill	twitching after chill	Puls.
Chill	twitching during chill	Acon., dig., jatr., lyc., nux-m., nux-v., op., ox-ac., stram., tab.
Chill	twitching in forearm during chill	Nux-m.
Chill	twitching in hand during chill	Nux-m., nux-v.
Chill	twitching in thigh during chilliness	Sep.
Chill	urine copious with amenorrhoea with chill	Lec.
Chill	urticaria after chill	Elat., hep.
Chill	urticaria before chill	Hep.
Chill	urticaria during chill	Apis., ars., ign., **Nat-m.**, **Rhus-t.**
Chill	violent chill with bluish, cold face and hands, mottled skin	**Nux-v.**, rhus-t.
Chill	violent chill with delirium	Arn., ars., bell., bry., cham., **Chin.**, **Nat-m.**, nux-v., puls., sep., stram., sulph., verat.
Chill	violent chill with red face and thirst	**Ferr.**, ign.
Chill	violent chill with unconsciousness (unable to see, hear, or otherwise sense what is going on, usually temporarily and often as a result of an accident or injury)	Ars., bell., camph., hep., lach., **Nat-m.**, nux-v., op., puls., stram., valer.
Chill	violent chill without subsequent heat	**Aran.**, bov., camph., hep., led., mez.
Chill	vomiting after chill	Phos.
Chill	vomiting during chill	Ail., ign., phos.
Chill	warm drinks are tolerated during chill	Ars., casc., cedr., eup-per., lyc., nux-v., rhus-t., sulph.
Chill	weakness before chill	Ars., chin., nat-m., thuj.
Chill	weakness during chill	Ant-t., Arn., ars., cann-i., chin., coc-c., ip., lach., nat-m., phos., psor., sep., thuj., verat.
Chill	weakness extending through back during chill	Thuj.
Chill	weakness in calf during chill	Thuj.
Chill	weakness in foot during chillinss	Hell.
Chill	weakness in hand during chill	Laur.
Chill	weakness in joints during chill	Raph.
Chill	weakness in thigh during chill	Verat.

Body part/Disease	Symptom	Medicines
Chill	weakness in upper limbs during chilliness	Gins., ph-ac.
Chill	yawning before chill	Aesc., ant-t., arn., ars., chin., elat., eup-per., ign., ip., nat-m., nicc., nux-v., rhus-t.
Chill	yawning before chill and mouth remains open for a long time	Ant-t.
Chill	yawning during chill	Ars-h., ars., bol., bry., calad., caps., caust., cimx., cina., cob., croc., **Elat., Eup-per.,** gamb., laur., lyc., mag-m., meny., merc., mez., mur-ac., murx., **Nat-m.,** nat-s., olnd., par., phos., ruta., sep., sil., thuj.
Chill	yawning with chilliness	Olnd., par., sep.
Chin	blotches on chin	Bry., carb-an., eupho., hep., mag-m., olnd.
Chin	boils under chin	Carb-v.
Chin	carbuncles on chin	Lyc.
Chin	comedones on chin and upper lip	Sulph.
Chin	comedones on chin	Dros., tub.
Chin	discolouration of chin	Plat.
Chin	eczema of chin	Bor., cic., graph., merc-i-r., phos., rhus-t., sep.
Chin	formication on chin	Stram.
Chin	itching of chin	Alum., am-c., benz-ac., berb., carb-an., chlor., con., Dulc., gamb., kali-c., lyc., nat-c., nat-m., nux-v., par., phos., sars., sep., stront., Sulph., ther.,thuj., trom., zinc.
Chin	leprous spots on chin	Calc.
Chin	nodosities on chin	Eupho.
Chin	pain in nose extending to chin	Chin.
Chin	rash on chin	Am-c.
Chin	rosacea on chin	Hydr., verat., viol-t.
Chin	swelling in chin	Carb-v., caust.
Chin	tingling in chin and nose	Ran-b., verat.
Chin	ulcer in chin	Cund., hep., merc., nat-m., nit-ac., sep.
Chin	veins of chin distended	Plat.
Chin	warts on chin	Lyc., Thuj.
Choking	choking (stop breathing through blockage of throat) of throat aggravated by clothing	Agar., ambr., apis., bell., cact., chel., elaps., kali-bi., kali-c., Lach., sep.
Choking	choking cough at midnight	Dros., ruta.
Choking	choking cough at night	Carb-v., hep., ip., ruta.
Choking	choking cough from inspiration	Cina.
Choking	choking cough in evening	Cina.
Choking	choking cough in morning after rising	Cina.
Choking	choking cough when lying on side	Kali-c.
Choking	choking of throat before menses	Puls.
Choking	choking of throat compelling to swallow	Bor., cact., lach., sep.
Choking	choking of throat during dinner	Bar-c.
Choking	choking of throat on coughing	Ars., coc-c., lach.

Body part/Disease	Symptom	Medicines
Choking	choking of throat on going to sleep	Bell., cench., crot-h., kali-c., lac-c., Lach., naja., Nux-v., sep., teucr., valer.
Choking	choking of throat on raising arm	Plb.
Choking	choking of throat on sight or thought of water	Anan., lyss.
Choking	choking of throat on swallowing liquids	Hyos., lyss., mag-p., nat-s., rhus-t.
Choking	choking of throat on swallowing solids	Carb-v., lach., Puls.
Choking	choking of throat on swallowing	Acon., ars., bar-c., bell., bry., cic., cupr., gent-c., graph., hyos., kali-c., laur., Lyc., mag-p., manc., meph., merc., mur-ac., nat-m., onos., par., plb., Puls., rhus-t., stry., tarent., verat., zinc.
Choking	choking of throat on waking	Agar.
Cholera	choking of throat paroxysmal	Verat.
Cholera	choking of throat upon bending the neck	Ph-ac.
Cholera	choking of throat upon lying down	Apis., kali-bi., ol-j.
Cholera	choking of throat when clearing the throat	Ambr., anac., Arg-n., bor., bry., calc-p., coc-c., ip., kali-c., Nux-v., osm., stann.
Cholera	choking of throat when drinking	Cimx., Hyos., iod., manc., meph., Nat-m., rhus-t.
Cholera	choking of throat when speaking	Manc., meph.
Cholera	choking of throat while eating	Kali-bi., kali-c., lach., meph., merc-c., nit-ac.
Cholera	contraction of muscles & tendons of fingers in cholera	Cupr.
Cholera	cramp in calf in cholera	Ant-t., camph., colch., **Cupr.**, jatr., kali-p., mag-p., **Sulph.**, **Verat.**
Cholera	cramp in fingers with cholera (an acute and often fatal intestinal disease that produces severe gastrointestinal symptoms and is usually caused by the bacterium Vibrio cholerae)	Colch., Cupr., sec., Verat.
Cholera	cramp in foot in cholera	**Cupr.**, sec., **Verat.**
Cholera	cramp in hand in cholera	Cupr., sec.
Cholera	cramp in sole at night in cholera	**Sulph.**
Cholera	diarrhoea during epidemic cholera	Camph., cupr., Ip., phos., puls.
Cholera	discolouration of face blue in cholera	Camph., Cupr., Verat.
Cholera	paralysis after cholera	Verat.
Cholera	retention of urine in cholera	Camph., canth., lach., op., Verat.
Cholera	suffocation during cholera	Hydr-ac., laur.
Cholera	suppression of urine in cholera	Ars., camph., carb-v., cupr., sec., verat.
Chorea	chorea (jerky spasmodic movements of the limbs, trunk, and facial muscles, common to various diseases of the central nervous system)	Acon., **Agar.**, ant-t., apis., arg-n., ars-i., ars., **Art-v.**, asaf., aster., bell., bufo., cact., **Calc.**, caul., **Caust.**, cedr., cham., chel., **Chin.**, chlol., **Cic.**, **Cimic.**, **Cina.**, cocc., coff., con., croc., crot-c., crot-h., cupr-ar., **Cupr.**, cypr., dios., dulc., ferr-ar., ferr-i., ferr., form., hipp., hyos., **Ign.**, iod., ip., kali-ar., kali-br., kali-c., kali-i., kali-p., lach., laur., lil-t., mag-p., merc., mez., **Mygal.**, nat-m., nit-ac., nux-m., nux-v., op., ph-ac., phos., plat., plb., psor., puls., rhod., rhus-t., sabin., samb., sec., sep., sil., stann., **Stram.**, sulph., **Tarent.**, thuj., verat-v., visc., zinc.

Body part/Disease	Symptom	Medicines
Chorea	chorea after coition	**Agar.**, agn., am-c., anac., anan., apis., arg-n., asaf., bar-c., bor., bov., calad., **Calc.**, canth., cedr., chin., con., graph., **Kali-c.**, **Kali-p.**, lyc., mag-m., mosch., nat-c., nat-m., nat-p., nit-ac., nux-v., petr., ph-ac., phos., plb., rhod., sel., **Sep.**, **Sil.**, staph., tarent., ther.
Chorea	chorea after coition in women	Agar., cedr.
Chorea	chorea after cold bath	Rhus-t.
Chorea	chorea after dinner	Zinc.
Chorea	chorea after eating	Ign.
Chorea	chorea after getting wet	Rhus-t.
Chorea	chorea after grief	Ign.
Chorea	chorea aggravated from coition	Cedr.
Chorea	chorea aggravated from wine	Zinc.
Chorea	chorea aggravated in afternoon	Zinc.
Chorea	chorea aggravated in clear weather	Acon., asar., bry., caust., hep., nux-v., plb., sabad., spong.
Chorea	chorea aggravated in cloudy weather	Am-c., bry., calc., cham., chin., dulc., mang., merc., nux-m., plb., puls., rhod., **Rhus-t.**, sep., sulph., verat.
Chorea	chorea ameliorated from exercise	Zinc.
Chorea	chorea ameliorated from loosening clothing	Am-c., arn., asar., bry., **Calc.**, cann-i., caps., carb-v., caust., chel., chin., coff., hep., **Lach.**, **Lyc.**, **Nit-ac.**, **Nux-v.**, olnd., op., puls., ran-b., sanic., sars., sep., spig., spong., stann., sulph.
Chorea	chorea ameliorated from lying on back	Cupr., ign.
Chorea	chorea ameliorated from sleep	**Agar.**, hell., ziz.
Chorea	chorea at day time	Art-v., tarent.
Chorea	chorea at night	Arg-n., caust.
Chorea	chorea before thunderstorm	Agar., rhod., sep.
Chorea	chorea begins in face and spreads to body	Sec.
Chorea	chorea during coition	Anac., asaf., bar-c., calad., canth., ferr., graph., kali-c., lyc., plat., sel., sep., thuj.
Chorea	chorea during menses	**Zinc.**
Chorea	chorea during pregnancy	Caust., cupr.
Chorea	chorea during rest	Zinc.
Chorea	chorea during thunderstorm	Phos.
Chorea	chorea from animal fluids	Chin.
Chorea	chorea from coal gas	Arn., bov., carb-s., carb-v.
Chorea	chorea from fright	Acon., agar., calc., **Caust.**, cupr., gels., ign., kali-br., laur., nat-m., op., phos., stram., zinc.
Chorea	chorea from imitation	Caust., cupr., mygal., tarent.
Chorea	chorea from onanism (masturbation)	Calc., chin.
Chorea	chorea from suppressed eruptions	Caust., **Sulph.**, zinc.
Chorea	chorea from worms	Calc., cina.
Chorea	chorea in afternoon	Nat-s.

Body part/Disease	Symptom	Medicines
Chorea	chorea in children who has grown too fast	Phos.
Chorea	chorea in dry weather	Caust.
Chorea	chorea in legs	Cocc., rhod., stict.
Chorea	chorea in morning	Mygal.
Chorea	chorea like motion of lower limbs	Agar., arg-n., coff., mygal.
Chorea	chorea of left side	Cimic., cupr., rhod.
Chorea	chorea of right side	Ars., caust., nat-s., phys., tarent.
Chorea	chorea on side lain on	Cimic.
Chorea	chorea one sided	Calc., cocc., cupr., nat-s., phys.
Chorea	chorea periodic	Cupr., nat-s.
Chorea	chorea when thinking of it	Caust.
Chorea	chorea with intolerance of clothing	Am-c., apis., **Arg-n.**, arn., asaf., asar., bov., bry., **Calc.**, caps., carb-s., carb-v., caust., chin., coff., con., **Crot-c.**, crot-h., graph., hep., ign., kali-bi., kali-c., kali-n., kreos., **Lach.**, **Lyc.**, nat-s., **Nux-v.**, olnd., **Onos.**, op., puls., ran-b., sanic., sars., sep., spig., **Spong.**, stann., sulph., tarent.
Chorea	chorea with intolerance of woolen clothing	Phos., psor., puls., sulph.
Chorea	constant disposition to swallow from chorea in throat	Agar.
Chorea	emotional chorea	Agar., ign., laur., op., phos.
Chorea	rheumatic chorea	**Caust.**, cimic., kali-i., rhus-t., stict.
Choroid	inflammation of eye due to choroid (a brownish membrane between the retina and the white of the eye that contains blood vessels and large pigmented cells)	Ars., aur., bell., Bry., cedr., coloc., gels., ip., jab., kali-chl., kali-i., merc-c., merc-d., merc., nux-v., phos., phyt., prun-s., psor., puls., ruta., sil., spig., sulph., thuj.
Cicatrice	cicatrices shining	Sil.
Cicatrice	old cicatrices (cause a wound to heal and form a scar) due to abscess in cervical region	Sil.
Cicatrice	old cicatrices in mammae	Carb-an., Graph., phyt.
Cicatrice	old cicatrices suppurating	Sil.
Cirrhosis	cirrhosis (a chronic progressive disease of the liver characterized by the replacement of healthy cells with scar tissue) of liver	Cupr., hep., hydr., mur-ac., phos., plb., sulph.
Clawing	clawing of leg in morning	Stront.
Clawing	clawing of thigh	Bry.
Clawing	clawing of upper limbs	Lach.
Clawing	clawing of wrist	Rhod.
Clawing	clawing sensation in chest	Samb., stront.
Clenching	clenched jaw (hold teeth or fist tightly together दांत लगना)	Acet-ac., acon., agar., ars., Bell., camph., cic., colch., crot-h., cupr., dig., dios., glon., hydr-ac., hyos., ign., laur., merc., nux-v., oena., op., ox-ac., phos., sil., staph., stram., sulph., tarent., verat., vip.
Clenching	clenched teeth firmly	Alum., bell., camph., cic., hyos., merc., podo., stram.
Clenching	clenching after fright	Ign.
Clenching	clenching at beginning of chill	Cimx.

Body part/Disease	Symptom	Medicines
Clenching	clenching covulsive	Glon., mag-p., nux-m., nux-v.
Clenching	clenching during sleep	Viol-t.
Clenching	clenching from epileptic covulsion	Lach., mag-p., oena.
Clenching	clenching from stretching out arms	Stry.
Clenching	clenching in noon	Am-c.
Clenching	clenching in rheumatism	Kali-i.
Clenching	clenching thumbs	Aeth., apis., ars., art-v., arum-t., bell., brach., bufo., camph., caust., cham., cic., cocc., Cupr., glon., hell., hyos., ign., lach., mag-p., Merc., oena., phyt., sec., stann., staph., stram., sulph., viol-t.
Clenching	clenching thumbs in epilepsy	Bufo., caust., cic., lach., stann., staph., sulph.
Clenching	clenching when seizing something	Arg-n., dros., stry.
Clenching	constant inclination to clench teeth together	Acet-ac., acon., agar., ambr., anan., bufo., camph., cann-i., caust., cob., cocc., cupr., hyos., iod., laur., lyc., mang., merc-i-f., nux-v., Phyt., podo., stry., tarent.
Climacteric	pain under nipples during climacteric	Cimic.
Climacteric	palpitation of heart during climacteric period (the time in a woman's life when menstruation diminishes and ceases, usually between the ages of 45 and 50)	Crot-h., Lach., tab.
Climaxis	congestion in chest at climaxis	Arg-n., Lach.
Clitoris	blotches prepuce (skin covering clitoris)	Sep.
Clitoris	burning prepuce	Caust., merc.
Clitoris	chancres in prepuce	Ail., arg-m., arg-n., ars-h., ars., aur-m-n., Aur-m., bor., caust., cinnb., cor-r., hep., kali-bi., Merc-c., merc-i-r., Merc., nit-ac., phos., sep., staph., sulph., thuj., viol-t.
Clitoris	herpetic eruption on prepuce	Ars., caust., dulc., graph., hep., kali-i., merc., nat-c., nit-ac., petr., ph-ac., rhus-t., sars., sep., thuj.
Clitoris	herpetic prepuce	Ars., caust., dulc., graph., hep., kali-i., merc., nat-c., nit-ac., petr., ph-ac., rhus-t., sars., sep., thuj.
Clitoris	induration of the prepuce	Lach., merc-i-r., sep., sulph.
Clitoris	inflammation of the inner surface of the prepuce	Crot-t., nit-ac.
Clitoris	inflammation of the prepuce	Apis., ars., calc., cann-s., Cinnb., con., cor-r., elaps., hep., jac-c., lach., lyc., Merc., mez., mur-ac., nat-a., nat-c., nit-ac., rhus-t., sabin., sep., sil., sulph., sumb.
Clitoris	irritation in clitoris (a sensitive erectile female sex organ at the front junction of the labia minora in the vulva)	Am-c.
Clitoris	itching at root of prepuce	Lyss., rhus-t.
Clitoris	itching in fraenum (a fold formed by union of labia minora on the under surface of clitoris)	Caust., hep., ph-ac.
Clitoris	itching in glans (small rounded at the end of penis or clitoris)	Agn., alum., ambr., ant-c., arn., ars-i., ars., aur-m., benz., calc., cann-i., cann-s., carb-ac., carb-v., caust., chel., chin., Cinnb., colch., Crot-t., dros., euphr., ferr-ma., gymn., hep., Ind., indg., iod., kali-bi., lyc., lyss., mang., merc., mez., nat-c., nat-m., nat-s., Nit-ac., nux-v., ph-ac., poth., psor., senec., sil., spong., Sulph., thuj.

Body part/Disease	Symptom	Medicines
Clitoris	itching in prepuce (skin covering clitoris)	Agar., aloe., berb., calc., cann-s., canth., carb-v., Caust., cham., Cinnb., colch., Con., eupho., gymn., hep., Ign., jac-c., lyc., merc., mez., nat-a., nat-m., nat-p., Nit-ac., nux-v., Petr., phos., puls., Rhus-t., sep., sil., sulph., sumb., thuj., viol-t., zinc., zing.
Clitoris	pain in penis from swelled prepuce	Rhus-t.
Clitoris	pain in prepuce	Calad., cor-r., cycl., lyc., osm., rhus-t., sabin., verat.
Clitoris	pain in prepuce during urination	Phos.
Clitoris	pimples on glans	Jac., lach., nit-ac., ph-ac.
Clitoris	pimples on prepuce	Arn., nit-ac., sil.
Clitoris	pinching pain in prepuce	Jac-c.
Clitoris	redness of glans	Ars., calad., cann-s., cor-r., crot-t., dor., merc., nat-m., rhus-t., sabin., sars.
Clitoris	redness of prepuce	Calc., cann-s., Cinnb., cor-r., lach., lyc., merc., prun-s., rhus-v., rumx., sil., sulph., sumb.
Clitoris	tingling sensation in prepuce	Jac., merc., ph-ac., seneg., tarax.
Clitoris	vesicles on prepuce	Ars-h., carb-v., caust., graph., merc., nit-ac.
Cobweb	cobwebs (spider web) sensation on face	Alum., bar-c., bor., brom., bry., calad., calc., carb-s., carl., con., Graph., laur., mag-c., mez., morph., ph-ac., plb., ran-s., sul-ac., sulph., sumb.
Cobweb	sensation of cobweb (a web of fine threads spun by a spider, especially when covered with dust) on hands	Bor.
Coition	Aching in lumbar region after coition	Cann-i.
Coition	ailments from onanism (act of masturbating)	Agar., alum., ambr., anac., ant-c., arg-m., ars., bov., bufo., calad., calc-s., **Calc.**, carb-v., **Chin.**, **Cocc.**, **Con.**, dig., ferr., **Gels.**, hyos., iod., kali-c., kali-p., lyc., mag-p., merc-c., merc., mosch., nat-c., nat-m., **Nat-p.**, nux-m., nux-v., **Orig.**, petr., **Ph-ac.**, phos., plb., puls., **Sel.**, **Sep.**, sil., spig., squil., **Staph.**, **Sulph.**
Coition	anxiety after coition	Sep.
Coition	anxiety from thought of coition in a woman	Kreos.
Coition	asthmatic after coition	Asaf., cedr., kali-bi.
Coition	asthmatic during coition	Aeth., ambr.
Coition	breathing difficult after coition	Cedr., dig.
Coition	breathing difficult during coition	Aeth., ambr., arund., asaf., con., sep., staph.
Coition	breathing difficult towards end of coition	Staph.
Coition	burning pain in back after coition	Mag-m.
Coition	burning pain in back in morning after coition aggravated by rest ameliorated by motion	Mag-m.
Coition	burning pain in urethra after coition	Berb., canth., nat-p., sep., sul-ac., Sulph.
Coition	burning pain in urethra ceases during coition	Anag.
Coition	burning pain in urethra during coition	Agar., ant-c., calc., canth., kreos., merc., sulph., thuj.
Coition	cheerful after coition	Nat-m.
Coition	chilliness after coition	Nat-m.

Body part/Disease	Symptom	Medicines
Coition	chorea after coition	**Agar.**, agn., am-c., anac., anan., apis., arg-n., asaf., bar-c., bor., bov., calad., **Calc.**, canth., cedr., chin., con., graph., **Kali-c.**, **Kali-p.**, lyc., mag-m., mosch., nat-c., nat-m., nat-p., nit-ac., nux-v., petr., ph-ac., phos., plb., rhod., sel., **Sep.**, **Sil.**, staph., tarent., ther.
Coition	chorea after coition in women	Agar., cedr.
Coition	chorea aggravated from coition	Cedr.
Coition	chorea during coition	Anac., asaf., bar-c., calad., canth., ferr., graph., kali-c., lyc., plat., sel., sep., thuj.
Coition	chorea from onanism (masturbation)	Calc., chin.
Coition	coldness in leg after coition	Graph.
Coition	constriction in chest after coition	Staph.
Coition	convulsion after coition	Agar.
Coition	convulsion after onanism	Bufo., calad., calc., dig., elaps., kali-br., lach., naja., nux-v., **Plat.**, plb., sep., sil., stram., sulph.
Coition	convulsion during coition	Bufo.
Coition	cough after coition	Tarent.
Coition	cramp in calf after coition	Coloc.
Coition	cramp in calf during coition	Cupr., graph.
Coition	cramp in calf on attempting to coition	Cupr.
Coition	cramp in foot in attempting to coition	Cupr.
Coition	disposition to masturbation after sexual excesses	Carb-v.
Coition	extreme enjoyment in sexual intercourse	Fl-ac., nat-m., nit-ac.
Coition	falling asleep during coition	Bar-c., lyc.
Coition	fever after coition	Graph., nux-v.
Coition	fever with dry heat at night after coition	Nux-v.
Coition	formication during sexual excitement	Mez., tarent.
Coition	heaviness in extremities after coition	Bufo.
Coition	hemorrhage from urethra during coition	Caust.
Coition	itching during coition	Sep.
Coition	itching in extremities after coition	Agar.
Coition	itching in urethra after coition	Nat-p.
Coition	itching in vagina after coition	Agar., Nit-ac.
Coition	lassitude after coition	**Calc.**
Coition	orgasm of blood after coition	Am-c., sep.
Coition	pain in back after coition (sexual inter course)	Cann-i., Nit-ac., sabal.
Coition	pain in bladder after coition	All-c.
Coition	pain in coccyx during coition	Kali-bi.
Coition	pain in extremities after coition	**Sil.**, tub.
Coition	pain in eye after coition (sexual intercourse)	Bart.
Coition	pain in heart after sexual intercourse	Dig.
Coition	pain in lumbar region during coition	Cann-i., nit-ac.

Body part/Disease	Symptom	Medicines
Coition	pain in prostate gland after sexual intercourse	All-c., alum., caps., psor., sel.
Coition	pain in sacral region from coition	Agar., calc-p., calc., kali-c., nat-c., petr., phos., Sep., Sil., staph.
Coition	pain in sacral region in morning during coition	Kali-bi.
Coition	pain in spine after coition	Nit-ac.
Coition	pain in thigh after coition	Nit-ac.
Coition	pain in uterus after coition	Plat.
Coition	pain in uterus during coition	Ferr-p., hep., merc-c.
Coition	palpitation of heart after coition	Am-c., dig., sep.
Coition	palpitation of heart after onanism (masturbation)	Dig., ferr., ph-ac.
Coition	palpitation of heart during coition	Calc., crot-t., lyc., ph-ac., Phos., visc.
Coition	paralysis after coition	Phos.
Coition	paralysis with hemiplegia from onanism	Stann.
Coition	perspiration after coition	Agar., calc., chin., eug., **Graph.**, nat-c., sel., **Sep.**
Coition	perspiration in chest after coition	Agar.
Coition	perspiration in shoulder after coition	Agar.
Coition	perspiration in upper limbs after coition	Agar.
Coition	profuse perspiration after coition	Agar.
Coition	prostate gland complaint of onanism (the act of masturbating)	Tarent.
Coition	seminal discharge (fluid ejaculated by male) failing during coition though the orgasm is present	Cann-i., graph.
Coition	skin burning after coition	Agar.
Coition	skin, burning after coition	Agar.
Coition	skin, heat after coition	Graph.
Coition	sleepiness after coition	Agar., sep.
Coition	sleepiness during coition	Bar-c., lyc.
Coition	sleeplessness after coition	Calc., cop., nit-ac., sep., sil.
Coition	sore bruised pain after coition	**Sil.**
Coition	trembling after coition	Agar.
Coition	trembling in leg after coition	**Calc.**
Coition	trembling in lower limbs after coition	**Calc.**
Coition	trembling in thigh after coition	**Calc.**
Coition	weakness after coition	Agar., berb., **Calc.**, chin., clem., con., dig., graph., kali-c., kali-p., lil-t., lyc., mosch., nat-m., nit-ac., petr., ph-ac., phos., **Sel.**, sep., sil., staph., tarent.
Coition	weakness in foot after coition	Calc-p.
Coition	weakness in hip from preventing finishing coition	All-c.
Coition	weakness in knee after coition	Agar., **Calc.**, con., kali-c., lyc., petr., sep., sil.
Coition	weakness in lower limbs after coition	Calc.
Coition	weakness in thigh after coition	Calc.
Coldness	cold & stiff on approaching warm stove	Laur.

Body part/Disease	Symptom	Medicines
Coldness	coldness after cold drinks	Ars., Chin., Elaps., rhus-t., sul-ac.
Coldness	coldness after eating	Carb-an., cist., crot-c., nit-ac.
Coldness	coldness after eating fruit	Ars., elaps.
Coldness	coldness after ice cream	Chin-s.
Coldness	coldness alternating with heat	Bell., lyc., stram.
Coldness	coldness ameliorated after loosening cloth	Chin-s.
Coldness	coldness ameliorated from motion	Acon.
Coldness	coldness at night in bed	Carb-an.
Coldness	coldness at night with heat at other side	Puls.
Coldness	coldness before eating	Cist.
Coldness	coldness beneath scapula	Agar.
Coldness	coldness between scapula	Abies-c., agar., am-c., am-m., arg-m., aur., Bol., cann-i., Caps., carl., caust., chel., eup-per., lac-d., lachn., led., nat-c., petr., puls., rhus-t., sarr., sep., sil., sulph., tab., viol-t.
Coldness	coldness between scapula as from cold water	Abies-c.
Coldness	coldness between scapula with cough	Am-m.
Coldness	coldness during diarrhoea	Nat-m., ptel.
Coldness	coldness during fever	Carb-an., kali-ar., sep., Stram.
Coldness	coldness during menses	Arn., calc., cham., sec., sil.
Coldness	coldness during stool	Sulph.
Coldness	coldness from excitement	Lach.
Coldness	coldness from mental exertion	Lach.
Coldness	Coldness in a spot of head	Croc.
Coldness	Coldness in a small spot of Vertex (The topmost point of the vault of the skull)	Mang.
Coldness	coldness in ankles	Acon., agar., berb., caust., chin., lach.
Coldness	coldness in ankles while walking in open air	Chin.
Coldness	coldness in back after afternoon rest	Cycl.
Coldness	coldness in back after dinner	Cedr., cycl.
Coldness	coldness in back after eating	Crot-c., sil.
Coldness	coldness in back after menses	Kali-c.
Coldness	coldness in back after stool	Fago., puls., sumb.
Coldness	coldness in back after urination	Sars.
Coldness	coldness in back aggravated from warmth	Apis.
Coldness	coldness in back ameliorated by lying down	Cast., kali-n., sil.
Coldness	coldness in back as if cold water has been sprayed with force	Caust., lyc., Puls.
Coldness	coldness in back at night	Ars., arum-t., chin-a., chin-s., chin., coc-c., lil-t., lyc., nat-a., nat-m., puls., stront., thuj.
Coldness	coldness in back at night on going to bed	Coc-c., lil-t.
Coldness	coldness in back before stool	Ars.
Coldness	coldness in back during eating	Raph.

Body part/Disease	Symptom	Medicines
Coldness	coldness in back during menses	Bell., kreos.
Coldness	coldness in back during stool	Colch., trom.
Coldness	coldness in back extending down as if cold water were flowing down in thin stream	Ars., caps., caust.
Coldness	coldness in back extending down as if cold water were poured down	Agar., alumn., anac., ars., lil-t., lyc., Puls., sabad., stram., vario., zinc.
Coldness	coldness in back extending down limbs	Gins.
Coldness	coldness in back extending down on motion	Rumx.
Coldness	coldness in back extending down lower limbs	Acon., ferr., ham.
Coldness	coldness in back extending down to feet	Croc.
Coldness	coldness in back extending down to feet	Croc.
Coldness	coldness in back extending into arms	Gins., verat.
Coldness	coldness in back extending over whole body	Amyg., bell., lyc.
Coldness	coldness in back extending to abdomen	Crot-t., phos., sec., spig.
Coldness	coldness in back from motion	Asaf., eup-pur., phys., sulph., thuj.
Coldness	coldness in back in afternoon	Alum., apis., asaf., cast., cic., cimic., cocc., fago., guai., hyos., lyc., nat-a., rumx., stram., thuj.
Coldness	coldness in back in evening	Ars., bapt., berb., caps., cast., cimic., cocc., coff., dulc., kreos., lyc., mur-ac., nat-m., nux-v., Puls., rhus-t., sang., sep., stann., Sulph., tab., thuj.
Coldness	coldness in back in forenoon	Ang., asaf., berb., cham., con., hydr., lyc.
Coldness	coldness in back in forenoon while walking in a room	Ang.
Coldness	coldness in back in forenoon while walking in open air	Hydr.
Coldness	coldness in back in morning	Arn., bry., con., ferr., mez., nit-s-d., Nux-v., sumb.
Coldness	coldness in back in morning after menses	Kali-c.
Coldness	coldness in back in noon	Arg-n., rhus-t.
Coldness	coldness in back near warm stove	Jug-c.
Coldness	coldness in back of hands	Anac., chin-s., naja., phos., rhus-t.
Coldness	coldness in back of hands in afternoon	Chin-s.
Coldness	coldness in back of hands with heat of palms	Anac., coff.
Coldness	coldness in back on waking	Dig.
Coldness	coldness in back when dressing	Anth.
Coldness	coldness in back while sitting	Brom.
Coldness	coldness in back while walking	Asaf., hyos., nit-s-d.
Coldness	coldness in back while walking in open air	Chin.
Coldness	coldness in calf	Ars., berb., bufo., chel., hyper., lach., mang., rumx.
Coldness	coldness in calf ameliorated while rising from sitting	Mang.
Coldness	coldness in calf in evening	Mang.
Coldness	coldness in calf in forenoon	Berb.
Coldness	coldness in cervical region	Calc., cann-i., carb-s., chel., chr-ac., dulc., fl-ac., ir-foe., kali-chl., laur., lyc., nat-s., op., ran-s., Sil., spong., zinc.

Body part/Disease	Symptom	Medicines
Coldness	coldness in cervical region extending to occiput	Chel.
Coldness	coldness in cervical region extending to sacrum on lying down	Thuj.
Coldness	coldness in dorsal region	Agar., croc., sil., spong., thuj.
Coldness	coldness in elbow	Agar., cedr., gins., graph., ir-f.
Coldness	coldness in elbow extending to hands towards noon	Cedr.
Coldness	coldness in finger joints	Chel.
Coldness	coldness in fingers alternating with headache	Cupr.
Coldness	coldness in fingers at night	Mur-ac.
Coldness	coldness in fingers extending to middle of upper arms	Graph.
Coldness	coldness in fingers extending to nape of neck	Coff.
Coldness	coldness in fingers extending to palms and soles	Dig.
Coldness	coldness in fingers in afternoon	Plan.
Coldness	coldness in fingers in evening	Sulph., thuj.
Coldness	coldness in fingers in morning	Chin-s., rat.
Coldness	coldness in fingers while sitting	Cham.
Coldness	coldness in first finger	Rhod.
Coldness	coldness in first toe	Ant-t., brom., iod., ran-b.
Coldness	coldness in foot after dinner	Cann-i., carb-v., sulph.
Coldness	coldness in foot after eating	Aloe., calc., camph., caps.
Coldness	coldness in foot after emission	Aloe., nux-v.
Coldness	coldness in foot after menses	Ferr.
Coldness	coldness in foot after motion	Cocc.
Coldness	coldness in foot after stool	Sulph.
Coldness	coldness in foot after supper	Lyc.
Coldness	coldness in foot after vomiting	Sin-a.
Coldness	coldness in foot after walking	Nit-ac.
Coldness	coldness in foot after wine	Lyc.
Coldness	coldness in foot ameliorated while lying	Phos.
Coldness	coldness in foot ameliorated after menses	Carb-v., chin-s.
Coldness	coldness in foot ameliorated before menses	Calc., hyper., lyc., nux-m.
Coldness	coldness in foot ameliorated during menses	Arg-n., calc., cop., crot-h., graph., nat-p., nux-m., phos., sabin., Sil.
Coldness	coldness in foot ameliorated in cold air	Camph., led.
Coldness	coldness in foot ameliorated in house	Mang.
Coldness	coldness in foot ameliorated while sitting	Mang.
Coldness	coldness in foot at day time	Hep., mag-s., nit-ac., phos., sep., sil., sulph.
Coldness	coldness in foot at day time during menses	Nat-p.
Coldness	coldness in foot at midnight	Calad.
Coldness	coldness in foot at midnight alternating with cold hands	Aloe., sep., zing.

Body part/Disease	Symptom	Medicines
Coldness	coldness in foot at midnight alternating with heat	Alum.
Coldness	coldness in foot at midnight alternating with heat with pain in limbs	Rhus-t.
Coldness	coldness in foot at night	Aloe., am-c., am-m., ant-c., aur., bov., bry., calad., Calc., carb-s., carb-v., chel., com., cop., ferr-i., ferr., iod., kali-ar., nit-ac., par., petr., phos., psor., raph., rhod., sars., sep., sil., sulph., thuj., verat., zinc.
Coldness	coldness in foot at night in bed	Am-m., aur., Calc., carb-v., chel., ferr., nit-ac., petr., phos., raph., rhod., sil., sulph., thuj., zinc.
Coldness	coldness in foot at night on waking	Nit-ac., zinc.
Coldness	coldness in foot during anxiety	Cupr., graph., puls., sulph.
Coldness	coldness in foot during dinner	Sulph.
Coldness	coldness in foot during excitement	during : Mag-c.
Coldness	coldness in foot during fever	Am-c., arn., ars., bar-c., bell., bufo., calad., calc., caps., carb-an., carb-v., chin., hell., ign., ip., iris., kali-c., kali-s., lach., meny., nux-v., petr., ptel., puls., ran-b., rhod., samb., stann., stram., sulph.
Coldness	coldness in foot during headache	Arg-n., ars., aur., bell., bufo., cact., calc., camph., carb-s., carb-v., chin., chr-ac., coca., dirc., ferr-p., ferr., Gels., lac-d., lach., laur., Meli., meny., naja., nat-m., phos., plat., psor., sars., Sep., stram., sulph., verat-v.
Coldness	coldness in foot during pregnancy	Lyc., Verat.
Coldness	coldness in foot during sleep	Samb., zinc.
Coldness	coldness in foot during sleep with heat of body	Samb.
Coldness	coldness in foot during supper	Ign.
Coldness	coldness in foot during urination	Dig.
Coldness	coldness in foot extending to calves	Aloe., crot-t.
Coldness	coldness in foot extending to knees	Aeth., chel., ign., meny., nat-m.
Coldness	coldness in foot from fast walking	Phos.
Coldness	coldness in foot from mental exertion	Agar., am-c., ambr., anac., Aur., bell., calc-p., Calc., carb-v., caust., chin., cocc., cupr., gels., kali-c., lach., lyc., Nat-c., nat-m., nit-ac., Nux-v., petr., ph-ac., Phos., psor., Puls., Sep., Sil.
Coldness	coldness in foot from walking in open air	Anac., bar-c., plan., plb.
Coldness	coldness in foot from walking in sun	Lach.
Coldness	coldness in foot in a warm room	Kali-br.
Coldness	coldness in foot in afternoon	Bar-c., chel., chin-s., coca., colch., gels., mez., nux-v., sang., sep., squil., sulph.
Coldness	coldness in foot in afternoon with hot face	Hura.
Coldness	coldness in foot in bed	Alum., ferr., kali-c., lach., naja., raph., rhod., thuj.
Coldness	coldness in foot in evening	Acon., aloe., am-br., am-c., ars., Calc., carb-an., carb-s., carb-v., cham., chel., chin., con., graph., hell., kali-s., lyc., mag-c., mang., nat-n., nux-v., ox-ac., petr., ph-ac., plan., puls., rhod., Sep., Sil., stront., sulph., til., verat., zinc.
Coldness	coldness in foot in evening ameliorated in bed	Sulph.

Body part/Disease	Symptom	Medicines
Coldness	coldness in foot in evening in bed	Aloe., Am-c., am-m., aur., Calc., carb-an., carb-s., carb-v., carl., chel., ferr-p., ferr., Graph., kali-ar., kali-c., kali-s., lyc., merc., nat-c., nit-ac., nux-v., par., petr., ph-ac., phos., raph., rhod., Sep., Sil., staph., sulph., thuj., zinc.
Coldness	coldness in foot in evening in the open air	Mang.
Coldness	coldness in foot in forenoon	Carb-an., chin-s., cop., fago., hura., mez., petr., sep.
Coldness	coldness in foot in hottest weather	Asar.
Coldness	coldness in foot in morning	Anac., caps., chel., coc-c., graph., hura., lyc., mag-m., merc., nux-v., Sep., spig., stram., sumb.
Coldness	coldness in foot in morning after breakfast	Verat.
Coldness	coldness in foot in morning during headache	Sep.
Coldness	coldness in foot in noon	Chin-s., nit-ac., zing.
Coldness	coldness in foot in noon during heat and redness of the face	Sep.
Coldness	coldness in foot in noon while the other one burns	Hura.
Coldness	coldness in foot on walking	Chel., samb., verat., zinc.
Coldness	coldness in foot while ameliorated walking	Aloe.
Coldness	coldness in foot while eating	Ign.
Coldness	coldness in foot while lying	Tell.
Coldness	coldness in foot while sitting	Ars., sep.
Coldness	coldness in foot while talking	Am-c.
Coldness	coldness in foot while walking	Anac., aran., asaf., chin., mang., mez., sil.
Coldness	coldness in foot while writing	Chin-s., sep.
Coldness	coldness in foot with burning soles	Cupr.
Coldness	coldness in foot with burning soles during chill	Ant-c., aur., ferr., Meny., phos., sep., Verat., zinc.
Coldness	coldness in foot with diarrhoea	Dig., lyc., nit-ac.
Coldness	coldness in foot with heat of face	Acon., asaf., cocc., gels., ign., ruta., samb., sep., Stram.
Coldness	coldness in foot with heat of feet ameliorated from bath	Glon.
Coldness	coldness in foot with heat of hands	Acon., calad., com., nux-m., sep.
Coldness	coldness in foot with heat of head	Alum., am-c., anac., arn., ars., aur., bar-c., bell., cact., calc., com., ferr., gels., laur., nat-c., ph-ac., sep., squil., thuj.
Coldness	coldness in foot with heat of one side of body	Ran-b.
Coldness	coldness in foot with heat of one side of body during sleep	Samb.
Coldness	coldness in foot with heat of thighs	Cocc., thuj.
Coldness	coldness in foot with one cold, the other hot	Chel., dig., ip., Lyc., puls.
Coldness	coldness in forearm (the part of the arm between the elbow and the wrist)	Arg-n., ars., brom., bry., calc., caust., cedr., con., crot-c., Graph., hydrc., kali-chl., nux-v., Phos., plb., rhus-t., verat-v.
Coldness	coldness in forearm during menses	Arg-n.
Coldness	coldness in forearm icy cold	Brom., rhus-t., thuj.
Coldness	coldness in forearm in morning after rising	Nux-v.
Coldness	coldness in forearm in morning	Nux-v.

Body part/Disease	Symptom	Medicines
Coldness	coldness in fourth finger	Lyc.
Coldness	coldness in gluteal (buttock muscle) region	Agar., calc.
Coldness	coldness in hands after breakfast	Verat.
Coldness	coldness in hands after dinner	Cann-i.
Coldness	coldness in hands after eating	Aloe., camph., caps., con.
Coldness	coldness in hands after emission	Merc.
Coldness	coldness in hands after motion	Alumn., cocc.
Coldness	coldness in hands after rising	Fago.
Coldness	coldness in hands after vexation	Phos.
Coldness	coldness in hands after wine	Verat.
Coldness	coldness in hands after writing	Agar.
Coldness	coldness in hands alternating with cold feet	Aloe., sep., zing.
Coldness	coldness in hands alternating with heat	Bell., chin., cimic., cocc., fago., par.
Coldness	coldness in hands ameliorated from lying down	Phos.
Coldness	coldness in hands at day time	Ars-m., phos.
Coldness	coldness in hands at night	Aur., bry., phos., sep., thuj.
Coldness	coldness in hands during chill	Aur., cact., camph., canth., carb-v., cedr., chel., colch., con., hep., ip., lyc., meny., Mez., nat-m., Nux-v., op., petr., Phos., plb., samb., Sec., stram., Verat.
Coldness	coldness in hands during cough	Rumx., sulph.
Coldness	coldness in hands during fever	Arn., asaf., canth., cycl., euphr., hell., ip., nit-ac., puls., ran-b., sabad.
Coldness	coldness in hands during menses	Aesc., arg-n., ferr., graph., kali-i., phos., sabin., sec., sulph., verat.
Coldness	coldness in hands during menses with pain	Calc., graph., sabin.
Coldness	coldness in hands during nausea	Gran.
Coldness	coldness in hands during pain in sacrum	Hura.
Coldness	coldness in hands during perspiration	Chin., dig., fago., lil-t., merc-c.
Coldness	coldness in hands during sleep	Ign., merc., samb.
Coldness	coldness in hands during urination	Dig.
Coldness	coldness in hands from diarrhoea	Apis., brom., dig., Phos.
Coldness	coldness in hands from excitement	Lil-t.
Coldness	coldness in hands from lying down	Kali-c.
Coldness	coldness in hands from mental exertion	Lach., ph-ac.
Coldness	coldness in hands in afternoon	Alumn., chin-s., gels., nux-v., sulph.
Coldness	coldness in hands in evening	Acon., agar., aloe., alumn., ambr., ars., aur., carb-an., carb-v., carl., chel., chin., colch., coloc., graph., hep., nat-c., ox-ac., phos., sulph., thuj., verat.
Coldness	coldness in hands in evening after heat	Thuj.
Coldness	coldness in hands in evening during heat	Sabad.
Coldness	coldness in hands in evening in bed	Aur., carb-an., colch.
Coldness	coldness in hands in evening in open air	Mang.

Body part/Disease	Symptom	Medicines
Coldness	coldness in hands in forenoon	Calc., chin., grat., mez., nat-m.
Coldness	coldness in hands in hottest weather	Asar.
Coldness	coldness in hands in morning	Chel., chin., cina., coloc., cycl., fago., gels., lyc., mang., spong., stram., sumb.
Coldness	coldness in hands in morning after rising	Coloc.
Coldness	coldness in hands in noon	Zing.
Coldness	coldness in hands in old people	Bar-c.
Coldness	coldness in hands in warm room	Nux-v., plan.
Coldness	coldness in hands numb & cold	Chel., lach., ox-ac.
Coldness	coldness in hands on walking	Dig.
Coldness	coldness in hands while reading	Lyc.
Coldness	coldness in hands while talking	Am-c., ph-ac.
Coldness	coldness in hands while walking	Asaf., camph., chin.
Coldness	coldness in hands while walking in open air	Phos., plb.
Coldness	coldness in hands while writing	Chin-s., mez.
Coldness	coldness in hands with cutting and tearing in abdomen	Ars.
Coldness	coldness in hands with heat in one side of body	Ran-b.
Coldness	coldness in hands with heat of body	Ars-m.
Coldness	coldness in hands with heat of thighs	Thuj.
Coldness	coldness in hands with hot face	Agar., Arn., ars., asaf., chin., con., eupho., hyos., ign., ruta., sabin., Stram., sumb., thuj.
Coldness	coldness in hands with hot feet	Aloe., calc., coloc., ph-ac., sep.
Coldness	coldness in hands with hot forehead	Ars., asaf., asar.
Coldness	coldness in hands with hot head	Arn., asaf., aur., Bell., Glon., hell., iod., nat-c., sumb.
Coldness	coldness in hands with internal heat	Arn.
Coldness	coldness in hands with vertigo (a condition in which somebody feels a sensation of whirling or tilting that causes a loss of balance)	Merc.
Coldness	coldness in hip	Agar., gad., gran., ham., hura., merc., merl., mez., morph., tax., ther., valer.
Coldness	coldness in hollow of knee at night	Agar., ars-h.
Coldness	coldness in joints	Camph., cinnb., nat-m., petr., rhus-t., sumb.
Coldness	coldness in joints in morning	Sumb.
Coldness	coldness in joints in morning in bed	Sumb.
Coldness	coldness in joints in open air	Nat-m.
Coldness	coldness in joints of second finger	Agar.
Coldness	coldness in knee at night	Carb-v., cop., euphr., Phos., raph., sep., verat.
Coldness	coldness in knee at night after walking in open air	Sil.
Coldness	coldness in knee at night as from wind	Benz-ac., cimx.
Coldness	coldness in knee at night as if cold water poured over	Verat.
Coldness	coldness in knee at night during chill	Apis., Carb-v., ign., Phos., sil.
Coldness	coldness in knee at night during menses	Cop.

Body part/Disease	Symptom	Medicines
Coldness	coldness in knee at night in bed	Phos., sep.
Coldness	coldness in knee at night in hottest weather	Asar.
Coldness	coldness in knee at night in while lying	Ars.
Coldness	coldness in knee at night on waking	Euphr.
Coldness	coldness in knee at night with swollen knee	Led.
Coldness	coldness in knee in evening	Agn., euphr.
Coldness	coldness in knee in evening on waking	Euphr.
Coldness	coldness in knee in forenoon	Thuj.
Coldness	coldness in left foot	Aeth., hydrc., pip-m., sumb., tub.
Coldness	coldness in left leg	Hyper., ol-an., sang., tub.
Coldness	coldness in left leg during chill	Carb-v., caust., thuj.
Coldness	coldness in left upper limbs	Ars., aster., carb-v., fl-ac., naja., nux-m., rhus-t., sumb.
Coldness	coldness in leg after coition	Graph.
Coldness	coldness in leg after dinner	Cedr.
Coldness	coldness in leg ameliorated from uncovering	Camph., med., Sec., tub.
Coldness	coldness in leg as from being in snow	Verat.
Coldness	coldness in leg as from wind	Bar-c., samb.
Coldness	coldness in leg at night	Agar., aloe., com., kali-ar., merc., thuj., verat.
Coldness	coldness in leg at night as from snow water	Verat.
Coldness	coldness in leg at night on waking	Nit-ac.
Coldness	coldness in leg before menses	Lyc.
Coldness	coldness in leg during fever	Carb-an., eup-pur., meph., sep., Stram.
Coldness	coldness in leg during menses	Arg-n., bufo., calc., lil-t., sec., sil.
Coldness	coldness in leg in afternoon	Aloe., alumn., nux-v.
Coldness	coldness in leg in evening	Aloe., chel., colch., euphr., puls., sang., sil., sulph.
Coldness	coldness in leg in evening in bed	Colch., ph-ac., sep., tub.
Coldness	coldness in leg in evening on waking	Euphr., nit-ac.
Coldness	coldness in leg in morning	Hep., hura.
Coldness	coldness in leg in open air	Ham.
Coldness	coldness in leg in warm room	Acon., meny., Sil.
Coldness	coldness in leg when dressing	Anth.
Coldness	coldness in leg while sitting	Camph., hyper., led.
Coldness	coldness in leg while standing	Nat-m., samb.
Coldness	coldness in leg while walking	Nit-ac., plan.
Coldness	coldness in leg with burning in thighs	Tab.
Coldness	coldness in leg with flushed face	Op.
Coldness	coldness in leg with heat of body	Tab.
Coldness	coldness in leg with heat on face	Arn.
Coldness	coldness in lower limbs alternates with heat in head	Sep.
Coldness	coldness in lower limbs at day time	Nat-c.
Coldness	coldness in lower limbs at night	Lac-c., petr., phos.

Body part/Disease	Symptom	Medicines
Coldness	coldness in lower limbs at night on waking	Nit-ac.
Coldness	coldness in lower limbs during mense	Bufo., calc., cham., lil-t., sec., sil.
Coldness	coldness in lower limbs during nausea	Arg-n.
Coldness	coldness in lower limbs icy cold	Apis., sep.
Coldness	coldness in lower limbs icy cold in spots	Agar., berb.
Coldness	coldness in lower limbs in forenoon	Rumx.
Coldness	coldness in lower limbs in forenoon until bed time	Sep.
Coldness	coldness in lower limbs in noon	Nit-ac.
Coldness	coldness in lower limbs in noon in bed	Chel., lyc., sars.
Coldness	coldness in lower limbs in painful limb	Led., merc.
Coldness	coldness in lower paralyzed limb	Ars., cocc., dulc., graph., nux-v., rhus-t.
Coldness	coldness in lumbar as if cold air passed over it	Sulph., sumb.
Coldness	coldness in lumbar at night	Nat-m., podo.
Coldness	coldness in lumbar at night during dinner	Hell.
Coldness	coldness in lumbar before stool	Nux-m.
Coldness	coldness in lumbar extending to abdomen after urinating	Sulph.
Coldness	coldness in lumbar region after stool	Puls.
Coldness	coldness in lumbar region aggravated from draft of cold air	Tarent.
Coldness	coldness in lumbar region aggravated from motion	Podo.
Coldness	coldness in lumbar region aggravated from walking	Camph.
Coldness	coldness in lumbar region ameliorated from warmth of stove	Hell.
Coldness	coldness in lumbar region in evening while sitting	Canth.
Coldness	coldness in lumbar region in morning	Cham., sumb.
Coldness	coldness in lumbar region right side	Med.
Coldness	coldness in lumbar while sitting	Chin.
Coldness	coldness in lumbar with cough	Carb-an.
Coldness	coldness in malleolus (protuberance at end of leg bone) in inner spots	Berb.
Coldness	coldness in nates	Agar., daph., hydr.
Coldness	coldness in nates at night in bed	Cench.
Coldness	coldness in nates during menses	Mang.
Coldness	coldness in olecranon (elbow bone)	Agar.
Coldness	coldness in one hand	Chin., dig., ferr., mosch.
Coldness	coldness in one hand one hot and pale , the other cold and red	Mosch.
Coldness	coldness in one hand one hot other cold	Chin., cocc., dig., ip., mosch., puls., tab.
Coldness	coldness in one hand with sweat of the other	j2
Coldness	coldness in open air	Chin.
Coldness	coldness in palms	Acon., dig., hyos., jatr.

Body part/Disease	Symptom	Medicines
Coldness	coldness in paralyzed limbs	Ars., caust., cocc., dulc., graph., nux-v., Rhus-t., zinc.
Coldness	coldness in patella at night	Aur., nat-m.
Coldness	coldness in right foot while walking	Bar-c.
Coldness	coldness in right foot	Ambr., bar-c., chel., lyc., sulph.
Coldness	coldness in right forearm	Med.
Coldness	coldness in right hand then left	Med.
Coldness	coldness in right hand with numbness of left	Ferr.
Coldness	coldness in right hand with warmth of left	Lact-ac., mez., mosch.
Coldness	coldness in right hand	Ant-t., cann-i., chel., ferr., gels., med., pall., sec.
Coldness	coldness in right hip	Bry., kali-bi., merl., rhus-t.
Coldness	coldness in right knee	Chel.
Coldness	coldness in right leg	Ambr., elaps., sabin.
Coldness	coldness in right leg during chill	Bry., chel., elaps., sabad., sep.
Coldness	coldness in right thigh	Camph.
Coldness	coldness in right upper limbs	Am-c., ant-t., berb., chel., dulc., hell., merl., pall.
Coldness	coldness in scapula	Camph., chin-s., croc., dios., phos., rhus-t.
Coldness	coldness in second finger	Mur-ac., phos., rhod.
Coldness	coldness in shoulder after eating	Arg-n.
Coldness	coldness in shoulder in epilepsy (disorder of the brain)	Caust.
Coldness	coldness in shoulder in epilepsy extending to small of back	Kreos.
Coldness	coldness in shoulder in evening after supper	Ran-b.
Coldness	coldness in shoulders	Arg-n., aur., bry., caust., cocc., hell., hydr., hyper., kali-bi., kreos., lyc., phos., sep., sil., spig., stry., tep., verat.
Coldness	coldness in shoulders in morning	Aur., sil.
Coldness	coldness in soles	Acon., ars., caust., chel., chin-s., colch., coloc., hyper., laur., lith., merc., nit-ac., nux-v., sulph.
Coldness	coldness in soles at night	Nit-ac.
Coldness	coldness in soles during menses	Calc., graph., nux-m., phos., sil., verat.
Coldness	coldness in soles in evening in bed	Aur., verat.
Coldness	coldness in soles in morning	Chin-s.
Coldness	coldness in soles in open air	Laur.
Coldness	coldness in spine	Am-m., cham., haem., ir-foe., meny.
Coldness	coldness in spine during stool	Trom.
Coldness	coldness in spine extending down	Canth., ruta., stry.
Coldness	coldness in spine from walking	Gins.
Coldness	Coldness in spot of Vertex	Mang., sulph.
Coldness	coldness in thigh at day time	Lyc., tax.
Coldness	coldness in thigh at night	Coc-c., cop., ign., merc., nux-v.
Coldness	coldness in thigh at night as if cold air blow on it	Camph.
Coldness	coldness in thigh at night during chill	Thuj.

Body part/Disease	Symptom	Medicines
Coldness	coldness in thigh at night during colic	Calc.
Coldness	coldness in thigh at night while sitting	Chin., ran-b.
Coldness	coldness in thigh at night while standing	Berb.
Coldness	coldness in thigh at night with convulsion	Calc.
Coldness	coldness in thigh in afternoon	Lyc.
Coldness	coldness in thigh in evening	Bry., calc.
Coldness	coldness in thigh in evening on rising from sitting	Rhod.
Coldness	coldness in thigh in morning	Arn.
Coldness	coldness in third finger	Rhod., sulph.
Coldness	coldness in third finger in evening	Sulph.
Coldness	coldness in tips of finger	Abrot., ant-t., arn., brom., caps., carb-v., carl., Chel., cist., coloc., hell., jatr., lac-d., lob., meny., merc., mur-ac., ph-ac., ran-b., sal-ac., sars., spig., sulph., sumb., tarax., thuj., zinc.
Coldness	coldness in tips of finger after writing	Carl.
Coldness	coldness in tips of finger during chill	Ran-b.
Coldness	coldness in tips of finger during heat	Caps.
Coldness	coldness in tips of finger in morning after rising	Coloc.
Coldness	coldness in tips of finger in open air	Ph-ac.
Coldness	coldness in tips of finger sensitive to cold	Sec.
Coldness	coldness in tips of finger with rest of body hot	Thuj.
Coldness	coldness in tips of toes	Aloe.
Coldness	coldness in toes	Acon., agar., card-m., carl., chel., chin-s., cinnb., coff., con., daph., dig., ferr., gels., lyc., med., meny., nux-v., ol-an., sec., sulph.
Coldness	coldness in toes after sitting	Carl.
Coldness	coldness in toes ameliorated while walking on	Bry.
Coldness	coldness in toes in morning	Chin-s.
Coldness	coldness in toes on touched	Ant-t.
Coldness	coldness in toes while sitting	Bry.
Coldness	coldness in upper arm	Coloc., graph., ign., mez., nat-m., ph-ac., puls., ran-b., rhus-t., sulph., sumb., tep.
Coldness	coldness in upper arm after dinner	Puls.
Coldness	coldness in upper arm after eating	Coloc.
Coldness	coldness in upper arm after supper	Ran-b.
Coldness	coldness in upper arm with burning	Graph.
Coldness	coldness in upper limbs after eating	Ars.
Coldness	coldness in upper limbs after fever	Sil.
Coldness	coldness in upper limbs as from cold wind	Aster.
Coldness	coldness in upper limbs as if dashed with cold water	Mez.
Coldness	coldness in upper limbs at night	Am-c.
Coldness	coldness in upper limbs before menses	Mang.

Body part/Disease	Symptom	Medicines
Coldness	coldness in upper limbs before menses	Mang.
Coldness	coldness in upper limbs during chill	Bell., dig., hell., mez.
Coldness	coldness in upper limbs during cough	Ars., calc., ferr., hep., kali-c., rhus-t., rumx., sil.
Coldness	coldness in upper limbs during menses	Mang.
Coldness	coldness in upper limbs during pain	Chel., fl-ac.
Coldness	coldness in upper limbs during rest	Dulc.
Coldness	coldness in upper limbs from cold air	Kali-c., lyss.
Coldness	coldness in upper limbs from cold air as if passing down to fingers	Fl-ac.
Coldness	coldness in upper limbs from lying on the back	Ign.
Coldness	coldness in upper limbs from walking in a warm room	Squil.
Coldness	coldness in upper limbs in afternoon	Nux-v., sil.
Coldness	coldness in upper limbs in evening	Nux-v.
Coldness	coldness in upper limbs in evening after lying down	Nux-v.
Coldness	coldness in upper limbs in forenoon	Berb.
Coldness	coldness in upper limbs in morning	Caust., chel., dulc., hep.
Coldness	coldness in upper limbs in paralyzed arms	Am-c., dulc., rhus-t.
Coldness	coldness in upper limbs in paralyzed arms from raising them	Verat.
Coldness	coldness in upper limbs in rheumatism	Sang.
Coldness	coldness in upper limbs while sitting	Chin.
Coldness	coldness in upper limbs with a cold thrill down arm	Lyss.
Coldness	coldness in upper limbs with stiffness & numbness	Aster., sulph.
Coldness	coldness in warm room	Brom.
Coldness	coldness in wrist	Gels., rhus-t., sang.
Coldness	coldness in wrist (joint at base of hand) from puerperal (blood poisoning following childbirth) fever	Puls.
Coldness	coldness like ice on spots	Agar.
Coldness	coldness like ice with pain	Bov., colch.
Coldness	coldness of face	Cham., chin., hell.
Coldness	coldness of face during heat	Cina., nat-c.
Coldness	coldness of feet during heat	Acon., calad., com., nux-m., sep.
Coldness	coldness of forehead ameliorated from walking	Gins.
Coldness	coldness of forehead ameliorated on lying	Calc.
Coldness	coldness of forehead ameliorated when covered	Aur., grat., kali-i., nat-m., sanic.
Coldness	coldness of forehead as from cold water	Cann-s., croc., cupr., glon., sabad., tarent.
Coldness	coldness of forehead as from ice	Agar., glon., laur.
Coldness	coldness of forehead as if a cold spot	Sulph.
Coldness	coldness of forehead during headache	Ars., sulph.
Coldness	coldness of forehead during menses	Ant-t., calc., mag-s., sep., sulph., verat.
Coldness	coldness of forehead during menses	Sulph.

Body part/Disease	Symptom	Medicines
Coldness	coldness of forehead even when covered	Mang.
Coldness	coldness of forehead from being heated	Carb-v.
Coldness	coldness of forehead which penetrates painfully	Zinc.
Coldness	coldness of forehead with heat	Chin., puls.
Coldness	coldness of forehead with pain	Gels., phos.
Coldness	coldness of forehead with perspiration	Merc-c.
Coldness	Coldness of head ameliorated by warmth	Lach.
Coldness	coldness of left arm during heat	Sep.
Coldness	Coldness of left side of head	Lach., phos.
Coldness	Coldness of occiput (Back of head)	Acon., agar., aloe., alum., berb., Calc-p., calc., cann-i., Chel., chin-s., coc-c.,dulc., echi., gels., gins., kali-n., nux-m., phos., plat., podo., sep., sil., tarent., thea., verat.
Coldness	Coldness of occiput as if frozen	Gels., nux-v., sep.
Coldness	Coldness of one side of head	Calc., con., lach.
Coldness	Coldness of right side of head but feels burning hot	Bar-c., calc.
Coldness	Coldness of right side of occiput	Form.
Coldness	Coldness of right side of temple	Berb., tarent.
Coldness	Coldness of sides of head above the ear	Asar.
Coldness	coldness of skin after eating	Camph., ran-b.
Coldness	coldness of skin after menses	Graph.
Coldness	coldness of skin after scratching	Agar., mez., petr.
Coldness	coldness of skin after stool	Crot-t.
Coldness	coldness of skin along painful nerves	Led., merc., sil.
Coldness	coldness of skin alternates with heat	Stram.
Coldness	coldness of skin at night	Ars., camph., carb-v., hyos., mosch.
Coldness	coldness of skin before menses	Sil.
Coldness	coldness of skin during convulsions	Anan., camph., caust., cic., hell., hyos., mosch., **Oena.**, op., stram., verat.
Coldness	coldness of skin during diarrhoea	Aeth., camph., jatr., laur., tab., verat.
Coldness	coldness of skin during exercise	Plb., sil.
Coldness	coldness of skin during fever	Camph., iod.
Coldness	coldness of skin during labor	Coff.
Coldness	coldness of skin during menses	Coff., dig., led., tab., thuj., verat.
Coldness	coldness of skin during pain	Ars.
Coldness	coldness of skin during pregnancy	Nux-m.
Coldness	coldness of skin in injured parts	**Led.**
Coldness	coldness of skin in spots	Agar., arg-m., berb., caust., mosch., par., petr., **Verat.**
Coldness	coldness of skin must uncover	Camph., sec.
Coldness	coldness of skin of suffering parts	Caps., caust., led., merc., mez., sil.
Coldness	coldness of skin of the upper part of body	Ip.
Coldness	coldness of skin on left side	Caust., dros., lach., sil.
Coldness	coldness of skin on left side before epilepsy	Sil.

Body part/Disease	Symptom	Medicines
Coldness	coldness of skin with internal heat	Bar-c., eupho., ferr., ign., iod., mosch., verat., zinc.
Coldness	coldness of skin with trembling	Mosch., op.
Coldness	Coldness of Temples	Bell., berb., gamb., merc-c., ol-an., ph-ac., plat., rhod., tarent.
Coldness	coldness of urethra	Clem.
Coldness	Coldness of Vertex	Agar., am-c., arn., arum-t., aur-m., bry., Calc-p., calc-s., calc., ferr-p., grat., kali-c., kali-i., kali-s., laur., mang., myric., nat-m., plat., psor., sep., sil., sulph., tarent., valer., Verat.
Coldness	Coldness of Vertex as from cold water	Tarent.
Coldness	Coldness of Vertex during menses	Sep., sulph., verat.
Coldness	Coldness of Vertex extending to sacrum	Acon.
Coldness	coldness on painful parts	Led., mez., sil.
Coldness	coldness while sitting	Kreos.
Coldness	coldness with convulsion	Aeth., Bell., cic.
Coldness	coldness with diarrhoea	Ars., Camph., carb-v., cop., laur., nux-m., podo., sec., tab., Verat.
Coldness	coldness with heat of body	Chin., colch., rhus-t.
Coldness	coldness with pain in abdomen	Ars.
Coldness	coldness yet warm bed unendurable	Camph., Led., mag-c., med., Sec.
Coldness	icy coldness in foot	Agar., apis., aur., cact., calad., Camph., Carb-v., cedr., Crot-c., cupr., dor., Elaps., eup-per., gels., graph., hep., Lach., lyc., manc., meny., merc-c., merc., nat-p., nux-m., par., Phos., psor., samb., sars., Sep., Sil., squil., sulph., Verat., zinc.
Coldness	icy coldness in leg	Apis., Calc., sep., sil., tab.
Coldness	icy coldness in leg while lying	Chin-s.
Coldness	icy coldness in soles at night	Nit-ac.
Coldness	icy coldness of forehead	Agar., ars., bar-c., calc-p., Calc., Ind., laur., nux-v., phos., sep., valer.
Coldness	icy coldness of skin	Ant-t., ars., cadm., calc., **Camph.**, **Carb-v.**, cupr., hell., lachn., nat-m., sec., tarent., verat.
Coldness	icy coldness of skin in spots	Agar., arg-m., bar-c., petr., **Verat.**
Coldness	icy coldness of the body	Acon-f., ant-t., **Ars.**, bism., bry., cadm., calc., **Camph.**, carb-s., **Carb-v.**, cic., con., **Cupr.**, hell., lachn., merc-c., nat-m., nat-s., nux-v., **Sec.**, sep., **Sil.**, stram., tarent., verat., zinc.
Coldness	icy coldness of the body as if lying on ice	Lyc.
Coldness	icy coldness of the body during menses	Sil.
Coldness	icy coldness of the body in single places	Ars., calad., camph., meny.
Coldness	icy coldness of the body in single spots	Arg-m., par., petr., verat.
Coldness	icy coldness of the body with clammy sweat & blueness , cannot bear to be covered	Sec.
Coldness	icy coldness of the body with desire to uncover	Camph., **Sec.**
Coldness	icy coldness of the body with skin dry & blue yet wants to be uncovered	Camph.

Body part/Disease	Symptom	Medicines
Coldness	icy coldness of the whole body with cold breath	**Carb-v.**, verat.
Coldness	icy coldness of Vertex	Agar., arn., laur., valer., verat.
Coldness	icy coldness of vertex even when covered	Valer.
Coldness	icy coldness running down back before epilepsy	Ars.
Collapse	collapse (sudden end to something)	Acet-ac., **Am-c.**, amyg., apis., ars-h., **Ars.**, bar-c., **Camph.**, cann-i., canth., carb-ac., **Carb-s.**, **Carb-v.**, cina., crot-h., crot-t., cupr-ar., cupr-s., cupr., dor., euon., hell., iod., jab., kali-n., laur., med., merc-c., merc., morph., naja., olnd., op., ox-ac., phos., phys., plb., sec., stram., sul-ac., tab., tax., verat., vip.
Collapse	collapse after diarrhoea	**Ars.**, **Camph.**, **Carb-v.**, **Verat.**
Collapse	collapse after vomitting	**Ars.**, lob., phys., verat.
Collapse	collapse as beginning of paralysis	Con.
Collapse	collapse during vomitting	Ars.
Collapse	congestive fever with threatened brain paralysis with collapse	Carb-v.
Collapse	sudden collapse	**Ars.**, phos.
Coma	comatose (coma) sleep after suppressed eruption	Zinc.
Coma	comatose sleep alternating with delirium	Plb.
Coma	comatose sleep alternating with delirium with sleeplessness	Camph.
Coma	comatose sleep beteen convulsions	Agar., aur., bufo., ign., **Oena.**, **Op.**, plb.
Coma	comatose sleep day & night	Bar-c.
Coma	comatose sleep during convulsions	Rheum.
Coma	comatose sleep during labor (process of childbirth)	Lach.
Coma	comatose sleep every other day	Sep.
Coma	comatose sleep in afternoon	Zing., Ant-t.
Coma	comatose sleep in evening	Ant-t., ars.
Coma	comatose sleep in forenoon	Ant-t.
Coma	comatose sleep in morning	Phos.
Coma	delirium with coma and somnolency (feeling sleepy or tending to fall asleep)	Plb., stram.
Coma	intermittent chronic fever occuring in old people with coma	Alum., nux-m., op.
Coma	respiration accelerated during coma	Stram.
Complexion	plethora (an excess of blood in a part of the body, especially in the facial veins, causing a reddish complexion)	Acon., alum., am-c., ambr., arn., ars., **Aur.**, bar-c., **Bell.**, bov., **Bry.**, **Calc.**, canth., carb-an., carb-s., carb-v., caust., cham., chel., chin., clem., cocc., coloc., con., croc., cupr., dig., dulc., ferr-ar., ferr-p., ferr., graph., guai., hep., **Hyos.**, ign., iod., ip., **Kali-bi.**, kali-c., kali-n., lach., led., **Lyc.**, mag-m., merc., mosch., nat-c., **Nat-m.**, nit-ac., nux-v., op., petr., ph-ac., **Phos.**, puls., rhod., rhus-t., sabin., sars., sec., sel., seneg., **Sep.**, **Sil.**, spig., spong., stann., staph., stram., stront., **Sulph.**, thuj., valer., verat., zinc.
Compression	compression (reduction in size) of ankle	Chlf., led., nat-m., nat-s., sep., thuj.

Body part/Disease	Symptom	Medicines
Compression	compression of ankle after walking in open air	Sep.
Compression	compression of calf	Jatr., led., sol-n.
Compression	compression of elbow	Chlor., nat-s.
Compression	compression of elbow in evening	Nat-s.
Compression	compression of first toe	Plat.
Compression	compression of foot	Ang., cimic.
Compression	compression of forearm	Led., nat-s.
Compression	compression of heel	Alum.
Compression	compression of hip	Tarent.
Compression	compression of joints	Coloc., merc.
Compression	compression of knee	Aur., led., nat-m., nat-s., plat., spig.
Compression	compression of knee while walking	Spig.
Compression	compression of left forearm	Led., nat-s.
Compression	compression of leg	Arg-n., led., nat-s.
Compression	compression of thigh	Plat., sabad., stront.
Compression	compression of thigh aggravated on motion	Sabad.
Compression	compression of thigh ameliorated on continued motion	Sabad.
Compression	compression of upper arm	Am-m., brom., led., nat-s.
Compression	compression of wrist	Led., nat-s.
Compression	convulsion from compression on spinal column	Tarent.
Condyle	arthritic (joint or joints, causing pain, swelling, and stiffness) nodosities (a lump, knob, knot, or other kind of swelling that sticks out) on condyles (rounded end of bone. The ball part of a ball-and-socket joint such as the hip or shoulder joint is a condyle) painful	Led.
Condyle	arthritic nodosities on condyles	Calc-p.
Condyle	arthritic nodosities on condyles above elbow	Mag-c.
Condyle	arthritic nodosities on condyles above elbow with stiffness	Lyc.
Condyle	arthritic nodosities on condyles on back of wrist	Petr.
Condyle	arthritic nodosities on condyles on finger joints	Aesc., agn., ant-c., Apis., Benz-ac., calc-f., calc-p., Calc., Caust., clem., colch., dig., Graph., hep., Led., Lith., Lyc., ox-ac., ran-s., rhod., sil., staph., sulph., urt-u.
Condyle	arthritic nodosities on condyles on first toe	Rhod.
Condyle	arthritic nodosities on condyles on foot	Bufo., kali-i., Led., nat-s.
Condyle	arthritic nodosities on condyles on forearm	Am-c.
Condyle	arthritic nodosities on condyles on hands	Ant-c., benz-ac., calc., carb-s., hep., led., plb.
Condyle	arthritic nodosities on condyles on knee	Bufo., calc., led., nux-v.
Condyle	arthritic nodosities on condyles on olecranon	Still.
Condyle	arthritic nodosities on condyles on shoulder	Calc., kali-i.
Condyle	arthritic nodosities on condyles on toes	Asaf., caust., graph., ran-s., sabin., sulph., thuj.

Body part/Disease	Symptom	Medicines
Condyle	arthritic nodosities on condyles on wrist	Benz-ac., calc., led., lyc., petr., rhod.
Condyle	arthritic nodosities on condyles pinching & cracking on motion	Led.
Condyle	arthritic nodosities on condyles pinching & cracking on motion in skin over joints	Led.
Condyle	arthritic nodositieson condyles on finger joints with stiffness	Carb-an., graph., Lyc.
Congestion	chill beginning in chest with violent congestion and suffocation in warm room	Apis.
Congestion	chill felt most severely in pit of stomach with violent congestion of head, cold body, with thirst and body feels bruised	**Arn.**
Congestion	congestion (condition of having an excessive amount of blood or fluid accumulate in an organ or body part) in chest after exertion	Spong.
Congestion	congestion in chest after exposure to cold air	Cimic., phos.
Congestion	congestion in chest after menses	Ign.
Congestion	congestion in chest after motion	Spong.
Congestion	congestion in chest after uterine haemorrhage	Aur-m., chin., phos.
Congestion	congestion in chest after writing	Am-c.
Congestion	congestion in chest at climaxis	Arg-n., Lach.
Congestion	congestion in chest at night	Ferr., puls.
Congestion	congestion in chest before menses	Kali-c.
Congestion	congestion in chest during menses	Glon.
Congestion	congestion in chest during pregnancy	Glon., nat-m., sep.
Congestion	congestion in chest during sleep	Mill., puls.
Congestion	congestion in chest in afternoon	Seneg.
Congestion	congestion in chest in morning	Elaps., pall.
Congestion	congestion in chest on walking	Lach.
Congestion	congestion in chest on walking in open air	Mag-m., phos.
Congestion	congestion in chest while walking rapidly	Nux-m.
Congestion	congestion in chest with weakness & nausea	Spong.
Congestion	congestion in convulsions	Glon.
Congestion	congestion in heart	Acon., asaf., cycl., Glon., hyper., lil-t., nux-m., puls., sulph.
Congestion	congestion in heart at night	Puls.
Congestion	congestion of chest alternating with congestion of head	Glon.
Congestion	congestion of face	Acon., agar., Aml-n., ant-t., apis., arg-n., Aur., bar-c., Bell., bry., cact., calc., cann-s., caust., chin., coc-c., coloc., cop., equis., eup-per., gels., Glon., hydr-ac., hyos., ign., Ind., iod., lach., lact-ac., lil-t., meli., merc-c., mit., morph., oena., op., paeon., phos., Puls., sabin., Stram., stry., tanac., thuj., ust., ziz.
Congestion	congestion of face, rubbing after	Aesc.

Body part/Disease	Symptom	Medicines
Congestion	congestive fever with threatened brain paralysis with paralysis of lungs	Ant-t., ars., carb-v., lyc., mosch., phos., sulph.
Congestion	congestive fever with threatened brain paralysis	Hell., lach., lyc., **Op.**, ph-ac., phos., tarent., zinc.
Congestion	congestive fever	Arn., bry., gels., glon., lach., sang., verat.
Consolation	Ameliorated from Consolation	Puls.
Consolation	angry when consoled	Ars., cham., nat-m.
Consolation	cough aggravated from consolation	Ars.
Consolation	Weeping aggravated from consolation	Bell., cact., calc-p., calc., chin., hell., ign., kali-c., lil-t., lyc., merc., Nat-m., nit-ac., nux-v., plat., Sep., Sil., staph., sulph., tarent., thuj.
Constipation	Aching in lumbar region when constipated	Kali-bi., tep.
Constipation	ameliorated in constipation	Calc., merc., psor.
Constipation	cheerful when constipated	Calc., psor.
Constipation	constipation after abuse of drugs	Agar., ant-c., bry., chin., Coloc., hydr., lach., Nux-v., op., ruta., sulph.
Constipation	constipation after menses	Dirc., graph., lac-c.
Constipation	constipation after wine	Zinc.
Constipation	constipation aggravated alternate days	Alum., nat-m.
Constipation	constipation can pass stool only when urinating	Aloe., alum.
Constipation	constipation during pregnancy	Agar., alum., ambr., ant-c., apis., bry., coll., coloc., con., Dol., hydr., lyc., Nat-s., Nux-v., op., Plat., Plb., podo., puls., Sep., sulph.
Constipation	constipation in aged people	Ant-c., bry., nux-v., op., phos.
Constipation	constipation must lean far back to pass stool	Med.
Constipation	constipation periodic	Kali-bi.
Constipation	constipation where stool recedes	Agn., eug., kali-s., lac-d., mag-m., mur-ac., nat-m., Op., sanic., Sil., sulph., thuj.
Constipation	constipation, passes stool easily in standing position	Caust.
Constipation	cramping pain in abdomen during constipation	Merc., op., plb., podo.
Constipation	distension of abdomen during constipation	Bry., ery-a., graph., hyos., iod., lach., mag-m., nit-ac., phos., ter.
Constipation	flatulence with constipation	Aur., iod., lyc., rhod., sulph.
Constipation	fullness during constipation (a condition in which a person has difficulty in eliminating solid waste from the body and the feces are hard and dry)	Bry., dios., ery-a., graph., hyos., iod., lach., nit-ac., nux-v., phos., ter.
Constipation	haemorrhage from urethra with constipation	Lyc.
Constipation	headache while constipated	Aloe., alum., Bry., calc-p., coff., coll., con., crot-h., ign., lac-d., lach., mag-c., merc., nat-m., nat-s., nux-v., op., petr., plb., podo., puls., verat., zinc.
Constipation	hemorrhage from urethra with constipation	Lyc.
Constipation	pain in abdomen from constipation	Ars., bell., con., cupr., kali-c., merc., op., plb., sil., sul-ac., thuj.
Constriction	breathing difficult due to constriction of trachea	Petr.

Body part/Disease	Symptom	Medicines
Constriction	breathing difficult due to tetanic constriction of larynx during convulsion	Mill.
Constriction	constricted cough from eating	Puls.
Constriction	constriction (feeling of tightness) in heart extending to back	Lil-t.
Constriction	constriction (process of narrowing) in cervical region	Agar., apis., asar., bell., chel., glon., lach., nux-m., sep.
Constriction	constriction as from band in lower part of chest	Agar., chlor., thuj.
Constriction	constriction in bladder	Alum., berb., cact., caps., caust., chel., cocc., cub., dig., hydrc., lyc., petr., ph-ac., puls., sars., thuj., verat.
Constriction	constriction in bladder after urination	Cub., nat-m.
Constriction	constriction in bladder during urination	Berb., bry., dig., petr., thuj.
Constriction	constriction in bones	Am-m., anac., aur., chin., cocc., coloc., con., graph., kreos., lyc., merc., nat-m., **Nit-ac.**, nux-v., petr., phos., **Puls.**, rhod., rhus-t., ruta., sabad., sep., sil., stront., **Sulph.**, zinc.
Constriction	Constriction in brain in morning	Agar., bry., cham., con., gamb., graph., kali-bi., nat-m., nux-m., sulph., sumb., tarax.
Constriction	Constriction in brain aggravated from bending forward	Asaf.
Constriction	Constriction in brain aggravated from sitting	Fl-ac.
Constriction	Constriction in brain aggravated from standing	Mag-c.
Constriction	Constriction in brain aggravated from stooping	Berb., coloc., dig., med., thuj.
Constriction	Constriction in brain aggravated in open air	Mang., merc., nat-m., valer.
Constriction	Constriction in brain aggravated in wet weather	Sulph.
Constriction	Constriction in brain ameliorated by heat of sun	Stront.
Constriction	Constriction in brain ameliorated from motion	Op., sulph., valer.
Constriction	Constriction in brain ameliorated from pressure	Aeth., anac., lach., meny., thuj.
Constriction	Constriction in brain ameliorated from uncovering head	Carb-v.
Constriction	Constriction in brain ameliorated from vomitting	Stann.
Constriction	Constriction in brain ameliorated from walking in open air	Ox-ac.
Constriction	Constriction in brain ameliorated from warmth	Stront.
Constriction	Constriction in brain ameliorated in morning	Glon.
Constriction	Constriction in brain ameliorated in open air	Berb., coloc., kali-i., lach., lyc.
Constriction	Constriction in brain ameliorated on lying	Nat-m.
Constriction	Constriction in brain ameliorated on rising	Dig., laur., merc.
Constriction	Constriction in brain at night	Merc., mez., nux-v.
Constriction	Constriction in brain extending to eyes and nose	Nit-ac.
Constriction	Constriction in brain from mental exertion	Iris., par., sulph.
Constriction	Constriction in brain from sleeping	Graph., merc.
Constriction	Constriction in brain in afternoon	Graph., mag-c., naja., nit-ac., phos.
Constriction	Constriction in brain in evening	Anac., asaf., hyper., kali-bi., merc., mur-ac., murx., phos., rhus-t., sep., stront., sulph., tab., tarent., valer.

Body part/Disease	Symptom	Medicines
Constriction	constriction in chest from inclination to cough	Sep.
Constriction	constriction in chest after breakfast	Agar., sulph.
Constriction	constriction in chest after coition	Staph.
Constriction	constriction in chest after dinner	Carb-s., hep., phel.
Constriction	constriction in chest after drinking	Cupr.
Constriction	constriction in chest after eating	Arn., carb-an., cupr., hep., phel., puls.
Constriction	constriction in chest after suppressed foot sweat	Sil.
Constriction	constriction in chest after talking	Hep.
Constriction	constriction in chest after vomiting	Verat-v.
Constriction	constriction in chest after waking	Dig., psor.
Constriction	constriction in chest aggravated after supper	Mez.
Constriction	constriction in chest aggravated from covering of bed	Ferr.
Constriction	constriction in chest aggravated from motion	Agar., ang., ars., ferr., led., lyc., nux-v., spong., verat.
Constriction	constriction in chest aggravated from touch	Arn., cupr.
Constriction	constriction in chest aggravated lying on left	Myric.
Constriction	constriction in chest aggravated lying on right	Lycps.
Constriction	constriction in chest aggravated lying quiet	Caps.
Constriction	constriction in chest alternating with pain in abdomen	Calc.
Constriction	constriction in chest alternating with sudden expansion	Sars.
Constriction	constriction in chest ameliorated after eating	Sulph.
Constriction	constriction in chest ameliorated during deep respiration	Sulph.
Constriction	constriction in chest ameliorated from bending backwards	Caust.
Constriction	constriction in chest ameliorated from drawing shoulders back	Calc.
Constriction	constriction in chest ameliorated from expectoration	Calc., manc.
Constriction	constriction in chest ameliorated from motion	Seneg.
Constriction	constriction in chest ameliorated from perspiration	Sulph.
Constriction	constriction in chest ameliorated from straightening up	Mez.
Constriction	constriction in chest ameliorated from warmth of bed	Phos.
Constriction	constriction in chest ameliorated from weeping	Anac.
Constriction	constriction in chest ameliorated while lying	Calc-p.
Constriction	constriction in chest ameliorated while lying head high	Ferr.
Constriction	constriction in chest ameliorated while sitting	Nux-v.
Constriction	constriction in chest ameliorated while sitting bent	Lach.
Constriction	constriction in chest ameliorated while standing	Mez.
Constriction	constriction in chest ameliorated while walking	Ferr.

Body part/Disease	Symptom	Medicines
Constriction	constriction in chest ameliorated while walking in open air	Alum., chel., dros., puls.
Constriction	constriction in chest as from band	Acon., aml-n., arg-n., ars., bry., Cact., chlor., led., lob., lyc., op., Phos., pic-ac., sil.
Constriction	constriction in chest asthmatic	Ang., coff., led., mez., naja., nux-v., sulph.
Constriction	constriction in chest at day time	Mez., phos.
Constriction	constriction in chest at night	Alum., aral., bry., coloc., ferr., kali-n., lach., mez., myric., puls., seneg., sep., sil., stram., tab.
Constriction	constriction in chest at night in bed	Ferr., nux-v.
Constriction	constriction in chest before menses	Phos.
Constriction	constriction in chest before vomiting	Cupr.
Constriction	constriction in chest convulsive	Asaf., Bell., Cupr.
Constriction	constriction in chest during chill	Ars., cimx., kali-c., Nux-v., phos.
Constriction	constriction in chest during cough	Calc., cham., cimx., con., cupr., form., hell., lyc., mag-p., merc., myrt., Phos., puls., stram., sulph.
Constriction	constriction in chest during deep respiration	Agar., aspar., caust., cham., cic., coc-c., dulc., euon., ferr., ham., kali-bi., kali-n., lact., lyc., mag-m., mosch., nat-c., nux-v., puls., sang., seneg., stry., sulph., tab., tarax., thuj.
Constriction	constriction in chest during expiring	Bor., caust., chel., kali-c.
Constriction	constriction in chest during inspiration	Agar., aspar., cham., chel., con., dros., mez., raph., sabad., seneg., sulph.
Constriction	constriction in chest during menses	Sep.
Constriction	constriction in chest during spasmodic cough	Mosch.
Constriction	constriction in chest during stool	Coloc.
Constriction	constriction in chest during whooping cough (an infectious bacterial disease that causes violent coughing mainly affects children)	Caust., mur-ac., spong.
Constriction	constriction in chest from anger	Cupr.
Constriction	constriction in chest from ascending	Ang., Ars., Calc., led., mag-c., nux-v.
Constriction	constriction in chest from becoming cold	Mosch., phos.
Constriction	constriction in chest from bending backwards	Nit-ac.
Constriction	constriction in chest from bending forward	Dig.
Constriction	constriction in chest from bringing arms together in front	Sulph.
Constriction	constriction in chest from cold air	Bry., phos., sabad.
Constriction	constriction in chest from cold bathing	Nux-m.
Constriction	constriction in chest from exertions	Ars., calc., ferr., nat-m., nux-v., spong., verat.
Constriction	constriction in chest from flatulance	Nux-v., rheum., sil.
Constriction	constriction in chest from manual labuor	Calc.
Constriction	constriction in chest from stooping	Alum., laur., merc., mez., seneg.
Constriction	constriction in chest from straightening up	Sars.
Constriction	constriction in chest from stretching	Nat-m.
Constriction	constriction in chest in afternoon	Bapt., eupi., lac-c., mag-c., nat-m., petr., sulph.

Body part/Disease	Symptom	Medicines
Constriction	constriction in chest in evening	Ars., bry., calc-p., carb-s., carb-v., hyper., puls., raph., rhus-t., stann., sulph., verb., zinc.
Constriction	constriction in chest in evening in bed	Ars., bell., berb.
Constriction	constriction in chest in hydrothorax (fluid in pleural cavity)	Apis., apoc., colch., lact., merc., psor., spig., stann.
Constriction	constriction in chest in morning	Arg-n., calc., carb-v., cycl., lyc., nat-m., phos., puls., sars., sep.
Constriction	constriction in chest in morning during fasting	Sulph.
Constriction	constriction in chest in morning on waking	Sep.
Constriction	constriction in chest in noon	Agar.
Constriction	constriction in chest on swallowing	Kali-c.
Constriction	constriction in chest on waking	Alum., dig., graph., Lach., lact., seneg., sep.
Constriction	constriction in chest one sided	Cocc., zinc.
Constriction	constriction in chest painful	Sulph., verat.
Constriction	constriction in chest preventing talking	Cact.
Constriction	constriction in chest spasmodic	Am-c., Asaf., aur., calc., carb-s., carb-v., caust., cupr., glon., hep., Ign., ip., kali-c., kali-p., lact., led., nat-m., op., phos., sars., sec., sep., spong., sulph., verat.
Constriction	constriction in chest when falling asleep	Bry., graph., lach.
Constriction	constriction in chest while cough	Carb-v., clem., dros., ip., mosch., samb., stram., sulph.
Constriction	constriction in chest while lying	Aral., lach., nat-m., nux-v.
Constriction	constriction in chest while rapid walking	Puls.
Constriction	constriction in chest while sitting	Agar., ars., mez., nit-ac.
Constriction	constriction in chest while standing	Verat.
Constriction	constriction in chest while walking	Am-c., anac., ang., Ars., dig., ferr., jug-c., kali-c., led., lyc., nux-v., puls., sulph., verat.
Constriction	constriction in chest while walking in open air	Am-c., calc., lith.
Constriction	constriction in ear	Thuj.
Constriction	constriction in heart after grief	Ign.
Constriction	constriction in heart aggravated from eating	Alum.
Constriction	constriction in heart ameliorated by bending chest forward	Lact-ac., lil-t.
Constriction	constriction in heart ameliorated from drinking water	Phos.
Constriction	constriction in heart at night	Lil-t.
Constriction	constriction in heart before epilepsy	Calc-ar., lach.
Constriction	constriction in heart from exertion	Asaf., bry.
Constriction	constriction in heart with grasping sensation	Arn., Cact., Iod., lach., laur., Lil-t., nux-m., rhus-t., spig., tarent.
Constriction	constriction in heart with inability to walk erect	Lil-t.
Constriction	constriction in heart with urging to stool	Calc-ar.
Constriction	constriction in larynx after anger	Sulph.
Constriction	constriction in larynx after drinking	Ars.

Body part/Disease	Symptom	Medicines
Constriction	constriction in larynx after eating	Puls.
Constriction	constriction in larynx aggravated on singing	Agar.
Constriction	constriction in larynx ameliorated aduring cough	Asar.
Constriction	constriction in larynx ameliorated from walking	Dros.
Constriction	constriction in larynx ameliorated in open air	Coloc.
Constriction	constriction in larynx at night	Phos., puls., rhus-t.
Constriction	constriction in larynx during cough	Agar., ars., bell., chel., Cor-r., Cupr., Dros., euphr., Hyos., ign., ip., puls., stram., sulph., verat.
Constriction	constriction in larynx from touch	Bell.
Constriction	constriction in larynx in bed	Ferr., naja.
Constriction	constriction in larynx in open air	Hep., kali-c.
Constriction	constriction in larynx on falling asleep	Kali-c., spong., sulph.
Constriction	constriction in larynx on inhaling	Hep.
Constriction	constriction in larynx on lying	Kali-bi., puls.
Constriction	constriction in larynx on swallowing	Dig.
Constriction	constriction in larynx on waking	Lach., manc., phos., thuj.
Constriction	constriction in larynx while sleeping	Agar., cench., coff., crot-h., kali-c., kali-i., Lach., naja., nit-ac., Nux-v., sep., sil., Spong., sulph., valer.
Constriction	constriction in larynx while talking	Dros., mang.
Constriction	constriction in larynx with choking cough	Agar., ars., bell., chel., Cor-r., Cupr., Dros., euphr., Hyos., ign., ip., puls., stram., sulph., verat.
Constriction	constriction in leg painful	Ant-c.
Constriction	constriction in lower part of chest aggravated from lying on right side	Lycps.
Constriction	constriction in lumbar region as from a tight band	Cina., Puls.
Constriction	constriction in neck of bladder	Ant-c., cact., canth., caps., colch., con., elaps., kali-i., mag-p., op., paeon., petr., phos., plb., ruta., sulph.
Constriction	constriction in neck of bladder after urination	Bry., cann-s., cub., sulph.
Constriction	constriction in neck of bladder during urination	Colch., kali-i., petr., polyg-h.
Constriction	constriction in orifces (opening, especially the mouth, anus, vagina, or other opening into a cavity or passage in the body)	Acon., alum., ars-i., ars., bar-c., **Bell.**, brom., **Cact.**, calc., carb-v., chel., cic., cocc., colch., con., crot-h., dig., dulc., ferr., form., graph., hep., hyos., ign., iod., ip., **Lach.**, lyc., merc-c., **Merc.**, mez., nat-m., **Nit-ac.**, nux-v., op., phos., plat., plb., rat., rhod., **Rhus-t.**, sabad., sars., sep., **Sil.**, staph., **Stram.**, sulph., sumb., tarax., thuj., verat-v., verat.
Constriction	constriction in pit on swallowing	Staph.
Constriction	constriction in right side of chest	Cocc., zinc.
Constriction	constriction in scapula	Mag-m.
Constriction	constriction in sternum (breastbone)	Acon., cann-s., lob., mur-ac., nux-m., phos., rhus-t., sabin., sulph., zinc.
Constriction	constriction in sternum on coughing	Phos.
Constriction	constriction in sternum on motion	Cact., op.
Constriction	constriction in sternum while eating	Led.

Body part/Disease	Symptom	Medicines
Constriction	constriction in stomach a night	Mag-c., rat.
Constriction	constriction in stomach after dinner	Gamb., nat-c.
Constriction	constriction in stomach after eating	Tab.
Constriction	constriction in stomach aggravated when inspirating deep	Bry.
Constriction	constriction in stomach ameliorated after eating	Rat., sep., thuj.
Constriction	constriction in stomach before menses	Sulph.
Constriction	constriction in stomach extendig to chest	Alum.
Constriction	constriction in stomach extendig to pharynx	Plb.
Constriction	constriction in stomach extendig to spine	Bor.
Constriction	constriction in stomach extendig to throat	Alum., kali-c.
Constriction	constriction in stomach in afternoon	Bar-c.
Constriction	constriction in stomach in evening	Nat-m., rat., zinc.
Constriction	constriction in stomach in forenoon	Nicc., osm.
Constriction	constriction in stomach in forenoon before eructations	Thuj.
Constriction	constriction in stomach in morning	Kali-bi., nat-m.
Constriction	constriction in stomach in morning after rising	Mang.
Constriction	constriction in stomach when fasting	Carl.
Constriction	constriction in stomach when inspiration	Viol-t.
Constriction	constriction in throat (the part of the airway and digestive tract between the mouth and both the esophagus and the windpipe) pit ameliorated from eating	Rhus-t.
Constriction	constriction in throat pit from anger	Staph.
Constriction	constriction in throat pit on going to sleep	Valer.
Constriction	constriction in trachea	Cocc., mosch., stann.
Constriction	constriction in trachea (the tube in air-breathing vertebrates that conducts air from the throat to the bronchi, strengthened by incomplete rings of cartilage)	Alum., Ars., bell., brom., calad., canth., cham., chel., cocc., hydr-ac., ign., ip., lach., laur., mag-c., mosch., phos., puls., sars., spong., stann., verat.
Constriction	constriction in trachea on lying down in evening	Ars.
Constriction	constriction in upper part of chest	Cham., phos., rhus-t.
Constriction	constriction in urethra	Cann-s., clem., lyc.
Constriction	constriction on going to sleep	Agar., arg-n., Lach., phos., spong., sulph.
Constriction	constriction while cough at night during first sleep while lying on the side	Kali-c., phos., spong.
Constriction	constriction while cough at night during sleep	Agar., lach., nit-ac., phos., sulph.
Constriction	constrictions	Alumn., arund., carb-s., chin., con., lyc., nit-ac., rhus-t.
Constriction	constrictions in ankles (joint between foot and leg)	Acon., cham., graph., helod., plat.
Constriction	constrictions in ankles as if tied with string	Acon., am-br.
Constriction	constrictions in bend of elbow	Elaps., rat.
Constriction	constrictions in big toe	Plat.

Body part/Disease	Symptom	Medicines
Constriction	constrictions in bones of upper limb	Con.
Constriction	constrictions in elbow	Agar., caust., lach., mang., petr., rat., sep.
Constriction	constrictions in elbow as with a cord	Rat.
Constriction	constrictions in elbow in morning	Petr.
Constriction	constrictions in elbow on bending	Rat.
Constriction	constrictions in fingers	Aeth., carb-an., croc., dros., elaps., lach., nux-v., phos., sep., spong.
Constriction	constrictions in fingers periodical	Phos.
Constriction	constrictions in foot	Anac., graph., nat-m., nit-ac., petr., stront.
Constriction	constrictions in forearm	Cupr., gins.
Constriction	constrictions in forearm from walking in open air	Mez.
Constriction	constrictions in hand	Cocc., cupr., nux-v., prun-s.
Constriction	constrictions in hips	Anac., anag., coloc., eug., lyc.
Constriction	constrictions in joints	Anac., aur., calc., carb-an., coloc., ferr., Graph., lyc., Nat-m., Nit-ac., petr., sil., stront.
Constriction	constrictions in knee	Anac., nat-m., nit-ac., plat., sil., sulph., zinc.
Constriction	constrictions in left elbow	Agar.
Constriction	constrictions in left shoulder	Agar.
Constriction	constrictions in leg	Anac., ars., benz-ac., Chin., guai., lyc., manc., nit-ac., petr., plat., stann., sul-ac., sulph.
Constriction	constrictions in leg as wih garter (an elastic band)	Alumn., ant-c., card-m., Chin., cocc., manc., raph.
Constriction	constrictions in lower limbs	Alum., alumn., ambr., anac., ars., carb-an., carb-s., chin., graph., Lyc., mur-ac., petr., phos., plat., stront., sul-ac., sulph.
Constriction	constrictions in nates	Plat., thuj.
Constriction	constrictions in right forearm (between the elbow and the wrist)	Cupr.
Constriction	constrictions in right upper arm	Alumn.
Constriction	constrictions in right upper arm above the elbow	Phys.
Constriction	constrictions in right upper limb	Cupr.
Constriction	constrictions in shoulder	Agar., Alumn., bov., cact., nit-ac., Alumn.
Constriction	constrictions in shoulder	Alumn.
Constriction	constrictions in tendons of wrist	Carb-v., ign., lach.
Constriction	constrictions in thigh	Acon., anac., carb-v., lyc., manc., mur-ac., nit-ac., Plat., sul-ac., sulph.
Constriction	constrictions in thigh as by a band	Coloc., sulph.
Constriction	constrictions in thigh as by a string	Am-br., lyc., manc.
Constriction	constrictions in thigh as from a tightly drawn bandage	Acon., Plat.
Constriction	constrictions in thigh while sitting	Plat.
Constriction	constrictions in thigh while walking	Lyc., olnd.
Constriction	constrictions in upper arm	Alumn., bism., manc., mez., phys.
Constriction	constrictions in upper limbs	Alumn., brom., chin., coloc., nit-ac., nux-m., raph.

Body part/Disease	Symptom	Medicines
Constriction	constrictions in wrist	Cocc., manc., sil.
Constriction	cramp like constrictions under nails	Elaps.
Constriction	impeded, obstructed breath from constriction of chest	Bell., brom., Cact., caps., chel., cic., cupr-ac.
Constriction	pain in back ascends with constriction of anus	Coloc.
Constriction	periodic Constriction of chest	Phos.
Constriction	respiration arreasted during constriction of chest	Hell., sep.
Constriction	spasmodic constrictions in right upper limb while writing	Sul-ac.
Contraction	clonic (rapid involuntary muscular contraction and relaxation in rapid succession) convulsion	Ars., atro., brom., carb-o., coc-c., cupr-s., cupr., ign., nux-m., op., phos., plb., Sec., stram., Stry., sul-ac.
Contraction	clonic convulsion of hand	Stry.
Contraction	clonic convulsion of lower limbs	Coc-c., plb., sep.
Contraction	contraction in stomach after coughing	Ars.
Contraction	contraction in stomach after coughing	Ars.
Contraction	contraction in stomach ameliorated while vomiting	Nat-c.
Contraction	contraction in stomach while vomiting	Crot-t., dig.
Contraction	contraction of extensor (a muscle that straightens or extends a part of the body, e.g. an arm or leg) muscles when writing	Nat-p.
Contraction	contraction of flexor tendons (muscle bending joint or limb)	Crot-h., sil.
Contraction	contraction of flexor tendons of hand	Plb.
Contraction	contraction of muscles & tendons at night	Plb.
Contraction	contraction of muscles & tendons during chill	Cimx.
Contraction	contraction of muscles & tendons from paralysis of extensors	Ars., Plb.
Contraction	contraction of muscles & tendons of bend of elbow	Caust., elaps., puls., sars., sulph.
Contraction	contraction of muscles & tendons of bend of thigh	Agar., carb-an., caust., rhus-t.
Contraction	contraction of muscles & tendons of calf of leg	Agar., agn., arg-n., ars., bov., calc-p., caps., caust., jatr., led., med., nat-c., nat-m., puls., sil.
Contraction	contraction of muscles & tendons of calf of leg while walking	Agar., lyc.
Contraction	contraction of muscles & tendons of calf of leg with cramp like pain	Ferr.
Contraction	contraction of muscles & tendons of elbow	Ars., glon., lyc., nux-v., tep.
Contraction	contraction of muscles & tendons of fingers after vomiting blood	Ars.
Contraction	contraction of muscles & tendons of fingers before chill	Cimx.
Contraction	contraction of muscles & tendons of fingers from abductors (a muscle that pulls the body or a limb away from a midpoint or midline)	Arg-n.
Contraction	contraction of muscles & tendons of fingers from flexors muscle	Ars., caust., cimx., sil.

Body part/Disease	Symptom	Medicines
Contraction	contraction of muscles & tendons of fingers in afternoon	Morph.
Contraction	contraction of muscles & tendons of fingers in cholera	Cupr.
Contraction	contraction of muscles & tendons of fingers in epilepsy	Lach., mag-p., merc.
Contraction	contraction of muscles & tendons of fingers in morning	Phos.
Contraction	contraction of muscles & tendons of fingers periodical	Phos.
Contraction	contraction of muscles & tendons of fingers when yawning	Crot-t., nux-v.
Contraction	contraction of muscles & tendons of fingers while grasping	Arg-n., dros., stry.
Contraction	contraction of muscles & tendons of fingers while lying on that side	Crot-t.
Contraction	contraction of muscles & tendons of first finger	Alum., cycl., graph.
Contraction	contraction of muscles & tendons of foot	Acon., cann-s., carb-an., caust., ferr-s., guare., Ind., merc-c., nat-c., nat-m., plat., sec., sep.
Contraction	contraction of muscles & tendons of forearm	Calc-ar., calc., caust., cina., coloc., con., hydrc., meny., mez., nat-c., plb., rheum., rhod., sep., stann., verat.
Contraction	contraction of muscles & tendons of forearm near the wrist	Sil.
Contraction	contraction of muscles & tendons of forearm while walking	Viol-t.
Contraction	contraction of muscles & tendons of fourth finger	Sabad., sulph.
Contraction	contraction of muscles & tendons of hamstrings (either of the two prominent common tendons of the muscles hamstring muscle behind the knee)	Acon., agar., am-m., ambr., ant-c., ant-t., asar., bar-c., calc-p., carb-an., Caust., cimx., graph., Guai., kali-ar., led., lyc., lyss., med., nat-c., Nat-m., nat-p., nit-ac., Nux-v., phos., phyt., puls., rhus-t., ruta., samb., sulph.
Contraction	contraction of muscles & tendons of hamstrings after abscess	Lach.
Contraction	contraction of muscles & tendons of hamstrings after menses	Nat-p.
Contraction	contraction of muscles & tendons of hamstrings during chill	Cimx.
Contraction	contraction of muscles & tendons of hamstrings while walking	Carb-an., Nux-v., pall., rhus-t.
Contraction	contraction of muscles & tendons of hand	Anac., ars., aur., bell., bism., calc., cann-s., carb-s., carb-v., caust., cina., cinnb., colch., coloc., euphr., ferr-s., hydr-ac., kali-bi., lyc., mag-s., merc-c., merc., mur-ac., nux-v., op., ph-ac., phos., sec., sil., sol-n., stann., sulph., tab., zinc.
Contraction	contraction of muscles & tendons of hand	Carb-v., caust., lach., sulph.
Contraction	contraction of muscles & tendons of hand alternating with feet	Stram.
Contraction	contraction of muscles & tendons of hand extending over forearm	Coloc.
Contraction	contraction of muscles & tendons of hand tearing	Sulph.

Body part/Disease	Symptom	Medicines
Contraction	contraction of muscles & tendons of heel	Colch., led., sep.
Contraction	contraction of muscles & tendons of hip	Am-m., carb-v., coloc., eupho., meny.
Contraction	contraction of muscles & tendons of hollow of knee	Am-m., ars., bell., berb., carb-an., carb-v., Caust., cimx., coloc., con., euphr., ferr., graph., Guai., kreos., lach., led., med., merc., mez., nat-c., Nat-m., nat-s., nit-ac., nux-v., ol-an., ox-ac., petr., phos., rhus-t., rhus-v., ruta., samb., staph., sulph., syph., tell., verat.
Contraction	contraction of muscles & tendons of hollow of knee during chill	Cimx.
Contraction	contraction of muscles & tendons of hollow of knee while lying on back	Nat-s.
Contraction	contraction of muscles & tendons of joints	Anac., aur., caust., colch., form., graph., merc., nat-m., nit-ac., petr., sec., stront.
Contraction	contraction of muscles & tendons of left foot	Cycl.
Contraction	contraction of muscles & tendons of left foot with cramp like pain	Nat-m., phos.
Contraction	contraction of muscles & tendons of leg	Am-c., Am-m., apoc., aster., bad., cann-i., canth., cedr., cic., ferr., merc-c., mez., nat-m., nux-v., ox-ac., phyt., puls., sulph.
Contraction	contraction of muscles & tendons of leg in evening	Cedr.
Contraction	contraction of muscles & tendons of leg in sciatica	Nux-v.
Contraction	contraction of muscles & tendons of leg while walking	Ferr.
Contraction	contraction of muscles & tendons of lower limbs	Aesc., Am-m., ambr., ars., aster., bar-c., bism., canth., Caust., coloc., guai., hydr-ac., nat-c., nat-m., nux-v., olnd., ph-ac., phos., puls., rhus-t., sec., sil., stry., tarent., tell., zinc.
Contraction	contraction of muscles & tendons of lower limbs during menses	Phos.
Contraction	contraction of muscles & tendons of lower limbs in evening	Olnd.
Contraction	contraction of muscles & tendons of lower limbs on rousing	Olnd.
Contraction	contraction of muscles & tendons of nates	Rhus-t.
Contraction	contraction of muscles & tendons of palm	Carb-an., caust., nux-v., sabad., stann., stry., verat.
Contraction	contraction of muscles & tendons of right thumb	Cycl.
Contraction	contraction of muscles & tendons of second finger	Cina., sil.
Contraction	contraction of muscles & tendons of shoulder	Brom., elaps., kali-c., mag-c., plb., rhod.
Contraction	contraction of muscles & tendons of shoulder extending to back	Mag-c.
Contraction	contraction of muscles & tendons of shoulder extending to back in morning	Mag-c.
Contraction	contraction of muscles & tendons of shoulder extending to hand	Elaps.
Contraction	contraction of muscles & tendons of shoulder in morning	Mag-c.

Body part/Disease	Symptom	Medicines
Contraction	contraction of muscles & tendons of skin	Cupr.
Contraction	contraction of muscles & tendons of sole	Berb., cham., nux-v., rhus-t., syph.
Contraction	contraction of muscles & tendons of tendo Achillis (An inelastic cord or band of tough white fibrous connective tissue that attaches a muscle to a bone or other part of heel)	Acon., calc., cann-s., carb-an., cimic., colch., euphr., graph., kali-c., sep., zinc.
Contraction	contraction of muscles & tendons of thigh	Ambr., asar., berb., carb-v., cham., mag-c., ol-an., plat., puls., rhus-t., ruta., sabin.
Contraction	contraction of muscles & tendons of thigh as if drawn together	Cann-s.
Contraction	contraction of muscles & tendons of thigh before menses	Cham.
Contraction	contraction of muscles & tendons of thigh when sitting down	Sabin.
Contraction	contraction of muscles & tendons of thigh while walking	Rhus-t., thuj.
Contraction	contraction of muscles & tendons of third finger	Sabad.
Contraction	contraction of muscles & tendons of thumb	Colch., hell., sec., staph.
Contraction	contraction of muscles & tendons of toes	Ars., asaf., crot-c., ferr-ar., ferr., gamb., gels., guare., jatr., kali-n., mag-s., merc., paeon., phyt., plat., sec.
Contraction	contraction of muscles & tendons of toes at night	Merc.
Contraction	contraction of muscles & tendons of toes at night while sitting	Kali-n.
Contraction	contraction of muscles & tendons of toes while sitting	Kali-n.
Contraction	contraction of muscles & tendons of toes while walking	Hyos.
Contraction	contraction of muscles & tendons of toes while yawning	Nux-v.
Contraction	contraction of muscles & tendons of toes with cramp like pain	Nux-v.
Contraction	contraction of muscles & tendons of upper arm	Caust.
Contraction	contraction of muscles & tendons of upper arm	Calc., nat-m., rhod., stram., sulph.
Contraction	contraction of muscles & tendons of Upper limbs	Agar., all-s., ant-t., ars., atro., bell., calc., cann-i., carb-s., ferr., hydr-ac., ip., lyc., merc-c., merc., nux-v., olnd., op., ox-ac., phos., plb., ran-b., rhod., rhus-t., sec., tab.
Contraction	contraction of muscles & tendons of Upper limbs during paralysis	Carb-s.
Contraction	contraction of muscles & tendons of Upper limbs on attempting to drink	Atro.
Contraction	contraction of muscles & tendons of wrist	Jatr.
Contraction	contraction of muscles & tendons of wrist with shortening of tendons	Carb-v., caust.
Contraction	contraction of muscles & tendons periodic	Sec.
Contraction	contraction of muscles & tendons stiff during exacerbation (severity of desease) of pains	Phos.

Body part/Disease	Symptom	Medicines
Contraction	contraction of muscles & tendons, sudden	Sec.
Contraction	contraction of opening of urethra after urination	Coc-c., thuj.
Contraction	contraction of scrotum	Acon., arn., berb., cann-s., clem., ferr-m., op., plb.
Contraction	contraction of urethra	Asar., canth., carb-an., carb-v., chin., clem., cop., dig., indg., nux-v., petr., phos., Puls., stram., verat., zinc.
Contraction	contraction of urethra after urination	Nux-v.
Contraction	contraction of urethra before stool & urination	Nat-m.
Contraction	contraction of urethra during erection	Canth.
Contraction	contraction of urethra during urination	Bry., clem., dig., indg.
Contraction	contraction of urethra from suppressed gonorrhoea	Puls.
Contraction	contraction of urethra in morning	Carb-v.
Contraction	contraction of urethra with urging to urinate	Nat-m.
Contraction	cramp in toes alternating with spasm (muscle contraction) of glottis (voice box)	Asaf.
Contraction	sensation of contraction in bladder	Ant-c., berb., carb-s., coc-c., hyos., kali-i., lyc., mez., op., petr., ruta., verat.
Contraction	sleepiness from contraction of eyelids	Ant-t., con., croc., kali-c.
Contraction	spasm (involuntary muscle contraction) of eyelids	Agar., alum., bell., calc-p., calc., camph., chin-a., croc., cupr., euphr., mag-p., merc-c., nat-m., nux-v., plat., plb., puls., ruta., sep., sil.
Contraction	spasmodic constrictions in right upper limb while writing	Sul-ac.
Contraction	spasmodic pain in arm	Agar., lact., mosch., olnd., valer.
Contraction	spasmodic yawning	Acon., agar., am-c., ang., ant-t., arn., bry., calc., cina., cocc., coloc., cor-r., croc., cupr., euphr., hep., ign., laur., mag-p., med., mosch., nat-m., nux-v., **Plat.**, **Rhus-t.**, sep., squil., staph., sulph., tarent.
Contraction	spasmodic yawning after stool	Anac., op.
Contraction	spasmodic yawning after supper	Coca., lyc., ruta.
Contraction	spasmodic yawning after walking in open air	Nat-m.
Contraction	spasmodic yawning ameliorated after wine	Nat-m.
Contraction	spasmodic yawning ameliorated while walking in open air	Plan.
Contraction	spasmodic yawning before supper	Merc.
Contraction	spasmodic yawning in evening	Am-c., ign., sulph.
Contraction	spasmodic yawning in morning	Ign.
Contraction	spasmodic yawning in warm bed	Chin-s.
Contraction	spasmodic yawning in warm rooms	Mez.
Contraction	spasmodic yawning while walking	Camph., chlf.
Contraction	spasmodic yawning while walking in open air	Eug., euphr., lycps., stann.
Contraction	spasmodically abducted convulsion of lower limbs	Lyc., merc.
Contraction	spasms (an involuntary sudden muscle contraction) of sides of neck	Carb-ac., med.

Body part/Disease	Symptom	Medicines
Contraction	spasms compelling him to retch	Graph., Merc-c.
Contraction	spasms compelling him to swallow liquids only	Bapt., bar-c., plb.
Contraction	spasms in back on touch	Acon.
Contraction	spasms in back while nursing	Arn., cham., puls.
Contraction	sudden contraction of muscles & tendons of shoulder	Alum.
Contraction	weakness in upper limbs after spasms	**Cic.**
Convulsion	anger before convulsion	Bufo.
Convulsion	Biting with convulsions (uncontrollable shaking)	Lyss.
Convulsion	breathing difficult due to constriction of larynx during convulsion	Lyss., op., stry., tanac.
Convulsion	breathing difficult due to tetanic constriction of larynx during convulsion	Mill.
Convulsion	cheerful after convulsions (uncontrollable shaking)	Sulph.
Convulsion	chill in evening followed by convulsion and heat lasting all night	Cina.
Convulsion	clenching covulsive	Glon., mag-p., nux-m., nux-v.
Convulsion	clenching from epileptic covulsion	Lach., mag-p., oena.
Convulsion	clonic (rapid involuntary muscular contraction and relaxation in rapid succession) convulsion	Ars., atro., brom., carb-o., coc-c., cupr-s., cupr., ign., nux-m., op., phos., plb., Sec., stram., Stry., sul-ac.
Convulsion	coldness in thigh at night with convulsion	Calc.
Convulsion	coldness of skin during convulsions	Anan., camph., caust., cic., hell., hyos., mosch., **Oena.,** op., stram., verat.
Convulsion	coldness with convulsion	Aeth., Bell., cic.
Convulsion	comatose sleep beteen convulsions	Agar., aur., bufo., ign., **Oena., Op.,** plb.
Convulsion	comatose sleep during convulsions	Rheum.
Convulsion	congestion in convulsions	Glon.
Convulsion	constriction in chest convulsive	Asaf., Bell., Cupr.
Convulsion	convulsion with falling	Agar., alum., am-c., ars., aster., **Bell.,** calc-p., calc., canth., caust., cedr., **Cham.,** cic., cina., cocc., con., **Cupr.,** dig., dulc., **Hyos.,** ign., iod., ip., laur., lyc., merc., nit-ac., **Oena.,** op., petr., ph-ac., phos., plb., sec., sep., sil., stann., staph., stram., sulph., verat., zinc.
Convulsion	convulsion (uncontrollable shaking) aggravated by coffee	Stram.
Convulsion	convulsion after anger	Bufo., **Cham.,** cina., kali-br., lyss., **Nux-v.,** op., plat., sulph.
Convulsion	convulsion after being unjustly accused	Staph.
Convulsion	convulsion after coition	Agar.
Convulsion	convulsion after coughing	Cupr., ip.
Convulsion	convulsion after drinking	Ars., bell., hyos.
Convulsion	convulsion after eating	Cina., grat., hyos.
Convulsion	convulsion after exertion	Alum., calc., glon., kalm., lach., lyss., nat-m., petr., sulph.

Body part/Disease	Symptom	Medicines
Convulsion	convulsion after grief	Art-v., hyos., ign., nat-m., op.
Convulsion	convulsion after hiccough	Bell.
Convulsion	convulsion after loss of sleep	Cocc.
Convulsion	convulsion after menses	Syph.
Convulsion	convulsion after mental exertion	Bell., glon.
Convulsion	convulsion after metastasis (spread of Cancer)	Cupr.
Convulsion	convulsion after midnight	Cupr.
Convulsion	convulsion after miscarriage	Ruta.
Convulsion	convulsion after mortification (death and decay of living tissue)	Calc.
Convulsion	convulsion after onanism	Bufo., calad., calc., dig., elaps., kali-br., lach., naja., nux-v., **Plat.**, plb., sep., sil., stram., sulph.
Convulsion	convulsion after palpitation	Glon.
Convulsion	convulsion after punishment	Cham., cina., **Ign.**
Convulsion	convulsion after running	Sulph.
Convulsion	convulsion after shocks	Op.
Convulsion	convulsion after suppressed foot sweat	**Sil.**
Convulsion	convulsion after suppressed milk	Agar.
Convulsion	convulsion after suppressed secretions and excretions	Ars., bufo., canth., lach., tarent.
Convulsion	convulsion after vaccination	**Sil.**
Convulsion	convulsion after vertigo on rising from a chair	Nux-v.
Convulsion	convulsion aggravated by draft	Ars., lyss., **Nux-v.**, **Stry.**
Convulsion	convulsion aggravated by motion	Cocc., nux-v.
Convulsion	convulsion aggravated from light	Bell., **Lyss.**, nux-v., op., **Stram.**
Convulsion	convulsion aggravated from motion	Ars., bell., cocc., graph., nux-v., stry.
Convulsion	convulsion aggravated from wiping perspiration from face	Nux-v.
Convulsion	convulsion alternating with excitement of mind	**Stram.**
Convulsion	convulsion alternating with rage	**Stram.**
Convulsion	convulsion alternating with trembling of body	Nux-v.
Convulsion	convulsion alternating with unconsciousness	Agar., aur.
Convulsion	convulsion ameliorated by bending elbow	Nux-v.
Convulsion	convulsion ameliorated during vomiting	Agar.
Convulsion	convulsion ameliorated from bending head backwards	**Nux-v.**
Convulsion	convulsion ameliorated from cold water	Caust.
Convulsion	convulsion ameliorated from diarrhoea	Lob.
Convulsion	convulsion ameliorated from eructations	Kali-c.
Convulsion	convulsion ameliorated from forceful extension of body	Nux-v., stry.
Convulsion	convulsion ameliorated from riding in carriage	Nit-ac.
Convulsion	convulsion ameliorated from rubbing	Phos., sec.

Body part/Disease	Symptom	Medicines
Convulsion	convulsion ameliorated from stretching limbs	Sec.
Convulsion	convulsion ameliorated from stretching out parts	Sec.
Convulsion	convulsion ameliorated from tight grasp	Nux-v.
Convulsion	convulsion ameliorated from tightly binding the body	Mez.
Convulsion	convulsion ameliorated from vinegar	Stram.
Convulsion	convulsion ameliorated from warm bath	Apis., glon., nat-m., op.
Convulsion	convulsion apoplectic (furious)	Bell., crot-h., cupr., lach., nux-v., stram.
Convulsion	convulsion at midnight	Bufo., cina., cocc., sant., zinc.
Convulsion	convulsion at night	Arg-n., ars., art-v., aur., bufo., calc-ar., calc., caust., cic., cina., cupr., dig., hyos., kali-c., kalm., lyc., merc., nit-ac., nux-v., oena., **Op.**, plb., sec., **Sil.**, stram., sulph., zinc.
Convulsion	convulsion at puberty	Caust.
Convulsion	convulsion at puerperal (relating to childbirth)	Ambr., apis., arg-n., ars., art-v., **Bell.**, canth., carb-v., caust., cham., **Cic.**, cimic., cocc., coff., crot-c., cupr., gels., glon., hell., hydr-ac., **Hyos.**, ign., ip., lach., laur., lyc., lyss., mag-p., merc-c., mosch., nux-m., nux-v., oena., op., plat., puls., sec., **Stram.**, ter., verat-v., verat., zinc.
Convulsion	convulsion at puerperal with blindness	Aur-m., cocc., cupr.
Convulsion	convulsion at puerperal with haemorrhage	Chin., hyos., plat., sec.
Convulsion	convulsion at sight of strange person	Lyss.
Convulsion	convulsion at sight of water	Bell., **Lyss.**, **Stram.**
Convulsion	convulsion before epilepsy with sensation of expansion of body	Arg-n.
Convulsion	convulsion before menses	Bufo., carb-v., caust., cupr., hyos., kali-br., oena., puls.
Convulsion	convulsion begin in arm	Bell.
Convulsion	convulsion begin in back	Sulph.
Convulsion	convulsion begin in face	Absin., bufo., cina., dulc., hyos., ign., lach., sant., sec.
Convulsion	convulsion begin in finger & toes	Cupr.
Convulsion	convulsion begin in the abdomen	Aran., bufo.
Convulsion	convulsion during attempt to swallow	**Lyss.**, mur-ac., nux-m., stram.
Convulsion	convulsion during chill	Ars., Lach., merc., nux-v.
Convulsion	convulsion during coition	Bufo.
Convulsion	convulsion during colic	Plb.
Convulsion	convulsion during cough	Cupr.
Convulsion	convulsion during dentition	Acon., aeth., art-v., bell., **Calc.**, **Cham.**, cic., cina., cupr., hyos., ign., kreos., merc., podo., stann., stram.
Convulsion	convulsion during emission of semen	Art-v., grat., nat-p.
Convulsion	convulsion during heat	Cic., cina., cur., hyos., **Nux-v.**, op., **Stram.**
Convulsion	convulsion during menses	Nux-m., tarent.
Convulsion	convulsion during nervous weakness	Sep.
Convulsion	convulsion during pregnancy	Cedr., cham., cic., cupr., hyos., lyc., mill.

Body part/Disease	Symptom	Medicines
Convulsion	convulsion during sleep	Bufo., caust., cic., cupr., hyos., ign., kali-c., lach., oena., op., sec., sil., stram.
Convulsion	convulsion during vomiting	Guar., op.
Convulsion	convulsion epileptic from heart	**Calc-ar.**, lach., naja.
Convulsion	convulsion epileptic from right heel to occiput	Stram.
Convulsion	convulsion epileptic from solar plexus (a point on the upper abdomen just below where the ribs separate)	Art-v., bell., bufo., calc., caust., **Cic.**, cupr., indg., **Nux-v.**, sil., **Sulph.**
Convulsion	convulsion epileptic in uterus to throat	Lach.
Convulsion	convulsion epileptic in uterus	Bufo.
Convulsion	convulsion epileptic knees	Cupr.
Convulsion	convulsion epileptic like a mouse running	**Bell.**, **Calc.**, ign., nit-ac., *sil.*, *sulph.*
Convulsion	convulsion epileptic with aura (warning sensation before epileptic episode) abdomen to head	Indg.
Convulsion	convulsion epileptic with coldness running down spine	Ars.
Convulsion	convulsion epileptic with drawing in limbs	Ars.
Convulsion	convulsion epileptic with jerk in nape	Bufo.
Convulsion	convulsion epileptic with nervous feeling	Arg-n., nat-m.
Convulsion	convulsion epileptic with numbness of brain	Bufo.
Convulsion	convulsion epileptic with sensation of cold air over spine and body	Agar.
Convulsion	convulsion epileptic with shocks	Ars., laur.
Convulsion	convulsion epileptic with warm air streaming up spine	Ars.
Convulsion	convulsion epileptic with waving sensation in brain	Cimic.
Convulsion	convulsion followed by paralysis	**Caust.**
Convulsion	convulsion from becoming cold	Bell., caust., cic., mosch., nux-v.
Convulsion	convulsion from bone in throat	Cic.
Convulsion	convulsion from bright light	Bell., lyss., nux-v., op., **Stram.**
Convulsion	convulsion from cerebral softening	Caust.
Convulsion	convulsion from cold air	Ars., bell., cic., merc., nux-v.
Convulsion	convulsion from cold drinks	Cupr.
Convulsion	convulsion from coldness of one side of the body	Sil.
Convulsion	convulsion from coldness of the body	Camph., caust., cic., hell., hyos., mosch., **Oena.**, op., stram., verat.
Convulsion	convulsion from compression on spinal column	Tarent.
Convulsion	convulsion from contradiction	Aster.
Convulsion	convulsion from disappointed love	Hyos.
Convulsion	convulsion from errors in diet	Cic.
Convulsion	convulsion from excitement	Acon., agar., aster., bell., cham., cic., cimic., coff., cupr., gels., **Hyos.**, ign., kali-br., nux-v., **Op.**, plat., puls., sec., tarent.
Convulsion	convulsion from fluids	Bell., canth., hyos., **Lyss.**, **Stram.**
Convulsion	convulsion from forcibly aroused from trance (dazed state)	Nux-m.

Body part/Disease	Symptom	Medicines
Convulsion	convulsion from fright	Acon., agar., apis., arg-n., art-v., bufo., **Calc.**, caust., cic., cupr., **Hyos.**, **Ign.**, **Indg.**, kali-br., lyss., **Op.**, plat., sec., stram., sulph., tarent., verat., zinc.
Convulsion	convulsion from indigestion	**Ip.**
Convulsion	convulsion from indignation (anger at unfairness)	Staph.
Convulsion	convulsion from injuries	Arn., art-v., cic., **Hyper.**, nat-s., oena., op., rhus-t., sulph., valer.
Convulsion	convulsion from laughing	Coff., graph.
Convulsion	convulsion from lying on side	Puls.
Convulsion	convulsion from lying on side convulsively turned on the back	Cic.
Convulsion	convulsion from mercurial vapours	Stram.
Convulsion	convulsion from nervousness	Arg-n.
Convulsion	convulsion from noise	Ant-c., arn., cic., ign., lyss., nux-v., stry.
Convulsion	convulsion from pressure on spine	Tarent.
Convulsion	convulsion from pressure on stomach	Canth., cupr., nux-v.
Convulsion	convulsion from sexual excitement	Bufo., lach., plat.
Convulsion	convulsion from shining objects	Bell., **Lyss.**, **Stram.**
Convulsion	convulsion from strong odors	Lyss.
Convulsion	convulsion from suppressed discharges	Asaf., cupr., stram.
Convulsion	convulsion from suppressed eruption	Agar., bry., calc., caust., cupr., stram., sulph., zinc.
Convulsion	convulsion from suppressed menses	Bufo., calc-p., cocc., cupr., gels., puls.
Convulsion	convulsion from thunderstorm	Agar., gels.
Convulsion	convulsion from vexation (Annoyance)	Ars., bell., calc., camph., **Cupr.**, ign., ip., nux-v., staph., sulph.
Convulsion	convulsion hysterical	Absin., alum., apis., ars., **Asaf.**, aur., bell., bry., calc-s., calc., cann-s., caust., cedr., cham., cic., cimic., cocc., coff., coll., **Con.**, croc., gels., hyos., **Ign.**, iod., ip., lach., lyc., mag-m., merc., **Mosch.**, nat-m., nit-ac., nux-m., nux-v., op., petr., phos., plat., plb., puls., sec., sep., staph., stram., sulph., sumb., tarent., valer., verat-v., verat., zinc.
Convulsion	convulsion in addison's disease (a wasting disease caused by failure of the adrenal glands to function normally and characterized by bronzing of the skin, low blood pressure, and weakness)	Calc.
Convulsion	convulsion in afternoon	Arg-m., stann.
Convulsion	convulsion in children	Acon., aeth., agar., ambr., apis., **Art-v.**, **Bell.**, bry., calc., camph., caust., cham., cic., **Cina.**, cocc., coff., crot-c., cupr., dol., gels., **Hell.**, hep., hydr-ac., hyos., ign., ip., kali-c., lach., laur., lyc., mag-p., nux-v., **Op.**, plat., sec., sil., **Stram.**, sulph., **Verat.**, **Zinc.**
Convulsion	convulsion in children from approach of strangers	Op.
Convulsion	convulsion in drunkards	Glon., nux-v., ran-b.
Convulsion	convulsion in evening	Alum., **Calc.**, caust., croc., gels., laur., merc-n., op., stann., stram., sulph.

Body part/Disease	Symptom	Medicines
Convulsion	convulsion in evening in open air	Caust.
Convulsion	convulsion in extensor muscles	**Cina.**
Convulsion	convulsion in left side of body	Calc-p., cupr., elaps., graph., ip., nat-m., plb., sulph.
Convulsion	convulsion in morning	Arg-n., art-v., calc., caust., cocc., crot-h., kalm., lyc., mag-p., nux-v., plat., sec., sep., Squil., sulph., tab.
Convulsion	convulsion in morning from 4.00 a.m. to 4.00 p.m.	Calc.
Convulsion	convulsion in right side of body	Bell., caust., **Lyc.**, nux-v.
Convulsion	convulsion instead of menses	Oena.
Convulsion	convulsion intermittent	Absin.
Convulsion	convulsion interrupted by painful shocks	Stry.
Convulsion	convulsion of calf	Berb., cupr., ferr-m.
Convulsion	convulsion of extensor muscles	Cina.
Convulsion	convulsion of first finger	Cycl.
Convulsion	convulsion of first toe	Apis.
Convulsion	convulsion of flexor muscles	Carb-o., cham.
Convulsion	convulsion of foot	Bar-m., calc., camph., cupr., iod., merc-c., nat-m., nux-v., op., phos., sec., stram., zinc.
Convulsion	convulsion of foot at night	Iod.
Convulsion	convulsion of foot during menses	Hyos.
Convulsion	convulsion of foot extending to knees	Stram.
Convulsion	convulsion of foot from touch	Nux-v.
Convulsion	convulsion of forearm	Chen., sec., zinc.
Convulsion	convulsion of hand	Acon., ambr., anac., arum-t., bar-m., bell., bism., calc., camph., cann-s., carb-s., carb-v., caust., coloc., dros., graph., iod., kali-bi., kali-i., merc., mosch., nat-m., paeon., plat., plb., sec., stram., stry., sul-ac., tab., zinc.
Convulsion	convulsion of hand during menses	Hyos.
Convulsion	convulsion of hand from taking hold of something	Ambr., dros., stry., sulph.
Convulsion	convulsion of hip	Phos.
Convulsion	convulsion of knee	Berb.
Convulsion	convulsion of left side	Ip.
Convulsion	convulsion of left upper limbs	Caust.
Convulsion	convulsion of leg	Acet-ac., ant-t., ars., cann-i., card-m., cupr-s., jatr., kali-i., merc-c., podo., sep., stram., stry., tab., tarent., tell.
Convulsion	convulsion of lower limbs	Ars., cann-i., cic., cina., cocc., crot-c., cupr., gamb., hydr-ac., hyos., ign., ip., lach., lyss., merc-c., mosch., nux-v., op., phos., plb., sec., spong., squil., stram., Stry., tab.
Convulsion	convulsion of lower limbs at night	Plb.
Convulsion	convulsion of nates	Bar-c., calc., nux-v., sep.
Convulsion	convulsion of radial (muscles of radius bone of the forearm) muscles	Merc.
Convulsion	convulsion of right leg	Acet-ac., podo., stram.

Body part/Disease	Symptom	Medicines
Convulsion	convulsion of right side	Chen-a.
Convulsion	convulsion of right side with left side paralyzed	Art-v.
Convulsion	convulsion of thigh	Ars., dig., podo.
Convulsion	convulsion of thumb	Aesc., arum-t., bell., cocc., cupr., cycl., nat-m.
Convulsion	convulsion of toes	Chel., cupr., sec.
Convulsion	convulsion of upper limb then the lower limbs	Phos.
Convulsion	convulsion of upper limbs after miscarriage	Ruta.
Convulsion	convulsion of upper limbs ameliorated from working hard with hands	Agar.
Convulsion	convulsion of upper limbs at night	Bell., nux-v., sulph.
Convulsion	convulsion of upper limbs extending to fingers	Acon.
Convulsion	convulsion of upper limbs extending to trunk (the main part of the body excluding the head, neck, and limbs)	Agar-ph.
Convulsion	convulsion of upper limbs from drawing limbs backwards	Am-c.
Convulsion	convulsion of upper limbs from epileptic starting	Sulph.
Convulsion	convulsion of upper limbs from right to left	Visc.
Convulsion	convulsion of upper limbs in prosopalgia (a disorder of the trigeminal nerve (the fifth cranial nerve) that causes episodes of sharp, stabbing pain in the cheek, lips, gums, or chin on one side of the face)	Plat.
Convulsion	convulsion of upper limbs in prosopalgia (a disorder of the trigeminal nerve (the fifth cranial nerve) that causes episodes of sharp, stabbing pain in the cheek, lips, gums, or chin on one side of the face)	Plat.
Convulsion	convulsion of upper limbs more than legs	Camph., stram.
Convulsion	convulsion of upper limbs one sided	Sabad.
Convulsion	convulsion on attempting to speak	Lyss.
Convulsion	convulsion on closing a door	Stry.
Convulsion	convulsion on left side before epilepsy	Sil.
Convulsion	convulsion on waking	Bell.
Convulsion	convulsion one side other side paralyzed	Apis., art-v., hell., stram.
Convulsion	convulsion one sided	Apoc., art-v., bell., calc-p., caust., dulc., elaps., gels., graph., hell., ip., plb.
Convulsion	convulsion paralyzed side	Phos., sec.
Convulsion	convulsion periodic	Agar., ars., bar-m., calc., cedr., chin-s., cupr., ign., indg., lyc., nat-m., sec., stram.
Convulsion	convulsion periodic every 14 days	Cupr., oena.
Convulsion	convulsion periodic every 7 days	Agar., chin-s., indg., nat-m.
Convulsion	convulsion syphilitic	Nit-ac.
Convulsion	convulsion tetanic (capable of producing muscle spasms such as those seen in tetanus)	Ars., hydr-ac., hyper., mill.

Body part/Disease	Symptom	Medicines
Convulsion	convulsion uremic (form of blood poisoning)	Apoc., crot-h., cupr-ar., cupr., dig., hydr-ac., kali-s., merc-c., mosch., plb., ter.
Convulsion	convulsion when eruptions fail to break out	Ant-t., **Cupr.**, **Zinc.**
Convulsion	convulsion when skin rash repelled or do not appear	Ant-t., bry., camph., cupr., gels., ip., stram., sulph., **Zinc.**
Convulsion	convulsion when small pox fails to break	**Ant-t.**
Convulsion	convulsion when touched	Acon., bell., carb-o., **Cic.**, cocc., lyss., nux-v., stram., stry.
Convulsion	convulsion when turning the head	Cic.
Convulsion	convulsion while eating	Plb.
Convulsion	convulsion while touching eyelids	Coc-c.
Convulsion	convulsion with aura	Calc., lach., sulph.
Convulsion	convulsion with consciousness	Ars., bell., calc., camph., canth., caust., **Cina.**, grat., hell., hyos., ip., kali-ar., kali-c., lyc., mag-c., merc., mur-ac., nat-m., nit-ac., nux-m., nux-v., phos., plat., plb., sec., sep., sil., **Stram.**, stry., sulph.
Convulsion	convulsion with downward spread	Cic., sec.
Convulsion	convulsion with falling backwards	Bell., canth., chin., cic., ign., ip., nux-v., oena., **Op.**, rhus-t., spig., stram.
Convulsion	convulsion with falling forward	Arn., aster., calc-p., canth., cic., cupr., ferr., rhus-t., sil., sulph., sumb.
Convulsion	convulsion with falling left side	Bell., caust., lach., sabad.
Convulsion	convulsion with falling right side	Bell.
Convulsion	convulsion with haemorrhage	Chin., hyos., plat., sec.
Convulsion	convulsion with paralysis	Arg-n., bell., **Caust.**, cic., cocc., cupr., hyos., lach., laur., nux-m., nux-v., phos., plat., plb., rhus-t., sec., stann., tab., vib., zinc.
Convulsion	convulsion with tetanic rigidity	Absin., acon., aesc., alum., am-c., anac., arn., ars., asaf., bell., camph., cann-i., cann-s., canth., carb-o., caust., cham., chin-s., chlol., **Cic.**, cocc., con., cupr-ar., cupr., cur., dros., gels., hell., hep., hydr-ac., hyos., **Hyper.**, ign., ip., kreos., lach., laur., led., lob., lyc., lyss., mag-p., merc., mosch., mur-ac., **Nux-v.**, oena., op., **Petr.**, phos., phys., phyt., **Plat.**, plb., puls., rhod., rhus-t., sec., seneg., **Sep.**, sol-n., stram., stry., sulph., teucr., ther., verat-v., verat., zinc.
Convulsion	convulsion with tetanic rigidity amelioratic from dashing cold water on face	Benz-n.
Convulsion	convulsion with tetanic rigidity with injured parts become cold as ice and spasms begin in the wound	**Led.**
Convulsion	convulsion with wounds in the soles, finger and palm	Bell., **Hyper.**, led.
Convulsion	convulsion without consciousness	Absin., acet-ac., acon., aeth., ant-t., **Arg-n.**, ars., aster., aur., bell., **Bufo.**, calc-ar., calc-s., **Calc.**, camph., **Canth.**, carb-ac., caust., cham., chin., **Cic.**, cina., cocc., crot-h., cupr., dig., ferr., glon., hydr-ac., **Hyos.**, ip., kali-c., lach., laur., led., lyc., merc., mosch., nat-m., nit-ac., nux-v., **Oena.**, op., phos., plat., **Plb.**, sec., sep., sil., staph., stram., sulph., tanac., tarent., verat., **Visc.**
Convulsion	convulsion, noise arrests the paroxysm	Hell.
Convulsion	convulsions interrupted by painful shocks	Stry.

Body part/Disease	Symptom	Medicines
Convulsion	convulsive contraction of muscles & tendons of heel in bed	Am-m.
Convulsion	convulsive motion	Absin., acon., agar-ph., **Agar.**, arg-n., aster., aur-m., **Bell.**, calc-p., cann-i., carb-s., caust., chlor., cocc., colch., crot-h., cupr., kali-c., lyc., merc-c., mygal., **Op.**, phos., plb., rhus-t., sant., sec., **Stram.**, sul-ac., verat., zinc., ziz.
Convulsion	convulsive motion ameliorated when lying on side	Calc-p.
Convulsion	convulsive motion of foot	zinc.
Convulsion	convulsive motion of hands	Apis., bell., kali-c., nat-m., op., plb., zinc.
Convulsion	convulsive motion of leg	Acet-ac., agar., caust., merc-c., mygal., op., plb., sul-ac.
Convulsion	convulsive motion of lower limbs	Merc-c., mygal., plb., stram.
Convulsion	convulsive motion of thumb	Calc-p., calc., coc-c., con., crot-c.
Convulsion	convulsive motion of upper limbs	Apis., arg-n., aur-m., bell., caust., con., merc-c., mez., mygal., op., plb., stram., sul-ac., tab., zinc-s.
Convulsion	convulsive motion when lying on back	Calc-p.
Convulsion	convulsive trembling	Acon., asaf., carb-h., crot-h., op.
Convulsion	convulsive trembling of first finger	Calc.
Convulsion	convulsive trembling of foot	Hyos., kali-cy.
Convulsion	convulsive trembling of hand	Colch., hyos., plb.
Convulsion	convulsive twitching of calf	Op.
Convulsion	convulsive twitching of hand	Brom., colch., nux-v., phyt.
Convulsion	convulsive twitching of leg	Ars., bad., phyt., stram.
Convulsion	cough with convulsions	Ars., bell., brom., calc., cham., cina., croc., Cupr., dros., hyos., led., meph., stram., sulph., verat.
Convulsion	covulsions beginning in face	Absin., bufo., cina., dulc., hyos., ign., sant., sec.
Convulsion	covulsions in left side of face	Lach.
Convulsion	covulsions in masseters (cheek muscle)	Ambr., ang., cocc., cupr., mang., nux-v.
Convulsion	covulsions of face before menses	Puls.
Convulsion	covulsions of face while speaking	Plb.
Convulsion	covulsions of lips	Ambr., caust., crot-c., kali-c., ran-b.
Convulsion	covulsions of right side of face	Agar.
Convulsion	cracking in joints during convulsions	Acon.
Convulsion	cursing during convulsions	Ars.
Convulsion	deep sleep after convulsions	Bufo., canth., caust., hell., hyos., ign., lach., **Nux-v.**, oena., **Op.**, plb., sec., sulph., tarent.
Convulsion	deep sleep between convulsions	Agar., bufo., ign., **Oena.**, **Op.**, plb.
Convulsion	delirium after convulsions	Absin., bell., kali-c., sec.
Convulsion	delirium before convulsions	Op.
Convulsion	delirium during convulsions	Ars., crot-h.
Convulsion	diplopia with convulsions	Bell., cic., hyos., nux-v., stram.
Convulsion	discoloration of skin yellow / jaundice with convulsion	Agar.
Convulsion	discoloration with blueness on hand with convulsion	Aesc.

Body part/Disease	Symptom	Medicines
Convulsion	discolouration of face blue with convulsions	Cic., Cupr., hyos., ip., oena., phys., stry.
Convulsion	distesion of abdomen, during convulsion	Cic.
Convulsion	extremities flexed during convulsion	Colch., hydr-ac., hyos., phos., plb.
Convulsion	fever with intense heat with convulsions	**Bell.**, cic., hyos., op., **Stram.**
Convulsion	formication after convulsion	Stry.
Convulsion	from stretching out limbs before convulsions	Calc.
Convulsion	hiccough convulsive	Aeth., ars., bell., Gels., mag-p., nux-v., ran-b., stram., tab.
Convulsion	involuntary urination during convulsion	Art-v., Bufo., caust., cocc., cupr., Hyos., nux-v., oena., plb., stry., zinc.
Convulsion	jerking as in convulsion	Acon., agar., alum., **Ambr.**, ant-c., arg-m., arn., ars., bell., bry., calc., camph., cann-s., caps., carb-v., **Caust.**, cham., chin., cic., coloc., cupr., dig., dros., dulc., hep., hyos., ign., ip., kali-c., lach., laur., lil-t., lyc., mag-c., meny., merc., mez., mur-ac., nat-c., **Nat-m.**, nit-ac., nux-v., op., petr., phos., plat., **Plb.**, ran-b., rhod., sabad., sec., sep., sil., squil., staph., stram., stront., sul-ac., sulph., thuj., verat., viol-t., zinc.
Convulsion	jerking of hand convulsive (uncontrollable shaking)	Bar-m., merc.
Convulsion	letting legs swing excites convulsion	Calc.
Convulsion	metrorrhagia with convulsion	Bell., chin., hyos., Sec.
Convulsion	motion between convulsions in fever	Arg-n.
Convulsion	numbness in fingers between convulsiions	Sec.
Convulsion	numbness in leg before convulsion	Plb.
Convulsion	pain in back with convulsions	Acon.
Convulsion	pain in extremities after convulsions	Plb.
Convulsion	pain in soles of foot from convulsions	Ars.
Convulsion	pain in spine after convulsion	Acon.
Convulsion	painful convulsion of lower limbs	Stry.
Convulsion	palpitation of heart before convulsion (a violent shaking of the body or limbs caused by uncontrollable muscle contractions, which can be a symptom of brain disorders and other conditions)	Cupr., glon.
Convulsion	palpitation of heart convulsive	Nux-v.
Convulsion	paralysis agitans after convulsions	Hyos.
Convulsion	perspiration after convulsions	Acon., ars., cedr., cupr., sec., stry.
Convulsion	perspiration cold during convulsions	Ferr., stram.
Convulsion	perspiration during convulsions	Ars., bell., **Bufo.**, camph., nux-v., op., sep.
Convulsion	perspiration on face during convulsions	Bufo., cocc.
Convulsion	pulse almost imperceptible during convulsions	Nux-v., olnd.
Convulsion	quick breath during convulsion	Tab.
Convulsion	respiration arreasted during convulsions	Cic., cina., coff., sant., sars., stry.
Convulsion	restlessness before convulsions	Bufo.
Convulsion	shocks like electric before convulsions	Bar-m., laur.

Body part/Disease	Symptom	Medicines
Convulsion	sighing (breathe long and loud) after convulsions	Cocc.
Convulsion	slow breath during convulsion	Op.
Convulsion	spasmodically abducted convulsion of lower limbs	Lyc., merc.
Convulsion	stertorous after convulsion	Oena., Op.
Convulsion	stiffness during convulsion	Acon., alum., am-c., arg-m., ars., asaf., bell., camph., canth., caust., cham., chin., cic., cina., cocc., coloc., dros., hell., hyos., ign., **Ip.**, kali-c., laur., led., lyc., merc., **Mosch.**, nit-ac., nux-m., oena., op., petr., phos., **Plat.**, plb., sec., sep., sil., stram., sulph., thuj., verat., zinc.
Convulsion	sudden convulsion	Stry.
Convulsion	suppression of urine with convulsion	Cupr., dig., hyos., stram.
Convulsion	tetanic convulsion	Anthr., camph., cann-s.
Convulsion	tetanic convulsion of fingers	Am-c., arn., ars., bell., calc., cann-s., cham., Chel., cic., clem., cocc., coff., cupr., dros., ferr., hell., ign., iod., ip., kali-n., lach., lyc., merc-c., mosch., nat-m., nux-v., phos., plb., sant., sec., stann., staph., sulph., tab., verat.
Convulsion	tetanic convulsion of foot	Camph., nux-v.
Convulsion	tetanic convulsion of forearm	Zinc.
Convulsion	tetanic convulsion of hand	Camph., zinc.
Convulsion	trembling in upper limbs during convulsions	Sulph.
Convulsion	twitching after convulsions	Nux-v.
Convulsion	twitching during convulsions	Op.
Convulsion	weakness after convulsions	Acon., ars., merc-c., sec., stry., tab.
Convulsion	weakness after epileptic convulsions	Camph.
Convulsion	weakness after hysterical (emotional instability caused by trauma) convulsions	Ars.
Corn	corns (a hardened or thickened, often painful, area of skin, usually on a toe, caused by friction or pressure)	Acet-ac., agar., am-c., Ant-c., arn., bar-c., bor., bov., bry., calc-s., calc., carb-an., caust., chin., coloc., cur., graph., hep., ign., Lyc., lyss., nat-c., nat-m., nit-ac., nux-v., rhus-t., Sep., Sil., staph., sulph., ter.
Corn	corns aching	Ant-c., lyc., sep., sil., sulph.
Corn	corns burning	Agar., alum., am-c., ant-c., arg-m., bar-c., bry., calc-s., calc., carb-v., caust., graph., hep., Ign., lith., lyc., meph., nat-m., nux-v., petr., ph-ac., phos., ran-b., ran-s., rhus-t., Sep., sil., sulph., thuj.
Corn	corns horny (hard or rough like horn)	Ant-c., graph., ran-b., sulph.
Corn	corns inflamed	Ant-c., calc., lyc., puls., sep., Sil., staph., Sulph.
Corn	corns jerks	Dios., phos., Sep., sul-ac., sulph.
Corn	corns on heel	Phos.
Corn	corns painful	Agar., alum., ambr., ant-c., arn., aster., bar-c., bov., bry., calad., calc-s., calc., caust., hep., ign., iod., kali-c., lach., lith., lyc., meph., nat-m., nit-ac., nux-v., phos., puls., ran-s., rhus-t., sep., sil., spig., Sulph.
Corn	corns painful from pressing	Agar., ant-c., bov., bry., calc-s., calc., carb-v., caust., graph., iod., Lyc., ph-ac., sep., sil., Sulph.

Body part/Disease	Symptom	Medicines
Corn	corns painful when touched	Bry., kali-c.
Corn	corns pulsating	Calc., kali-c., lyc., sep., sil., sulph.
Corn	corns sore	Aesc., agar., ambr., ant-c., arn., bar-c., bry., calc-s., calc., camph., Carb-an., fl-ac., graph., hep., Ign., lith., Lyc., med., nat-c., nat-p., nux-v., petr., phos., puls., ran-b., ran-s., rhus-t., sep., Sil., spig., sulph., thuj., verat.
Corn	corns stinging	Agar., Alum., am-c., ant-c., bar-c., bor., bov., Bry., calad., Calc-s., Calc., carb-an., caust., hep., ign., kali-c., lyc., mag-m., Nat-c., Nat-m., nat-p., petr., ph-ac., phos., ptel., puls., ran-s., rhod., Rhus-t., rumx., sep., sil., staph., sul-ac., Sulph., thuj., verat.
Corn	corns tearing	Am-c., arn., bry., calc-s., calc., cocc., kali-c., Lyc., sep., Sil., sul-ac., Sulph., thuj.
Corn	corns with pinching pain	Bar-c.
Corn	corns with shooting pain	Bov., Nat-m.
Corn	horny corns (hardened uncomfortable area on foot) on soles	Ant-c., ars., calc., kali-ar., sil.
Cornea	Cancer, epithelioma of cornea	Hep.
Cornea	opacity (material through which light cannot pass) of left cornea with arcus senilis (an opaque circle around the cornea of the eye that can develop late in life)	Acon., ars., cocc., coloc., kali-bi., merc-c., merc., mosch., Puls., Sulph., zinc.
Cornea	opacity of left cornea	Hep., sulph.
Cornea	opacity of right cornea	Lyc., sil.
Coryza	burning pain in nose during coryza	Aesc., all-c., aloe., am-c., Ars., calad., caust., gels., mez., senec., seneg., sulph.
Coryza	catarrh (runny nose) alternating with diarrhoea	Seneg.
Coryza	catarrh extends to antrum (a cavity within a bone, especially a sinus cavity)	Berb., kali-c., kali-i., merc.
Coryza	catarrh go back from eruption	Sep.
Coryza	catarrh in old people	Ammc., ant-t., Bar-c., chin., nat-s., phel., Seneg., tub.
Coryza	catarrh of old age	Alum., am-c., bar-c., eup-per., kali-s., kreos., merc-i-f., poth.
Coryza	coryza	Avena Sat.Q (15-20 drops)
Coryza	coryza with cough and expectoration	Euphr.
Coryza	coryza after a bath	Calc-s.
Coryza	coryza aggravated in cold	Calc-p., coff., dulc., graph., hyos., kali-ar., mang., Merc., Ph-ac.
Coryza	coryza aggravated in warm yet dreads cold	Apis., merc.
Coryza	coryza during diphtheria	Am-c., ars., Arum-t., carb-ac., chlor., crot-h., ign., Kali-bi., kali-ma., lac-c., lach., lyc., merc-c., merc-cy., merc-i-f., mur-ac., Nit-ac.
Coryza	coryza from cutting hair	Bell., Nux-v., puls., sep.
Coryza	coryza from least contact of cold air	Dulc.
Coryza	coryza from uncovering the head	Hep., nat-m.
Coryza	coryza in aged people	Am-c.

Body part/Disease	Symptom	Medicines
Coryza	coryza in bed	Kali-c.
Coryza	coryza in diphtheria	Am-c., hydr., kali-bi., lyc., merc-c., merc-cy., nit-ac., petr.
Coryza	coryza in warm	Ant-c., apis., Merc.
Coryza	coryza with hunger	All-c., hep., sul-ac.
Coryza	coryza with inflammation of larynx during scarlatina	Ail., all-c., am-c., Arum-t., caps., mur-ac., nit-ac., phos., phyt., rhus-t.
Coryza	coryza with inflammation of larynx with sore throat	Calc-p., carb-an., cimic., lach., Merc., Nit-ac., Nux-v., Phos., phyt.
Coryza	coryza with intermittent inflammation of larynx	Nat-c.
Coryza	coryza with periodical attacks of inflammation of larynx	Graph., sil.
Coryza	coryza with soreness beneath and on margin of nose	Brom., iod.
Coryza	coryza with sudden attacks of inflammation of larynx	Agar., alum., apis., cycl., fl-ac., iod., plan., spig., staph., thuj., zinc.
Coryza	coryza, after getting wet	Sep.
Coryza	coryza, ameliorated in warm room	Ars., calc-p., coloc., dulc., sabad.
Coryza	coryza, caused by cold, dry wind	Acon., spong.
Coryza	coryza, constant	Bar-c., calc., carb-s., graph., kali-n., nat-c., sil.
Coryza	coryza, extending to chest	All-c., carb-v., euphr., ip., merc., nux-v.
Coryza	coryza, extending to frontal sinuses	Ars., calc-p., cimx., kali-i., sil., stict.
Coryza	coryza, in changeable weather	Gels., hep.
Coryza	coryza, left	Agar., all-c., Arum-t., bad., berb., cist., cop., jug-c., mang., thlaspi., thuj., zinc.
Coryza	coryza, left to right	Agar., all-c.
Coryza	coryza, right	Ars., brom., calc-s., euphr., kali-bi., merc-i-r., sang., sars., tarent.
Coryza	coryza, right to left	Brom., carb-v., chel., euphr., lyc.
Coryza	coryza, violent attacks	Alum., Ars., Arum-t., bry., calc., carb-v., chlor., cocc., cycl., Lyc., mag-c., mez., nat-c., nit-ac., sil., staph., thuj.
Coryza	coryza, with croup	Acon., ars., cub., hep., nit-ac., spong.
Coryza	cough with coryza	Cub., graph.
Coryza	dry cough during coryza	Bell., graph., merc., nat-m., nit-ac., sel., sep.
Coryza	dry cough during coryza in evening	Dig.
Coryza	frontal sinuses from chronic coryza	Ars., kali-bi., sang., Sil., thuj.
Coryza	itching in eye during coryza	Caps.
Coryza	lachrymation during coryza	agar., All-c., alum., anac., anan., arg-n., ars-i., ars., carb-ac., Carb-v., chin., dulc., Euphr., iod., jab., kali-c., lach., lyc., Nux-v., phos., phyt., puls., ran-s., sabad., sang., sin-n., spig., staph., Tell., verb.
Coryza	pain, burning in larynx during coryza	Am-m., seneg.
Coryza	sneezing, without coryza	Acon., aesc., agar., alum., am-m., ars., Calc., carb-v., caust., cic., cist., con., dig., dros., euphr., hell., hyos., iod., kali-c., lyc., meny., merc., mur-ac., nat-c., nicc., nit-ac., phos., sep., sil., stann., staph., sulph., teucr., zinc.

Body part/Disease	Symptom	Medicines
Coryza	stiffness in cervical region during coryza	Ars., bell., dulc., Lach., lachn., lyc., nux-v., rhus-t., sulph.
Coryza	urine copious with amenorrhoea with coryza	All-c., calc., verat.
Coryza	vertigo ameliorated after coryza	Aloe.
Cough	Aching between scapula on coughing	Calc., kali-bi., stram.
Cough	Aching in back on coughing	Am-c., kali-n., merc., puls., sep.
Cough	Aching in cervical region on coughing	Bell.
Cough	Aching in lumbar region during cough	Arund., kali-n., merc., tell.
Cough	anger from cough	Acon., ant-t., arn., bell., cham.
Cough	anxiety before attack of whooping cough	Cupr.
Cough	anxiety before cough	Ars., cupr., iod., lach.
Cough	anxiety from coughing	Arund., merc-c., nit-ac., stram.
Cough	anxiety on coughing	Arund.
Cough	asthma aggravated from coughing	Meph.
Cough	asthma catching after cough	Arn., ars., bry., hep., nat-m., puls.
Cough	asthma catching from cough	Bry., cina.
Cough	barking cogh	Acon., all-c., ant-t., aur-m., Bell., brom., caps., cimx., clem., coc-c., cor-r., cub., Dros., dulc., Hep., hipp., kali-bi., lac-c., lact., lyc., lyss., merc., mur-ac., nit-ac., nux-m., phos., phyt., rumx., Spong., stann., stict., Stram., sulph., verat.
Cough	barking cogh ameliorated from drinking cold water	Coc-c.
Cough	barking cogh day & night	Spong.
Cough	barking cogh in evening	Nit-ac.
Cough	barking cogh in morning	Kali-bi., thuj.
Cough	barking cogh like a dog	Bell., lyss.
Cough	barking cough during sleep	Hipp., lyc., nit-ac.
Cough	barking cough loud	Acon., aur-m., kali-bi., lyc., stann., verat.
Cough	bleeding from mouth in whooping cough	Cor-r., dros., ip., nux-v.
Cough	boring pain in lumbar from coughing	Rhus-t.
Cough	boring pain in sacrum with cough	Phos.
Cough	boring pain in sacrum with cough	Phos.
Cough	breathing difficult during cough	Meph.
Cough	burning pain in trachea with cough	Caust., ferr., gels., mag-s., phyt., Spong.
Cough	cannot lie dow & sits bent forward during cough	Iod.
Cough	cardiac croup (an inflammatory condition of the larynx and trachea, especially in young children, marked by a cough, hoarseness, and difficulty in breathing)	Spong.
Cough	child becomes stiff & blue on face with suffocative cough	Cupr., Ip.
Cough	child coughs at sight of strangers	Ambr., ars., bar-c., phos.
Cough	chill causes cough	Cimx., psor.

Body part/Disease	Symptom	Medicines
Cough	chill from coughing	Ars., bry., calc., carb-v., con., cupr., hyos., mez., nat-c., nux-v., phos., **Puls.**, rhus-t., sabad., sep., sulph., verat.
Cough	choking cough at midnight	Dros., ruta.
Cough	choking cough at night	Carb-v., hep., ip., ruta.
Cough	choking cough from inspiration	Cina.
Cough	choking cough in evening	Cina.
Cough	choking cough in morning after rising	Cina.
Cough	choking cough when lying on side	Kali-c.
Cough	choking of throat on coughing	Ars., coc-c., lach.
Cough	chronic cough in old people at night	Hyos.
Cough	chronic cough in old people in morning	Alumn.
Cough	chronic cough in old people in winter	Kreos., psor.
Cough	chronic dry cough in scrofulous (diseased, or shabby in appearance due to tuberculosis of the lymph glands, especially of the neck) children	Bar-m.
Cough	coldness between scapula with cough	Am-m.
Cough	coldness in hands during cough	Rumx., sulph.
Cough	coldness in lumbar with cough	Carb-an.
Cough	coldness in upper limbs during cough	Ars., calc., ferr., hep., kali-c., rhus-t., rumx., sil.
Cough	constricted cough from eating	Puls.
Cough	constriction in chest from inclination to cough	Sep.
Cough	constriction in chest during cough	Calc., cham., cimx., con., cupr., form., hell., lyc., mag-p., merc., myrt., Phos., puls., stram., sulph.
Cough	constriction in chest during spasmodic cough	Mosch.
Cough	constriction in chest during whooping cough (an infectious bacterial disease that causes violent coughing mainly affects children)	Caust., mur-ac., spong.
Cough	constriction in chest while cough	Carb-v., clem., dros., ip., mosch., samb., stram., sulph.
Cough	constriction in larynx ameliorated aduring cough	Asar.
Cough	constriction in larynx during cough	Agar., ars., bell., chel., Cor-r., Cupr., Dros., euphr., Hyos., ign., ip., puls., stram., sulph., verat.
Cough	constriction in larynx with choking cough	Agar., ars., bell., chel., Cor-r., Cupr., Dros., euphr., Hyos., ign., ip., puls., stram., sulph., verat.
Cough	constriction in sternum on coughing	Phos.
Cough	constriction while cough at night during first sleep while lying on the side	Kali-c., phos., spong.
Cough	constriction while cough at night during sleep	Agar., lach., nit-ac., phos., sulph.
Cough	contraction in stomach after coughing	Ars.
Cough	convulsion after coughing	Cupr., ip.
Cough	convulsion during cough	Cupr.
Cough	coryza with cough and expectoration	Euphr.
Cough	cough 6 a.m. to 6 p.m.	Calc-p.
Cough	cough after 1 hour of sleep	Aral., arn., calc.

Body part/Disease	Symptom	Medicines
Cough	cough after bath in morning	Calc-s.
Cough	cough after chicken pox (a highly infectious viral disease, especially affecting children, characterized by a rash of small itching blisters on the skin and mild fever)	Ant-c.
Cough	cough after coition	Tarent.
Cough	cough after dancing	Puls.
Cough	cough after dinner	Aeth., agar., anac., arg-n., bar-c., bry., calc-f., carb-v., coc-c., ferr., hep., kali-bi., lach., mur-ac., nux-v., phos., sil., sulph., syph., tab., tax., thuj., zinc.
Cough	cough after heat	Bell.
Cough	cough after irritation	Acon., ant-t., ars., bry., Cham., chin., cina., Ign., iod., nat-m., nux-v., ph-ac., sep., Staph., verat.
Cough	cough after measles	Ant-c., arn., bry., calc., camph., carb-v., cham., chel., chin., coff., con., cop., cupr., Dros., dulc., eup-per., gels., hep., hyos., ign., kali-c., murx., nat-c., nux-v., Puls., squil., stict., sulph.
Cough	cough after midnight	Acon., cocc., Mag-m.
Cough	cough after midnight every half hour	Acon.
Cough	cough after parturition	Rhus-t.
Cough	cough after scarlet fever	Ant-c., con., hyos.
Cough	cough after sleeping	Apis., aral., caust., kali-bi., Lach., lachn., nit-ac., puls., sep., sulph.
Cough	cough after supper (the main meal of the day when taken in the evening)	Nat-a.
Cough	cough after suppressed gonorrhoea (a sexually transmitted bacterial disease that causes inflammation of the genital mucous membrane, burning pain when urinating, and a discharge)	Benz-ac., med., sel., thuj.
Cough	cough after suppressed itch	Psor.
Cough	cough after taking meat	Staph.
Cough	cough after vaccination (a preparation containing weakened or dead microbes of the kind that cause a disease, administered to stimulate the immune system to produce antibodies against that disease)	Thuj.
Cough	cough after variola (a highly contagious disease marked by high fever and the formation of scar-producing pustules)	Calc.
Cough	cough after vinegar	Alum., ant-c., sep., sulph.
Cough	cough aggravated by crying	Ant-t., Arn., ars., bell., cham., cina., dros., ferr., guare., hep., lyc., phos., samb., sil., sulph., verat.
Cough	cough aggravated from acids	Ant-c., brom., con., lach., mez., nat-m., nux-v., sep., sil., sulph.
Cough	cough aggravated from all kinds of smoke	Euphr., ment.
Cough	cough aggravated from bathing	Ant-c., ars., calc-f., calc-s., calc., caust., dulc., lach., nit-ac., nux-m., psor., Rhus-t., sep., stram., sul-ac., sulph., verat., zinc.

Body part/Disease	Symptom	Medicines
Cough	cough aggravated from becoming warm in bed	Ant-t., brom., Caust., cham., dros., led., merc., naja., nat-m., nux-m., nux-v., Puls., verat.
Cough	cough aggravated from beer	Mez., nux-v., rhus-t., spong.
Cough	cough aggravated from bending head backward	Bry., cupr., hep., kali-bi., lyc., psor., rumx., sil., spong.
Cough	cough aggravated from bending head forward	Caust., dig.
Cough	cough aggravated from brandy	Ferr.
Cough	cough aggravated from bread	Kali-c.
Cough	cough aggravated from close air	Brom., nat-a.
Cough	cough aggravated from coffee	Caps., caust., cham., cocc., ign., nux-v., sul-ac.
Cough	cough aggravated from consolation	Ars.
Cough	cough aggravated from eating hastily	Sil.
Cough	cough aggravated from eating high seasoned food	Sulph.
Cough	cough aggravated from elongated (to make something longer) uvula (a small fleshy "V"-shaped extension of the soft palate that hangs above the tongue at the entrance to the throat) in morning	Brom.
Cough	cough aggravated from elongated uvula	Alum., bapt., brom., hyos., merc-i-r., nat-m.
Cough	cough aggravated from entering in warm room from cold air or vice versa (the position being reversed)	Acon., all-c., carb-v., lach., nat-c., nux-v., Phos., rumx., sep., verat-v.
Cough	cough aggravated from fog (condensed water vapor in the air at or near ground level)	Sep.
Cough	cough aggravated from fruit	Arg-m., mag-m.
Cough	cough aggravated from happy surprise	Acon., merc.
Cough	cough aggravated from hot tea	Spong.
Cough	cough aggravated from lying and ameliorated from sitting	Hyos., laur., Puls., rhus-t., sang., Sep.
Cough	cough aggravated from milk	Ambr., ant-c., ant-t., brom., kali-c., spong., sul-ac., zinc.
Cough	cough aggravated from motion	Arn., ars-i., ars., bar-c., bell., brom., bry., bufo., calc., carb-o., carb-v., chin-a., chin., cina., coc-c., cur., dros., eup-per., ferr-ar., Ferr., form., iod., ip., kali-ar., kali-bi., kali-c., kali-n., kreos., lach., laur., led., lob., lyc., merc., mez., mosch., mur-ac., nat-m., nat-s., nit-ac., nux-v., osm., phos., plan., psor., pyrog., seneg., sep., sil., spong., squil., stann., staph., sul-ac., zinc.
Cough	cough aggravated from motion of arms	Ars., calc., ferr., kali-c., led., lyc., Nat-m., nux-v.
Cough	cough aggravated from motion of chest	Anac., bar-c., Chin., cocc., dros., lach., mang., merc., mur-ac., nat-m., Nux-v., phos., sil., Stann.
Cough	cough aggravated from mucous in upper chest	Anac., bar-c., Chin., cocc., dros., lach., mang., merc., mur-ac., nat-m., Nux-v., phos., sil., Stann.
Cough	cough aggravated from music	Ambr., calc., cham., kali-c., kreos., ph-ac.
Cough	cough aggravated from other person approaching or passing	Carb-v.
Cough	cough aggravated from other person coming into room	Phos.

Body part/Disease	Symptom	Medicines
Cough	cough aggravated from potatoes	Alum.
Cough	cough aggravated from raising the arms	Bry., ferr., lyc., ol-j.
Cough	cough aggravated from reading aloud	Ambr., cina., dros., mang., meph., nit-ac., nux-v., par., Phos., stann., tub., verb.
Cough	cough aggravated from reading aloud in evening	Phos.
Cough	cough aggravated from rinsing (flush mouth with water)	Coc-c.
Cough	cough aggravated from running	Cina., iod., merc., seneg., sil., stann., sul-ac.
Cough	cough aggravated from sensation from sulphur fumes or vapour	Am-c., aml-n., Ars., asaf., brom., bry., calc., carb-v., chin., cina., Ign., ip., kali-chl., lach., Lyc., mosch., par., Puls.
Cough	cough aggravated from singing	Alum., arg-m., arg-n., dros., hyos., mang., meph., phos., rhus-t., rumx., sil., spong., stann., stram.
Cough	cough aggravated from sitting bent	Rhus-t., spig., stann.
Cough	cough aggravated from sitting long	Coc-c., ph-ac.
Cough	cough aggravated from standing	Acon., aloe., euphr., ign., mag-s., nat-m., nat-s., sep., stann., sulph., zinc.
Cough	cough aggravated from sugar	Zinc.
Cough	cough aggravated from sun	Ant-t., coca.
Cough	cough aggravated from swallowing	Aesc., Brom., cupr., eug., kali-ma., lyc., lyss., nat-m., op., phos., puls., sul-ac.
Cough	cough aggravated from tea	Ferr., spong.
Cough	cough aggravated from tight clothing	Stann.
Cough	cough aggravated from turning left to right side in bed	Kreos.
Cough	cough aggravated from uncovering feet or head	Sil.
Cough	cough aggravated from uncovering hands	Bar-c., Hep., Rhus-t., sil.
Cough	cough aggravated in dark room	Bry.
Cough	cough aggravated where many persons are present	Ambr.
Cough	cough alternating with eruptions	Ars., crot-t., mez., psor., sulph.
Cough	cough alternating with sciatica (pain and tenderness extending from the back of the hip down to the calf, usually caused by a protrusion of vertebral disk substance pressing on the roots of the sciatic nerve) in summer	Staph.
Cough	cough ameliorated after breakfast	Alumn., aspar., bar-c., coc-c., kali-c., lach., murx.
Cough	cough ameliorated at daybreak	Syph.
Cough	cough ameliorated by developing eruptions of measles	Cupr.
Cough	cough ameliorated by diarrhoea	Bufo.
Cough	cough ameliorated by expectoration	Ail., alum., alumn., bell., calc., carb-an., caust., guai., hep., iod., ip., kali-n., kreos., lach., lob., meli., mez., phos., phyt., plan., sang., sep., sulph., zinc.
Cough	cough ameliorated by lying down in noon	Mang.
Cough	cough ameliorated during day time	Bell., caust., con., dulc., euphr., ign., lach., lyc., merc., nit-ac., sep., spong.
Cough	cough ameliorated from becoming warm in bed	Cham., kali-bi.

Body part/Disease	Symptom	Medicines
Cough	cough ameliorated from bending head forward	Eup-per., spong.
Cough	cough ameliorated from cold	Calc-s., coc-c., kali-s.
Cough	cough ameliorated from cold milk	Am-caust., bor., brom., caps., Caust., coc-c., Cupr., euphr., glon., iod., ip., kali-c., kali-s., onos., op., sulph., verat.
Cough	cough ameliorated from deep breath	Lach., puls., verb.
Cough	cough ameliorated from eating	All-s., am-c., ammc., anac., carb-an., euphr., ferr-m., ferr., kali-c., sin-n., Spong., tab.
Cough	cough ameliorated from empty swallowing	Bell.
Cough	cough ameliorated from eructations	Sang.
Cough	cough ameliorated from frequent stools	Bufo.
Cough	cough ameliorated from kneeling with face towards pillow	Eup-per.
Cough	cough ameliorated from lying	Mang.
Cough	cough ameliorated from motion	Ambr., arg-n., ars., caps., coc-c., dros., dulc., eupho., euphr., grat., hyos., kali-i., mag-c., mag-m., nux-v., ph-ac., phos., psor., puls., rhus-r., rhus-t., sabad., samb., sep., sil., stann., sulph., verb., zinc.
Cough	cough ameliorated from passing flatus	Sang.
Cough	cough ameliorated from rising	Mag-c., mag-s., rhus-t.
Cough	cough ameliorated from sitting bent	Iod.
Cough	cough ameliorated from smoking at night	Tarent.
Cough	cough ameliorated from sneezing	Osm.
Cough	cough ameliorated from standing	Mag-s.
Cough	cough ameliorated from sugar	Sulph.
Cough	cough ameliorated from swallowing	Apis., eug., spong.
Cough	cough ameliorated from turning left to right side	Ars., kali-c., phos., rumx., sep., thuj.
Cough	cough ameliorated from vomiting	Mez.
Cough	cough ameliorated from warm fluids	Alum., Ars., bry., eupi., Lyc., Nux-v., Rhus-t., Sil., spong., verat.
Cough	cough ameliorated from warm food	Spong.
Cough	cough ameliorated from warming abdomen	Sil.
Cough	cough ameliorated from wine	Sulph.
Cough	cough ameliorated in frosty (very cold) weather	Spong.
Cough	cough ameliorated in morning	Agar., coc-c., grat.
Cough	cough ameliorated while sitting still	Verat.
Cough	cough as after intermittent fever	Nat-m.
Cough	cough as before intermittent fever in spells	Eup-per., rhus-t., samb.
Cough	cough as from dust in throat pit	Ign.
Cough	cough as from dust in trachea	Ferr-ma.
Cough	cough as from mucous in trachea while ascending or descending	Coc-c.
Cough	cough as from vapour of carbon	Arn., puls.
Cough	cough at 2.00 a.m.	Cocc.

Body part/Disease	Symptom	Medicines
Cough	cough at beginning of menses	Phos.
Cough	cough at day time	Anac.
Cough	cough at midnight	Cocc.
Cough	cough at night	Anac., con., laur., lyc., med., Sep., stict., stront., zinc.
Cough	cough at night	Acon., cocc., merc.
Cough	cough at Same hour every day	Lyc., sabad.
Cough	cough at the same hour	Lyc., sabad.
Cough	cough before an attack of gout	Led.
Cough	cough before breakfast	Alumn., kali-c., murx., seneg., sulph.
Cough	cough before dinner	Arg-n.
Cough	cough before menses	Arg-n., graph., hyos., lac-c., plat., sulph., zinc.
Cough	cough before menses at day time	Graph., sulph., zinc.
Cough	cough before menses in early morning	Graph.
Cough	cough before menses in evening	Sulph., zinc.
Cough	cough before menses in evening ameliorated by sitting up in bed	Sulph.
Cough	cough before menses in morning	Graph., Zinc.
Cough	cough before rising	Ail., Nux-v.
Cough	cough before sleeping	Coc-c., lyc., merc., Sulph.
Cough	cough before storm	Phos.
Cough	cough before stove	Coc-c.
Cough	cough before thunder	Phos., sil.
Cough	cough compels to sit up as soon as cough commences	Ars., bry., caust., coc-c., colch., Con., hep., lach., plan.
Cough	cough croaking (rough voice)	Acon., ant-t., lach., nit-ac., ruta., spong.
Cough	cough croupy after eating	Anac.
Cough	cough croupy aggravated after midnight	Ars.
Cough	cough croupy at night	Ars., carb-ac., hep., ip., phyt., spong.
Cough	cough croupy in evening	Cinnb.
Cough	cough croupy in morning	Calc-s.
Cough	cough croupy in winter alternating with sciatica (pain and tenderness extending from the back of the hip down to the calf, usually caused by a protrusion of vertebral disk substance pressing on the roots of the sciatic nerve) in summer	Staph.
Cough	cough croupy on expiration	Acon.
Cough	cough croupy only after waking	Calc-s.
Cough	cough croupy with sopor (deep sleep) stertorous (noisy snoring) breathing and wheezing, with open mouth and head thrown back; the child starts up, kicks about, is on point of suffocating, turns black and blue in face, after which cough with rattling breathing sets in again, suffocations and paralysis, of lungs appear unavoidable	Samb.
Cough	cough day & night	Ign., lyc., nat-m., phos., spong., squil.

Body part/Disease	Symptom	Medicines
Cough	cough day or night	Squil.
Cough	cough deep sounding	Aloe., kali-bi., mang., Stram., verb.
Cough	cough deep sounding at night	Verb.
Cough	cough disturbing sleep	Agar., alum., calad., mez., nux-v., ol-j., phos., rhod., rhus-t., sang., spong., squil., stict., Sulph., syph., zinc.
Cough	cough during breakfast	Alum., alumn., seneg.
Cough	cough during dentiton (the type, number, and arrangement of a set of teeth)	Calc-p., calc., cham., cina., hyos., kreos., podo., rhus-t.
Cough	cough during east wind	Acon., cham., cupr., Hep., samb., sep., spong.
Cough	cough during lactation	Ferr.
Cough	cough during measles	Coff., cop., eup-per., spong., squil.
Cough	cough during measles at day time	Cupr.
Cough	cough during menses	Am-m., atro-s., bry., cact., calc-p., cast., cham., coff., cop., cub., cur., graph., iod., lac-c., lachn., nat-m., phos., rhod., senec., sep., sulph., thuj., zinc.
Cough	cough during menses in every evening	Sulph.
Cough	cough during menses in morning	Cop.
Cough	cough during north wind	Acon., cham., cupr., Hep., sep., spong.
Cough	cough during pregnancy	Calc., caust., con., ip., kali-br., nux-m., phos., puls., sabin., sep., vib.
Cough	cough during pregnancy at night	Con.
Cough	cough during remittent fever	Podo.
Cough	cough during sleep in noon	Euphr.
Cough	cough during supper	Carb-v.
Cough	cough during variola	Plat.
Cough	cough every fourth night	Cocc.
Cough	cough every other day	Anac., lyc., nux-v.
Cough	cough every other day	Anac., lyc., nux-v., sep.
Cough	cough every other night	Merc.
Cough	cough every third day	Anac., lyc.
Cough	cough every three hours	Anac., dros.
Cough	cough excited from closing eyes at night	Hep.
Cough	cough excited from eructations	Ambr., bar-c., lact-ac., sol-t-ae., staph.
Cough	cough excited from rawness in larynx	Acon., alum., ambr., bar-c., brom., bry., cast., coc-c., dulc., hep., kali-i., laur., Nux-v., ol-an., Phos., Rumx., sang., sil., Sulph.
Cough	cough exhausting at day time	Lyc.
Cough	cough exhausting at noon	Arg-n.
Cough	cough exhausting in evening ameliorated on sitting	Nat-c.
Cough	cough exhausting in evening disturbing sleep	Puls.
Cough	cough exhausting in evening	Arg-n., ip., kali-c., lyc., rhod., sil., still.
Cough	cough exhausting in evening	Caust., nat-c., Puls., rhod., tarent.
Cough	cough exhausting in morning	Rhod., squil., sulph., thuj.
Cough	cough exhausting in morning after waking	Mag-s., thuj.

Body part/Disease	Symptom	Medicines
Cough	cough exhausting on going to sleep	Lyc.
Cough	cough following difficult labour or abortion, with backache and sweat	Kali-c.
Cough	cough following scarlatina (bacterial infection marked by fever, a sore throat, and a red rash, mainly affecting children)	Ant-c., con., hyos.
Cough	cough from air of basement	Ant-t., nux-m., sep., stram.
Cough	cough from anger	Acon., ant-t., arg-m., arg-n., arn., ars., bry., caps., cham., chin., coloc., ign., nux-v., sep., staph., verat.
Cough	cough from as if pepper in larynx	Crot-h.
Cough	cough from ascending stairs	Arg-m., arg-n., ars., bar-c., bry., cench., iod., kali-n., lyc., mag-c., mag-m., merc., nux-v., seneg., sep., spong., squil., stann., staph., zinc.
Cough	cough from becoming feet cold	Bar-c., bufo., sil., sulph.
Cough	cough from burning in larynx	Acon., aphis., arg-n., ars., bell., bov., brom., bufo., caust., mag-s., ph-ac., phos., phyt., seneg., spong., stict., tarent., urt-u., zing.
Cough	cough from burning in throat pit	Ars.
Cough	cough from burning in trachea	Acon., ars., euphr.
Cough	cough from change of weather	Dulc., erig., lach., nit-ac., phos., rumx., sil., spong., verat., verb.
Cough	cough from cold food	Am-m., carb-v., dros., hep., lyc., mag-c., ph-ac., rhus-t., sil., thuj., verat.
Cough	cough from cold milk	Ant-t.
Cough	cough from cold wind on chest	Phos., rumx.
Cough	cough from company	Ambr., bar-c.
Cough	cough from cramps in chest	Bell.
Cough	cough from damp cold	Ant-t., bar-c., calc., carb-an., carb-v., chin., cur., Dulc., iod., lach., mag-c., merc., mosch., mur-ac., nit-ac., nux-m., phyt., rhus-t., sep., sil., sul-ac., sulph., verat., zinc.
Cough	cough from draft of cold	Acon., calc., caps., caust., chin., ph-ac., sep.
Cough	cough from dryness in chest	Bell., benz-ac., kali-chl., lach., laur., merc., puls.
Cough	cough from dryness in fauces (the passage between the back of the mouth and the pharynx)	Dros., mez., phyt.
Cough	cough from dryness in larynx (the cartilaginous box-shaped part of the respiratory tract between the level of the root of the tongue and the top of the trachea) in morning	Phyt.
Cough	cough from dryness of air passages	Carb-an., lach., merc., petr., puls.
Cough	cough from eating fish	Lach.
Cough	cough from eating until he vomits	Mez.
Cough	cough from empty swallowing	Caust., lyc., nat-m., op.
Cough	cough from entering in warm room from open air	Acon., all-c., Ant-c., anth., bov., brom., bry., carb-v., coc-c., com., con., cupr., dig., med., nat-c., nat-m., nux-v., puls., sep., squil., sulph., verat., verb.

Body part/Disease	Symptom	Medicines
Cough	cough from exposure to snowfall in children	Sep.
Cough	cough from fasting	Kali-c., mag-m.
Cough	cough from fat food	Mag-m.
Cough	cough from fright	Acon., bell., ign., rhus-t., samb., stram.
Cough	cough from fullness of chest	Chin-a., sulph.
Cough	cough from fullness of chest in morning	Chin-a., sulph.
Cough	cough from gastric	Bor., card-m., ferr., ip., kali-ar., lob., nux-v.
Cough	cough from going from cold to warm room	Acon., carb-v., nat-c., nux-v., phos., Rumx., sang., sep.
Cough	cough from going on bed	Acon., ars., bar-c., bry., calc-s., canth., carb-an., carb-v., chel., cocc., con., euphr., ferr-p., ign., Lach., mag-s., nat-s., phos., plb., sep., sul-ac., tarent., thuj., verat.
Cough	cough from grief	Arn., asar., cham., ph-ac., phos.
Cough	cough from heart burn	Carb-s.
Cough	cough from icy cold air in air passages	Cor-r.
Cough	cough from lifting heavy weight	Ambr.
Cough	cough from liquid touching back part of mouth	Am-c.
Cough	cough from loss of animal fluid	Chin., cina., ferr., ph-ac., staph.
Cough	cough from lump in throat	Bell., calc., coc-c., lach.
Cough	cough from malignant tumour/cancer with the sound of croup	Cupr.
Cough	cough from manual labour	Led., nat-m.
Cough	cough from odor of coffee	Sul-ac.
Cough	cough from pain in larynx	Acon., ang., arg-m., bry., calad., caust., chin-s., euphr., ferr., grat., hep., iod., kali-c., sars., spong., stann.
Cough	cough from pain in trachea	Acon., ang., arg-m., bry., calad., eupho., grat., hep., indg., ip., sars., spong., stann.
Cough	cough from pressing pain in larynx	Agar.
Cough	cough from pressure in chest	Iod., op.
Cough	cough from pressure in goitre (enlargement of thyroid gland)	Psor.
Cough	cough from pressure in larynx	Apis., bell., chin., cina., crot-h., ferr., Lach., rumx., tarax.
Cough	cough from pressure in stomach	Calad.
Cough	cough from pressure in trachea	Bell., hydr., lach., rumx.
Cough	cough from pressure on throat-pit	Rumx.
Cough	cough from prickling in trachea (wind pipe)	Hydr-ac.
Cough	cough from putting out tongue	Lyc.
Cough	cough from raising the voice	Arg-n.
Cough	cough from riding	Staph., sul-ac., sulph.
Cough	cough from roughness in larynx	Alum., ang., aur-m., bar-c., bry., carb-an., carb-s., carb-v., cast., caust., coloc., con., dig., graph., kali-c., kali-i., kalm., kreos., lach., laur., mang., nat-s., Nux-v., ol-an., plb., puls., rhod., rhus-t., sabad., sars., seneg., spong., stront., sulph., verat-v.

Body part/Disease	Symptom	Medicines
Cough	cough from roughness in throat	Cast.
Cough	cough from roughness in trachea	Bar-c., carb-an., dig., kreos., laur., sabad.
Cough	cough from salty food	Alum., con., lach.
Cough	cough from scratching in larynx	Acon., alum., alumn., am-c., ang., arg-n., arn., bart., dig., kreos., mag-m., nux-m., petr., phos., psor., puls., sabad., sil., staph., sul-ac., zing.
Cough	cough from scratching in trachea	Acon., agar., cimx., dig., kreos., puls.
Cough	cough from sea wind	Cupr., mag-m.
Cough	cough from sensation as of a plug moving up & down in trachea	Calc.
Cough	cough from sensation of crawling in bronchia	Aeth.,Eupi., kreos.
Cough	cough from sensation of crawling in chest	Cahin., caust., con., kreos., nux-m., rhus-t., squil.
Cough	cough from sensation of crawling in larynx	Am-m., ant-t., bry., calc-p., carb-v., caust., colch., Con., dros., eupho., iod., Kali-c., kreos., lach., lact., led., mag-m., nux-m., prun-s., psor., rhus-t., sabin., sang., stann., stict., sulph.
Cough	cough from sensation of crawling in throat-pit	Apis., kreos., mag-m., Sang.
Cough	cough from sensation of crawling in trachea	Anac., arn., carb-v., caust., kreos., prun-s., rhus-t.
Cough	cough from sensation of foreign bodies in larynx	Am-caust., arg-m., Bell., brom., dros., hep., lach., lob., phos., ptel., rumx., sil.
Cough	cough from sensation of heat in bronchia	Aeth., eup-per.
Cough	cough from sensation of heat in chest	Carb-v.
Cough	cough from sensation of plug in larynx	Spong.
Cough	cough from sensation of smoke in larynx	Ars., bry., nat-a.
Cough	cough from sneezing	Seneg.
Cough	cough from sour food	Ant-c., brom., lach., nat-m., nux-v., sep., sulph.
Cough	cough from south wind	Euphr.
Cough	cough from speaking or smoking	Atro.
Cough	cough from spirit drinking	Arn., ferr., ign., lach., led., spong., stann., stram., zinc.
Cough	cough from sprinkle food with pepper	Alum., cina.
Cough	cough from standing in cold water	Nux-m.
Cough	cough from stinging in larynx	Agar., aphis., bufo.
Cough	cough from stitching in chest	Acon., bry., nit-ac., nux-v.
Cough	cough from stitching in larynx	Acon., agar., aphis., bufo., cham., cist., hydr-ac., indg., kali-c., naja., ox-ac., sol-t-ae., stann.
Cough	cough from stitching in trachea	Arg-m., lach., stann.
Cough	cough from stooping	All-s., arg-m., arg-n., arn., bar-c., Caust., chel., dig., hep., kali-c., laur., lyc., phos., seneg., sil., spig., spong., staph., verat.
Cough	cough from straining (Make extreme effort)	Aspar., caust., chel., cocc., croc., cupr., ip., lach., led., nux-v., par., phos., rhod., rhus-t., sel., thuj.
Cough	cough from sun set to sun rise	Aur.
Cough	cough from suppressed eruptions	Dulc.

Body part/Disease	Symptom	Medicines
Cough	cough from suppressed menses	Mill., puls.
Cough	cough from suppression of intermittent (Occurring at irregular intervals) fever	Eup-per.
Cough	cough from swallowing liquid at night	Sul-ac.
Cough	cough from swollen feeling in larynx	Ars., ox-ac.
Cough	cough from swollen larynx	Kali-i.
Cough	cough from thinking of it	Bar-c., nux-v., ox-ac.
Cough	cough from tingling in chest	Sep., squil.
Cough	cough from to cutting, stinging in larynx	Ang., arg-m.
Cough	cough from to cutting, stinging in thyroid gland (an endocrine gland located in the neck of human beings and other vertebrate animals that secretes the hormones responsible for controlling metabolism and growth.Excessive action of the thyroid gland can cause Graves' disease, while underactivity can cause myxedema)	Arg-n.
Cough	cough from troubles of spleen	Card-m.
Cough	cough from violent hunger	Kali-c., mag-c.
Cough	cough from warm fluids	Ambr., ant-t., caps., coc-c., ign., laur., mez., phos., stann.
Cough	cough from warm food	Bar-c., coc-c., kali-c., laur., mez., puls.
Cough	cough from wine	Acon., ant-t., arn., bor., ferr., ign., lach., led., stann., stram., Zinc.
Cough	cough from writing	Cina.
Cough	cough from yawning	Arn., asaf., cina., mur-ac., nux-v., puls., staph.
Cough	cough has a whispering sound	Card-b.
Cough	cough in afternoon after bath	Calc-s.
Cough	cough in autumn	Caps., cina., iod., kreos., lact-ac., verat.
Cough	cough in autumn & spring	Cina., kreos., lact-ac.
Cough	cough in child which must be raised that gets blue in face cannot exhale	Meph.
Cough	cough in cold wind	Coca., Hep., lyc., lycps.
Cough	cough in damp weather	Bar-c., calc., carb-v., cur., dulc., iod., lach., mang., nat-s., phyt., rhus-t., sil., spong., sulph.
Cough	cough in dry wind	Acon., cham., Hep., spong.
Cough	cough in evening	Acon., caust., cub., Puls.
Cough	cough in forenoon	Agar., alum., am-c., am-m., bell., bry., camph., chin-s., coc-c., dios., dros., glon., grat., hell., kali-c., lact., mag-c., nat-a., nat-c., nat-m., rhus-t., sabad., sars., seneg., sep., sil., stann., staph., sul-ac., sulph., zing.
Cough	cough in hot weather	Lach.
Cough	cough in morning	Cupr-s., phel., Stram.
Cough	cough in noon	Agar., arg-n., arund., bell., euphr., naja., sil., staph., sulph.
Cough	cough in old men	Am-c., kreos.

Body part/Disease	Symptom	Medicines
Cough	cough in old people	Alum., alumn., am-c., ambr, ammc., ant-c., ant-t., bar-c., camph., con., hydr., hyos., ip., kreos., psor., seneg.
Cough	cough in pleurisy (inflammation of the membrane pleura surrounding the lungs, usually involving painful breathing, coughing, and the buildup of fluid in the pleural cavity)	Acon., ars., bry., ip., lyc., sulph.
Cough	cough in series	Phos., sumb.
Cough	cough in stormy weather	Mag-m., phos., rhod., sep., sil., sulph.
Cough	cough in tall slender, gracefully and attractively thin) tuberculous subjects	Phos.
Cough	cough in the spring	Ambr., cina., gels., kreos., lact-ac., verat.
Cough	cough in the spring & autumn	Cina., kreos., lact-ac.
Cough	cough in warm wet weather	Iod.
Cough	cough in winter	Acon., cham., coc-c., dulc., eupi., kreos., nit-ac., plan., psor., rumx., stann., staph.
Cough	cough in winter alternating with sciatica in summer	Staph.
Cough	cough of drunkards	Ars., coc-c., lach., stram.
Cough	cough of students	Nux-v.
Cough	cough on becoming warm	Caust., laur., nit-ac., nux-m., puls.
Cough	cough on being spoken to	Ars.
Cough	Cough on crying	Arnica
Cough	cough on descending	Lyc.
Cough	cough on falling to sleep	Med.
Cough	cough on getting wet	Ant-c., calc-s., calc., dulc., lach., nit-ac., psor., rhus-t., sep., sulph.
Cough	cough on going out in evening	Naja.
Cough	cough on going to sleep	Lyc.
Cough	cough on going to sleep after midnight	Con., hep., ign., Lyc.
Cough	cough on playing violine	Kali-c.
Cough	cough on rising in morning & continuing until lying down	Euphr.
Cough	cough on rising in morning & in evening after lying down	Thuj.
Cough	cough on touching the canal of ear	Agar., arg-n., carb-s., kali-c., lach., mang., psor., sil., sulph., tarent.
Cough	cough on waking	Sep.
Cough	cough only at night	Merc.
Cough	cough remittent during intermittent fever	Podo.
Cough	cough seems to come from stomach	All-s., ant-t., bell., Bry., cann-s., ery-a., lach., merc., nux-v., puls., Sep.
Cough	cough short after dinner	Agar.
Cough	cough short after drinking tea	Ars.
Cough	cough short after eating	Anac., caust., ter.

Body part/Disease	Symptom	Medicines
Cough	cough short after midnight	Acon., ars.
Cough	cough short after rest in afternoon	Rhus-t.
Cough	cough short after rising	Am-br., arn.
Cough	cough short aggravated from inspiration	Nat-a.
Cough	cough short aggravated in open air	Ang., seneg., spig.
Cough	cough short aggravated on smoking	Thuj.
Cough	cough short ameliorated from sitting up	Arg-n., cinnb., nat-c.
Cough	cough short at night	Arg-n., bell., calc., mez., rhus-t.
Cough	cough short at night in bed	Arg-n., calc.
Cough	cough short before midnight	Rhus-t.
Cough	cough short during day time	Arg-m., kali-bi., nat-c., phos.
Cough	cough short during day time & night	Mez.
Cough	cough short frequent	Fl-ac.
Cough	cough short from breathing deep	Aesc.
Cough	cough short from irritation in larynx	Am-c., seneg., spong.
Cough	cough short from swallowing	Aesc.
Cough	cough short from tickling in larynx	Acon., agar., ang., cimic., graph., iris., kali-bi., laur., led., mez., spong.
Cough	cough short from walking fast	Seneg.
Cough	cough short from walking fast in open air	Ang.
Cough	cough short in afternoon	Anac., chin-s., laur., nat-m.
Cough	cough short in evening	Alum., bar-c., bell., carb-v., chel., cimic., Ign., kali-bi., lyc., phos., sep., sulph., thuj.
Cough	cough short in evening in bed	Lyc., sep.
Cough	cough short in forenoon	Agar., alum., coc-c., rhus-t.
Cough	cough short in morning	Agar., am-br., arn., ars., croc., kali-bi., lyc., nit-ac., thuj.
Cough	cough short on lying after eating	Caust., ter.
Cough	cough short on undressing	Chel.
Cough	cough short on waking	Dig.
Cough	cough short wakens before midnight	Rhus-t.
Cough	cough short when moving	Carb-o.
Cough	cough short when smoking	Coca., thuj.
Cough	cough short while sleeping	Sulph.
Cough	cough short while talking	Ant-t.
Cough	cough suffocation	Meli., Lach.
Cough	cough until evening	Nux-m.
Cough	cough until midnight	Bell., sulph.
Cough	cough when playing piano	Ambr., Calc., cham., kali-c., kreos., ph-ac.
Cough	cough when sleeping	Puls., staph.
Cough	cough which makes the boy quite breathless at night	Nat-m.
Cough	cough while ameliorated from sitting erect	Ant-t.

Body part/Disease	Symptom	Medicines
Cough	cough while brushing teeth	Coc-c., staph.
Cough	cough while dressing in morning	Seneg.
Cough	cough while dressing in morning & at night	Caust.
Cough	cough while lying down	Sep., zinc.
Cough	cough while sitting	Agar., aloe., alum., astac., euphr., ferr., guai., hell., kali-c., mag-c., mag-m., mur-ac., nat-c., nat-p., ph-ac., phos., puls., rhus-t., sabad., seneg., sep., spig., stann., zinc.
Cough	cough while sitting erect	Kali-c., nat-m., spong.
Cough	cough while sitting still	Coca., rhus-t.
Cough	cough with burning in chest	Am-c., caust., coc-c., eupho., euphr., led., mag-m., ph-ac.
Cough	cough with convulsions	Ars., bell., brom., calc., cham., cina., croc., Cupr., dros., hyos., led., meph., stram., sulph., verat.
Cough	cough with copious greenish salty expectorations aggravated in morning	Stann.
Cough	cough with coryza	Cub., graph.
Cough	cough with expectoration	Dulc., sil.
Cough	cough with feeling as if stomach turned inside out	Puls., ruta., tab.
Cough	cough with heart affection	Lach., laur., Naja., tab.
Cough	cough with hysterical attack followed by crying	Form.
Cough	cough with loss of consciousness	Cadm., cina., cupr.
Cough	cough with mucous in chest	Ant-t., arg-m., ars., arum-t., asar., bar-c., calc., caust., cham., cina., euphr., graph., guare., iod., ip., Kali-bi., kali-n., kreos., med., nat-m., plb., Puls., sep., spong., Stann., sulph.
Cough	cough with mucous in larynx	Aesc., am-br., am-c., am-caust., arg-m., arg-n., arum-t., asaf., asar., atro., brom., caust., cham., chin-s., cina., coc-c., cocc., crot-t., cupr., dig., dulc., euphr., grat., hyos., Kali-bi., kreos., Lach., laur., mang., nux-v., osm., par., phel., plan., raph., seneg., stann., stram., zinc.
Cough	cough with mucous in trachea	Arg-m., arum-t., caust., cham., cina., crot-t., cupr., dulc., euphr., gels., hyos., nux-v., seneg., spong., squil., Stann.
Cough	cough with noisy snoring	Cact.
Cough	cough with noisy snoring at night	Cact.
Cough	cough with oppression (trouble) in epigastrium (the upper middle part of the abdomen	Kali-bi.
Cough	cough with perspiration at night	Chin., dig., eug., kali-bi., lyc., merc., nat-c., nit-ac., psor., sulph.
Cough	cough with sensation as if larynx were tickled by a feather in evening before sleep	Lyc.
Cough	cough with shrill (making a high-pitched penetrating sound)	Ant-t., sol-t-ae., stram.
Cough	cough with sibilant & dry, like a saw driven through a pine board	Spong.

Body part/Disease	Symptom	Medicines
Cough	cough with sibilant (producing hissing sound as if escaping from a tyre)	Kreos., prun-s., spong.
Cough	cough with sneezing	All-c., alum., anac., ant-t., aspar., bad., bell., bry., carb-an., carb-v., chin., cina., con., eup-per., hep., iod., kali-c., kreos., lob., merc., nat-m., nit-ac., nux-v., osm., sal-ac., sep., sil., squil., staph., sulph.
Cough	cough with snoring	Ant-t., arg-m., bell., caust., ip., nat-c., nat-m., nux-v., puls., sep.
Cough	cough with strong odors	Phos., sul-ac.
Cough	cough with violent hunger	Nux-v., sul-ac.
Cough	cramp in leg during cough	Dros.
Cough	cramps in chest on coughing	Kali-c., laur.
Cough	crawling in larynx from cough	Kreos.
Cough	crawling in larynx from cough	Kreos.
Cough	crawling in trachea from cough	Colch., mag-m.
Cough	croup after eating	Anac.
Cough	croup after exposure to dry cold air	Acon., Hep., kali-bi.
Cough	croup after night	Spong.
Cough	croup aggravated after sleep	Lach., spong.
Cough	croup aggravated on lying	Hep.
Cough	croup before midnight	Spong.
Cough	croup during whooping cough	Brom.
Cough	croup extending to fauces	Brom.
Cough	croup extending to trachea	Iod., Kali-bi., kali-chl., phos.
Cough	croup from being heated	Brom.
Cough	croup gangrenous	Ars.
Cough	croup paroxysmal	Hep., kali-br.
Cough	croup recurrent	Calc-s., calc., Hep.
Cough	croup sequelæ (disease resulting from another)	Calc., carb-v.
Cough	crowing , violent, spasmodic cough, commencing with gasping for breath, and continuing with repeated crowing (to give the loud shrill cry of a rooster) inspirations till face becomes black or purple and patient exhausted, aggravated at night and after a meal	Cor-r.
Cough	discharges of blood from ear during cough	Bell.
Cough	discolouration of face blue during cough	Apis., bell., caust., coc-c., cor-r., Dros., Ip., mag-p., verat.
Cough	discolouration of face blue in whooping cough	Ars., coc-c., cor-r., crot-h., dros., ip., nux-v.
Cough	discolouration of face blue in croup	Brom., carb-v.
Cough	dry cough after dinner	Aeth., agar., kali-bi., lach., nux-v.
Cough	dry cough after drinking	Ars., hyos., kali-c., nux-m., phos., staph.
Cough	dry cough after drinking loose after eating	Nux-m., staph.
Cough	dry cough after dry chill	Nux-m., samb.
Cough	dry cough after every sleep	Puls.

Body part/Disease	Symptom	Medicines
Cough	dry cough after measles	Cham., dros., hyos., ign.
Cough	dry cough after measles before menses	Graph., hyos., lac-c., plat., sulph., Zinc.
Cough	dry cough after measles before menses in morning	Zinc.
Cough	dry cough after measles during menses	Bry., cast., cop., cur., graph., lac-c., phos., Zinc.
Cough	dry cough after measles during menses with profuse sweat	Graph.
Cough	dry cough after midnight	Ars., bell., calc., hyos., lec., nicc., Nux-v.
Cough	dry cough after suppressed gonorrhoea	Benz-ac., sel.
Cough	dry cough aggravated from heat of room	Coc-c., nat-a.
Cough	dry cough almost constant	Alum., arn., eupho., ign.
Cough	dry cough ameliorated after dinner	Bar-c.
Cough	dry cough ameliorated after drinking	Brom., bry., caust., coc-c., iod., kali-c., op., Spong.
Cough	dry cough ameliorated by discharge of flatus up and down and must sit up	Sang.
Cough	dry cough ameliorated from eating	Spong.
Cough	dry cough ameliorated from lying down	Sep.
Cough	dry cough ameliorated from open air	Iod., lil-t.
Cough	dry cough ameliorated on motion	Kali-c., phos.
Cough	dry cough ameliorated while lying	Am-c., Mang., sep., zinc.
Cough	dry cough ameliorated while sitting	Arg-n., cinnb., sang.
Cough	dry cough as if from stomach	Bry., Sep.
Cough	dry cough at day time	Alum., bar-c., bell., calc., chel., coloc., con., eupho., gamb., ign., kali-bi., lyc., op., phos., puls., sep., sol-t-ae., Spong., sulph.
Cough	dry cough at midnight	Am-c., grat., nicc., nux-v., phos.
Cough	dry cough at midnight ameliorated from lying on side	Nux-v.
Cough	dry cough at midnight from lying on back	Nux-v.
Cough	dry cough at midnight until daybreak	Nux-v.
Cough	dry cough at night & loose by day	Acon., anac., ars., bry., calc., carb-an., caust., cham., chin., con., euphr., hep., hyos., kali-c., lach., lyc., mag-c., mag-m., merc., nit-ac., nux-v., phos., puls., sabad., samb., sil., Sulph., verat., zinc.
Cough	dry cough at night aggravated from inspiration	Nat-a.
Cough	dry cough at night aggravated from lying	Con., hyos., kali-br., laur., ol-j., phyt., puls., Sulph., zinc.
Cough	dry cough at night aggravated from lying on right side	Carb-an.
Cough	dry cough at night aggravated from motion	Bell., seneg.
Cough	dry cough at night ameliorated from sitting up	Hyos., Puls., sang.
Cough	dry cough at night ameliorated from smoking	Tarent.
Cough	dry cough at night followed by profuse salty expectoration with pain as if something were torn loose from larynx	Calc.
Cough	dry cough at night from waking from sleep	Graph., puls., sil., Sulph.

Body part/Disease	Symptom	Medicines
Cough	dry cough at night on falling asleep	Med.
Cough	dry cough before dry chill	Mag-c., Rhus-t., samb., tub.
Cough	dry cough before intermittent fever	Eup-per., rhus-t., tub.
Cough	dry cough before midnight	Arg-n., Calc., lyc., nit-ac., phos., rhus-t., stann.
Cough	dry cough before midnight during sleep	Nit-ac., rhus-t.
Cough	dry cough disturbing sleep	Alum., calad., kali-c., nux-v., ol-j., phos., rhod., rhus-t., sang., spong., squil., stict., sulph., syph., zinc.
Cough	dry cough during coryza	Bell., graph., merc., nat-m., nit-ac., sel., sep.
Cough	dry cough during coryza in evening	Dig.
Cough	dry cough during day time and loose at night	Caust., sep., staph.
Cough	dry cough during day time before menses	Graph.
Cough	dry cough during dry chill	Ferr., rhus-t.
Cough	dry cough during fever	Acon., ang., ant-c., apis., arn., ars., bell., brom., Bry., calc., carb-v., caust., cham., chin-a., chin., cina., coff., Con., cupr., dros., hep., hyos., ign., Ip., Kali-c., kali-p., lach., lyc., Nat-m., nit-ac., nux-m., Nux-v., op., petr., Phos., plat., puls., rhus-t., Sabad., samb., sep., spig., spong., squil., staph., sul-ac., sulph., tarent., verat., verb.
Cough	dry cough during sleep	Cham., coff., mag-s., nit-ac., rhus-t., sep.
Cough	dry cough from change of temperature	Acon.
Cough	dry cough from cold air	Kali-c., phos., sang., seneg.
Cough	dry cough from cold drinks	Sil.
Cough	dry cough from constriction of throat	Aesc.
Cough	dry cough from dry cold air	Crot-h.
Cough	dry cough from dryness in larynx	Ant-t., atro., bell., bry., calc., carb-an., carb-o., caust., colch., con., cop., crot-h., dros., eug., ip., kali-c., kali-chl., kalm., lach., lachn., laur., mang., nux-v., petr., phyt., plan., puls., raph., rhus-t., Sang., seneg., spong., stann., stram., sulph., verat-v., verat.
Cough	dry cough from eating	Aeth., agar., all-s., ferr-ma., hyos., kali-c., nux-v., sep., sulph., ter.
Cough	dry cough from eating at night	Ter.
Cough	dry cough from inhaling smoke	Kali-bi.
Cough	dry cough from open air	Coff., kali-c., mag-arct., seneg., spig.
Cough	dry cough from reading aloud	Mang., meph., Phos.
Cough	dry cough from scrapping of larynx	Alumn., aur-m-n., bell., bov., Brom., bry., chel., coc-c., con., dig., gamb., hep., hydr-ac., laur., led., mang., naja., nit-ac., nux-v., op., osm., Puls., sabad., seneg., til.
Cough	dry cough from smoking	Acon., all-s., atro., coc-c., coca., hell., petr., thuj.
Cough	dry cough from smoking and sneezing	Cina.
Cough	dry cough from sunset to sunrise	Aur.
Cough	dry cough from suppressed measles	Cop.

Body part/Disease	Symptom	Medicines
Cough	dry cough from tickling in larynx	Agar., am-m., arg-n., asaf., aur-m-n., aur-m., bar-c., bell., bov., brom., cact., calc-f., carb-ac., carb-an., caust., cimic., coca., colch., coloc., Con., crot-c., cycl., hydr-ac., hydr., iod., ip., ir-foe., iris., kali-bi., kali-c., lach., lachn., led., Lyc., mang., mez., nat-m., nat-s., nit-ac., nux-v., op., ox-ac., phyt., psor., Puls., rat., rumx., sang., seneg., sep., zinc., zing.
Cough	dry cough from violent exertion	Ox-ac.
Cough	dry cough from walking in sharp cold air	Verat.
Cough	dry cough going from warm room to open air	Acon., con.
Cough	dry cough in afternoon	Am-m., anth., calc-p., cench., chel., kali-bi., mez., nat-c., nat-m., nux-m., phel., sang., sulph., thuj.
Cough	dry cough in afternoon on entering warm room	Anth., nat-c.
Cough	dry cough in afternoon while walking	Thuj.
Cough	dry cough in damp weather	Cur.
Cough	dry cough in early morning	Alum., am-m., ant-c., chin., graph., grat., lyc., nux-v., ol-an., op., rhod., stann., sul-ac., verat.
Cough	dry cough in early morning & loose in afternoon	Am-m.
Cough	dry cough in early morning & loose in evening	Arn., bov., chin., cina., crot-t., dig., ign., iod., nux-v.
Cough	dry cough in emaciated boys	Lyc.
Cough	dry cough in evening & loose in morning	Acon., alum., ambr., ant-c., ant-t., bar-c., bry., Calc., carb-v., cupr., dros., eupho., ferr., Hep., hyos., ip., kali-c., lach., led., lyc., mag-c., mag-m., mez., mur-ac., nat-m., nit-ac., nux-v., ph-ac., phos., puls., rhus-t., seneg., sep., sil., spong., Squil., stann., stram., sul-ac., sulph., zinc.
Cough	dry cough in evening aggravated from inspiring	Dig.
Cough	dry cough in evening ameliorated on lying down	Am-m., zinc.
Cough	dry cough in evening and night and can neither sleep nor lie down	Stict.
Cough	dry cough in evening from smoking	Thuj.
Cough	dry cough in evening on entering warm room	Nat-c., puls.
Cough	dry cough in evening on going to sleep	Hep., sulph.
Cough	dry cough in evening on lying down	Alumn., bell., bor., caps., carb-v., ferr., indg., Kali-c., nat-m., nicc., nux-v., Ph-ac., Puls., Sang., Sep., stict., Sulph., teucr.
Cough	dry cough in evening until midnight	Hep., phos., rhus-t., sep., stann.
Cough	dry cough in forenoon	Agar., alum., am-m., camph., coc-c., sars., zing.
Cough	dry cough in morning after rising	Alum., ang., arg-m., arn., bar-c., bor., bov., carb-an., chin., dig., grat., nat-s., plb.
Cough	dry cough in morning before menses	Graph., Zinc.
Cough	dry cough in morning from suppressed menses	Cop.
Cough	dry cough in morning on waking	Caust., ign., mag-s., sil.
Cough	dry cough in noon	Arg-n., naja., sulph.
Cough	dry cough loose after midnight	Calc.
Cough	dry cough on deep inspiration	Aesc., brom., dig., ferr-p., hep., nat-a., plb., squil.
Cough	dry cough on entering a warm room	Anth., com., nat-c.

Body part/Disease	Symptom	Medicines
Cough	dry cough on inspiration	Bell., brom., dig., hep., lach., nat-a., plb., rumx.
Cough	dry cough on inspiration in sleep	Sep.
Cough	dry cough on motion	Bell., iod., seneg.
Cough	dry cough on rising	Grat.
Cough	dry cough on talking	Atro., bell., cimic., crot-h., dig., hep., hyos., lach., mang., rumx., stann.
Cough	dry cough on walking	Agar., bry., calc., caust., coc-c., dig., ign., mag-s., puls., sang., sil., sol-t-ae., Sulph., thuj.
Cough	dry cough while sitting	Agar., lach., phos., rhus-t.
Cough	dry cough with discharge of blood	Zinc.
Cough	dry cough with discharge of blood ends in raising black blood	Elaps.
Cough	dry cough with expectoration only in morning	Alum., am-c., bell., bry., calc., carb-v., coc-c., eupho., ferr., hep., kali-c., led., lyc., mag-c., mang., mur-ac., nat-c., nat-m., nit-ac., nux-v., ph-ac., phos., Puls., sep., sil., Squil., stann., sul-ac.
Cough	dry cough with expectoration only in morning on hawking later copious green sputum	Carb-v.
Cough	dry cough with irritation in larynx	Aphis., bell., carb-ac., cimic., kali-i., lach., lith., lyc., rumx., seneg., sulph., tab., thuj., zinc.
Cough	dry cough with sudden loss of breath	Nux-m.
Cough	ecchymosis in eye from coughing	Arn., bell.
Cough	expectoration bloody in evening when coughing	Nat-c.
Cough	expectoration bloody on coughing	Bell., sep.
Cough	expectoration copious after each paroxysmal cough	Agar., alumn., anan., arg-n., Coc-c., kali-bi., sulph.
Cough	expectoration easier after each cough	Aspar.
Cough	faintness during cough	Ars., coff.
Cough	falls asleep during dry cough	Mag-s.
Cough	feeling of tightness in abdomen during cough	Lach.
Cough	feels as though larynx would be torn at every cough	All-c.
Cough	fever with cough which increases the heat	Am-c., ambr., ant-t., arn., ars., bell., carb-v., hep., hyos., iod., ip., kreos., lach., led., lyc., mag-m., nat-c., nux-v., phos., puls., sabad., squil., sulph.
Cough	fever with dry heat at night with spasmodic gagging (choking)	**Cimx.**
Cough	food regurgitate after coughing	Raph., sul-ac.
Cough	gasping for air at 2.a.m. with cough	Chin-s.
Cough	gasping for air before cough	Ant-t., brom., bry., coc-c.
Cough	gasping for air during cough	Ant-t., cor-r., sul-ac.
Cough	gouty pain in joints increses as cough diminishes	Coloc.
Cough	grasping throat during cough	Acon., all-c., ant-t., bell., dros., hep., iod., lach.
Cough	hacking (a repeated cough that is short, dry, and rasping) cough after dinner	Agar., calc-f., Hep.

Body part/Disease	Symptom	Medicines
Cough	hacking cough after eating	Anac., hep.
Cough	hacking cough after rising	Arg-m., arn., chin., eupho., ferr., lach., nit-ac., ox-ac., par., staph., thuj.
Cough	hacking cough after the appearance of hemorrhoids	Berb., euphr., sulph.
Cough	hacking cough aggravated from heat	Hyper.
Cough	hacking cough aggravated in cold air	All-c., hyper.
Cough	hacking cough ameliorated in open air	Lil-t.
Cough	hacking cough ameliorated from holding pit of stomach	Con., Croc., dros.
Cough	hacking cough ameliorated from rising on	Rhus-t.
Cough	hacking cough ameliorated in evening after lying down	Am-m.
Cough	hacking cough at beginning of menses	Phos.
Cough	hacking cough at day time	Calc., com., gamb., nat-m., sumb.
Cough	hacking cough at night	Aeth., calc., cina., con., graph., kali-bi., kali-c., mag-s., nat-m., phyt., senec., sil.
Cough	hacking cough at night & day	Eupho.
Cough	hacking cough from crawling in the larynx	Carb-v., caust., colch., eupho., lach., prun-s.
Cough	hacking cough from deep inspiration	Nat-a.
Cough	hacking cough from dryness in larynx	Carb-an., Con., dros., kali-c., laur., mang., plan., puls., Sang., seneg., spong.
Cough	hacking cough from irritation in larynx	Hep., hyper., seneg., sumb., thuj., trom.
Cough	hacking cough from motion	Osm., seneg.
Cough	hacking cough from mucous	Laur.
Cough	hacking cough from rawness in larynx	Alum., bry., caust., coc-c., dulc., kali-bi., kali-i., laur., phos., rumx., sil., stront., sulph.
Cough	hacking cough from rising on	Benz-ac.
Cough	hacking cough from sensation of hair in trachea	Sil.
Cough	hacking cough from smoking	Clem., coc-c., coloc., hell., ign., lach., nux-v., petr.
Cough	hacking cough from talking	Sumb.
Cough	hacking cough from walking fast in open air	Ang.
Cough	hacking cough in afternoon	Calc-f., calc-p., cench., kali-c., laur., Sang.
Cough	hacking cough in evening after lying down	Caps., Ign., kali-bi., phyt., rhus-t., rumx., Sang., Sep., sil.
Cough	hacking cough in evening in bed	Bry., carb-an., Ign., lact., nit-ac., rhus-t., Sep., sulph.
Cough	hacking cough in forenoon	Am-m.
Cough	hacking cough in morning	All-c., ant-t., arg-m., arn., ars., calc., cina., con., iris., kali-c., kali-i., laur., mang., nit-ac., ol-an., par., phos., sil., sumb., thuj.
Cough	hacking cough in noon	Arg-n., naja.
Cough	hacking cough in open air	Osm., seneg.
Cough	hacking cough in warm room	Com.
Cough	hacking cough on waking	Phos., sil.

Body part/Disease	Symptom	Medicines
Cough	hacking cough wakening at midnight	Ruta.
Cough	hacking cough when going to sleep	Agar., arn., brom., hep., lach., lyc., nit-ac., sep., sulph.
Cough	hacking cough while eating	Nit-ac., sang.
Cough	hacking cough while lying down	Ars., bry., con., Hyos., ign., lach., nat-m., par., phos., rhus-t., rumx., Sang., sep., sil., stann., sulph., vesp.
Cough	hacking cough with suffocative (to die from lack of air) feeling	Asaf.
Cough	headache alternating with cough	Lach., psor.
Cough	heaviness of Head on coughing	Euphr., tax.
Cough	hissing (to make a sound like a loud continuous "s") cough	Ant-t., caust.
Cough	holds chest with hands during cough	Arn., bor., Bry., cimic., Dros., eup-per., kreos., merc., nat-m., nat-s., phos., sep.
Cough	impeded, obstructed breath during cough	Cupr-s., cupr., dig., ferr., ign., ip., nux-m., sil., squil.
Cough	inability to cough from pain	Nat-s.
Cough	inability to cough from pain ameliorated by pressure of hand on pit of stomach	Dros.
Cough	involuntary urination during cough	Alum., anan., ant-c., Apis., bell., bry., caps., carb-an., Caust., cench., colch., dulc., ferr-p., ferr., hyos., ign., kreos., lach., laur., lyc., mag-c., murx., Nat-m., nit-ac., nux-v., ph-ac., Phos., psor., Puls., rhod., rhus-t., rumx., seneg., sep., spong., Squil., staph., sulph., tarent., thuj., verat., vib., zinc.
Cough	irregular breath during cough	Clem., cupr-s.
Cough	irritation in air passages increases when more one coughs	Cist., Ign., raph., squil., teucr.
Cough	irritation in larynx ameliorated from suppressing the cough	Hyos.
Cough	itching in throat when coughing	Ambr.
Cough	jerking in knee upward during cough	Ther.
Cough	jerking in lower limb with coughing while sitting	Stram.
Cough	lachrymation with cough	Acon., agar., aloe., brom., bry., calc., carb-ac., carb-v., cench., chel., cina., cycl., eup-per., eupho., Euphr., graph., hep., ip., kali-c., kali-ma., kreos., merc., Nat-m., op., phyt., Puls., rhus-t., sabad., sil., Squil., staph., sulph.
Cough	loose cough after breakfast	Coc-c.
Cough	loose cough after eating	Bell., nux-m., phos., sanic., sil., staph., thuj.
Cough	loose cough after eating & dry after drinking	Nux-m., staph.
Cough	loose cough after midnight	Calc., hep.
Cough	loose cough aggravated from exercise & warm room	Brom.
Cough	loose cough ameliorated by sitting up	Phos.
Cough	loose cough ameliorated from drinking cold water	Coc-c.
Cough	loose cough at day & night	Dulc., sil.
Cough	loose cough at day time & dry at night	Calc., euphr., lyc., puls.
Cough	loose cough at midnight	Phos., sep.

Body part/Disease	Symptom	Medicines
Cough	loose cough at night	Am-m., calc., eug., eup-per., puls., sep., sil., stict.
Cough	loose cough at night & less free during day	Stict.
Cough	loose cough at night while lying	Arum-d.
Cough	loose cough during fever	Alum., anac., apis., arg-m., Ars., bell., bism., brom., bry., Calc., carb-v., chin., cic., cub., dig., dros., dulc., ferr., iod., Kali-c., kreos., lyc., ph-ac., phos., puls., ruta., seneg., sep., sil., spong., squil., stann., staph., sulph., thuj.
Cough	loose cough from sensation of skin hanging in throat	Alum.
Cough	loose cough from tickling deep in chest	Graph.
Cough	loose cough in afternoon	Am-m.
Cough	loose cough in afternoon & dry in morning	Am-m.
Cough	loose cough in evening	Bov., eug., mur-ac.
Cough	loose cough in evening & dry in morning	Bov.
Cough	loose cough in forenoon	Stann.
Cough	loose cough in morning & tight in afternoon	Bad.
Cough	loose cough without expectoration	Am-c., arn., arum-t., brom., caust., con., crot-t., dros., kali-s., lach., phos., sep., stann., sulph.
Cough	mucus flies from mouth when coughing	Bad., chel.
Cough	mucus in larynx after each paroxysmal of cough	Agar., Coc-c., kali-bi., nat-m., seneg., sulph.
Cough	must hold chest with both hands while whooping cough	Arn., bor., Bry., cimic., Dros., eup-per., kreos., merc., nat-m., nat-s., phos., sep.
Cough	nausea during cough	Ant-t., ars., aspar., bry., calc., caps., coc-c., coloc., cupr., dros., elaps., hep., hydr., ign., Ip., kali-ar., kali-bi., kali-c., kali-p., kali-s., lach., merc., nat-a., nat-c., nat-m., nat-p., nit-ac., nux-v., petr., ph-ac., Puls., ruta., sars., sep., squil., thuj., verat.
Cough	numbness in tips of finger during whooping cough	Spong.
Cough	oppressive cough	Ail., phel.
Cough	pain between scapula during cough	Calc., stram., sul-ac.
Cough	pain in abdomen from coughing	Am-c., apoc., arn., ars., arund., bell., Bry., cadm., calc., camph., chin-a., chin., chlor., cor-r., dros., hell., hyos., ip., kali-bi., lach., lob., Lyc., mang., nit-ac., nux-v., phos., puls., rhus-t., rumx., ruta., sabad., sep., sil., squil., Stann.
Cough	pain in back when coughing	Acon., am-c., arn., arund., Bell., Bry., calc-s., calc., caps., carb-an., chin-s., chin., cocc., cor-r., kali-bi., kali-c., kali-n., kreos., merc., nit-ac., ph-ac., phos., puls., rhus-t., rumx., seneg., sep., stram., sulph., tell.
Cough	pain in bladder when coughing	Caps.
Cough	pain in calf on coughing	Nux-v.
Cough	pain in cervical glands when couging	Nat-m.
Cough	pain in cervical region on coughing	Alum., bell., caps., lact., Sulph.
Cough	pain in chest during cough	Apis., arn., ars., bell., Bry., calc-s., calc., caps., caust., chel., coff., con., kali-n., lact., lyc., Merc., nat-s., phos., psor., puls., rhus-t., sabad., seneg., sep., Squil., stram., Sulph., tarent., verat., zinc.

Body part/Disease	Symptom	Medicines
Cough	pain in clavicle on coughing	Apis.
Cough	pain in dorsal region on coughing	Calc., caps., kali-bi., merc., sil., stram.
Cough	pain in heart on coughing	Tarent.
Cough	pain in hip on coughing	Arg-m., bell., **Caust.**, rhus-t., sulph., valer.
Cough	pain in joints when cough diminishes	Coloc.
Cough	pain in kidneys on coughing	Bell.
Cough	pain in knee during cough	Bry., caps.
Cough	pain in larynx grasps the larynx on coughing	Acon., All-c., ant-t., bell., dros., Hep., iod., lach., phos.
Cough	pain in larynx on coughing	Acon., All-c., arg-m., Bell., bor., brom., bry., calc., carb-v., caust., chel., chin., coc-c., dros., hep., iod., kali-bi., kali-c., lach., med., nat-m., osm., phos., puls., rumx., sars., spong., stann.
Cough	pain in left shoulder during cough	Ferr., rhus-t.
Cough	pain in leg during cough	Bell., caps., nux-v., sulph.
Cough	pain in lumbar region to testes on coughing	Osm.
Cough	pain in lumbar region when coughing	Am-c., arn., bell., bor., bry., calc-s., calc., caps., kali-bi., kali-n., merc., nit-ac., ph-ac., puls., sep., sulph.
Cough	pain in mammae during cough	Con.
Cough	pain in nose when coughing	Nit-ac.
Cough	pain in pharynx during cough	Mag-m.
Cough	pain in region of heart after hawking	Spig.
Cough	pain in region of scapula on coughing	Apis.
Cough	pain in sacral region when coughing	Am-c., bry., chel., merc., nit-ac., sulph., tell.
Cough	pain in shoulder during cough	Am-c., ars., bry., chin., dig., ferr., lach., phos., puls., rhus-t., sang., thuj., xan.
Cough	pain in spermatic cord during cough	Nat-m.
Cough	pain in spine during cough	Bell.
Cough	pain in sternum when coughing	Bell., Bry., Caust., chel., chin., cina., cor-r., daph., euphr., hep., Kali-bi., kali-i., kali-n., kreos., osm., ox-ac., ph-ac., phos., phyt., psor., rumx., sang., staph., sulph., thuj.
Cough	pain in teeth aggravated from coughing	Bry., lyc., sep.
Cough	pain in throat after coughing	Coc-c., naja.
Cough	pain in throat on coughing	Acon., ambr., Arg-m., arum-t., calc., camph., Caps., carb-an., carb-s., carb-v., chin-s., chin., cist., coc-c., cycl., fl-ac., hep., iod., kali-bi., kalm., lach., lyc., mag-s., nat-m., nux-v., phos., psor., ran-s., sep., sil., spong., sulph., tarent.
Cough	pain in trachea on coughing	Bell., Bry., camph., Caust., chel., chin., cor-r., ign., Kali-bi., kali-i., kali-n., kreos., laur., nat-m., nux-v., osm., ox-ac., ph-ac., Phos., phyt., psor., puls., rumx., sang.,spong., staph., sulph., thuj.
Cough	pain in upper limb during cough	Dig., puls.
Cough	pain in uvula after cough	Cast., coc-c., hep., mag-m., mur-ac., ph-ac., phos., sulph.
Cough	pain in uvula when hawking	Lyc., sep.

Body part/Disease	Symptom	Medicines
Cough	pain of face during cough	Kali-bi.
Cough	pain under left scapula during cough	Stict.
Cough	pain under left scapula when coughing	Cor-r., sulph.
Cough	pain under nipples during cough	Mosch.
Cough	pain under scapula when coughing	Seneg.
Cough	pain, burning in larynx during cough	Ars., bell., bufo., carb-v., caust., cham., chel., coc-c., dros., gels., iod., mag-m., phos., pyrog., rumx., seneg.
Cough	pain, burning in trachea during cough	Ant-c., carb-v., caust., cina., iod., lach., mag-m., pyrog., Spong., sulph., zinc.
Cough	pain, burning in trachea on coughing	All-c., staph., sulph.
Cough	painful cough	Aur.
Cough	painful cough at midnight before waking	Rhus-t.
Cough	painful cough at night	Caust., rhus-t.
Cough	painful cough in bed in evening	Bry.
Cough	palpitation of heart during cough	Agar., calc-p., calc., cupr., kali-n., nat-m., psor., puls., stram., sulph.
Cough	panting (take short fast shallow breaths) cough	Calad., dulc., mur-ac., phos., rhus-t., sul-ac.
Cough	panting cough preventing sleep	Calad.
Cough	paroxysmal cough at 11.00 p.m. after lying down	Rumx.
Cough	paroxysmal convulsive stretching Cough	Bell., carb-h., chin., cina., hydr-ac., lyc.
Cough	paroxysmal cough after dinner	Aeth., calc-f., phos.
Cough	paroxysmal cough ameliorated at at day time	Bell., ign., lyc., spong.
Cough	paroxysmal cough ameliorated from lying hand on pit of stomach	Croc.
Cough	paroxysmal cough ameliorated from rinsing mouth with cold water	Coc-c.
Cough	paroxysmal cough ameliorated from sitting up	Cinnb.
Cough	paroxysmal cough at 1.30 p.m.	Phel.
Cough	paroxysmal cough at 11.00 p.m.	Ant-t., bell., lach., Rumx., spong., squil.
Cough	paroxysmal cough at 11.00 p.m. after sleep	Aral., lach.
Cough	paroxysmal cough at 2.00 a.m	Dros.
Cough	paroxysmal cough at 2.00 a.m and 3.30 a.m.	Coc-c.
Cough	paroxysmal cough at 2.00 p.m.	Ol-an.
Cough	paroxysmal cough at 4.00 p.m.	Chel., coca.
Cough	paroxysmal cough at 5.00 p.m.	Cupr.
Cough	paroxysmal cough at 5.00 p.m. to 9.00 p.m.	Caps.
Cough	paroxysmal cough at day time	Agar., euphr., hep., nit-ac., staph.
Cough	paroxysmal cough at midnight	Cham., dig., mosch., naja., phos., sulph.
Cough	paroxysmal cough at midnight ameliorated by swallowing mucous	Apis.
Cough	Paroxysmal cough at night	Nat-m.

Body part/Disease	Symptom	Medicines
Cough	paroxysmal cough at night after becoming warm in bed	Coc-c., naja.
Cough	paroxysmal cough at night before going to bed	Coc-c.
Cough	paroxysmal cough consisting of a few coughs	Bell., calc., laur.
Cough	paroxysmal cough consisting of long coughs	Ambr., carb-v., Cupr., ip., lob.
Cough	paroxysmal cough consisting of short coughs	Alum., ant-t., asaf., bell., calc., carb-v., coc-c., cocc., cor-r., dros., kali-bi., kali-c., lact., squil.
Cough	paroxysmal cough consisting of three coughs	Carb-v., cupr., phos., stann.
Cough	paroxysmal cough consisting of two coughs	Agar., cocc., grat., laur., merc., phos., plb., puls., sul-ac., sulph., thuj.
Cough	paroxysmal cough consisting of two coughs in quick succession	Merc-sul.
Cough	paroxysmal cough follow one another quickly	Agar., ant-t., cina., coff., cor-r., Dros., hep., ip., merc., sep., sulph.
Cough	paroxysmal cough followed by copious (produced or existing in large quantities) mucous	Agar., alumn., anan., arg-n., Coc-c., kali-bi., seneg., stann., sulph.
Cough	paroxysmal cough from crawling in larynx	Psor.
Cough	paroxysmal cough from eating bread or cake	Kali-n.
Cough	paroxysmal cough from walking in cool wind	Coca.
Cough	paroxysmal cough from walking in hot sun	Coca.
Cough	paroxysmal cough in aterafnoon	Agar., all-c., bad., bell., bry., caps., chel., coca., cupr., mosch., mur-ac., ol-an., phel.
Cough	paroxysmal cough in evening after lying down	Nux-v.
Cough	paroxysmal cough in evening at 6.15 p.m.	Ol-an.
Cough	paroxysmal cough in evening at 7.00 p.m.	Grat.
Cough	paroxysmal cough in evening at 7.00 p.m. till midnight	Bar-c., carb-v., ferr., hep., led., mag-c., mez., nit-ac., puls., rhus-t., sep., stann., zinc.
Cough	paroxysmal cough in evening in bed	Cocc., nat-m.
Cough	paroxysmal cough in evening in cool wind	Coca.
Cough	paroxysmal cough in forenoon	Agar., cact., coc-c., grat., sabad., sep.
Cough	paroxysmal cough in morning after rising	Ant-c., ferr-p.
Cough	paroxysmal cough in morning after waking	Agar., ambr., Rumx., thuj.
Cough	paroxysmal cough in morning ameliorated by eating	Ferr.
Cough	paroxysmal cough in morning in bed	Coc-c., ferr., Nux-v.
Cough	paroxysmal cough in noon until midnight	Mosch.
Cough	paroxysmal cough not ceasing until masses of offensive sputa are raised	Carb-v.
Cough	paroxysmal cough while smoking	All-s.
Cough	paroxysmal cough with sneezing	Agar., carb-v., lyc.
Cough	paroxysmal cough with ssudden suffocation in swallowing	Brom.
Cough	persistent (continuing) cough	Acon., am-caust., Bell., cact., crot-t., cub., Cupr., dios., hyos., ip., jatr., kali-n., lyc., mag-p., merc., mez., nux-v., rumx., sang., squil.

Body part/Disease	Symptom	Medicines
Cough	persistent cough at midnight aggravated from lying on back and ameliorated from lying on side	Nux-v.
Cough	perspiration from coughing	Acon., ant-c., ant-t., apis., arg-n., **Ars.**, bell., brom., bry., calc., caps., carb-an., carb-s., carb-v., caust., cham., chin-a., chin., cimx., dig., dros., eug., eupi., ferr-ar., ferr., guare., **Hep.**, ip., kali-c., kali-n., lach., lyc., merc., nat-a., nat-c., nat-m., nat-p., nux-v., ph-ac., **Phos.**, psor., puls., rhus-t., sabad., **Samb.**, sel., seneg., **Sep.**, sil., spong., squil., sulph., tab., thuj., verat.
Cough	perspiration from coughing at night	Chin., dig., eug., kali-bi., lyc., merc., nat-c., nit-ac., psor., sulph.
Cough	perspiration from fetid odor after coughing	Hep.
Cough	perspiration from offensive odor after cough	Hep., merl.
Cough	perspiration in hand on coughing	Ant-t.
Cough	Phthisis of larynx with short hacking cough and loss of voice	Stann.
Cough	pulsation at night from coughing	Calc.
Cough	pulsation during cough	Calc.
Cough	pulsation in head from coughing	Arn., aur., dirc., ferr., hep., hipp., ip., iris., kali-c., led., Lyc., nat-m., nit-ac., ph-ac., phos., seneg., sep., sil., spong., sulph.
Cough	pulsation on back aggravated from coughing	Nit-ac.
Cough	rasping (harsh grating sound) cough	Calc., Spong., stram.
Cough	Resonant (deep in sound) cough	Kali-bi.
Cough	respiration accelerated during paroxysms of cough	Dros.
Cough	respiration arreasted during cough	Nat-m.
Cough	retching with cough	Agar., ambr., ant-t., apis., arg-n., ars-i., ars., aspar., bell., bor., brom., bry., bufo., carb-s., Carb-v., caust., cench., cham., chin-a., chin., chlor., cimx., Cina., coc-c., crot-h., crot-t., cupr., daph., Dros., dulc., ferr-m., hell., Hep., hyos., ign., iod., ip., kali-ar., kali-bi., kali-c., kali-i., kali-s., kreos., lach., lob., lyc., mag-m., mag-p., merc., mez., nat-m., Nit-ac., nux-v., ol-j., plan., Puls., ruta., sabad., sang., seneg., sep., sil., squil., stann., sul-ac., sulph., tab., tarent., thuj., verat.
Cough	ringing (a clear, continuing, usually high-pitched sound) cough	Acon., all-c., apis., ars., asaf., dol., Dros., kali-bi., lac-c., spong., stram.
Cough	sawing respiration between coughs	Spong.
Cough	sciatic pain in lower limb aggravated from coughing	Caps., caust., sep., tell.
Cough	sensation as though he could not cough, to start mucus deep enough	Ars., bell., Caust., dros., lach., med., mez., rumx.
Cough	sensation of crawling in throat causing cough	Bry., carb-v., eupho., kali-c., lach., prun-s., stann.
Cough	sensation of emptyness in chest after cough	Ill., kali-c., nat-s., sep., stann., zinc.
Cough	sensation of emptyness in chest during cough	Sep., stann., sulph.
Cough	sleepiness after coughing	Ign.
Cough	sleepiness with cough	Ant-c., **Ant-t.**, ip., kreos., op.
Cough	slow breath during cough	Clem.

Body part/Disease	Symptom	Medicines
Cough	sneezing ends in cough	Agar., arg-n., bad., bell., bry., carb-v., hep., lyc., psor., seneg., squil., sulph.
Cough	stiffness before cough	**Cina.**
Cough	stiffness during cough	Bell., caust., cina., cupr., ip., led., mosch.
Cough	stitching pain in larynx during cough	Aloe., bufo., dros., kali-c., mur-ac., phos., sulph.
Cough	stitching pain in trachea on coughing	All-c., bell., bor., calc., cist., med., phos., staph.
Cough	suffocative cough after eating & drinking	Bry.
Cough	suffocative cough during sleep	Aral., carb-an., Lach.
Cough	suffocative cough from inspiration	Cina.
Cough	suffocative cough from walking	Ars.
Cough	suffocative cough on swallowing	Brom.
Cough	suffocative cough while lying	Spong.
Cough	Supports larynx on coughing	Acon., All-c., ant-t., bell., dros., hep., iod., lach.
Cough	sweating on forehead during cough	Ant-t., chlor., ip., verat.
Cough	tearing cough at night	Bell., senec.
Cough	tearing cough during menses	Senec.
Cough	three coughs in succession	Carb-v., cupr., phos., stann.
Cough	tight cough at day time	Nat-a.
Cough	tight cough in evening	Calc-s.
Cough	toneless (lifeless) cough	Calad., card-b., cina., dros.
Cough	trembling from coughing	Bell., cupr., phos.
Cough	twitching in hand when coughing	Cina.
Cough	unconsciousness between attacks of cough	Ant-t., cadm.
Cough	vertigo on coughing	Acon., ant-t., calc., coff., cupr., kali-bi., led., mosch., naja., nux-v.
Cough	vomiting blood with cough	Anan.
Cough	vomiting from cough	Anac., anan., ant-t., Bry., coc-c., dig., dros., ferr., Ip., kali-c., laur., mez., nat-m., nit-ac., ph-ac., puls., sep.
Cough	waking from cough	Alum., ars., bism., calc., caust., coc-c., graph., hep., **Hyos.**, mag-m., mang., nit-ac., nux-v., op., psor., **Puls.**, rhus-t., sep., sil., stront., **Sulph.**, tab., thuj.
Cough	waking from cough during menses	Zinc.
Cough	weakness from cough & expectoration	Nux-v.
Cough	weakness in chest from cough	Graph., nit-ac., ph-ac., psor., ruta., sep., Stann.
Cough	weakness in chest from cough before menses	Graph.
Cough	wheezing (breathe with hoarse whistling sound) or whistling cough, while lying on back, or on either side	Med.
Cough	whistling (to make a shrill or musical sound by forcing the breath through a small gap between the lips or the teeth) cough	Acon., ars., brom., carb-v., chlor., hep., kali-bi., kali-i., kali-p., kreos., laur., lyc., prun-s., samb., sang., seneg., spong.
Cough	whistling breath during cough	Lyc.
Cough	whistling respiration in whooping cough	Brom., carb-v., cupr., hep., samb., spong.
Cough	yawning after coughing	Ant-c., **Ant-t.**, ip., **Kreos.**, op.

Body part/Disease	Symptom	Medicines
Cough	yawning when coughing	Bell.
Crack	chapped (to become sore and cracked by exposure to wind or cold) fingers	Nat-m.
Crack	chapped face	Arum-t., graph., lach., petr., sil.
Crack	chapped hand	Aesc., alum., am-c., anan., apis., arn., aur., Calc., Calen., carb-ac., Graph., ham., Hep., hydr., kali-c., kreos., lyc., mag-c., merc., nat-c., nat-m., Petr., puls., Rhus-t., Sars., Sep., sil., Sulph, zinc.
Crack	chapped hand from working in water	Alum., ant-c., Calc., cham., hep., merc., rhus-t., sars., sep., Sulph.
Crack	chapped lips	Agar., Alum., am-m., ant-t., apis., arn., ars., Arum-t., bov., Calc., Carb-v., cham., chel., chin., colch., cor-r., fl-ac., graph., guare., hep., kali-bi., kali-c., kali-i., kreos., mag-m., Nat-m., ol-an., ph-ac., phos., sel., staph., Sulph., tab., tarax., zinc.
Crack	chapped nails	Nat-m.
Crack	chapped nose	Arum-t., carb-an.
Crack	chapped nostril	Aur.
Crack	chapped tips of fingers	Bar-c.
Crack	cracked , dry and rough scurfs (thin dry flaking scales of skin, usually as a result of a skin condition such as dandruff) on scrotum	Chel.
Crack	cracked corners of mouth	Am-c., ambr., ant-c., apis., Arum-t., calc., caust., cinnb., Cund., eup-per., Graph., hell., hydr., Ind., merc., mez., nat-a., nat-m., Nit-ac., sep., Sil., zinc.
Crack	cracked gums	Plat.
Crack	cracked lower lips	Apis., cham., cimic., nat-c., nit-ac., phos., Sep.
Crack	cracked lower middle lips	Agar., am-c., aur-m., cham., dros., hep., nat-m., puls.
Crack	cracked mouth	Ambr., bism., bufo., cocc., lach., ph-ac., phos.
Crack	cracked nipples	Arn., Cast-eq., Caust., cur., fl-ac., Graph., hydr., lyc., merc-c., mill., Phyt., Rat., sep., sil., sulph.
Crack	cracked painful nipples	Graph., phyt.
Crack	cracked ulcer in hand	Merc.
Crack	cracked upper lips	Bar-c., hell., kali-c., nat-c., nat-m., tarax.
Crack	cracked upper middle lips	Hep., nat-m., sel.
Crack	cracks behind ears	Chel., Graph., hep., hydr., lyc., petr., sep., sulph.
Crack	cracks between fingers	Ars., aur-m., graph., sulph., zinc.
Crack	cracks between toes	Aur-m., carb-an., eug., graph., lach., nat-m., sars., Sil.
Crack	cracks between toes with violent itching	Nat-m.
Crack	cracks in axilla	Hep.
Crack	cracks in back of hands	Merc., nat-c., petr., rhus-t., sanic., Sep.
Crack	cracks in ball of hands	Hep.
Crack	cracks in corner of eye	Alum., Graph., iod., Lyc., merc., nat-m., nit-ac., petr., phos., plat., sep., sil., sulph., zinc.

Body part/Disease	Symptom	Medicines
Crack	cracks in fingers	Am-m., bar-c., Calc., cist., hep., kali-c., mag-c., merc., Petr., phos., Sars., sil., zinc.
Crack	cracks in first finger	Sil.
Crack	cracks in joints of fingers	Graph., mang., merc., phos., sanic.,sulph.
Crack	cracks in joints of fingers that ulcerate	Merc.
Crack	cracks in meatus of urethra	Nat-c., nit-ac., ph-ac., phos., thuj.
Crack	cracks in palms of hands	Cist., merc-i-r., petr., sulph.
Crack	cracks in septum (a thin partition or membrane dividing or separating the nostrils)	Merc.
Crack	cracks of hands from wetting	Alum., ant-c., Calc., cist., kali-c., nit-ac., puls., rhus-t., rhus-v., sars., Sep., Sulph., zinc.
Crack	cracks of hands in winter	Alum., Calc., cist., merc., Petr., psor., sanic., Sep., Sulph.
Crack	cracks of skin	Aesc., aloe., alum., am-c., ant-c., arn., aur., bad., bar-c., bry., calc-s., **Calc.**, carb-an., **Carb-s.**, carb-v., cham., com., cycl., **Graph.**, hep., hydr., iris., kali-c., kali-s., kreos., lach., lyc., mag-c., mang., merc., nat-c., nat-m., nit-ac., olnd., osm., paeon., **Petr.**, phos., psor., **Puls.**, rhus-t., ruta., **Sars.**, **Sep.**, sil., **Sulph.**, teucr., viol-t., zinc.
Crack	cracks of skin after washing	Alum., ant-c., bry., calc-s., **Calc.**, cham., kali-c., lyc., nit-ac., puls., rhus-t., sars., **Sep.**, **Sulph.**, zinc.
Crack	cracks of skin in winter	Alum., calc-s., **Calc.**, **Carb-s.**, graph., **Petr.**, psor, **Sep.**, **Sulph.**
Crack	cracks of skin itching	Merc., petr.
Crack	cracks of skin painful	Graph., mang., zinc.
Crack	cracks of skin ulcerated	Bry., merc.
Crack	cracks of skin with burning	Petr., sars., zinc.
Crack	cracks of skin yellow	Merc.
Crack	cracks on bends & joints of skin	Graph., hippoz.
Crack	cracks on feet	Aur-m., com., hep., Sars., sulph.
Crack	cracks on hands	Aesc., Alum., am-c., anan., ant-c., arn., aur-m., aur., bar-c., Calc., carb-s., cench., cist., cycl., Graph., hep., kali-c., kali-s., kreos., lach., lyc., mag-c., maland., merc., nat-c., nat-m., Nit-ac., Petr., phos., psor., puls., rhus-t., rhus-v., ruta., sanic., Sars., sec., sep., Sil., Sulph., Zinc.
Crack	cracks on hands burning	Petr., sars., zinc.
Crack	cracks on hands from cold	Sanic., zinc.
Crack	cracks on heel	Lyc.
Crack	cracks on lower limbs	Alum., aur-m., aur., bar-c., calc., Hep., lach., merc., nat-c., nat-m., petr., sulph., zinc.
Crack	cracks on nails	Ant-c., ars., nat-m., sil.
Crack	cracks on shoulder	Petr.
Crack	cracks on soles	Ars.
Crack	cracks on surface of abdomen	Sil.
Crack	cracks on thumb	Sars.
Crack	cracks on tips of nails	Aur-m., bar-c., Graph., Petr.

Body part/Disease	Symptom	Medicines
Crack	cracks on upper limbs	Kali-ar., sil.
Crack	cracks on wrist	Kali-ar.
Crack	cracks under toes	Sabad.
Crack	deep and bleeding cracks on hands	Alum., merc., Nit-ac., Petr., sanic., sars.
Crack	deep bloody cracks of skin	Merc., **Nit-ac., Petr.,** puls., sars., sulph.
Crack	deep cracks between toes	Hydr.
Crack	eruption, cracked in hands	Alum., lyc., merc., petr.
Crack	eruption, cracked in upper limbs	Phos.
Crack	eruption, cracked	Phos.
Crack	eruption, cracks in back of hands	Merc.
Crack	eruption, crusty & full of cracks in hands	Anthr., **Graph.,** petr., sanic.
Crack	eruption, fissures (a break in the skin lining the anal canal, usually causing pain during bowel movements and sometimes bleeding. Anal fissures occur as a consequence of constipation or sometimes of diarrhoea) in bend of elbow	Kali-ar.
Crack	eruption, fissures in wrists	Kali-ar.
Crack	eruption, pustules cracked	Rhus-t.
Crack	fetid cracks of skin	Merc.
Crack	horny callosities with deep cracks	Cist., graph.
Crack	horny excrescences on hand cracked at base	Thuj.
Crack	humid cracks of skin	Aloe.
Crack	itching in cracks of hands	Merc., petr.
Crack	mercurial cracks of skin	Hep., nit-ac., sulph.
Crack	new cracks of skin with burning	Sars.
Crack	tongue fissured across	Cob.
Crack	tongue fissured in all directions	Fl-ac., Nit-ac.
Crack	tongue fissured in centre	Bapt., bufo., cob., cub., lept., mez., nit-ac., raph., rhus-v., sin-n.
Crack	tongue fissured on edges painful with hard margins	Clem.
Crack	tongue fissured on edges	Anan., clem., lach., nux-v.
Crack	tongue fissured on left side	Bar-c.
Crack	tongue fissured on tip of tongue	Lach.
Crack	urticaria vesicular cracked	Bry., crot-h., lach., phos., vip.
Cracking	cracking cervical region	Agar., agn., aloe., anac., aur-m-n., chel., chin., cocc., nat-c., nicc., nit-ac., nux-v., ol-an., petr., puls., raph., spong., stann., sulph., thuj.
Cracking	cracking in ankle from bending side to side	Caust.
Cracking	cracking in ankle from bending	Ant-c.
Cracking	cracking in ankle from false step	Caust.
Cracking	cracking in ankle in evening	Am-c.
Cracking	cracking in ankle on stretching	Ant-c., thuj.

Body part/Disease	Symptom	Medicines
Cracking	cracking in ankle while walking	Carb-s., nit-ac., nux-v., sulph.
Cracking	cracking in ankle	Am-c., ant-c., aster., camph., Canth., carb-s., caust., hep., kali-bi., mag-s., nit-ac., nux-v., petr., ph-ac., sep., sulph., thuj.
Cracking	cracking in elbow	Am-c., ant-c., brom., cinnb., con., dios., kalm., merc., mur-ac., nat-m., sulph., tep., thuj., zinc., zing.
Cracking	cracking in elbow from stretching	Thuj.
Cracking	cracking in elbow in afternoon	Kalm.
Cracking	cracking in finger from closing the hand	Ars-m.
Cracking	cracking in finger joints	Ars-m., caps., carb-an., kali-n., merc., sulph.
Cracking	cracking in foot	Caust., petr., ph-ac., sars., sulph., thuj.
Cracking	cracking in hip	Aloe., anac., camph., cocc., croc., glon., nat-m.
Cracking	cracking in hip in morning on rising	Aloe.
Cracking	cracking in joints during convulsions	Acon.
Cracking	cracking in joints in morning	Brom.
Cracking	cracking in joints in morning after rising	Brom.
Cracking	cracking in joints of lower limbs	Benz-ac., brach., bry., camph., caust., cham., cocc., con., led., nux-v., petr., puls., ran-b., sel., sep., tab., thuj.
Cracking	cracking in joints of lower limbs from stepping	Euphr., mag-s.
Cracking	cracking in joints of lower limbs from stooping	Croc.
Cracking	cracking in joints of lower limbs from walking	Bry.
Cracking	cracking in joints of upper limbs	Ant-t., benz-ac., brach., chin-s., croc., kali-bi., merc., mur-ac., thuj.
Cracking	cracking in joints when turning	Caul.
Cracking	cracking in joints while walking	Am-c., bry., caul., cocc.
Cracking	cracking in knee	Acon., alum., am-c., ars., aster., benz-ac., bry., calad., calc., camph., caps., Caust., cham., cocc., con., cop., croc., gins., glon., hura., ign., lach., led., mag-s., mez., nat-a., nat-m., nit-ac., nux-v., petr., podo., puls., raph., sel., sep., Sulph., tab., tep., thuj., verat.
Cracking	cracking in knee as if cartilage slipped	Petr.
Cracking	cracking in knee from ascending stairs	Hura.
Cracking	cracking in knee from descending stairs	Caust., hura.
Cracking	cracking in knee from extending limb	Nat-a.
Cracking	cracking in knee when flexing	Calad., nat-a., sel.
Cracking	cracking in knee when lying down	Sel.
Cracking	cracking in knee when stretching	Cop., mag-s., ran-b., rhus-t., thuj.
Cracking	cracking in knee while walking	Alum., ars., bry., calad., calc., Caust., glon., hura., led., mag-s., nat-m., nit-ac., nux-v., tab.
Cracking	cracking in knee, painless	Acon.
Cracking	cracking in left knee	Aster., calad.
Cracking	cracking in patella	Con., ran-b.
Cracking	cracking in right knee	Mez.
Cracking	cracking in right shoulder	Carb-s.

Body part/Disease	Symptom	Medicines
Cracking	cracking in right shoulder from elevation of arm	Kali-c., nat-a.
Cracking	cracking in right shoulder from stretching	Sabad.
Cracking	cracking in right shoulder in bed at night	Mez.
Cracking	cracking in right shoulder in morning	Aloe.
Cracking	cracking in shoulder	Aloe., anac., ant-t., bar-c., brach., calc., carb-s., cic., cinnb., croc., ferr., gins., kali-c., merc., mez., nat-a., nat-m., phos., sabad., sars., thuj.
Cracking	cracking in sternum in region of heart	Nat-c.
Cracking	cracking in sternum on bending chest backwards	Am-c.
Cracking	cracking in sternum on motion	Nat-m., sulph.
Cracking	cracking in third joint of finger	Hydr., phos.
Cracking	cracking in thumb	Nux-v.
Cracking	cracking in upper limbs when leaning on arm	Thuj.
Cracking	cracking in wrist	Arn., cic., con., kali-bi., merc., ox-ac., phos., sel., tep.
Cracking	cracking in wrist from stretching	Sel.
Cracking	cracking in wrist in evening	Con.
Cracking	cracking in wrist with tearing in hands	Sel.
Cracking	cracking of cervical region from stooping on	Spong.
Cracking	cracking of cervical region rising from stooping on	Nicc.
Cracking	cracking of lumbar region extending to anus	Sulph.
Cracking	cracking of lumbar region when stooping	Agar., rhus-t.
Cracking	cracking of lumbar region while walking	Zinc.
Cracking	cracking of scapula on lifting arm	Anac.
Cracking	cracking of spine on moving	Agar., cocc., kali-bi.
Cracking	crackling (a network of fine cracks created as decoration) of gums on pressure	Daph.
Cramp	cramp in right hip	Sul-ac.
Cramp	cramp (Painful muscle contraction) in bladder	Berb., caps., carb-s., carb-v., coc-c., mag-p., nux-v., ph-ac., plb., prun-s., ruta., sars., sep., zinc.
Cramp	cramp (painful muscle contraction) in right lower limbs	Bufo.
Cramp	cramp after exertion	Mag-p.
Cramp	cramp aggravated from cold air	Bufo.
Cramp	cramp aggravated from pressure	Zinc.
Cramp	cramp at night	Merc.
Cramp	cramp during chill	Cupr., sil.
Cramp	cramp during stool	Bell.
Cramp	cramp from discharge of semen	Bufo.
Cramp	cramp in urethra	Chel., nit-ac., phos.
Cramp	cramp in afternoon	Sulph.
Cramp	cramp in ankle	Agar., calc-p., carl., cupr., plat., sel.
Cramp	cramp in ankle extending over heel	Agar.
Cramp	cramp in ankle extending to calf	Cupr.

Body part/Disease	Symptom	Medicines
Cramp	cramp in ankle feeling as if extremities were going to sleep	Plat.
Cramp	cramp in ankle in evening	Sel.
Cramp	cramp in ankle in evening while lying	Sel.
Cramp	cramp in anterior part of forearm (part of the human arm between the elbow and the wrist)	Berb., plat., plb.
Cramp	cramp in back	Bell., calc-p., iod., kali-bi., lyc., naja., nux-v., plb.
Cramp	cramp in back of hand at night in bed	Anac.
Cramp	cramp in ball of hand	Plat.
Cramp	cramp in biceps (a muscle that has two points of attachment at one end, especially one biceps brachii in the upper arm and one biceps femoris in the back of the thigh)	Ruta., valer.
Cramp	cramp in bladder	Berb., caps., carb-s., carb-v., coc-c., mag-p., nux-v., ph-ac., plb., prun-s., ruta., sars., sep., zinc.
Cramp	cramp in bladder after urination	Caust., nat-m.
Cramp	cramp in bladder during urination	Carb-s.
Cramp	cramp in buttock muscles	Agar., bell., gels., hyos., hyper.
Cramp	cramp in calf after coition	Coloc.
Cramp	cramp in calf after mortification (the death and decaying of a part of a living body, e.g. because the blood supply to it has been cut off)	Coloc.
Cramp	cramp in calf after stool	Ox-ac., trom.
Cramp	cramp in calf after walking	Carb-an., plat., **Rhus-t.**
Cramp	cramp in calf ameliorated on motion	Arg-m., bry., ferr., rhus-t.
Cramp	cramp in calf at day time	Graph., petr.
Cramp	cramp in calf at night	Ambr., anac., arg-n., ars., berb., bry., Calc., carb-an., carb-v., caust., coca., cocc., dig., eupi., ferr-m., ferr., graph., kali-c., Lyc., lyss., mag-c., mag-m., med., nit-ac., nux-m., nux-v., petr., plb., rhus-v., sars., sep., stann., Sulph., zinc.
Cramp	cramp in calf at night from bending foot	Chin.
Cramp	cramp in calf before menses	Phos.
Cramp	cramp in calf before sleep	Nux-m.
Cramp	cramp in calf during coition	Cupr., graph.
Cramp	cramp in calf during labor	Nux-v.
Cramp	cramp in calf during menses	Cupr., phos., verat.
Cramp	cramp in calf during pregnancy	Sep.
Cramp	cramp in calf during sleep	Ant-t., graph., inul., kali-c., nat-m., tep.
Cramp	cramp in calf from ascending	Berb.
Cramp	cramp in calf from lifting the foot	Agar.
Cramp	cramp in calf in afternoon	Ant-t., elaps.
Cramp	cramp in calf in bed	Ars., bov., Calc., Carb-s., caust., eupi., ferr-m., ferr., graph., hep., ign., kali-c., lachn., lact-ac., mag-c., nux-v., phys., Rhus-t., sep., sil., Sulph.

Body part/Disease	Symptom	Medicines
Cramp	cramp in calf in bed on flexing thigh	Nux-v.
Cramp	cramp in calf in cholera	Ant-t., camph., colch., **Cupr.**, jatr., kali-p., mag-p., **Sulph.**, **Verat.**
Cramp	cramp in calf in evening	Kali-n., mag-c., nux-v., sel., sulph.
Cramp	cramp in calf in evening in bed	Ars., mag-c., puls.
Cramp	cramp in calf in evening on going to sleep	Berb., nux-m.
Cramp	cramp in calf in forenoon	Nat-m., sulph.
Cramp	cramp in calf in morning	Bry., carb-an., lach., nit-ac.
Cramp	cramp in calf in morning in bed	Bov., caust., graph., hep., ign., lach., lact-ac., nit-ac., sil., sulph.
Cramp	cramp in calf in morning on rising	Ferr., lact-ac.
Cramp	cramp in calf in morning on waking	Lob.
Cramp	cramp in calf on attempting to coition	Cupr.
Cramp	cramp in calf on bending knee	Cocc., hep., ign.
Cramp	cramp in calf on crossing feet	Alum.
Cramp	cramp in calf on descending	Coca.
Cramp	cramp in calf on drawing up knee	Coff.
Cramp	cramp in calf on drawing up leg	Kali-c., nit-ac.
Cramp	cramp in calf on flexing leg	Cocc., coff., kali-c., nux-v.
Cramp	cramp in calf on motion	Bapt., bufo., calc., coca., hyos., ign., lyc., nux-m.
Cramp	cramp in calf on pulling boot	Calc.
Cramp	cramp in calf on rising from a bed	Ferr., mag-c.
Cramp	cramp in calf on rising from a seat	Alum., anac.
Cramp	cramp in calf on standing long	Euphr.
Cramp	cramp in calf on standing	Euphr., ferr., nat-m.
Cramp	cramp in calf on stepping	Sulph.
Cramp	cramp in calf on waking	Graph., lob., staph., verat-v.
Cramp	cramp in calf on walking	Agar., am-c., **Anac.**, arg-m., arg-n., ars., berb., **Calc-p.**, cann-s., coca., dulc., ign., lact., lyc., mag-m., nat-m., nit-ac., puls., sul-ac., **Sulph.**
Cramp	cramp in calf when stretching foot after waking	Aspar.,Chin., nit-ac., thuj.
Cramp	cramp in calf when stretching foot in bed after waking	**Calc.**, carl., cham., lyss., nat-c., pin-s., sulph.
Cramp	cramp in calf when stretching leg	Bar-c., bufo., **Calc.**, carl., lyc., nux-v., sep., sulph.
Cramp	cramp in calf when thinking about it	Spong., staph.
Cramp	cramp in calf when turning foot while sitting	Nat-m.
Cramp	cramp in calf when turning over in bed	Mag-c.
Cramp	cramp in calf while dancing	Sulph.
Cramp	cramp in calf while lying	Bry., led., mag-c., sel.
Cramp	cramp in calf while sitting bent	Lyc.
Cramp	cramp in calf while sitting	Ign., lyc., olnd., plat., **Rhus-t.**
Cramp	cramp in calf while walking	Phos.

Body part/Disease	Symptom	Medicines
Cramp	cramp in extensor muscle of forearm	Merc.
Cramp	cramp in fifth toe	Coc-c.
Cramp	cramp in fifth toe at night	Coc-c.
Cramp	cramp in fifth toe at night on lying	Coc-c.
Cramp	cramp in fingers at midnight in bed	Nux-v.
Cramp	cramp in fingers at night in bed	Ars.
Cramp	cramp in fingers during parturition (act of giving birth)	Cupr., Dios.
Cramp	cramp in fingers from playing piano or violin	Mag-p.
Cramp	cramp in fingers in evening	Ars.
Cramp	cramp in fingers in morning	Tab.
Cramp	cramp in fingers on moving	Merc.
Cramp	cramp in fingers when stretching them	Ars.
Cramp	cramp in fingers while sewing	Kali-c.
Cramp	cramp in fingers while shoe making	Stann.
Cramp	cramp in fingers while writing	Brach., cycl., mag-p., Stann., tril.
Cramp	cramp in fingers with cholera (an acute and often fatal intestinal disease that produces severe gastrointestinal symptoms and is usually caused by the bacterium Vibrio cholerae)	Colch., Cupr., sec., Verat.
Cramp	cramp in fingers, on attempting to pick a small object	Stann.
Cramp	cramp in fingers, periodical	Phos.
Cramp	cramp in first finger	Cycl., kali-chl., nat-p.
Cramp	cramp in first finger while writing	Cycl.
Cramp	cramp in first toe	Calc-p., coloc., gamb., kali-c., nux-v., psor., sil., tarent.
Cramp	cramp in first toe in bed	Gamb
Cramp	cramp in first toe on stretching out foot	Psor.
Cramp	cramp in first toe while walking	Gamb., sil.
Cramp	cramp in flexor muscle of forearm	Chin-s.
Cramp	cramp in flexor tendons (tough band connecting muscle to bone)	Dios.
Cramp	cramp in foot at day time	Ox-ac., petr., sep.
Cramp	cramp in foot at night alternating with dim vision	Bell.
Cramp	cramp in foot during chill	Cupr., elat., nux-v.
Cramp	cramp in foot during menses	Lachn., sulph.
Cramp	cramp in foot in attempting to coition	Cupr.
Cramp	cramp in foot in bed	Bry., graph., sanic.
Cramp	cramp in foot in cholera	**Cupr.**, sec., **Verat.**
Cramp	cramp in foot in evening on drawing up limbs	Ferr.
Cramp	cramp in foot in morning	Lachn.
Cramp	cramp in foot on going to sleep	Hyper.
Cramp	cramp in foot on motion	Calc., ph-ac.
Cramp	cramp in foot on motion after resting	Plb.

Body part/Disease	Symptom	Medicines
Cramp	cramp in foot on sitting	Eupho.
Cramp	cramp in foot on stretching	Caust., verat.
Cramp	cramp in foot when standing	Eupho.
Cramp	cramp in foot while walking	Verat.
Cramp	cramp in forearm	Am-c., anac., arn., berb., calc-p., calc., cina., coloc., corn., ferr-ma., kali-i., lyc., mur-ac., ph-ac., plat., plb., ruta., sep.
Cramp	cramp in forearm aggravated from motion	Kali-i., plb.
Cramp	cramp in forearm at night in bed	Anac.
Cramp	cramp in forearm from flexing arm	Arn., mur-ac.
Cramp	cramp in forearm in afternoon	Lyc.
Cramp	cramp in forearm in morning	Calc.
Cramp	cramp in forearm while walking	Sep.
Cramp	cramp in fourth finger	Cocc., com., sulph.
Cramp	cramp in fourth finger while writing	Cocc.
Cramp	cramp in fourth toe	Coc-c.
Cramp	cramp in fourth toe at night	Coc-c.
Cramp	cramp in fourth toe at night on lying	Coc-c.
Cramp	cramp in hand after flexing	Merc.,
Cramp	cramp in hand after resting	Plb.
Cramp	cramp in hand aggravated from extending	Plb.
Cramp	cramp in hand alternating with cramps in feet	Stram.
Cramp	cramp in hand alternating with dim vision	Bell.
Cramp	cramp in hand ameliorated on motion	Acon.
Cramp	cramp in hand at night	Calc.
Cramp	cramp in hand at night in bed	Plb.
Cramp	cramp in hand from exertion	Plat., sec., sil.
Cramp	cramp in hand from grasping	Ambr., Dros., graph., lyc., nit-ac., plat., stann.
Cramp	cramp in hand from grasping a cold stone	Nat-m.
Cramp	cramp in hand from writing	Alum-sil., anac., cycl., eupho., gels., Mag-p., nat-p., pic-ac., plat., sil.
Cramp	cramp in hand in afternoon	Calc-s., dios.
Cramp	cramp in hand in cholera	Cupr., sec.
Cramp	cramp in hand in evening	Lyc.
Cramp	cramp in hand in morning	Calc.
Cramp	cramp in hand on closing hand	Chin.
Cramp	cramp in hand on motion	Ars., merc., sec.
Cramp	cramp in hand transversely across	Ruta.
Cramp	cramp in heel	Anac., bry., crot-c., eug., led., mag-c., sel.
Cramp	cramp in hip	Ang., arg-m., aur., bell., cann-s., carb-v., caust., cimic., coloc., cop., cur., jug-c., nat-m., ph-ac., phos., ruta., sep., sul-ac., valer.

Body part/Disease	Symptom	Medicines
Cramp	cramp in hip at night	Jug-c.
Cramp	cramp in hip during labor	Cimic.
Cramp	cramp in hip during menses	Form.
Cramp	cramp in hip while eating	Ph-ac.
Cramp	cramp in hip while sitting	Ph-ac.
Cramp	cramp in hollow of knee	Bell., berb., calc., cann-s., caust., kali-n., lyc., paeon., petr., phys., plb., sulph.
Cramp	cramp in inner side of biceps muscles	Sulph.
Cramp	cramp in joints	Anac., ang., aur., bell., bry., Calc., camph., canth., caust., cic., cocc., hyos., ign., lach., laur., merc., op., par., ph-ac., Plat., plb., rhus-t., sec., stram., sulph., verat.
Cramp	cramp in knee	Ang., arg-m., arn., arund., berb., bry., cadm., calc., carb-an., carb-v., coloc., crot-t., dios., hep., hyper., lach., led., petr., plb., sulph., tab., zinc.
Cramp	cramp in knee alternating with each other	Sulph.
Cramp	cramp in knee at night	Bry.,Sulph.
Cramp	cramp in knee from stretching leg	Calc.
Cramp	cramp in knee in afternoon	Dios.
Cramp	cramp in knee in morning	Dios.
Cramp	cramp in knee on waking	Lach.
Cramp	cramp in knee when stamping foot	Berb.
Cramp	cramp in knee while sitting	Bry., paeon.,Chin.
Cramp	cramp in knee while sitting long after	Chin.
Cramp	cramp in knee while standing	Ang.
Cramp	cramp in knee while walking	Ang., carb-an., chin., petr.
Cramp	cramp in left hand	Calc., euphr., nat-p., sulph.
Cramp	cramp in left hip	Jug-c.
Cramp	cramp in left thigh	Cina., rhus-t.
Cramp	cramp in left upper limb	Cact.
Cramp	cramp in left upper limb after midnight on waking	Sulph.
Cramp	cramp in left upper limb at midnight on waking	Caust.
Cramp	cramp in left upper limb in evening	Lyc.
Cramp	cramp in left upper limb in morning	Fl-ac.
Cramp	cramp in left wrist	Sulph.
Cramp	cramp in leg ameliorated from pressing upon flexors muscle	Ox-ac., rhus-t.
Cramp	cramp in leg ameliorated from sitting	Cina.
Cramp	cramp in leg at day time	Ferr-m., ox-ac.
Cramp	cramp in leg at night	Ambr., carb-an., carb-v., Lyc., merc-d., merc., nat-m., pall., sulph.
Cramp	cramp in leg at night in bed	Dios., nux-v., plb., puls., rhus-t.
Cramp	cramp in leg during chill	Cupr., elat., nux-v.

Body part/Disease	Symptom	Medicines
Cramp	cramp in leg during cough	Dros.
Cramp	cramp in leg during labor	Cupr., mag-p.
Cramp	cramp in leg during menses	Gels., graph.
Cramp	cramp in leg during pregnancy	Gels., ham., vib.
Cramp	cramp in leg during stool	Colch., cupr., sulph., verat.
Cramp	cramp in leg from physical exertion	Alum.
Cramp	cramp in leg from pressing upon flexors muscle	Lyc.
Cramp	cramp in leg in afternoon while in bed	Rhus-t.
Cramp	cramp in leg in evening	Orig., sep.
Cramp	cramp in leg in evening after lying down	Puls.
Cramp	cramp in leg in morning	Arum-t., crot-h.
Cramp	cramp in leg in morning on waking	Arum-t.,Bufo.
Cramp	cramp in leg on extension	Calc., plb.
Cramp	cramp in leg on motion	Verat-v.
Cramp	cramp in leg when going to sleep	Hyper.
Cramp	cramp in leg when lifting	Calc., iod.
Cramp	cramp in leg when stretching out the feet	Sulph.
Cramp	cramp in leg while lying	Am-c.
Cramp	cramp in leg while walking	Carb-an., carb-v., cina., gels.
Cramp	cramp in lower limbs after sitting	Nit-ac.
Cramp	cramp in lower limbs at night	Ambr., ars., bry., calad., carb-v., eug., eup-per., iod., ip., lachn., lyc., mag-c., mag-m., nit-ac., nux-v., rhus-t., sec., sep., staph., sulph.
Cramp	cramp in lower limbs from bending foot forward	Coff.
Cramp	cramp in lower limbs from crossing limbs	Alum.
Cramp	cramp in lower limbs from extending leg	Bar-c., calc.
Cramp	cramp in lower limbs in evening	Jatr., sil.
Cramp	cramp in lower limbs in morning	Bov., bry., nit-ac.
Cramp	cramp in lower limbs when lifting legs	Coff.
Cramp	cramp in lower limbs when stepping out	Alum.
Cramp	cramp in lower limbs while descending stairs	Arg-m.
Cramp	cramp in lower limbs while sitting	Olnd., paeon., rhus-t.
Cramp	cramp in lower limbs while sitting after walking	Rhus-t.
Cramp	cramp in lower limbs while standing	Eupho., euphr.
Cramp	cramp in lower limbs while walking	Eupho., euphr.
Cramp	cramp in lower limbs with colic	Coloc.
Cramp	cramp in nates	Bell., bry., cann-s., caust., graph., rhus-t., sep.
Cramp	cramp in nates at night in bed	Sep.
Cramp	cramp in nates while standing	Rhus-t.
Cramp	cramp in nates while stooping	Cann-s.
Cramp	cramp in oesophagus	Op.

Body part/Disease	Symptom	Medicines
Cramp	cramp in palms	Coloc., mur-ac., naja., stry., zing.
Cramp	cramp in pregnancy	Cupr., verat., vib.
Cramp	cramp in region of tibia	Am-c.
Cramp	cramp in right calf	Agar., kali-c., lyss., trom.
Cramp	cramp in right hand	Acon., merc-i-r., plb., sabad.
Cramp	cramp in right thigh	Sulph., tarent.
Cramp	cramp in right upper limb	Bufo.
Cramp	cramp in right wrist	Hura., staph.
Cramp	cramp in second finger	Am-m., hura., lil-t., plb., sulph.
Cramp	cramp in second toe	Sep.
Cramp	cramp in shoulder	Cimic., elaps., lil-t., naja., plat.
Cramp	cramp in shoulder extending to hand	Elaps.
Cramp	cramp in side of external throat	Bar-c.
Cramp	cramp in sole after walking	Calc.
Cramp	cramp in sole ameliorated while walking	Verb.
Cramp	cramp in sole at day time	Nux-v.
Cramp	cramp in sole at day time on trying to rise	Nux-v.
Cramp	cramp in sole at night	Agar., calad., calc., med., nit-ac., nux-v., petr., **Sulph.**
Cramp	cramp in sole at night from drawing up limbs	Kali-c., nux-v.
Cramp	cramp in sole at night in cholera	**Sulph.**
Cramp	cramp in sole at night when lying down	Bry.
Cramp	cramp in sole at night when rising	Plat.
Cramp	cramp in sole at night while lying down	Sel.
Cramp	cramp in sole during menses	Sulph.
Cramp	cramp in sole during pregnancy	**Calc.**
Cramp	cramp in sole from drawing on boot	Calc.
Cramp	cramp in sole from hanging foot down	Berb.
Cramp	cramp in sole from smoking	Calad.
Cramp	cramp in sole from standing	Verb.
Cramp	cramp in sole in bed	Bell., carb-v., sep., thuj.
Cramp	cramp in sole in bed aggravated from putting foot out of bed	Chel.
Cramp	cramp in sole in evening	Hipp., nat-m., zing.
Cramp	cramp in sole in evening after lying down	Carb-v.
Cramp	cramp in sole in intermittent fever	Elat.
Cramp	cramp in sole in intermittent fever	Elat.
Cramp	cramp in sole in morning	Ferr., form.
Cramp	cramp in sole on moving	Eug., petr.
Cramp	cramp in sole on stepping	Chel., sulph.
Cramp	cramp in sole on stretching	Caust.
Cramp	cramp in sole on the side lain on	Staph.

Body part/Disease	Symptom	Medicines
Cramp	cramp in sole preceding colic	Plb.
Cramp	cramp in sole when dancing	Bar-c.
Cramp	cramp in sole while riding in a carriage	Thuj.
Cramp	cramp in sole while sitting	Bry., hipp., stann.
Cramp	cramp in sole while walking	Bar-c., petr., sil., sulph., vib.
Cramp	cramp in sole while walking in open air	Carb-v.
Cramp	cramp in tendo	Calc., caust.
Cramp	cramp in tendo (an inelastic cord or band of tough white fibrous connective tissue that attaches a muscle to a bone or other part) achillis (heel) in bed at night	Caust.
Cramp	cramp in thigh at night	Ambr., carb-an., hep., ip., kali-c.
Cramp	cramp in thigh during day time	Petr.
Cramp	cramp in thigh during menses	Wies.
Cramp	cramp in thigh during sleep	Kali-c.
Cramp	cramp in thigh in evening	Bell.
Cramp	cramp in thigh in evening in bed	Ars.
Cramp	cramp in thigh on going to sleep	Tep.
Cramp	cramp in thigh while ascending stairs	Carb-v.
Cramp	cramp in thigh while sitting	Iod., plat.
Cramp	cramp in thigh while walking	Sep.
Cramp	cramp in thigh while walking in open air	Verb.
Cramp	cramp in third finger	Hura., sep., sulph.
Cramp	cramp in third finger from extending to elbow	Sep., sulph.
Cramp	cramp in third finger in evening	Sep., sulph.
Cramp	cramp in third toe	Coc-c., iod.
Cramp	cramp in third toe at night	Coc-c.
Cramp	cramp in third toe at night on lying	Coc-c.
Cramp	cramp in throat	Acon., ars., chel., gels., graph., kali-i., phos., sars., sep., sul-ac.
Cramp	cramp in thumb	Agar., aml-n., asaf., mang., nat-m., valer.
Cramp	cramp in thumb while writing	Aml-n., brach., cycl.
Cramp	cramp in thumb with twitching	Valer.
Cramp	cramp in toes alternating with spasm (muscle contraction) of glottis (voice box)	Asaf.
Cramp	cramp in toes at midnight in bed	Nux-v.
Cramp	cramp in toes at night	Calc., coc-c.
Cramp	cramp in toes at night in bed	Ars., merc-i-f.
Cramp	cramp in toes during labor	Cupr.
Cramp	cramp in toes during menses	Sulph.
Cramp	cramp in toes during pregnancy	Calc.
Cramp	cramp in toes from stretching out foot	Psor., sulph.
Cramp	cramp in toes in evening in bed	Ars.

Body part/Disease	Symptom	Medicines
Cramp	cramp in toes in morning in bed	Nicc.
Cramp	cramp in ulnar (the longer of the two bones in the human forearm, situated on the inner side) side of hand	Cocc., puls.
Cramp	cramp in upper arm	Agar., arg-m., bell., com., kali-bi., lil-t., lyc., mur-ac., petr., ph-ac., rhus-t., sulph., valer.
Cramp	cramp in upper arm on exertion	Mur-ac.
Cramp	cramp in upper arm on holding something in hand	Rhus-t., valer.
Cramp	cramp in upper arm on raising arm	Arg-m.
Cramp	cramp in urethra	Chel., nit-ac., phos.
Cramp	cramp in wrist	Aml-n., anac., calc-p., cina., cit-v., com., euphr., hura., nat-p., ph-ac., plb., staph., sulph.
Cramp	cramp in wrist from coldness in part	Plb.
Cramp	cramp in wrist on motion	Calc-p.
Cramp	cramp in wrist when arm is outstretched	Cina.
Cramp	cramp in wrist while writing	Aml-n., brach.
Cramp	cramp like twitching of calf	Jatr.
Cramp	cramp like constrictions under nails	Elaps.
Cramp	cramp like numbness in lower limb during exertion	Alum.
Cramp	cramp like numbness in upper arm during exertion	Alum.
Cramp	cramp like stiffness of forearm	Plat., stann.
Cramp	cramp like stiffness of hand	Plat., stann.
Cramp	cramp like stiffness of thigh	Bry.
Cramp	cramp like twitching of forearm	Asaf.
Cramp	cramp on motion	Nux-v.
Cramp	cramp, compelling him to bend double	Prun-s.
Cramp	cramping (painful muscle contraction) pain in abdomen after breakfast	Agar., eupi., grat., ham., kali-bi., nux-m., stront., Zinc.
Cramp	cramping pain in abdomen after fruit	Calc-p., chin., coloc., puls.
Cramp	cramping pain in abdomen after ice cream	Ars., calc-p., ip., puls.
Cramp	cramping pain in abdomen after menses	Am-c., cocc., kreos., merl., puls.
Cramp	cramping pain in abdomen after milk	Cupr., lac-d., mag-s., raph.
Cramp	cramping pain in abdomen after sour food	Asaf.
Cramp	cramping pain in abdomen after taking cold	All-c., alumn., Asaf., dulc.
Cramp	cramping pain in abdomen ameliorated by warm milk	Crot-t., op.
Cramp	cramping pain in abdomen ameliorated from hot milk	Crot-t.
Cramp	cramping pain in abdomen ameliorated from kneading abdomen	Nat-s.
Cramp	cramping pain in abdomen ameliorated from passing flatus	Acon., am-c., cimx., coloc., con., echi., graph., hydr., lyc., mag-c., merc-c., nat-a., nat-m., nux-m., ol-an., psor., rumx., sil., spong., squil., sulph.
Cramp	cramping pain in abdomen ameliorated while lying	Cupr., ferr.
Cramp	cramping pain in abdomen ameliorated while lying on the abdomen	Am-c., chion., coloc., dor.

Body part/Disease	Symptom	Medicines
Cramp	cramping pain in abdomen before menses	Aloe., alum., am-c., bar-c., bell., brom., calc-p., carb-v., caust., cham., chin., cinnb., cocc., coloc., croc., cupr., cycl., hyper., ign., Kali-c., lach., mag-c., mag-p., manc., nux-v., ph-ac., plat., puls., sep., spong.
Cramp	cramping pain in abdomen before menses from hip to hip	Thuj.
Cramp	cramping pain in abdomen during constipation	Merc., op., plb., podo.
Cramp	cramping pain in abdomen during fever	Caps., carb-v., elat., rhus-t., rob.
Cramp	cramping pain in abdomen from fasting	Dulc.
Cramp	cramping pain in abdomen from melons	Zing.
Cramp	cramping pain in extremities at night	Phos.
Cramp	cramps in axilla	Com., hura., iod.
Cramp	cramps in chest after eating	Nat-m.
Cramp	cramps in chest after exertion	Plb.
Cramp	cramps in chest aggravated from motion	Ferr., sulph.
Cramp	cramps in chest ameliorated on lying down	Sulph.
Cramp	cramps in chest at night	Nat-a.
Cramp	cramps in chest during menses	Cocc.
Cramp	cramps in chest in evening in warm room	Sulph.
Cramp	cramps in chest in evening while riding	Phos.
Cramp	cramps in chest in open air	Iod.
Cramp	cramps in chest in warm room	Sulph.
Cramp	cramps in chest on coughing	Kali-c., laur.
Cramp	cramps in chest on walking	Ferr.
Cramp	cramps in chest with eructations	Dig.
Cramp	cramps in heart	Anan., ars., bry., cupr., kali-bi., kali-c., Lach., mez., myric., sep., tarent., thuj., zinc.
Cramp	cramps in heart from soft music	Thuj.
Cramp	cramps in lungs after walking	Arum-t.
Cramp	cramps in lungs from drinking cold water	Thuj.
Cramp	cramps in lungs	Mosch., zinc.
Cramp	cramps in mammae gradually increasing and decreasing	Plat.
Craving	craving for Alcohol	China
Craving	desires acidic fruit	Ars., calc-s., calc., chin., cist., cub., ign., thuj., Verat.
Craving	desires alcoholic drinks before menses	Sel.
Craving	desires almonds	Cub.
Craving	desires apples	Aloe., ant-t., guai., sulph., tell.
Craving	desires aromatic drinks	Anan.
Craving	desires ashes	Tarent.
Craving	desires bananas	Ther.
Craving	desires bitter drinks	Acon., dig., nat-m., ter.

Body part/Disease	Symptom	Medicines
Craving	desires bitter food	Dig., nat-m.
Craving	desires boiled eggs	Calc.
Craving	desires boiled milk	Abrot., nat-s.
Craving	desires bread	Abrot., aloe., am-c., ars., aur., bell., bov., cina., coloc., con., cub., ferr-ar., ferr., grat., hell., hydr., ign., mag-c., merc., nat-a., nat-c., nat-m., op., plb., puls., sec., sil., staph., stront., sumb.
Craving	desires bread & butter	Agar., bell., ferr., grat., hell., hydr., ign., mag-c., Merc., puls.
Craving	desires burnt coffee	Alum., chin.
Craving	desires butter	All-s., merc.
Craving	desires cayenne pepper (a very hot-tasting red powder made from the dried and ground fruit and seeds of several kinds of chili. Use: in cooking and as a gastric astringent)	Merc-c.
Craving	desires charcoal	Alum., cic., con., nit-ac., nux-v.
Craving	desires cheese	Arg-n., aster., cist., ign., mosch., puls.
Craving	desires cherries	Chin.
Craving	desires chocolate	Lepi., lyss.
Craving	desires cider (non alcoholic fresh apple drink)	Benz., sulph.
Craving	desires cloves	Alum., chlor.
Craving	desires coal	Alum., calc., cic.
Craving	desires coffee	Alum., Ang., arg-m., arg-n., ars., aster., aur., bry., calc-p., caps., carb-v., cham., chel., chin., colch., con., gran., lach., lec., lob., mez., mosch., nat-m., nux-m., nux-v., ph-ac., sabin., sel., sol-t-ae., sulph.
Craving	desires coffee which nauseates	Caps.
Craving	desires cold food	Am-c., ant-t., cupr-ar., cupr., kali-s., lyc., merc-c., nat-m., Phos., Puls., sil., thuj., verat., zinc.
Craving	desires cold milk	Ph-ac., phel., phos., rhus-t., sabad., staph., tub.
Craving	desires cucumbers	Abies-n., ant-c., verat.
Craving	desires death during convalescence	Absin., aur., lac-c., sep.
Craving	desires dry food	Alum.
Craving	desires dry rice	Alum., ter.
Craving	desires eggs	Calc., hydr., nat-p., ol-an.
Craving	desires fat	Ars., hep., Nit-ac., nux-v., sulph.
Craving	desires fat	Ars.
Craving	desires fish	Nat-m., nat-p., phos.
Craving	desires food containig starch	Lach., nat-m., sabad., sumb.
Craving	desires fried eggs	Nat-p.
Craving	desires fried food	Plb.
Craving	desires fruit	Aloe., alum., alumn., ant-t., ars., calc-s., chin., cist., cub., gran., hep., ign., lach., mag-c., nat-m., Ph-ac., puls., sul-ac., Verat.

Body part/Disease	Symptom	Medicines
Craving	desires green fruit	Calc-s., med.
Craving	desires highly seasoned fruit	Chin., fl-ac., hep., lac-c., nux-v., Phos., puls., sang., sep., Sulph., tarent.
Craving	desires honey	Sabad.
Craving	desires hot milk	Calc., chel., graph., hyper.
Craving	desires ice	Elaps., med., merc-c., nat-s., Verat.
Craving	desires ice cream	Calc., eup-per., Phos., tub., verat.
Craving	desires indigestible things	Alum., alumn., bell., bry., calc-p., calc., cycl.
Craving	desires indistinct knows not what	Bry., chin., Ign., ip., lach., mag-m., Puls., sang., sil., ther.
Craving	desires juicy things	Aloe., gran., nat-a., Ph-ac., puls., sabin., sars., verat.
Craving	desires lemonade (drinks made from lemons)	Bell., calc., cycl., eup-pur., jatr., nit-ac., puls., sabin., sec., sul-i.
Craving	desires lemons	Ars., benz., verat.
Craving	desires lime, slate pencils, earth, chalk, clay, etc.	Alum., calc., cic., ferr., nat-m., Nit-ac., nux-v.
Craving	desires liquid food	Ang., bell., bry., calc-ar., caps., ferr., merc., ph-ac., staph., sulph., verat.
Craving	desires many things	Cina., kreos., phos.
Craving	desires meat	Abies-c., aloe., aur., canth., cycl., ferr-m., ferr., graph., hell., iod., kreos., lil-t., mag-c., meny., merc., nat-m., sabad., sanic., sulph., tub.
Craving	desires milk	Anac., apis., ars., aur., bapt., bor., bov., bry., calc., chel., elaps., kali-i., lac-c., mag-c., mang., merc., nat-m., nux-v., ph-ac., phel., Rhus-t., sabad., sabin., sil., staph., stront., sulph.
Craving	desires mustard	Ars., cocc., colch., hep., mez., mill., nicc.
Craving	desires nuts	Cub.
Craving	desires oranges	Cub., elaps., med., sol-t-ae., ther.
Craving	desires oysters	Apis., brom., bry., calc., Lach., lyc., nat-m., rhus-t.
Craving	desires pastry	Bufo., calc., chin., plb.
Craving	desires pepper	Lac-c.
Craving	desires pickles	Abies-c., ant-c., ham., hep., hyper., lach., nat-a., sul-i., sulph., verat.
Craving	desires pig's meat	Calc-p., cench., mez., sanic., tub.
Craving	desires plums	Sul-ac.
Craving	desires plums sauce	Arg-n.
Craving	desires pork	Crot-h., tub.
Craving	desires potatoes	Nat-c., ol-an.
Craving	desires puddings	Sabad.
Craving	desires pungent things	Ars., aster., cist., fl-ac., hep., lac-c., nat-p., ph-ac., sang.
Craving	desires raw food	Ail., sil., Sulph., tarent.
Craving	desires raw ham (meat from pig's thigh)	Uran.
Craving	desires raw onions	All-c., cub.
Craving	desires raw potatoes	Calc.

Body part/Disease	Symptom	Medicines
Craving	desires salads	Elaps.
Craving	desires salty sands	Tarent.
Craving	desires salty things	Aloe., Arg-n., atro., calc-p., calc-s., calc., Carb-v., caust., cocc., con., cor-r., Lac-c., lyss., manc., med., meph., merc-i-f., merc-i-r., Nat-m., nit-ac., Phos., plb., sanic., sel., sulph., tarent., teucr., thuj., tub., Verat.
Craving	desires sands	Tarent.
Craving	desires sardines (tiny oceon fish)	Cycl., verat.
Craving	desires smoked meat	Calc-p., Caust., kreos., Tub.
Craving	desires smoked things	Calc-p., Caust., kreos.
Craving	desires smoking	Calad., carb-an., card-m., eug., glon., ham., led., lyc., ther.
Craving	desires snow	Crot-c.
Craving	desires snuff (tobacco in the form of powder, taken by sniffing it up the nostrils)	Bell.
Craving	desires soft boiled eggs	Calc., ol-an.
Craving	desires soup	Calc-ar.
Craving	desires sour milk	Mang.
Craving	desires sour, acids	Alum., alumn., am-c., am-m., ant-c., ant-t., apis., arg-n., arn., ars., arund., bell., bol., bor., brom., bry., calc-s., calc., carb-an., carb-s., carb-v., cham., chel., chin-a., chin., cist., con., conv., Cor-r., corn., cub., cupr., dig., elaps., ferr-ar., ferr-m., ferr-p., ferr., fl-ac., gran., Hep., hipp., ign., kali-ar., kali-bi., kali-c., kali-p., kali-s., kreos., lach., mag-c., mang., med., merc-i-f., nat-m., phel., phos., plb., podo., psor., ptel., puls., rhus-t., sabad., sabin., sec., sep., squil., stram., sul-i., sulph., thea., ther., thuj., ust., Verat., ziz.
Craving	desires starch	Alum., calc., cic., nit-ac., nux-v.
Craving	desires strange things	Bry., calc-p., calc., chel., cycl., hep., manc.
Craving	desires strange things during pregnancy	Chel., Lyss., mag-c.
Craving	desires strange things during pregnancy	Chel., Lyss., mag-c.
Craving	desires strong cheese	Arg-n., aster.
Craving	desires sugar	Am-c., Arg-n., calc., kali-c., sec.
Craving	desires sweets	Am-c., arg-m., Arg-n., ars., bar-c., bry., bufo., calc-s., calc., carb-v., chin-a., Chin., elaps., ip., kali-ar., kali-c., kali-p., kali-s., Lyc., mag-m., med., merc., nat-a., nat-c., nat-m., nux-v., op., petr., plb., rheum., rhus-t., sabad., sec., sep., Sulph., tub.
Craving	desires tea	Aster., calc-s., hep., hydr., pyrus.
Craving	desires tobacco	Bell., carb-ac., daph., eug., kreos., manc., nat-c., nux-v., ox-ac., plat., plb., staph., Tab., ther., thuj.
Craving	desires tomatoes	Ferr.
Craving	desires tonics	Aloe., carb-ac., carb-an., caust., cocc., nux-v., ph-ac., puls., rheum., rhus-t., sul-ac., valer.
Craving	desires vegetables	Alum., alumn., ars., calc-s., carb-an., cham., mag-c., mag-m.

Body part/Disease	Symptom	Medicines
Craving	desires vinegar	Apis., arn., ars., chel., Hep., kali-p., lepi., sep., sulph.
Craving	desires warm drinks	Ang., Ars., bell., Bry., calad., carb-v., casc., cast-v., cedr., chel., cupr., eup-per., eup-pur., graph., hyper., kali-ar., kreos., Lac-c., lyc., merc-c., pyrus., sabad., sulph.
Craving	desires warm drinks during chill	Ars., cedr., eup-per.
Craving	desires warm drinks during fever	Casc., cedr., eup-per., lyc.
Craving	desires warm food	Ang., Ars., chel., cocc., cupr., cycl., ferr., lyc., ph-ac., sabad., sil.
Craving	desires warm milk	Bry.
Craving	desires warm soup	Bry., calc-ar., ferr., nat-m., phel.
Crawling	burning pain & crawling in first finger	Agar.
Crawling	cough from sensation of crawling in bronchia (relating to or affecting the tubes bronchi that carry air from the windpipe into the lungs)	Aeth.,Eupi., kreos.
Crawling	cough from sensation of crawling in chest	Cahin., caust., con., kreos., nux-m., rhus-t., squil.
Crawling	cough from sensation of crawling in larynx	Am-m., ant-t., bry., calc-p., carb-v., caust., colch., Con., dros., eupho., iod., Kali-c., kreos., lach., lact., led., mag-m., nux-m., prun-s., psor., rhus-t., sabin., sang., stann., stict., sulph.
Crawling	cough from sensation of crawling in throat-pit	Apis., kreos., mag-m., Sang.
Crawling	cough from sensation of crawling in trachea	Anac., arn., carb-v., caust., kreos., prun-s., rhus-t.
Crawling	crawling in corner of eye	Plat.
Crawling	crawling in eye	Agar., asar., bell., chin., cina., colch., nat-c., nat-s., seneg., sep., spig., sulph., verat.
Crawling	crawling in gums	Arn., graph., kali-c., Sec.
Crawling	crawling in larynx after eating	Nit-ac.
Crawling	crawling in larynx after lying	Caps.
Crawling	crawling in larynx at night	Lyc.
Crawling	crawling in larynx from cough	Kreos.
Crawling	crawling in larynx from cough	Kreos.
Crawling	crawling in larynx in evening	Carb-v.
Crawling	crawling in larynx in morning	Iod.
Crawling	crawling in larynx when swallowing	Staph.
Crawling	crawling in larynx while sitting	Psor.
Crawling	crawling in larynx	Am-m., ant-t., arn., bov., bry., calc-s., caps., carb-v., caust., colch., Con., dros., graph., iod., Kali-c., kreos., lach., laur., led., lyc., mag-m., Nat-m., nit-ac., prun-s., psor.,rhus-t., sabin., sang., sep., stann., stram., stront., sulph., thuj., zinc.
Crawling	crawling in palate	Acon., carb-v., grat., sabad.
Crawling	crawling in tongue	Plat.
Crawling	crawling in trachea after lying down in evening	Caps.
Crawling	crawling in trachea from cough	Colch., mag-m.

Body part/Disease	Symptom	Medicines
Crawling	crawling in trachea	Anac., arn., caps., colch., lach., led., lyc., mag-m., nit-ac., nux-m., ruta., seneg., spong., stann.
Crawling	crawling in urethra	Agar., berb., chin., ferr-i., ign., junc., lyc., merl., mez., petros., ph-ac., ran-s., tarent., thuj., tus-p.
Crawling	crawling in urethra after urinating	Canth., lyc.
Crawling	crawling in urethra when not urinating	Ph-ac.
Crawling	crawling in urethra when urinating	Ign., petros., ph-ac.
Crawling	crawling in urethra when urinating	Ign., petros., ph-ac.
Crawling	crawling of worm in forehead	Alum.
Crawling	crawling on floor	Lach.
Crawling	despair (hopelessness) from crawling on skin	**Psor.**
Crawling	feeling of insects crawling on Occiput	Ars., brom., sep., thuj.
Crawling	feeling of insects crawling on vertex	Calc-p., cann-i., cupr., lil-t., nat-s.
Crawling	feeling of insects crawling on forehead	Apis., arn., arund., benz-ac., chel., cic., colch., glon., kali-c., laur., manc., nux-v., ph-ac., rhus-t., rhus-v., tarax., zinc.
Crawling	feeling of insects crawling on skin after emission	Ph-ac.
Crawling	feeling of insects crawling on skin of glans	Alum., chel., merc., nat-m., ph-ac.
Crawling	feeling of insects crawling on skin of glans after urination	Puls.
Crawling	feeling of insects crawling on skin of penis	Acon., alum., carl., coloc., puls., Sec., tab., valer.
Crawling	feeling of insects crawling on skin of scrotum in evening in bed	Chin.
Crawling	feeling of insects crawling on skin of scrotum	Carb-v., carl., chel., chin., com., merc., nit-ac., ph-ac., plat., rhus-v., Sec., Sil., staph., thuj.
Crawling	feeling of insects crawling on skin of testis	Agn., berb., carb-v., euphr., hipp., merc., rhod., thuj., zinc.
Crawling	feeling of insects crawling on skin	Acon., berb., clem., Plat., Sec., tarent.
Crawling	formication (feeling of insects crawling)	Acon., agar., alum., arg-n., ars-h., ars., bar-c., cact., camph., caps., carb-ac., carb-s., carl., caust., crot-c., hep., hipp., hydr-ac., ign., kali-ar., kali-c., lach., laur., **Lyc.**, mez., nux-v., **Ph-ac.**, phos., plb., psor., puls., rhod., **Rhus-t.**, sabad., **Sec.**, stram., stry., **Tarent.**, teucr., verat., zinc.
Crawling	formication after abuse of mercury	Hep.
Crawling	formication after convulsion	Stry.
Crawling	formication after emission	Ph-ac.
Crawling	formication aggravated from heat of bed	Rhod.
Crawling	formication aggravated from scratching	Dulc.
Crawling	formication ameliorated from rubbing	Zinc.
Crawling	formication ameliorated from scratching	Croc., zinc.
Crawling	formication ameliorated from warmth	Acon.
Crawling	formication at night	Bar-c., cist., mag-m., sulph.
Crawling	formication at night after lying down	Cist., ph-ac.
Crawling	formication at night during chill	Gamb.
Crawling	formication at night on waking	Carb-v.

Body part/Disease	Symptom	Medicines
Crawling	formication at root of nose	Teucr.
Crawling	formication at tip of nose	Con.
Crawling	formication beginning at feet and extending upwards	Nat-m.
Crawling	formication between the shoulders	Carl., laur., viol-t.
Crawling	formication during chill	Gamb.
Crawling	formication during erection	Tarent.
Crawling	formication during menses	Graph.
Crawling	formication during perspiration	Rhod.
Crawling	formication during sexual excitement	Mez., tarent.
Crawling	formication during urination	Hep.
Crawling	formication from walking	Graph.
Crawling	formication in ankles	Ars-i., meph., pall., rhus-v.
Crawling	formication in axilla	Berb., con.
Crawling	formication in back at night	Bar-c., bov., zinc.
Crawling	formication in back extending to fingers and toes	Sec.
Crawling	formication in back extending to limbs	Phos.
Crawling	formication in back in afternoon	Asaf., mag-s.
Crawling	formication in back in evening	Lyc., mag-s., osm.
Crawling	formication in back in morning	Ars-m.
Crawling	formication in back of fingers	Bar-ac., ran-b.
Crawling	formication in bones of lower limb	Guai.
Crawling	formication in calf	Agar., alum., ant-c., bar-c., cast., caust., cham., coloc., ip., lach., nux-v., onos., plb., rhus-v., sang., sol-n., spig., sul-ac., sulph., zinc.
Crawling	formication in calf after walking in open air	Nux-v.
Crawling	formication in calf in evening	Alum.
Crawling	formication in calf while sitting	Bar-c.
Crawling	formication in calf while standing	Verat.
Crawling	formication in calf while walking	Sul-ac.
Crawling	formication in cervical region on entering a house	Phos.
Crawling	formication in cervical region	Arund., carl., dulc., lac-c., phos., sabin., sec., spong.
Crawling	formication in chest from warm food	Mez.
Crawling	formication in chest in warm room	Mez.
Crawling	formication in chest on entering house	Phos.
Crawling	formication in day time	Arg-n.
Crawling	formication in dorsum (the back or upper surface of a part of the body such as the hand or foot)	Con.
Crawling	formication in ear in morning	Zinc.
Crawling	formication in ear while eating	Lachn.
Crawling	formication in evening	Gent-c., Nat-c., mag-c., **Sulph.**
Crawling	formication in evening on bed	Osm., Sulph., thuj.

Body part/Disease	Symptom	Medicines
Crawling	formication in evening while lying	Cist.
Crawling	formication in female private parts	Elaps., plat.
Crawling	formication in fifth toe	Crot-t., phos.
Crawling	formication in fingers	**Acon.**, aeth., agar., alum., ars., brom., calc., caust., colch., gins., graph., hep., kali-c., kreos., lach., **Lyc.**, mag-c., mag-s., mez., mur-ac., nat-c., nat-m., nit-ac., op., paeon., phos., plat., plb., psor., ran-b., rhod., rhus-t., samb., sep., sil., staph., sul-ac., thuj., verat.
Crawling	formication in fingers as from anxiety	Verat.
Crawling	formication in fingers in evening	Alum., ars., colch.
Crawling	formication in fingers in morning in bed	Psor.
Crawling	formication in fingers while writing	Acon.
Crawling	formication in first finger	Croc., mag-s., phos., tab.
Crawling	formication in first toe	Alum., brom., caust., chin., gins., jatr., phos., plat., plb.
Crawling	formication in first toe as freezing after	Alum.
Crawling	formication in first toe at night	Brom., mez.
Crawling	formication in first toe in evening	Nit-ac.
Crawling	formication in first toe on waking	Brom.
Crawling	formication in first toe with twitching	Crot-t.
Crawling	formication in foot	Acon., aeth., **Agar.**, alum., am-c., ang., ant-c., apis., arn., ars-h., ars-i., ars., arund., bell., bor., canth., caps., carb-an., carb-s., carl., caust., chel., cic., clem., coloc., con., croc., crot-c., dulc., eupho., graph., guai., hep., hyper., ign., jatr., kali-c., kali-n., kreos., lyc., mag-c., manc., mang., mez., nat-c., nat-m., nat-p., nux-v., op., par., phos., plb., rhod., rhus-t., rhus-v., sars., **Sec.**, sep., spong., stann., stram., stront., sulph., tarax., tax., zinc.
Crawling	formication in foot after heat	Sulph.
Crawling	formication in foot ameliorated from open air	Bor., zinc.
Crawling	formication in foot at night	Phos.
Crawling	formication in foot during chill	Canth.
Crawling	formication in foot extending over body	Caps., nat-m.
Crawling	formication in foot in morning	Hyper., nat-c.
Crawling	formication in foot in morning in bed	Rhus-t.
Crawling	formication in foot in morning on stepping	Puls.
Crawling	formication in foot while sitting	Carl.
Crawling	formication in foot while standing	Mang., sep.
Crawling	formication in forearm	Acon., alum., arn., carb-an., carb-s., caust., chin., chlor., con., lach., merc., plb., sec.
Crawling	formication in forenoon	Mag-c., sars.
Crawling	formication in fourth finger	Agar., aran., mag-s., phos., rhod.

Body part/Disease	Symptom	Medicines
Crawling	formication in hand	**Acon.**, agn., arn., ars-h., ars., arund., atro., bar-c., bry., canth., carb-s., caust., chel., cupr., dulc., graph., guare., hyos., hyper., kali-n., kreos., lach., lact-ac., lyc., mez., nux-v., op., ph-ac., phos., plat., rhod., **Sec.**, seneg., spig., sulph., thuj., verat.
Crawling	formication in hand after putting them in water	Sulph.
Crawling	formication in hand after writing	Agar.
Crawling	formication in hand at night	Ars.
Crawling	formication in hand during chill	Canth.
Crawling	formication in hand during menses	Graph.
Crawling	formication in hand in evening	Lact-ac.
Crawling	formication in hand in morning	Hyper., nat-c.
Crawling	formication in hand in ulnar side	Agar.
Crawling	formication in hand while yawning in open air	Phos.
Crawling	formication in heel	Agar., am-c., bell., caust., ferr-ma., graph., nat-c., par., phos., stront., sulph., zing.
Crawling	formication in heel in morning in bed	Graph.
Crawling	formication in joints	Arn., carl., ip., sec.
Crawling	formication in kidneys	Hydrc.
Crawling	formication in knee	Apis., crot-t., cycl., gent-l., kali-c., rat., rhus-t., zinc.
Crawling	formication in leg	Agar., alum., amyg., apis., arg-n., arn., ars., aster., bar-c., bov., calc-p., calc., caps., carb-o., carb-s., caust., graph., guai., hep., jatr., kali-c., kreos., lach., lact-ac., lil-t., morph., naja., nicc., **Nux-v.**, op., pall., ph-ac., phos., pic-ac., plat., puls., rhod., **Sec., Sep.**, stann., staph., stram., sul-ac., sulph., tab., tarent., tax., verat., zinc.
Crawling	formication in leg at night in bed	Zinc.
Crawling	formication in leg in evening	Lact-ac., plat.
Crawling	formication in leg in evening while walking	Graph.
Crawling	formication in leg while sitting	Ol-an., plat.
Crawling	formication in lower limb after sitting	Calc-p., sep.
Crawling	formication in lower limb while riding	Calc-p., rumx.
Crawling	formication in lower limbs	Aesc., arn., ars., aster., bov., calc-p., **Calc.**, caps., caust., euphr., graph., helod., hep., lachn., nit-ac., op., plat., rhod., rumx., sabad., **Sec.**, sep., stry., sulph.
Crawling	formication in lower limbs at night in bed	Helod.
Crawling	formication in lower limbs during menses	Graph., puls.
Crawling	formication in lower limbs in evening in bed	Sulph.
Crawling	formication in lumbar region extending to face	Arund.
Crawling	formication in lumbar region extending to shoulders	Arund.
Crawling	formication in lumbar region while sitting	Canth.
Crawling	formication in lumbar region	Acon., ars., arund., bufo-s., canth., crot-t., meny., merc-c., ph-ac., stann., tarax., thuj.

Body part/Disease	Symptom	Medicines
Crawling	formication in mammae	Calc., con., mang., ran-s.
Crawling	formication in morning in bed	Teucr.
Crawling	formication in morning	Ferr., mag-c.
Crawling	formication in nates	Ars.
Crawling	formication in nose	Am-c., aur., carb-v., con., mez.
Crawling	formication in palm	Bar-c., berb., ol-an., par., seneg., spig., vip.
Crawling	formication in paralysis	**Phos.**
Crawling	formication in paralyzed lower limb	Nux-v.
Crawling	formication in paralyzed parts	Phos., plb.
Crawling	formication in region of clavicle	Alum., arund., mez.
Crawling	formication in region of kidneys	Dirc.
Crawling	formication in rough weather	Rhod.
Crawling	formication in sacrum	Bor., crot-t., ph-ac., sars.
Crawling	formication in scapula	Anac., sil., zinc.
Crawling	formication in second finger	Acon., mag-s., mez., tab.
Crawling	formication in sole of foot	Agar., am-c., bell., berb., calc-p., **Caust.**, cic., coloc., con., fl-ac., hep., hura., kali-c., laur., mag-m., nat-m., pic-ac., plb., raph., sep., spong., staph., vip., zing.
Crawling	formication in sole of foot aggravated from rest	Sep.
Crawling	formication in sole of foot in evening	Zing.
Crawling	formication in sole of foot in evening while sitting	Zing.
Crawling	formication in sole of foot while sitting	Mag-m., staph.
Crawling	formication in sole of foot while standing	Plb., zing.
Crawling	formication in sole of foot while walking	Con., plb., spong.
Crawling	formication in spine	Acon., Agar., ars., arund., con., kali-p., lach., nat-c., sal-ac.
Crawling	formication in sternum	Ran-s.
Crawling	formication in teeth	Bar-c.
Crawling	formication in thigh	Acon., ars., caust., eupho., guai., hydr-ac., nat-c., nit-ac., pall., phos., **Sec.**, sep., spig., staph., stram., sul-ac.
Crawling	formication in thigh extending to abdomen	Ars.
Crawling	formication in thigh extending to toes	Sep.
Crawling	formication in third finger	Aran., caust., mag-s., sulph., tab.
Crawling	formication in thumb	Alum., chel., mez., phos., plb., rhod., zinc.
Crawling	formication in tip of first finger	Graph., nat-m.
Crawling	formication in tip of second finger	Kali-c.
Crawling	formication in tip of thumb	Am-m., cina., nat-m.
Crawling	formication in tips of fingers	**Am-m.**, cann-s., cupr., glon., graph., hep., mag-s., morph., **Nat-m.**, nat-s., plat., **Sec.**, sep., spig., stry., sulph., tep., thuj.
Crawling	formication in tips of fingers in afternoon	Am-m.
Crawling	formication in tips of fingers in evening	Nat-c.
Crawling	formication in tips of toes	Acon., agar., **Am-m.**, colch.

Body part/Disease	Symptom	Medicines
Crawling	formication in toes	Agar., alum., am-c., am-m., ars., berb., caust., chel., cic., colch., con., eupho., euphr., guai., hep., jatr., kali-c., lach., lyc., mag-c., mag-m., nat-c., nat-m., nicc., phos., plat., plb., ran-s., rhod., sec., sep., stram., sulph., thuj., zinc., zing.
Crawling	formication in toes at night	Nicc.
Crawling	formication in toes in evening	Ars., lyc., puls.
Crawling	formication in toes in evening while walking	Lyc.
Crawling	formication in upper arm	Sep., thuj.
Crawling	formication in upper limbs	**Acon.**, alum., apis., arn., arum-t., arund., atro., bell., cact., caps., carb-s., caust., chin., cic., cocc., con., graph., guare., hep., kali-n., lach., nat-c., nat-m., nat-p., nux-m., pall., phos., plat., plb., rhod., rhus-v., rumx., sarr., **Sec.**, stry., sulph., urt-u., vip.
Crawling	formication near anus at night	Nux-v.
Crawling	formication on chin	Stram.
Crawling	formication on entering house	Phos.
Crawling	formication on external throat	Rhus-v.
Crawling	formication on lips menses during	Graph.
Crawling	formication on lips	Ant-c., berb., bor., calc., caust., graph., nat-m., ph-ac., stront.
Crawling	formication on lower jaw	Alumn., bufo-s., grat., ol-an., Plat.
Crawling	formication on lying down	Rumx.
Crawling	formication on right side of face	Alum., plat.
Crawling	formication on right side	Agar., hipp.
Crawling	formication on shoulder	Ars-h., arund., berb., caust., chin-s., cocc., fl-ac., lac-c., lyc., mag-c., osm., sarr., thuj., urt-u.
Crawling	formication on shoulder in morning	Mag-c.
Crawling	formication on waking	Puls.
Crawling	formication on waking on side lain on	Puls.
Crawling	formication over abdomen	Aloe., ars., calad., calc., camph., carb-v., caust., colch., coloc., crot-t., cycl., dulc., mag-m., paeon., pall., pic-ac., Plat., stann., zinc.
Crawling	formication painful in teeth	Bar-c.
Crawling	formication up and down the back	Crot-h., lach., manc.
Crawling	formication while sitting	Kali-c., teucr.
Crawling	formication while waking before midnight	Caust.
Crawling	formication while walking	Graph.
Crawling	formication with numbness	Euphr.
Crawling	formicationin ball of first toe	Caust.
Crawling	hacking cough from crawling in the larynx	Carb-v., caust., colch., eupho., lach., prun-s.
Crawling	itching in hand with crawling	Berb.
Crawling	itching in upper arm with crawling	Thuj.
Crawling	itching in upper limbs with crawling	Berb., thuj.
Crawling	itching of Scalp with crawling sensation	Arg-n., lach., sil.

Body part/Disease	Symptom	Medicines
Crawling	painful sensation of crawling through whole body if he knocks against any part	Spig.
Crawling	sensation of crawling in eruption in upper limbs	Lach.
Crawling	sensation of crawling in oesophagus	Anan., plb., zinc.
Crawling	sensation of crawling in throat as if worm were squimmering in	Hyper., merc., puls.
Crawling	sensation of crawling in throat causing cough	Bry., carb-v., eupho., kali-c., lach., prun-s., stann.
Crawling	sensation of crawling in throat on swallowing	Tab.
Crawling	sensation of formication in bones	Acon., arn., cham., colch., merc., nat-c., nat-m., nux-v., ph-ac., plat., plb., puls., rhod., rhus-t., sabad., sec., sep., spig., sulph., zinc.
Crawling	sensation of formication in glands	Acon., arn., bell., calc., cann-s., canth., **Con.**, ign., laur., merc., nat-c., ph-ac., plat., puls., rhod., rhus-t., sabin., sep., spong., sulph., zinc.
Crawling	sensation of mouse running down lower limbs	Calc., Lyss., sep., **Sulph.**
Crawling	sensation of mouse running up limbs	Calc., sep., sil., sulph.
Crawling	sensation of mouse running up upper limbs	**Bell.**, calc., sulph.
Crawling	sensation of mouse running up upper limbs before epilepsy	**Bell.**, **Sulph.**
Crawling	skin, crawling after eating	Calc-p.
Crawling	skin, crawling after eating meat	Ruta.
Crawling	skin, crawling after exertion	Nat-m.
Crawling	skin, crawling aggravated from perspiration	**Mang.**, merc., rhod.
Crawling	skin, crawling ameliorated from heat of stove	Rumx., **Tub.**
Crawling	skin, crawling ameliorated from lying	Urt-u.
Crawling	skin, crawling before nausea	Sang.
Crawling	skin, crawling before nausea must scratch until he vomits	Ip.
Crawling	skin, crawling during fever	Kali-br.
Crawling	skin, crawling during jaundice	Hep.
Crawling	skin, crawling during jerking	Calc., carb-s., caust., lyc., nat-m., puls., rhus-t.
Crawling	skin, crawling during menses	Graph., kali-c., phos.
Crawling	skin, crawling from mental exertion	Agar.
Crawling	skin, crawling in drunkards	Carb-v., lach., nux-v., sulph.
Crawling	skin, crawling in old people	Mez.
Crawling	skin, crawling in painful parts	Carb-s., ign., thuj.
Crawling	skin, crawling in paralyzed parts	Phos.
Crawling	skin, crawling in parts lain on	Chin.
Crawling	skin, crawling in perspiring parts	All-s., am-c., benz-ac., calc., cann-s., cedr., cham., coloc., fl-ac., ip., led., lyc., **Mang.**, op., par., rhod., rhus-t., sabad., spong., sulph.
Crawling	skin, crawling must scratch until it bleeds	Agar., alum., arg-m., **Ars.**, bar-c., bov., carb-v., chlol., led., med., psor., puls.

Body part/Disease	Symptom	Medicines
Crawling	skin, crawling must scratch until it is raw	Agar., alum., am-c., ant-c., arn., bar-c., bov., calc., carb-s., caust., chin., dros., **Graph.**, hep., kali-c., kreos., lach., lyc., mang., merc., olnd., **Petr.**, phos., plb., psor., puls., rhus-t., ruta., sabin., sep., sil., squil., sul-ac., sulph., til.
Crawling	skin, crawling when over heated	Ign., lyc.
Crawling	skin, crawling when pain ceases	Ign., lyc., stront.
Crawling	skin, crawling without eruption	**Alum.**, **Ars.**, cist., dol., gels., lach., med., merc., **Mez.**, petr., psor., sulph.
Crawling	skin, swelling & crawling	Acon., arn., caust., chel., colch., con., lach., merc., nat-c., nux-v., ph-ac., puls., **Rhus-t.**, sec., sep., spig., sulph.
Crawling	sleeplessness from formication of leg	Zinc.
Crawling	toes hot with crawling	Berb.
Crawling	twitching in foot while crawling	Thuj.
Crawling	ulcer with crawling	Acon., ant-t., **Arn.**, bell., caust., cham., clem., colch., con., croc., graph., hep., kali-c., lach., merc., nat-c., nat-m., nat-p., nux-v., ph-ac., plb., puls., ran-b., **Rhus-t.**, sabin., sec., **Sep.**, spong., staph., sul-ac., sulph., thuj.
Crawling	urination after crawling	Lyc.
Croup	coryza, with croup (inflammatory condition of the larynx and trachea, especially in young children, marked by a cough, hoarseness, and difficulty in breathing)	Acon., ars., cub., hep., nit-ac., spong.
Crust	eruption, blisters forming scabs in wrists	Am-m.
Crust	eruption, bluish hard lump oozing with scabs in upper limbs	Calc-p.
Crust	eruption, crusts (a dry hardened outer layer of blood, pus, or other bodily secretion that forms over a cut or sore) in bend of elbow	Cupr., mez., **Psor.**
Crust	eruption, crusts in forearm	Mez.
Crust	eruption, crusts in thighs	Anac., clem., graph., ph-ac.
Crust	eruption, crusty & full of cracks in hands	Anthr., **Graph.**, petr., sanic.
Crust	eruption, crusty in hollow of knee	Bov.
Crust	eruption, crusty in knee	Psor., sil.
Crust	eruption, elevated white scabs in lower limbs	Mez.
Crust	eruption, scabs (crust over healing wound)	Arn., ars., cit-v., ir-f., kali-br., **Kali-s.**, mez., mur-ac., phos., plb., podo., rhus-t., rhus-v., **Sil.**, staph., sul-ac., zinc.
Crust	eruption, scabs in back of hands	Mur-ac., plb., sep., sul-ac., sulph.
Crust	eruption, scabs in calf	Kali-br.
Crust	eruption, scabs in foot	Calc., rhus-v., sil.
Crust	eruption, scabs in hollow of knee	Puls.
Crust	eruption, scabs in joints	Staph.
Crust	eruption, scabs in legs	Arn., calc-p., ir-f., kali-br., lach., **Nit-ac.**, ph-ac., podo., sep., staph., **Sulph.**, zinc.
Crust	eruption, scabs in legs with scales in spots	Merc., zinc.
Crust	eruption, scabs in lower limbs	Arn., ars., bov., calc., ir-f., kali-br., lach., mez., podo., rhus-v., sabin., sil., staph., zinc.

Body part/Disease	Symptom	Medicines
Crust	eruption, scabs in nates	Chel., graph., psor.
Crust	eruption, scabs in shoulder	Ars.
Crust	eruption, scabs in toes	**Sil.**
Crust	eruption, scabs in upper limbs	Alum., am-m., ars., calc., cit-v., jug-c., jug-r., mez., mur-ac., phos., plb., podo., rhus-t., rhus-v., sep., staph., sul-ac., sulph.
Crust	eruption, scabs in upper limbs	Rhus-t., rhus-v.
Crust	eruption, scabs in wrists	Am-m., mez., rhus-t.
Crust	eruption, scabs itching in upper limbs	Sep.
Crust	eruption, scabs moist in upper limbs	Alum., staph.
Crust	eruption, scabs white in upper limbs	Mez.
Crust	eruption, scabs yellowish brown in upper limbs	Rhus-t.
Crust	eruption, with crusts in wrists	Mez.
Crust	eruption, yellow crusts in back of hands	Merc., mez.
Crust	eruptions carbuncle crusty brown	Am-c., ant-c., berb.
Crust	eruptions carbuncle crusty burning	Am-c., ant-c., calc., cic., puls., sars.
Crust	eruptions carbuncle crusty dry	Ars-i., ars., **Aur-m.**, **Aur.**, bar-c., calc., chin-s., graph., lach., led., merc., ran-b., sulph., thuj., viol-t.
Crust	eruptions carbuncle crusty over whole body	Ars., **Dulc.**, psor.
Crust	eruptions herpetic crusty	Alum., am-c., ambr., anac., ars., aur-m., aur., bar-c., bell., bov., bry., **Calc.**, caps., carb-an., carb-v., cic., clem., **Con.**, cupr., dulc., **Graph.**, hell., hep., kali-c., kreos., lach., led., **Lyc.**, mag-c., **Merc.**, mez., mur-ac., nat-m., nit-ac., nux-v., olnd., par., petr., ph-ac., phos., plb., puls., ran-b., **Rhus-t.**, sars., sep., sil., squil., staph., **Sulph.**, thuj., verat., viol-t., zinc.
Crust	eruption, pimples with crusts	Calc., merc., squil.
Crust	eruption, pimples with green crusts	Calc.
Crust	eruption, pimples with pain like splinter	Arn., hep., nit-ac.
Crust	eruptions, crusts in nails of fingers	Ars.
Crust	eruptions, scabs in fingers	Anag., cit-v., kali-bi., lyc., mur-ac., rhus-v., thuj.
Curvature	curvature of cervical bone	Calc., phos., syph.
Curvature	curvature of dorsal bone	Bar-c., bufo., calc-s., calc., con., lyc., plb., puls., rhus-t., sil., sulph., syph., thuj.
Curvature	curvature of spine	Bar-m., Calc-f., calc-p., Calc-s., Calc., carb-s., carb-v., con., lyc., Merc-c., merc., op., Ph-ac., phos., psor., puls., Sil., Sulph., tarent., thuj.
Curvature	curvature of spine lies knees drawn up	Merc-c.
Curvature	curvature of spine with pain	Aesc., Lyc., Sil.
Cyanosis	cyanosis (condition in which the skin and mucous membranes take on a bluish color because there is not enough oxygen in the blood)	Acon., agar., alum., am-c., ant-c., ant-t., arg-n., arn., ars., asaf., asar., aur., bar-c., bell., bism., bry., calc., **Camph.**, carb-an., **Carb-v.**, caust., cedr., cham., chel., chin-a., chin., cic., cina., cocc., con., **Cupr.**, **Dig.**, dros., ferr., hep., hyos., ign., ip., kali-chl., **Lach.**, **Laur.**, led., lyc., mang., merc., mosch., mur-ac., naja., nat-m., nit-ac., nux-m., nux-v., **Op.**, ph-ac., phos., plb., puls., ran-b., rhus-t., ruta., sabad., samb., sars., sec., seneg., sil., spong., staph., stram., sul-ac., sulph., thuj., **Verat.**, xan.

Body part/Disease	Symptom	Medicines
Cyanosis	cyanosis in chest	Ant-t., bor., carb-an., dig., ip., Lach., Laur.
Cyanosis	cyanosis in infants	Arn., ars., bor., cact., camph., carb-v., chin., **Dig., Lach., Laur.,** naja., op., phos., psor., rhus-t., sec., sulph.
Cyanosis	cyanosis in region of clavicle	Thuj.
Cyanosis	discoloration, cyanosis in thigh	Ars.
Cyanosis	discoloration, cyanosis on legs	Con., elaps.
Cyst	Blood Cyst on the scalp	Calc-f., merc., sil.
Cyst	Blood Cyst on the scalp	Calc-f., merc., sil.
Cyst	bluish black vesicles (fluid-filled cyst) above the eyes	Ran-b.
Cyst	burning vesicles (a very small blister filled with clear fluid serum) on chest	Alum.
Cyst	burning vesicles on penis	Caust., merc.
Cyst	cicatrices with vesicals around	Fl-ac.
Cyst	cysts	Cann-s., caust., graph., iod., kali-br., sil., sulph.
Cyst	cysts (a protective covering around a parasite, produced by a host or by the parasite itself) in female	Sabin.
Cyst	eruption on female gentialia with vesicles	Graph., lyc., nat-s., Rhus-t., sep., staph., sulph.
Cyst	eruption on female gentialia with vesicles	Graph., lyc., nat-s., Rhus-t., sep., staph., sulph.
Cyst	eruption, small red vesicles in upper limbs	Nat-m.
Cyst	eruption, vesicles between second and third fingers	Sulph.
Cyst	eruption, vesicles yellow in back of hands	Arg-n.
Cyst	eruption, black vesicles discharging acrid serum in upper limbs	Rhus-t.
Cyst	eruption, black vesicles in elbow	Ars.
Cyst	eruption, black vesicles in foot	**Ars.,** nat-m.
Cyst	eruption, black vesicles in hands	Sec.
Cyst	eruption, black vesicles in thighs	Anthr.
Cyst	eruption, black vesicles in upper limbs	Ars.
Cyst	eruption, black vesicles periodical every 4 to 6 weeks in upper limbs	Sulph.
Cyst	eruption, black vesicles with itching in upper limbs	Daph.
Cyst	eruption, burning vesicles between the fingers	Canth.
Cyst	eruption, burning vesicles in back of hands	Mez.
Cyst	eruption, burning vesicles in forearm	Sil.
Cyst	eruption, burning vesicles in hands	Canth., rhus-v.
Cyst	eruption, burning vesicles in lower limbs	Verat.
Cyst	eruption, burning vesicles in thighs	Verat.
Cyst	eruption, burning vesicles in wrists	Am-m., bufo., mez.
Cyst	eruption, corroding (destroy progressively by chemical action) vesicles in sole of foot	Ars., sulph.

Body part/Disease	Symptom	Medicines
Cyst	eruption, corroding vesicles in nates	Bor.
Cyst	eruption, greenish vesicles in knee	Iod.
Cyst	eruption, inflamed vesicles in hands	Rhus-t.
Cyst	eruption, itching vesicles in back of hands	Cic., kali-chl., **Mez.**, phos.
Cyst	eruption, itching vesicles in hands	**Carb-ac.**
Cyst	eruption, itching vesicles in knee	Carb-v.
Cyst	eruption, itching vesicles in lower limbs	Calc., carb-v.
Cyst	eruption, itching vesicles in palms	Kali-c., rhus-t.
Cyst	eruption, itching vesicles in thighs	Aster., clem.
Cyst	eruption, itching vesicles in wrists	Am-m., bufo., calc-p., kali-i., nat-m.
Cyst	eruption, large vesicles in palms	Anthr.
Cyst	eruption, moist vesicles in back of hands	Mez.
Cyst	eruption, phagedenic (rapidly spreading ulcer) vesicles in foot	Con., sel., sulph., zinc.
Cyst	eruption, red vesicles (Fluid filled Cyst) in back of hands	Psor.
Cyst	eruption, red vesicles in bend of elbow	Nat-c.
Cyst	eruption, red vesicles in lower limbs	Calc.
Cyst	eruption, spreading vesicles in sole of foot	**Ars.**, calc.
Cyst	eruption, spreading vesicles in toes	Graph., nit-ac.
Cyst	eruption, stinging vesicles in forearm	Rhus-t.
Cyst	eruption, stinging vesicles in knee	Rhus-t.
Cyst	eruption, suppurating vesicles in elbow	Sulph.
Cyst	eruption, suppurating vesicles in foot	Con., graph., nat-c., sel.
Cyst	eruption, transparent vesicles in forearm	Rhus-t.
Cyst	eruption, transparent vesicles in palms	Merc.
Cyst	eruption, ulcerating vesicles in sole of foot	**Ars.**, calc., psor., sulph.
Cyst	eruption, ulcerative vesicles in back of foot	Zinc.
Cyst	eruption, vesicles after scratching in forearm	Sars.
Cyst	eruption, vesicles after scratching in lower limbs	Sars., sep.
Cyst	eruption, vesicles after scratching in thighs	Sars.
Cyst	eruption, vesicles become ulcer in thighs	Aster.
Cyst	eruption, vesicles between index finger and thumb	Grat., nat-s., **Sulph.**
Cyst	eruption, vesicles between the fingers	Anag., apis., calc., canth., hell., iod., laur., nat-m., olnd., phos., **Psor.**, puls., rhus-t., rhus-v., ruta., sel., **Sulph.**
Cyst	eruption, vesicles between thighs	Carb-v., hep., nat-m., nat-s., petr., puls., sel.
Cyst	eruption, vesicles between third and fourth fingers	Mag-c.
Cyst	eruption, vesicles between toes	Hell., sil.
Cyst	eruption, vesicles between toes from walking	Sil.
Cyst	eruption, vesicles burning after scratching in shoulder	Mag-c., mang.

Body part/Disease	Symptom	Medicines
Cyst	eruption, vesicles burning in shoulder	Am-m.
Cyst	eruption, vesicles healing new vesicles appear in hands	Anag.
Cyst	eruption, vesicles in ankle	Aster., rhus-v., sel.
Cyst	eruption, vesicles in back of foot	Aster., bov., carb-o., lach., zinc.
Cyst	eruption, vesicles in back of hands	Anac., arg-n., brom., calc., canth., cic., graph., indg., kali-chl., kali-s., mez., phos., psor., **Rhus-t.**, rhus-v., sol-n., **Sulph.**, zinc.
Cyst	eruption, vesicles in back of hands discharging acid fluid	Sol-n.
Cyst	eruption, vesicles in back of hands discharging yellow fluid	Sol-n.
Cyst	eruption, vesicles in back of hands from taking cold	Zinc.
Cyst	eruption, vesicles in bend of elbow	Calc., nat-c., rhus-v., sulph.
Cyst	eruption, vesicles in calf	Caust., sars., sep.
Cyst	eruption, vesicles in elbow	Ars., calad., nat-p., sulph.
Cyst	eruption, vesicles in foot	Ars., aster., carb-o., caust., con., elaps., graph., lach., manc., nit-ac., phos., rhus-v., sec., sel., sep., sulph., tarax., vinc., vip.
Cyst	eruption, vesicles in foot from rubbing	Caust.
Cyst	eruption, vesicles in forearm	Anac., ant-t., arn., ars., calad., carb-o., caust., chin., cit-v., hura., merc., petr., phos., rhus-r., rhus-t., rhus-v., sars., sil., spong., staph., sulph.
Cyst	eruption, vesicles in hands	Anag., ant-c., aran., arn., ars., bor., bov., **Carb-ac.**, carb-s., caust., chin., clem., cocc., com., hell., hep., kali-ar., kali-bi., kali-c., kali-i., kali-s., lach., lact-ac., mag-c., mag-m., merc., merl., mez., nat-m., nat-s., petr., phos., plan., psor., ptel., ran-b., rhus-t., rhus-v., ruta., sanic., sars., sec., sel., sep., sil., spig., squil., sulph., ter., vip.
Cyst	eruption, vesicles in hollow of knee	**Ars.**, bov., bry., calc., carb-s., chin., dulc., **Graph.**, hep., kali-c., led., merc., nat-m., petr., phos., psor., sars., sep., tep., zinc.
Cyst	eruption, vesicles in hollow of knee	Chin., iod., phos., puls., sars., sep.
Cyst	eruption, vesicles in joints	Nat-p., phos., **Rhus-t.**
Cyst	eruption, vesicles in knee	Ant-c., arn., carb-v., caust., iod., iris., nat-p., phos., rhus-t., sabad., sars., sep.
Cyst	eruption, vesicles in knee after scratching	Sars., sep.
Cyst	eruption, vesicles in legs	Ant-c., bov., **Caust.**, com., dulc., hyos., kali-bi., kali-c., mang., psor., **Rhus-t.**, sec., staph., stram., sulph., vip.
Cyst	eruption, vesicles in lower limbs	Acon., am-c., ant-c., apis., arn., **Ars.**, aster., bell., bov., bufo., calc., cann-s., carb-o., carb-v., **Caust.**, chin., clem., cupr., elaps., graph., hyos., iod., kali-ar., kali-bi., lach., lachn., manc., **Nat-c., Nat-m.**, nat-p., **Nit-ac.**, petr., ph-ac., phos., **Rhus-t.**, rhus-v., sabad., sars., sec., sel., sep., sil., **Sulph.**, verat., zinc.
Cyst	eruption, vesicles in nates	Bor., cann-s., carb-an., crot-t., iris., olnd., ph-ac., rhus-t.

Body part/Disease	Symptom	Medicines
Cyst	eruption, vesicles in palms	Anthr., bufo., canth., caust., kali-c., mag-c., merc., ran-b., rhus-t., rhus-v., ruta.
Cyst	eruption, vesicles in patches in hands	Rhus-t.
Cyst	eruption, vesicles in shoulder	Am-m., ant-c., chlor., crot-h., lach., mag-c., mang., merc., rhus-t., vip.
Cyst	eruption, vesicles in sole of foot	Ars., bell., bufo., calc., kali-bi., kali-c., manc., nat-m., sulph.
Cyst	eruption, vesicles in spots in back of hands	Rhus-t.
Cyst	eruption, vesicles in spots in hands	Cic.
Cyst	eruption, vesicles in thighs	Ant-c., aster., cann-s., caust., clem., crot-t., kali-c., lach., nat-c., olnd., sars., sel., sulph., verat., vip.
Cyst	eruption, vesicles in toes	Caust., cupr., graph., lach., nat-c., nit-ac., petr., ph-ac., rhus-v., sel., sulph., zinc.
Cyst	eruption, vesicles in upper limbs	Am-m., anac., anag., ant-c., ant-t., arn., ars., asc-t., bell., bov., brom., bruc., bufo., calad., calc-p., calc., canth., caust., chin., chlor., cinnb., cit-v., com., crot-h., cupr-ar., cycl., daph., dulc., elaps., fl-ac., hipp., hura., indg., iod., iris., kali-ar., kali-bi., kali-c., kali-chl., kali-i., lach., mag-c., mang., merc-c., merc., mez., nat-c., nat-m., phos., psor., puls., ran-b., **Rhus-t.**, rhus-v., ruta., sars., **Sep.**, sil., sol-n., spong., staph., sulph., ter., vip.
Cyst	eruption, vesicles in upper limbs after scratching	Calc.
Cyst	eruption, vesicles in upper limbs aggravated from washing in cold water	Clem.
Cyst	eruption, vesicles in upper limbs change into ulcer	Calc.
Cyst	eruption, vesicles in wrists	Am-m., bufo., calad., calc-p., crot-h., hep., iris., kali-i., merc., mez., nat-m., rhus-t., rhus-v., sulph.
Cyst	eruption, vesicles in wrists burning when scratched	Am-m.
Cyst	eruption, vesicles in wrists containing clear & transparent water	Rhus-t.
Cyst	eruption, vesicles in wrists containing white water	Calad.
Cyst	eruption, vesicles in wrists containing yellow water	Rhus-t., sulph.
Cyst	eruption, vesicles in wrists scurfy from scratching	Am-m.
Cyst	eruption, vesicles like red areola in hands	Bov., ruta.
Cyst	eruption, vesicles on ulnar side of palms	Ant-c., lach., sel.
Cyst	eruption, vesicles phagadenic (rapidly spreading ulcer) in patches in hands	Graph., kali-c., mag-c., nit-ac., sil.
Cyst	eruption, vesicles putrid (decaying with disgusting smell) in upper limbs	Ars.
Cyst	eruption, vesicles spreading in lower limbs	Nit-ac.
Cyst	eruption, vesicles stinging in lower limbs	Rhus-t.
Cyst	eruption, vesicles ulcerating in lower limbs	Sulph., zinc.
Cyst	eruption, vesicles varioloid in lower limbs	Ant-c.
Cyst	eruption, vesicles watery in back of hands	Calc., rhus-v.
Cyst	eruption, vesicles watery in hands	Anag., ars., nat-c., psor., rhus-t., ruta.

Body part/Disease	Symptom	Medicines
Cyst	eruption, vesicles white in lower limbs	Mez., thuj.
Cyst	eruption, vesicles white in lower limbs	Agar.
Cyst	eruption, vesicles white with red areola in hands	Sanic., uran.
Cyst	eruption, vesicles white with red border in lower limbs	Corn-s.
Cyst	eruption, vesicles white	Agar.
Cyst	eruption, vesicles with bloody serum in lower limbs	Nat-m.
Cyst	eruption, vesicles with bloody serum in sole of foot	Nat-m.
Cyst	eruption, vesicles with fetid water in sole of foot	Ars.
Cyst	eruption, vesicles with fetid water in lower limbs	Ars.
Cyst	eruption, vesicles with red areola in thighs	Sulph.
Cyst	eruption, vesicles with shooting pain in upper limbs	Mag-c.
Cyst	eruption, vesicles with yellow fluid in lower limbs	Ars., bufo.
Cyst	eruption, vesicles with yellow fluid in sole of foot	Ars., bufo.
Cyst	eruption, vesicles yellowish in hands	Rhus-v., sulph.
Cyst	eruption, vesicular in hips	Calc.
Cyst	eruption, watery vesicles in foot	Rhus-v.
Cyst	eruption, watery vesicles in toes	Rhus-v.
Cyst	eruption, white vesicles in elbow	Sulph.
Cyst	eruption, white vesicles in foot	Cycl., graph., lach., sulph.
Cyst	eruption, white vesicles in forearm	Calad.
Cyst	eruption, white vesicles in toes	Graph.
Cyst	eruption, white vesicles in upper limbs	Agar., kali-c., kali-chl., merc., nat-m.
Cyst	eruption, white vesicles with red border in thighs	Cann-s.
Cyst	eruption, yellow vesicles in palms	Anthr., bufo., rhus-t., rhus-v.
Cyst	eruption, yellowish vesicles in elbow	Sulph.
Cyst	eruptions carbuncle purple with small vesicles around	Crot-c., **Lach.**
Cyst	eruption, pustules mixed with vesicles	Ant-t.
Cyst	eruptions, burning vesicles in fingers	Ran-b.
Cyst	eruptions, itching vesicles in fingers	Ran-b.
Cyst	eruptions, vesicles becoming ulcer in fingers	Calc., graph., kali-c., mag-c., nit-ac., ran-b., sil.
Cyst	eruptions, vesicles in fingers on becoming cold	Bell., bor., calc., cit-v., clem., cupr-ar., cupr., cycl., fl-ac., graph., hep., kali-c., kali-s., lach., mag-c., mang., mez., nat-c., nat-m., nat-s., nit-ac., ph-ac., phos., plb., puls., ran-b., rhus-t., rhus-v., sars., sel., sep., sil., sulph.
Cyst	eruptions, vesicles in first finger	Calc., kali-c., mag-c., nat-c., sil., sulph.
Cyst	eruptions, vesicles in first finger discharging water	Kali-c.
Cyst	eruptions, vesicles in fourth finger	Graph.
Cyst	eruptions, vesicles in nails of fingers	Ail., nat-c.
Cyst	eruptions, vesicles in thumb	Hep., lach., mez., nat-c., nat-s., nit-ac., ph-ac., sep.
Cyst	eruptions, vesicles in tip of thumb	Ail., nit-ac.
Cyst	eruptions, vesicles in tips of fingers	Ail., ars., cupr., nat-c.

Body part/Disease	Symptom	Medicines
Cyst	eruptions, vesicles in tips of fingers filled with blood	**Ars.**
Cyst	erysipelas on skin, vesicular (fluid-filled cyst/blister)	Am-c., anac., ars., astac., bar-c., bell., bry., canth., carb-an., carb-s., com., crot-t., **Eupho.**, graph., hep., kali-chl., kali-s., lach., mez., petr., phos., puls., ran-b., **Rhus-t.**, rhus-v., sabad., sep., staph., stram., sulph., urt-u.
Cyst	gangrenous vesicles on ears	Ars.
Cyst	itching vesicles (Fluid filled cyst) on penis	Calc., hep., Nit-ac., ph-ac.
Cyst	periodic ranula (cyst under tongue)	Chr-ac., lyss.
Cyst	pimples pointed with whitish semi-transparent vesicles on chest	Bry.
Cyst	purulent vesicles on ears	Ptel.
Cyst	ranula (cyst under tongue)	Ambr., Calc., canth., cham., fl-ac., hippoz., lac-c., lach., merc., mez., nat-m., nit-ac., plb., psor., sacc., staph., thuj., verat.
Cyst	skin wens (cyst containing material secreted by a sebaceous gland of the skin, usually on the scalp or genitals)	Agar., am-c., anac., ant-c., **Bar-c.**, **Calc.**, coloc., **Graph.**, hep., kali-c., nit-ac., ph-ac., rhus-t., sabin., sil., spong., sulph., thuj.
Cyst	tumours cystic (a protective covering around a parasite, produced by a host or by the parasite itself)	Agar., apis., **Bar-c.**, brom., calc-s., calc., **Graph.**, hep., nit-ac., sil., sulph.
Cyst	ulcer in skin surrounded by vesicles (filled with fluid serum)	Ars., bell., caust., fl-ac., hep., **Lach.**, merc., **Mez.**, nat-c., nat-m., petr., phos., rhus-t., sep., thuj.
Cyst	urticaria vesicular (fluid filled cyst) after scratching	Am-c., am-m., ant-c., ars., bar-c., bell., bry., calc., caust., chin., cycl., dulc., graph., grat., hep., kali-ar., kali-c., kreos., **Lach.**, laur., mang., merc., nat-c., nat-m., nicc., ol-an., phos., ran-b., **Rhus-t.**, sabin., sars., sel., sep., spong., sulph.
Cyst	urticaria vesicular aggravated from washing	Canth., **Clem.**, dulc., hydr., mez., phos., psor., sars., **Sulph.**, urt-u.
Cyst	urticaria vesicular aggravated from washing in cold water	**Clem.**, dulc., sulph.
Cyst	urticaria vesicular around a wound	Lach., rhus-t.
Cyst	urticaria vesicular as from heat of sun	Clem.
Cyst	urticaria vesicular black	Anthr., arg-n., **Ars.**, **Lach.**, nat-c., petr., vip.
Cyst	urticaria vesicular bluish	Anthr., **Ars.**, bell., con., **Lach.**, **Ran-b.**, rhus-t., vip.
Cyst	urticaria vesicular brown	Anag., ant-c., carb-v., lyc., mez., nit-ac., phos., sep., thuj.
Cyst	urticaria vesicular burning	Agar., am-c., am-m., anac., anag., ars., aur., bar-c., bov., calc., caust., crot-t., graph., guare., hep., lach., mag-c., mag-m., mang., merc., mez., mur-ac., nat-c., nat-m., nit-ac., phos., plat., ran-b., seneg., sep., sil., spig., spong., staph., sulph.
Cyst	urticaria vesicular close to each other	Ran-b., rhus-t., verat.
Cyst	urticaria vesicular covered with spots	Dulc., iod., lach., merc., rhus-t., spong.
Cyst	urticaria vesicular cracked	Bry., crot-h., lach., phos., vip.
Cyst	urticaria vesicular cutting	Graph.
Cyst	urticaria vesicular dry	Rhus-t.

Body part/Disease	Symptom	Medicines
Cyst	urticaria vesicular filled with blood	Ail., **Ars.**, aur., bry., camph., canth., carb-ac., fl-ac., graph., kali-p., **Lach.**, nat-c., nat-m., sec., sulph.
Cyst	urticaria vesicular forming on denuded (removed) surface	Anag., rhus-t., staph.
Cyst	urticaria vesicular from cold air	Dulc.
Cyst	urticaria vesicular from exposure to sun	Camph.
Cyst	urticaria vesicular gangrenous	Ars., bell., bufo., camph., carb-v., **Lach.**, mur-ac., ran-b., sabin., sec., sil.
Cyst	urticaria vesicular grape shaped	Bufo., rhus-t.
Cyst	urticaria vesicular grouped	Rhus-v., sulph.
Cyst	urticaria vesicular hard	Lach., ph-ac., sil.
Cyst	urticaria vesicular humid	Hell., hep., lach., mang., merc., phos., ran-b., ran-s., **Rhus-t.**, sulph., vip.
Cyst	urticaria vesicular in winter	Aloe., alum., calc., dulc., hep., kali-c., mang., merc., mez., petr., psor., **Rhus-t.**, sep., stront., sulph.
Cyst	urticaria vesicular inflammed	Am-m., anac., bar-c., bell., crot-t., dulc., kali-n., rhus-t., rhus-v.
Cyst	urticaria vesicular itching	Aeth., am-m., anac., ant-c., ant-t., apis., ars-h., bry., **Calc.**, canth., carb-ac., caust., crot-t., daph., fl-ac., graph., jug-r., lach., mag-c., mez., nat-c., rhus-t., rumx., sel., sep., sil., sulph., tell.
Cyst	urticaria vesicular itching around old scars	Fl-ac.
Cyst	urticaria vesicular itching at night	Graph.
Cyst	urticaria vesicular itching in cold air	Rumx.
Cyst	urticaria vesicular itching in evening	Kali-c.
Cyst	urticaria vesicular itching in warm bed	Aeth.
Cyst	urticaria vesicular itching in warm room	Apis.
Cyst	urticaria vesicular itching when uncovered	Rumx.
Cyst	urticaria vesicular painful	Clem.
Cyst	urticaria vesicular painful	Bell., clem., kali-c., phos.
Cyst	urticaria vesicular painful as if ulcerated	Mez., mur-ac.
Cyst	urticaria vesicular painless	Stront., sulph.
Cyst	urticaria vesicular peeling off	Bry., puls., rhus-t.
Cyst	urticaria vesicular rapidly spreading	Am-c., ars., bor., *calc.,* caust., cham., clem., graph., hep., kali-c., *mag-c.,* merc., nat-c., *nit-ac., petr.,* sep., *sil., sulph.*
Cyst	urticaria vesicular red	Ant-c., calc-p., cic., crot-h., cycl., fl-ac., lach., mang., merc., nat-c., nat-m., ol-an., sil., valer.
Cyst	urticaria vesicular red areola	Anac., calc., cann-s., crot-h., crot-t., kali-c., kali-chl., nat-c., sil., sulph., tab., vip.
Cyst	urticaria vesicular scurfy	Anac., hell., kali-bi., nat-c., nat-m., nit-ac., ran-b., sil., sulph.
Cyst	urticaria vesicular small	Am-m., cann-s., fl-ac., graph., hell., lach., mang., merc., nat-m., nit-ac., rhus-t., thuj.

Body part/Disease	Symptom	Medicines
Cyst	urticaria vesicular smarting	Con., graph., hell., mag-c., mang., nat-c., ph-ac., phel., plat., rhod., rhus-t., rhus-v., sil., staph., thuj.
Cyst	urticaria vesicular spots leaving	Caust.
Cyst	urticaria vesicular stinging	Am-c., calc., cham., crot-t., nat-m., **Nit-ac.,** sil., spong., staph., tell.
Cyst	urticaria vesicular suppurating (oozing pus)	Am-m., aur., bov., calc., carb-v., graph., mag-c., nat-c., nit-ac., petr., phos., puls., ran-b., ran-s., rhus-t., sars., sulph., vip., zinc.
Cyst	urticaria vesicular transparent	Kali-c., lach., mag-c., mag-m., mang., merc., ran-b.
Cyst	urticaria vesicular ulcerated	Calc., caust., clem., cupr-ar., graph., merc., nat-c., **Sulph.,** zinc.
Cyst	urticaria vesicular watery	Bell., bov., canth., clem., cupr., graph., kali-c., kali-n., merc., nat-c., ol-an., plat., plb., rhus-t., rhus-v., sec., sulph., tab., vip., zinc.
Cyst	urticaria vesicular white	Am-c., berb., cann-s., caust., clem., graph., hell., hep., kali-chl., lach., merc., mez., nat-c., phos., sabad., sulph., thuj., valer.
Cyst	urticaria vesicular whitish	Agar., anan., ant-c., ars-i., **Ars.,** bor., bov., bry., com., ip., merc., mez., phos., puls., sulph., thuj., valer., zinc.
Cyst	urticaria vesicular with shooting pain	Nat-c.
Cyst	urticaria vesicular yellow	Agar., am-m., anac., anag., ant-c., anthr., ars., bufo., calc-p., carb-s., chel., cic., clem., com., crot-h., crot-t., **Dulc.,** euphr., hydr., kali-n., kreos., lach., manc., merc., mur-ac., nat-c., nat-s., ph-ac., psor., ran-b., ran-s., raph., **Rhus-t.,** rhus-v., sep., sulph., tab., vip.
Cyst	urticaria vesicular yellow	Agar., anac., ant-c., ars., aur., bar-c., bar-m., bufo., cadm., calc-s., chel., cic., cocc., cupr., dulc., eupho., hell., kali-c., kali-chl., kreos., lach., led., lyc., **Merc.,** nat-c., nat-s., nit-ac., par., ph-ac., ran-s., raph., rhus-t., sep., spong., tab., valer.
Cyst	vesicles (a painful swelling on the skin containing fluid serum) upon inguinal (area between thigh and abdomen) region	Nat-c.
Cyst	vesicles ameliorates by cold things	Nat-s.
Cyst	vesicles becoming ulcer	Carb-an., clem., merc.
Cyst	vesicles below ears	Ptel.
Cyst	vesicles between scrotum & the thighs	Hep., nat-m., petr., puls., rhus-t.
Cyst	vesicles between the shoulders	Sep.
Cyst	vesicles between the shoulders surrounded by red areola (circular area)	Crot-h.
Cyst	vesicles discharging water from ears	Ptel.
Cyst	vesicles forming ulcer in meatus of urethra	Nit-ac.
Cyst	vesicles gangrenous	Sec.
Cyst	vesicles in cervical region	Calc-caust., camph., clem., mag-c., naja., nat-h., nat-p., petr., zinc-s.
Cyst	vesicles in front of ears	Cic.

Body part/Disease	Symptom	Medicines
Cyst	vesicles in margins of ears	Nicc.
Cyst	vesicles in meatus	Nicc.
Cyst	vesicles in meatus of urethra	Stann.
Cyst	vesicles in mouth painful	Anac., apis., berb., caust., kali-c., nux-v.
Cyst	vesicles in mouth suppurating	Phos.
Cyst	vesicles in pharynx	Ant-t., canth.
Cyst	vesicles in throat	Ant-t., apis., ars., rhus-t., sep.
Cyst	vesicles in tonsils	Aur-m-n., iris., nit-ac.
Cyst	vesicles menses before	Mag-c.
Cyst	vesicles on a red elevated base	Kali-bi.
Cyst	vesicles on abdomen	Clem., mag-c., ph-ac., sep., vip.
Cyst	vesicles on back	Ars., bov., clem., crot-h., kali-bi., olnd., psor., sep., sulph., tell., tep.
Cyst	vesicles on back when warm	Cocc., stram.
Cyst	vesicles on chest	Alum., arund., calc-s., calc., camph., carb-s., caust., graph., kali-i., led., merc., rhus-t., sep., stram., sulph.
Cyst	vesicles on ears	Alum., ars., meph., olnd., phos., ptel., rhus-v., sep., tell.
Cyst	vesicles on ears extending to face	Graph., sep.
Cyst	vesicles on ears extending to scalp	Hep.
Cyst	vesicles on ears filled with serum (liquid part of blood)	Rhus-v.
Cyst	vesicles on ears surrounded by inflamed base	Ars.
Cyst	vesicles on eyelids	Berb., cimic., crot-t., mez., pall., psor., rhus-t., rhus-v., sars., sel.
Cyst	vesicles on face burning	Agar., anac., aur., caust., cic., nat-m., ran-b.
Cyst	vesicles on face itching	Anac., ant-c., ars., cic., mez., sep.
Cyst	vesicles on glans	Ars-h., caust., merc., ph-ac., rhus-t., stann., thuj.
Cyst	vesicles on gums burning	Bell., mag-c., mez.
Cyst	vesicles on gums	Bell., canth., daph., iod., kali-c., mag-c., merc., mez., nat-s., petr., rhus-v., sep., Sil., zing.
Cyst	vesicles on mammae	Aeth., Graph.
Cyst	vesicles on palate	Iod., mag-c., manc., nat-s., nit-ac., phos., rhus-t.
Cyst	vesicles on prepuce	Ars-h., carb-v., caust., graph., merc., nit-ac.
Cyst	vesicles on scapula	Am-c., am-m., ant-c., caust., cic., lach., vip.
Cyst	vesicles on scrotum	Ars., bell., chel., Crot-t., cupr-ar., petr., psor., rhus-t., rhus-v.
Cyst	vesicles on sides	Alum.
Cyst	vesicles on sides from ear discharge	Tell.
Cyst	vesicles on tip of tongue	Am-c., am-m., aphis., apis., bar-c., bell., berb., calc-p., carb-an., Caust., cycl., Graph., hydr., indg., kali-i., kali-n., lach., Lyc., merc-i-r., Nat-m., nat-p., nat-s., puls., sal-ac.
Cyst	vesicles on tongue becoming ulcer	Calc., clem., lach.
Cyst	vesicles on tongue bleeding from slightest touch	Mag-c.

Body part/Disease	Symptom	Medicines
Cyst	vesicles on tongue burning like fire on right side	Phel.
Cyst	vesicles on tongue frenum (restraining fold of tissue)	Plb.
Cyst	vesicles on tongue painful	Ars., canth., Caust., graph., kali-c., mag-c., sal-ac., zinc.
Cyst	vesicles on tongue suppurating	Mag-c.
Cyst	vesicles under the tongue	Am-c., bar-c., bell., cham., chin., graph., ham., lach., rhod., rhus-v.
Cyst	vesicles, varioloid like	Ant-c.
Cyst	vesicular	Ant-t., carb-v., chin-s., Crot-t., cupr-ar., merc., nat-c., nat-p., Nit-ac., petr., ph-ac., Rhus-t., rhus-v., sep.
Cyst	vesicular (a small sac or hollow organ in the body, especially one containing fluid) on hairy parts	Lach.
Cyst	wens (a cyst containing material secreted by a sebaceous gland of the skin) on hands	Ph-ac., plb., sil.
Cyst	Wens (cysts)	Agar., bar-c., calc., Graph., hep., kali-c., lob., lyc., nat-c., sil.

Body part/Disease	Symptom	Medicines
Dandruff	dandruff White	Kali-chl., mez., Nat-m., phos., Thuj.
Dandruff	dandruff yellow	Kali-s.
Dandruff	eruption, scurfy (thin dry flaking scales of skin, usually as a result of a skin condition such as dandruff) brownish in upper limbs	Am-m., cinnb.
Dandruff	eruption, scurfy brownish	Am-m., bar-m., cinnb., merc.
Dandruff	eruption, scurfy in foot	Sil.
Dandruff	eruption, scurfy in hands	Sars., sep.
Dandruff	eruption, scurfy in legs	Ars., calc., kali-bi., sabin., sep., staph., zinc.
Dandruff	eruption, scurfy in lower limbs	Bar-m., merc., petr.
Dandruff	eruption, scurfy in nates	Calc-p.
Dandruff	eruption, scurfy in spots in lower limbs	Merc.
Dandruff	eruption, scurfy in spots in thighs	Merc.
Dandruff	eruption, scurfy in thighs	Bar-m., merc., mez.
Dandruff	eruption, scurfy tetters in palms	Cinnb., lyc., nat-s., sulph.
Dandruff	eruption, vesicles in wrists scurfy from scratching	Am-m.
Dandruff	eruption, with brownish scurfs in wrists	Am-m.
Dandruff	eruption, pustules scurfy	Anac., ant-c., ant-t., bov., crot-t., dulc., kali-chl., merc.
Dandruff	eruption, tubercles scurfy	Sulph.
Dandruff	scurfy (thin dry flaking scales of skin, usually as a result of a skin condition such as dandruff) eruptions on mammae	Lyc., petr.
Dandruff	scurfy in margins of ears	All-s., Lyc., psor.
Dandruff	scurfy of ears	Aur-m., bov., calc., com., graph., hep., iod., lach., Lyc., mur-ac., Psor., puls., sars., sil.
Dandruff	scurfy on eyelids	Mez., Petr., Sep., tub.
Dandruff	scurfy scales, black	Calc-p.
Dandruff	scurfy scales, dry	Bar-c.
Dandruff	scurfy scales, moist	Alum., anan., bar-c., calc., graph.
Dandruff	scurfy scales, serpiginous (resembling snake)	Calc., clem., psor., sars.
Dandruff	scurfy scales, spots	Ars., kali-c., mosch., zinc.
Dandruff	scurfy scales, suppurating	Ars., bar-m., calc-s., cic., clem., graph., hep., lyc., mez., psor., rhus-t., sep., staph., Sulph., vinc.
Dandruff	scurfy scales, white	Nat-m.
Deafness	vision, dimness alternating with deafness	Cic.

Body part/Disease	Symptom	Medicines
Decay	pain in lumbar region after mortification (the death and decaying of a part of a living body, e.g. because the blood supply to it has been cut off)	Nux-v.
Decay	ulcer in face putrid (decaying with disgusting smell)	Merc.
Delirium	blindness, during delirium (temporary mental disturbance caused by fever, poisoning, or brain injury)	Phos.
Delirium	comatose sleep alternating with delirium	Plb.
Delirium	comatose sleep alternating with delirium with sleeplessness	Camph.
Delirium	Constant Delirium	Bapt., con., lach.
Delirium	deep sleep after delirium	Bry., phos.
Delirium	deep sleep with delirium	Cocc., plb., stram., vip.
Delirium	delirium (Extreme restlessness / hallucination) after convulsions	Absin., bell., kali-c., sec.
Delirium	delirium after epilepsy	Arg-m., plb.
Delirium	delirium after hæmorrhage	Arn., ars., chin., ign., lach., lyc., ph-ac., phos., sep., squil., sulph., verat.
Delirium	delirium after miscarriage	Ruta.
Delirium	delirium aggravated from heat	Stram.
Delirium	delirium almost hysterical	Bell., ign., tarent., verat.
Delirium	delirium alternating with laughing, singing, whistling, crying, etc.	Stram.
Delirium	delirium ameliorated from eating	Anac., bell.
Delirium	delirium at day break	Bry., con.
Delirium	delirium attacks people with knife	Hyos.
Delirium	delirium before convulsions	Op.
Delirium	delirium before menses	Ars., bell., hyos., lyc.
Delirium	delirium bellows like a calf	Cupr.
Delirium	delirium blames himself for his folly	Op.
Delirium	delirium changing subjects rapidly	Lach.
Delirium	delirium during convulsions	Ars., crot-h.
Delirium	delirium during epilepsy	Op.
Delirium	delirium during headache	Acon., agar., ars., colch., glon., mag-c., mosch., sec., tarent., verat.
Delirium	delirium during menses	Acon., apis., bell., cocc., hyos., lyc., nux-m., puls., stram., verat.
Delirium	delirium during nap	Nux-v.
Delirium	delirium flies from her own children	Lyc.
Delirium	delirium flies from his wife	Ars., nat-s., plat., staph.
Delirium	delirium in dark	Calc-ar., carb-v., cupr., stram.
Delirium	delirium in evening	Bell., bry., canth., croc., lach., lyc., phos., plb., sulph.
Delirium	delirium in morning	Ambr., bry., con., dulc., hell., hep., merc., nat-c.
Delirium	delirium intermittent	Con.

Body part/Disease	Symptom	Medicines
Delirium	delirium occurring at irregular intervals staring fixed on one point	Art-v., bov., camph., canth., cupr., ign., ran-b., stram.
Delirium	delirium recognizes no one	Bell., calad., hyos., merc., nux-v., op., stram., tab., verat.
Delirium	delirium repeats the same sentence	Camph.
Delirium	delirium talks of fire	Calc.
Delirium	delirium with anger	Cocc.
Delirium	delirium with coma and somnolency (feeling sleepy or tending to fall asleep)	Plb., stram.
Delirium	delirium with fear of men	Bell., plat.
Delirium	fever in evening with delirium (state marked by extreme restlessness, confusion, and sometimes hallucinations, caused by fever, poisoning, or brain injury)	Psor.
Delirium	fever with dry heat at night with delirium	**Ars., Bell.,** bry., chin-s., coff., lach., lyc., phos., **Rhus-t.**
Delirium	fever with intense heat with delirium	Ant-t., apis., **Ars., Bell.,** bry., carb-v., chin-s., chin., chlor., coff., hep., hyos., iod., **Nat-m.,** nux-v., **Op., Puls.,** sarr., sec., **Stram.**
Delirium	profuse perspiration during delirium (temporary mental disturbance)	Carb-ac., stram.
Delirium	shaking chill maniacal (so uncontrolled as to appear to be affected by mania) delirium (a state marked by extreme restlessness, confusion, and sometimes hallucinations, caused by fever, poisoning, or brain injury)	Cimx., tarent.
Delivery	Aching in back after confinement (the period of time or the process of giving birth, beginning when a woman goes into labor and ending when a child is born)	Hyper.
Delivery	Birth of dead babies	Actea Race. 1X
Delivery	blindness, during parturition	Aur-m., caust., cocc., cupr.
Delivery	convulsion at puerperal (relating to childbirth)	Ambr., apis., arg-n., ars., art-v., **Bell.,** canth., carb-v., caust., cham., **Cic.,** cimic., cocc., coff., crot-c., cupr., gels., glon., hell., hydr-ac., **Hyos.,** ign., ip., lach., laur., lyc., lyss., mag-p., merc-c., mosch., nux-m., nux-v., oena., op., plat., puls., sec., **Stram.,** ter., verat-v., verat., zinc.
Delivery	convulsion at puerperal with blindness	Aur-m., cocc., cupr.
Delivery	convulsion at puerperal with haemorrhage	Chin., hyos., plat., sec.
Delivery	cough after parturition	Rhus-t.
Delivery	cramp in fingers during parturition (act of giving birth)	Cupr., Dios.
Delivery	excessive flow of blood in brain from suppressed lochia (the normal vaginal discharge of cell debris and blood after childbirth) from the vagina	Acon., bell., bry., cimic.
Delivery	lochia (vaginal discharge after childbirth) acrid	Bapt., carb-an., con., Kreos., lil-t., merc., plat., pyrog., rhus-t., sep., sil.
Delivery	lochia after least motion	Erig.

Body part/Disease	Symptom	Medicines
Delivery	lochia bloody	Acon., bry., calc., caul., cham., rhus-t., sil.
Delivery	lochia brown	Carb-v., kreos., sec.
Delivery	lochia cadaveric (thick toxic colorless liquid with an extremely unpleasant smell, produced when flesh rots)	Stram.
Delivery	lochia copious	Acon., bry., calc., carb-an., cham., chin., coff., con., croc., erig., hep., lil-t., mill., nat-c., plat., puls., rhus-t., sec., senec., sulph., tril., ust., xan.
Delivery	lochia dark	Cham., chin., croc., Kreos., plat., Sec., ust.
Delivery	lochia from anger	Coloc.
Delivery	lochia gushing	Plat.
Delivery	lochia hot	Bell.
Delivery	lochia ichorous	Carb-an., rhus-t., sec.
Delivery	lochia intermittent	Calc., kreos., plat., rhus-t.
Delivery	lochia lumpy	Cimic., Kreos.
Delivery	lochia milky	Calc., puls., sep.
Delivery	lochia offensive	Acon., bapt., bell., bry., carb-ac., carb-an., carb-v., chin., crot-h., Kali-p., Kreos., lach., nux-v., pyrog., rhus-t., Sec., sep., sil., stram., sulph.
Delivery	lochia protracted (lasting or drawn out for a long time)	Bapt., bell., benz-ac., calc., Carb-ac., caul., chin., croc., helon., hep., kreos., lil-t., Nat-m., plat., rhus-t., Sec., Senec., sep., sulph., tril., ust.
Delivery	lochia red	Acon., bry., calc., chin., psor., sil., sulph.
Delivery	lochia scanty (not much, and less than is needed)	Acon., bell., bry., coloc., dulc., nux-v., Puls., pyrog., Sec., stram., sulph.
Delivery	lochia suppressed	Acon., alet., aral., bell., Bry., camph., caul., cham., chin., cimic., coloc., dulc., hyos., mill., nux-v., op., plat., psor., Puls., Pyrog., sec., stram., Sulph., verat., zinc.
Delivery	lochia thin	Bell., carb-an., cimic., lach., pyrog., rhus-t., sec., ust.
Delivery	lochia when child nurses	Sil.
Delivery	milk leg (leg swelling after childbirth)	All-c., ant-c., apis., arn., ars., bell., **Bry.**, bufo., **Calc.**, carb-s., cham., chin., crot-h., graph., ham., hep., iod., kali-c., **Lach.**, led., lyc., merc., nat-s., nux-v., puls., rhod., **Rhus-t.**, sep., sil., sulph., verat.
Delivery	milk leg (leg swelling after childbirth) with contraction	Sil.
Delivery	pain in coccyx after confinement (process or time of giving birth)	Tarent.
Delivery	pain in extremities after giving birth	Rhod.
Delivery	pain in heart during parturition (act of giving birth)	Cimic.
Delivery	pain in hip after confinement	**Hyper.**
Delivery	pain in hip after instrumental delivery	Hyper.
Delivery	pain in hip during parturition	Cimic.
Delivery	pain in sacral region after instrumental delivery	Hyper.
Delivery	paralysis of lower limb after parturition	Caust., plb., **Rhus-t.**

Body part/Disease	Symptom	Medicines
Delivery	placenta retained	Agn., ars., art-v., bell., Canth., caul., cimic., croc., gels., ip., nux-v., puls., sabin., sec., Sep.
Delivery	puerperal (relating to child birth) fever	Apis., arg-n., arn., ars., bapt., bell., bry., **Carb-s.**, cham., cimic., coff., coloc., **Echi.**, ferr., gels., hyos., ign., ip., kali-c., **Lach.**, **Lyc.**, mill., mur-ac., nux-v., op., phos., plat., **Puls.**, **Pyrog.**, **Rhus-r.**, **Rhus-t.**, sec., sil., **Sulph.**, verat-v., verat.
Delivery	puerperal fever from suppressed lochia (vaginal discharge after childbirth)	Lyc., mill., puls., **Sulph.**
Delivery	retention of urine at the time of giving birth	Arn., Ars., bell., canth., Caust., equis., hyos., ign., lyc., nux-v., op., puls., rhus-t., sec., sep., stann., staph., stram.
Delivery	unconsciousness during parturition	Cimic., coff., Nux-v., puls., sec.
Delivery	urine albuminous during and after delivery	Merc-c., ph-ac., pyrog.
Delivery	weakness in leg after giving birth	Caust., rhus-t.
Delivery	weakness in lower limbs after parturition	Rhus-t.
Dentition	convulsion during dentition	Acon., aeth., art-v., bell., **Calc.**, **Cham.**, cic., cina., cupr., hyos., ign., kreos., merc., podo., stann., stram.
Dentition	cough during dentiton (the type, number, and arrangement of a set of teeth)	Calc-p., calc., cham., cina., hyos., kreos., podo., rhus-t.
Dentition	dentition (the process of developing and cutting new teeth) difficult	Calc-p., Calc., Cham., cic., cupr., hep., hyos., ign., kreos., phyt., podo., rheum., sec., sep., Sil., stann.
Dentition	dentition slow	Calc-p., Calc., fl-ac., mag-c., mag-m., Sil.
Dentition	stammering during dentition	Stram.
Deposit	tumours atheroma (fatty deposit in artery like cholesterol)	Bar-c.
Desire	avarice (an unreasonably strong desire to obtain and keep money)	Ars., bry., calc-f., calc., cina., coloc., lyc., meli., nat-c., puls., rheum., sep.
Desire	desire diminished in female	Agn., alum., ambr., bar-c., bell., berb., bor., camph., cann-s., carb-an., Caust., ferr-p., ferr., graph., helon., hep., kali-i., lyc., mag-c., mur-ac., nat-m., ph-ac., phos., rhod., sep., sil., sulph.
Desire	desire for Amusement	Lach., pip-m.
Desire	desire for cold bathing	Aster., meph., nat-m., phyt.
Desire	Desire for friend	Plb.
Desire	desire for open air	Acon., agn., alum., am-m., ambr., anac., ant-c., ant-t., apis., arg-m., arg-n., arn., ars-i., ars., asaf., asar., aster., **Aur-m.**, **Aur.**, bar-c., bar-m., bor., bov., brom., bry., bufo., **Calc-i.**, calc-s., carb-an., carb-h., carb-s., **Carb-v.**, caust., **Croc.**, dig., elaps., fl-ac., gels., graph., hell., **Iod.**, kali-c., **Kali-i.**, kali-n., **Kali-s.**, lach., laur., lil-t., **Lyc.**, mag-c., mag-m., mang., meny., mez., mur-ac., nat-c., nat-m., nat-s., op., ph-ac., phos., plat., ptel., **Puls.**, rhus-t., sabin., sanic., sars., sec., seneg., sep., spig., spong., stann., stram., **Sulph.**, tab., tarax., tarent., tell., teucr., thuj., viol-t., zinc.
Desire	desire increased during metrorrhagia (excessive discharge of blood from the womb)	Plat., sabin.

Body part/Disease	Symptom	Medicines
Desire	desire increased during pregnancy	Bell., lach., merc., plat., puls., stram., verat.
Desire	desire increased in female	Am-c., ant-c., apis, arg-n., ars-i., ars., asaf., aster., aur., bar-c., bar-m., bell., bov., cact., calad., Calc-p., Calc., Camph., cann-i., cann-s., Canth., carb-v., chin., coff., Con., cub., cur., dulc., Fl-ac., form., gels., Grat., Hyos., ign., iod., kali-br., kali-p., kreos., lac-c., Lach., lil-t., lyc., lyss., merc., mosch., murx., mygal., nat-a., nat-c., nat-m., nat-p., nit-ac., Nux-v., op., orig., Phos., pic-ac., Plat., plb., Puls., raph., sabin., sil., stann., staph., stram., sul-ac., tarent., thuj., Verat., zinc.
Desire	desire increased in female after menses	Kali-p.
Desire	desire increased in female during headache	Sep.
Desire	desire increased in female during menses	Agar., bell., bufo., camph., canth., chin., cina., coff., dulc., hyos., kali-br., lach., Lyc., mosch., nux-v., orig., plat., Puls., sul-ac., tarent., verat.
Desire	desire increased in old women	Mosch.
Desire	desire increased in virgins	Con., Plat.
Desire	desire increased in widows	Apis., Orig.
Desire	Desire to be alone while Aggravated	Ambr., Ars., bov., brom., cadm., calc., camph., con., dros., elaps., kali-c., lyc., mez., pall., Phos., rat., sil., stram., tab., zinc.
Desire	Desire to Break things	Apis., hura., stram., tub.
Desire	desire to close eyes	Agar., ant-t., bell., calc., caust., chel., con., dios., elaps., gels., lact-ac., med., ox-ac., sil.
Desire	desire to leave home	Elat.
Desire	desire to rub eye	All-c., apis, bor., carb-ac., caust., con., croc., fl-ac., gymn., kali-bi., mez., morph., nat-c., op., plb., puls., rat., squil., sulph.
Desire	desire to talk to some one	Arg-m., arg-n., caust., lil-t., petr.
Desire	desire to talk to some one alternating to quarrelsomeness	Con.
Desire	desire to travel	Anan., aur., Calc-p., cimic., cur., elaps., hipp., iod., lach., merc., sanic., tub.
Desire	desires death during chill	Kali-chl., spig.
Desire	desires death during convalescence	Absin., aur., lac-c., sep.
Desire	desires death during menses	Berb.
Desire	desires death in afternoon	Ruta.
Desire	desires death in evening	Aur., ruta.
Desire	desires death in forenoon	Apis
Desire	desires death in morning on waking	Nat-c., phyt.
Desire	desires solitude (the state of being alone, separated from other people, whether considered as a welcome freedom from disturbance or as an unhappy loneliness) to indulge her fancy (to find somebody sexually desirable)	Lach.
Desire	desires solitude to lie with closed eyes	Sep.
Desire	desires solitude to practice masturbation	Bufo., ust.

Body part/Disease	Symptom	Medicines
Desire	desires to be carried	Acet-ac., acon., ant-t., ars., benz-ac., brom., carb-v., Cham., cina., ign., kali-c., lyc., puls., rhus-t., sanic., staph., sulph., verat.
Desire	desires to be carried fast	Ars., bell., brom., rhus-t., verat.
Desire	desires to be carried slowly	Puls.
Desire	desires to be killed	Ars., bell., coff-t., stram.
Desire	desires to be uncovered while perspiration	Acon., calc., camph., ferr., iod., **Led.**, mur-ac., nat-m., op., **Sec.**, spig., staph., verat., zinc.
Desire	desires to beat children	Chel.
Desire	desires to cut others	Lyss.
Desire	desires to extend the arm	Am-c., bell., sabad., tab., verb.
Desire	desires to have children	Ox-ac.
Desire	desires to kill the person that contradicts	Merc.
Desire	desires to remain in bed	Alum., alumn., arg-n., con., hyos., merc., psor., rob., verat-v.
Diabetes	Diabetes	Ars.Brom Q
Diabetes	sugar in urine	Acet-ac., all-s., alumn., am-c., aml-n., arg-m., ars., benz-ac., Bov., calc-p., calc., camph., carb-ac., carb-v., chel., chin-a., chin., coff., colch., conv., cupr., cur., elaps., ferr-m., Helon., hep., iris., kali-chl., kali-n., kali-p., kreos., lac-d., lach., lact-ac., lec., lith., Lyc., lycps., lyss., mag-s., med., morph., mosch., nat-s., nit-ac., op., petr., Ph-ac., Phos., pic-ac., Plb., podo., rat., sal-ac., sec., sil., sul-ac., sulph., Tarent., Ter., thuj., Uran., zinc.
Diarhoea	appetite, increased with diarrhoea	Aloe., asaf., calc., coch., fl-ac., iod., lyc., olnd., Petr., stram., sulph., verat., zinc.
Diarhoea	asthma alternating with nocturnal diarrhoea	Kali-c.
Diarhoea	bloody discharge from urethra in chronic diarrhoea	Eupho.
Diarhoea	catarrh (runny nose) alternating with diarrhoea	Seneg.
Diarhoea	chest symptoms alternating with diarrhoea and bronchitis	Seneg.
Diarhoea	chill during diarrhoea	Aloe., ambr., apis., kali-n., sulph.
Diarhoea	chill in afternoon after diarrhoea	Ox-ac.
Diarhoea	coldness during diarrhoea	Nat-m., ptel.
Diarhoea	coldness in foot with diarrhoea	Dig., lyc., nit-ac.
Diarhoea	coldness in hands from diarrhoea	Apis., brom., dig., Phos.
Diarhoea	coldness of skin during diarrhoea	Aeth., camph., jatr., laur., tab., verat.
Diarhoea	coldness with diarrhoea	Ars., Camph., carb-v., cop., laur., nux-m., podo., sec., tab., Verat.
Diarhoea	collapse after diarrhoea	**Ars., Camph., Carb-v., Verat.**
Diarhoea	convulsion ameliorated from diarrhoea	Lob.
Diarhoea	cough ameliorated by diarrhoea	Bufo.
Diarhoea	diarrhoea after abuse of Aloe	Mur-ac., sulph.
Diarhoea	diarrhoea after acids	Aloe., ant-c., apis., ars., brom., bry., cist., coloc., lach., nux-v., ph-ac., sulph.

Body part/Disease	Symptom	Medicines
Diarhoea	diarrhoea after acute diseases	Carb-v., chin., psor., sulph.
Diarhoea	diarrhoea after alcoholic drinks	Ant-t., ars., lach., Nux-v., sulph.
Diarhoea	diarrhoea after anger	Acon., aloe., ars., bar-c., bry., calc-p., cham., Coloc., ip., nux-v., staph.
Diarhoea	diarrhoea after artificial food	Alum., calc., mag-c., sulph.
Diarhoea	diarrhoea after bathing	Calc., podo., rhus-t., sars.
Diarhoea	diarrhoea after beer	Aloe., chin., gamb., Ind., kali-bi., lyc., mur-ac., Sulph.
Diarhoea	diarrhoea after cabbage	Bry., petr., podo.
Diarhoea	diarrhoea after chocolate	Bor., lith.
Diarhoea	diarrhoea after cold bathing	Ant-c.
Diarhoea	diarrhoea after cucumbers	Verat.
Diarhoea	diarrhoea after eggs	Chin-a.
Diarhoea	diarrhoea after exposure to cold wind	Acon., dulc.
Diarhoea	diarrhoea after exposure to east wind	Psor.
Diarhoea	diarrhoea after fatty food	Ant-c., carb-v., cycl., kali-chl., puls., thuj.
Diarhoea	diarrhoea after fish	Chin-a.
Diarhoea	diarrhoea after fright	Acon., arg-n., Gels., ign., kali-p., op., ph-ac., phos., puls., verat.
Diarhoea	diarrhoea after fruit	Acon., aloe., ant-t., Ars., bor., Bry., calc-p., calc., carb-v., chin-a., Chin., cist., Coloc., crot-t., ferr., ip., iris., lach., lith., lyc., mag-c., mur-ac., Nat-s., olnd., ph-ac., podo., Puls., rheum., rhod., sul-ac., trom., Verat.
Diarhoea	diarrhoea after grief	Calc-p., coloc., gels., ign., merc., op., ph-ac.
Diarhoea	diarrhoea after hair cut	Bell.
Diarhoea	diarrhoea after ice cream	Arg-n., Ars., bry., calc-p., carb-v., dulc., puls.
Diarhoea	diarrhoea after injuries	Arn.
Diarhoea	diarrhoea after lemonade	Cit-ac., phyt.
Diarhoea	diarrhoea after loss of fluid	Carb-v., chin., ph-ac.
Diarhoea	diarrhoea after measles	Carb-v., chin., merc., puls., squil.
Diarhoea	diarrhoea after meat	Caust., ferr., lept., sep.
Diarhoea	diarrhoea after milk	Aeth., ars., bry., Calc., con., kali-ar., kali-c., lyc., mag-c., Mag-m., Nat-a., Nat-c., nicc., nit-ac., nux-m., podo., Sep., sil., sulph.
Diarhoea	diarrhoea after onion	Lyc., nux-v., puls., thuj.
Diarhoea	diarrhoea after oranges	Ph-ac.
Diarhoea	diarrhoea after pain in chest	Sang.
Diarhoea	diarrhoea after pastry	Arg-n., ip., kali-chl., lyc., nat-s., ph-ac., phos., Puls.
Diarhoea	diarrhoea after pears	Bor., bry., verat.
Diarhoea	diarrhoea after pork	Ant-c., cycl., nux-m., puls.
Diarhoea	diarrhoea after potatoes	Alum., coloc., sep., verat.
Diarhoea	diarrhoea after rich food	Arg-n., ip., kali-chl., nat-s., phos., Puls.
Diarhoea	diarrhoea after solid food	Bapt., olnd., Ph-ac., podo.

Body part/Disease	Symptom	Medicines
Diarhoea	diarrhoea after sour fruit	Ant-c., cist., ip., lach., ph-ac.
Diarhoea	diarrhoea after sugar	Arg-n., calc., crot-t., merc., ox-ac., sulph., trom.
Diarhoea	diarrhoea after suppressed eruptions	Bry., dulc., hep., lyc., mez., psor., Sulph., urt-u.
Diarhoea	diarrhoea after unripe fruit	Aloe., ip., rheum., sul-ac.
Diarhoea	diarrhoea after washing the head	Podo., tarent.
Diarhoea	diarrhoea aggravated by cold food	Ant-c., Ars., carb-v., cocc., coloc., Dulc., hep., lyc., nat-s., nit-ac., nux-m., nux-v., ph-ac., puls., rhus-t., sep., sul-ac.
Diarhoea	diarrhoea alternating with erruptions	Calc-p., crot-t.
Diarhoea	diarrhoea alternating with headache	Podo.
Diarhoea	diarrhoea alternating with rheumatism	Cimic., dulc., kali-bi.
Diarhoea	diarrhoea ameliorated after acidic food	Arg-n.
Diarhoea	diarrhoea ameliorated after breakfast	Bov., nat-s., trom.
Diarhoea	diarrhoea ameliorated after eructations	Arg-n., carb-v., grat., hep., lyc.
Diarhoea	diarrhoea ameliorated after external heat	Ars., hep.
Diarhoea	diarrhoea ameliorated after ice cream	Phos.
Diarhoea	diarrhoea ameliorated by cold food	Phos.
Diarhoea	diarrhoea ameliorated from cold drinks	Phos.
Diarhoea	diarrhoea ameliorated from riding in train	Nit-ac.
Diarhoea	diarrhoea ameliorated from wine	Chel., dios.
Diarhoea	diarrhoea ameliorated in damp weather	Alum., asar.
Diarhoea	diarrhoea ameliorates all symptoms	Zinc.
Diarhoea	diarrhoea ameliotated after hot milk	Chel., crot-t.
Diarhoea	diarrhoea as soon as boils begin to heal	Rhus-v.
Diarhoea	diarrhoea during epidemic cholera	Camph., cupr., Ip., phos., puls.
Diarhoea	diarrhoea during hectic fever	Aesc.
Diarhoea	diarrhoea during intermittent fever	Ars., chin-a., Cina., cocc., con., gels., puls., rhus-t., thuj.
Diarhoea	diarrhoea during jaundice	Chion., dig., lycps., merc., nat-s., nux-v., sep., sulph.
Diarhoea	diarrhoea during measles	Squil.
Diarhoea	diarrhoea during pregnancy	Alum., am-m., ant-c., apis., cham., chel., chin., dulc., ferr., hell., hyos., lyc., nux-m., nux-v., petr., Phos., puls., sep., sulph.
Diarhoea	diarrhoea during small pox	Ant-t., ars., Chin., thuj.
Diarhoea	diarrhoea from bad news	Gels.
Diarhoea	diarrhoea from change of least diet	All-s., nux-v.
Diarhoea	diarrhoea from exciting news	Gels.
Diarhoea	diarrhoea from melons	Zing.
Diarhoea	diarrhoea from riding in train	Med.
Diarhoea	diarrhoea from soup	Mag-c.
Diarhoea	diarrhoea from spices	Phos.
Diarhoea	diarrhoea from wine	Lach., lyc., zinc.
Diarhoea	diarrhoea immediately after drinking water	Arg-n., cina., crot-t., podo.
Diarhoea	diarrhoea in old drunkards	Ant-t., apis., ars., chin., Lach., nux-v., phos.

Body part/Disease	Symptom	Medicines
Diarhoea	diarrhoea in school girls	Calc-p., ph-ac.
Diarhoea	diarrhoea in summer	Carb-v., nat-s., Nux-m., verat.
Diarhoea	diarrhoea periodical on alternate days	Alum., carb-ac., Chin., dig., fl-ac., iris., nit-ac.
Diarhoea	diarrhoea while eating	Ars., chin., crot-t., Ferr., kali-p., podo., puls., trom.
Diarhoea	diarrhoea without weakness	Ph-ac., puls., sulph., tub.
Diarhoea	dropsy (a buildup of excess serous fluid between tissue cells) due to ascites (an accumulation of fluid serous fluid in the peritoneal cavity, causing abdominal swelling) with chronic diarrhoea	Apoc., oena.
Diarhoea	emptyness of abdomen, with diarrhoea	Fl-ac., lyc., petr., stram., sulph.
Diarhoea	eruptions on skin alternating with diarrhoae	Calc-p.
Diarhoea	faintness after diarrhoea	Ars.
Diarhoea	faintness before diarrhoea	Ars., sulph., sumb.
Diarhoea	fullness during diarrhoea (frequent and excessive discharging of the bowels producing thin watery feces, usually as a symptom of gastrointestinal upset or infection)	Nat-s.
Diarhoea	headache alternating with diarrhœa	Podo., sec.
Diarhoea	headache ameliorated during diarrhœa	Agar., alum., apis., lachn.
Diarhoea	headache with diarrhœa	Aeth., agar., aloe., ambr., apis., con., glon., graph., Ind., jatr., kali-n., stram., verat.
Diarhoea	inflammation of bronchial tubes (network of airways to and within the lungs) alternates with diarrhoea	Seneg.
Diarhoea	pain in leg from diarrhoea	Manc.
Diarhoea	perspiration in foot during diarrhoea	Sulph.
Diarhoea	perspiration with diarrhoea	Acon., con., sulph., **Verat.**
Diarhoea	profuse perspiration with diarrhoea & copious flow of urine	Acon.
Diarhoea	prolapsus of anus during diarrhoea	Calc., Dulc., gamb., mag-m., Merc., mur-ac., Podo.
Diarhoea	retching during diarrhoea	Arg-n., crot-t., cupr.
Diarhoea	rheumatic pain in extremities alternating with diarrhoea	Cimic., dulc., kali-bi.
Diarhoea	rheumatic pain in extremities following diarrhoea	Kali-bi.
Diarhoea	rheumatic pain in extremities from checked diarrhoea	Abrot.
Diarhoea	rheumatic pain in extremities in chronic diarrhoea	Nat-s.
Diarhoea	rumbling in abdomen during diarrhoea	Crot-t., glon., hyos., iris., kali-c.
Diarhoea	sleepiness after diarrhoea	Nux-v.
Diarhoea	sweating on forehead during diarrhœa	Sulph.
Diarhoea	unconsciousness after diarrhœa	Ars.
Diarhoea	vomiting during diarrhoea	Aeth., ant-c., apis., arg-m., Arg-n., Ars., asar., bell., bism., carb-ac., chin., colch., coloc., crot-t., cupr-ar., cupr., cycl., dios., dulc., elaps., Gamb., gnaph., gran., graph., grat., hell., indg., iod., ip., jatr., kali-n., kreos., lach., merc-c., merc., phos., phyt., plb., podo., puls., rob., sang., seneg., sep., stann., stram., sulph., tab., Verat.

Body part/Disease	Symptom	Medicines
Diarhoea	weakness from diarrhoea	Alum., ambr., apis., **Ars.**, bor., both., bry., carb-v., **Chin.**, coloc., con., dulc., ferr., gnaph., graph., hura., hydr., iod., ip., iris., kali-c., kali-chl., lil-t., mag-c., merc-cy., merc., **Nat-s.**, **Nit-ac.**, nux-v., **Olnd.**, op., ox-ac., petr., **Phos.**, phyt., **Pic-ac.**, **Podo.**, sec., senec., sep., **Sil.**, sul-ac., tab., tarent., **Verat.**, zinc.
Diarhoea	weakness in joints after diarrhoea	Bor.
Diarhoea	weakness in leg after diarrhoea	Bov.
Diarhoea	yawning after diarrhoea	Nux-v.
Diphtheria	coryza during diphtheria	Am-c., ars., Arum-t., carb-ac., chlor., crot-h., ign., Kali-bi., kali-ma., lac-c., lach., lyc., merc-c., merc-cy., merc-i-f., mur-ac., Nit-ac.
Diphtheria	coryza in diphtheria	Am-c., hydr., kali-bi., lyc., merc-c., merc-cy., nit-ac., petr.
Diphtheria	obstruction in nose in diphtheria	Am-c., hydr., kali-m., lyc., merc-cy.
Diphtheria	paralysis agitans after diphtheria (a serious infectious disease that attacks the membranes of the throat and releases a toxin that damages the heart and the nervous system. The main symptoms are fever, weakness, and severe inflammation of the affected membranes)	Ars., caust., **Cocc.**, con., crot-h., gels., hyos., lac-c., lach., nat-m., nux-v., phos., phyt., plb., sec., sil.
Diphtheria	post diphtheritic paralysis of pharynx	Apis., Ars., caust., cocc., gels., Lac-c., Lach., Naja., nat-m., plb., Sec., sil.
Diphtheria	urine albuminous (the presence of albumin in urine, usually an indication of kidney disease) after diphtheria	Apis., ars., carb-ac., hell., hep., kali-chl., lach., lyc., merc-c., merc-cy., phyt.
Diphtheria	vision, dimness after diphtheria	Apis., gels., Lach., nux-v., phys., Phyt., sil.
Discharge	bloody discharge from ear after measles	Bov., cact., carb-v., colch., crot-h., lyc., merc., nit-ac., Puls., sulph.
Discharge	bloody discharge from ear threatening caries	Asaf., Aur., calc-f., calc-s., calc., caps., nat-m., Sil., sulph.
Discharge	bloody discharge from urethra	Arg-n., bell., Calc-s., cann-s., Canth., caps., cop., cub., cur., kali-i., lith., lyc., merc-c., merc., mill., mur-ac., nit-ac., psor., puls., thuj., zinc.
Discharge	bloody discharge from urethra painful to touch	Caps.
Discharge	clear discharge from urethra	Brom., cann-i., cann-s., canth., cub., elaps., lyc., mez., nat-m., nit-ac., petros., ph-ac., phos.
Discharge	colourless discharge from urethra	Canth., nat-m., nit-ac., petros.
Discharge	constant discharge from nose	Agar., hydr., iod., kali-bi., lac-c., phos., teucr.
Discharge	convulsion from suppressed discharges	Asaf., cupr., stram.
Discharge	cramp from discharge of semen	Bufo.
Discharge	cream like discharge from urethra	Caps.
Discharge	discharge clear from urethra	Brom., cann-i., cann-s., canth., cub., elaps., lyc., mez., nat-m., nit-ac., petros., ph-ac., phos.
Discharge	discharge colourless from urethra	Canth., nat-m., nit-ac., petros.
Discharge	discharge from ears after scarlet fever	Apis., asar., aur., bar-m., bov., brom., calc-s., Carb-v., crot-h., graph., hep., kali-bi., Lyc., merc., nit-ac., Psor., puls., sulph., tell., verb.

Body part/Disease	Symptom	Medicines
Discharge	discharge from left nose	All-c., kali-s., lach., sep., teucr.
Discharge	discharge from nipple	Phel., phos., phyt.
Discharge	discharge from nose aggravated from stooping	Am-c.
Discharge	discharge from nose blood streaked	Phos.
Discharge	discharge from nose brownish	Kali-s., thuj.
Discharge	discharge from nose, constant glue like	Merc-c., psor., sel., stict., sulph.
Discharge	discharge from nose, gummy	Sumb.
Discharge	discharge from nose, hot	Acon.
Discharge	discharge from nose, one sided	Calc-s., hippoz.
Discharge	discharge from nose, purulent from left nostrils	Uran.
Discharge	discharge from nose, purulent from right nostrils	Kali-c., puls.
Discharge	discharge from nose, watery from left nostrils	Am-br., chlor.
Discharge	discharge from right nose	Crot-c., kali-bi., kali-c., kali-p., lyc., puls., sang.
Discharge	discharge from umbilicus (the area of the abdomen that surrounds the navell)	Abrot., calc-p., calc., kali-c., lyc., nat-m., nux-m., stann.
Discharge	discharge from urethra albuminous	Canth., nit-ac., petros.
Discharge	discharge from urethra bloody	Canth., Nit-ac., puls.
Discharge	discharge from urethra spotting linen	Nat-m.
Discharge	discharge from urethra sticky	Nat-m., thuj.
Discharge	discharge gleety (a discharge of purulent mucus from the penis or vagina resulting from chronic gonorrhoea) from urethra with impotency	Agn.
Discharge	discharge jelly - like from urethra	Kali-bi.
Discharge	discharge milky white from urethra	Kali-chl.
Discharge	discharge of blood from nose in morning	Am-c., arum-t., calc., kali-c., lach., lyc., petr., sulph.
Discharge	discharge of blood from one side on blowing nose	Asc-t.
Discharge	discharge of blood on blowing nose	Calad., caust., chel., graph., lach., nit-ac., puls., sulph., thuj., zinc.
Discharge	discharge of bloody fluid from umbilicus	Calc-p., calc., nux-m.
Discharge	discharge of bloody mucous from urethra	Canth., Nit-ac., puls.
Discharge	discharge of bloody water from nipple	Lyc., phyt.
Discharge	discharge of bloody wax from ear	Am-m., anac., hep., kali-c., lyc., merc., mosch., nat-m., nit-ac., phos., puls.
Discharge	discharge of clear blood from ear	Bry.
Discharge	discharge of copious blood from ear	Bar-m.
Discharge	discharge of drop of pus from urethra before urination	Tus-p.
Discharge	discharge sticky from urethra before urination	Mez.
Discharge	discharge stringy from urethra	Kali-bi.
Discharge	discharge thick and sticky from urethra	Agar., agn., bov., dig., ham., nit-ac., nux-v., ph-ac., phos.
Discharge	discharge thick from urethra	Alum., anan., arg-m., arg-n., cann-s., caps., clem., cub., ferr., hep., hydr., kali-i., med., merc-c., merc., nat-s., nux-v., psor., puls., sil., sulph.

Body part/Disease	Symptom	Medicines
Discharge	discharge thin from urethra	Apis., caps., kali-s., lyc., med., merc-c., nat-m., nit-ac., nux-v.
Discharge	discharge transparent from urethra	Cann-s., mez., petros., phos.
Discharge	discharge white from urethra	Ant-ox., arg-n., cann-i., cann-s., canth., caps., chim., cinnb., cob., cop., cupr-ar., ferr., gels., iod., kali-c., kali-chl., lach., med., merc., mez., Nat-m., nit-ac., petr., petros., ph-ac., Sep., sulph., thuj., zinc.
Discharge	discharge yellow from urethra	Agar., agn., Alum., anan., Arg-m., ars-s-f., bar-c., bell., calc-s., calc., cann-s., canth., caps., con., cop., cub., cur., fl-ac., hep., hydr., kali-bi., kali-s., lyc., med., Merc., nat-m., Nit-ac., petr., petros., psor., Puls., sars., Sel., Sep., sil., sulph., Thuj., tus-p., zing.
Discharge	discharge yellow from urethra with spots on linen	Alum., nat-m., psor.
Discharge	discharge, watery from right nostrils	Alum., calc-s., kali-bi., nit-ac.
Discharge	discharges from ear every seven days	Sulph.
Discharge	discharges from ear in warm bed	Merc.
Discharge	discharges from ear with putrid meat like smell	Kali-p., Psor., thuj.
Discharge	discharges from left ear	Ferr., graph., psor.
Discharge	discharges from right ear	Aeth., elaps., lyc., nit-ac., sil., thuj.
Discharge	discharges of blood from ear	Am-c., arn., arund., asaf., bell., Both., bry., bufo., chin., cic., colch., con., Crot-h., elaps., ery-a., ham., merc., mosch., op., petr., Phos., puls., rhus-t., tell.
Discharge	discharges of blood from ear instead of menses	Bry., phos.
Discharge	discharges of blood from ear after prolonged suppuration (discharge of pus as a result of an injury or infection)	Chin.
Discharge	discharges of blood from ear during cough	Bell.
Discharge	discharges of mucous or pus from eye at night	Alum.
Discharge	discharges of mucous or pus from eye in evening	Kali-p.
Discharge	discharges of mucous or pus from eye in morning	Arg-n., ars., cinnb., kali-bi., mag-c., plb., sep., sil., staph., sulph.
Discharge	discharges, acrid from eye	Am-c., ars-i., ars., calc., carb-s., cham., coloc., euphr., fl-ac., graph., hep., kali-ar., merc., nit-ac., sulph.
Discharge	discharges, bloody from eye	Ars., asaf., carb-s., carb-v., caust., cham., hep., kali-c., kreos., lach., lyc., merc., mez., nat-m., petr., ph-ac., phos., puls., rhus-t., sep., sil., sulph., thuj.
Discharge	discharges, from corner of eye	Ant-c., bell., berb., bism., dig., eupho., kali-bi., nat-c., nat-m., nux-v., pic-ac., psor.
Discharge	discharges, from lachrymal sac (bone of eye socket)	Ars., arum-t., con., hep., iod., merc., nat-m., Petr., puls., sil., stann., sulph.
Discharge	discharges, like acrid water from eye	Clem.
Discharge	discharges, milky-white from eye	Kali-chl.
Discharge	discharges, of pus from corner of eye	Cham., graph., kali-bi., kali-c., kali-i., led., Nux-v., ph-ac., ran-b., zinc.

Body part/Disease	Symptom	Medicines
Discharge	discharges, purulent from eye	Ail., alumn., arg-m., Arg-n., Calc., carb-s., carb-v., caust., cham., chlor., ery-a., eupho., ferr-i., graph., grin., Hep., kali-i., lach., led., Lyc., lyss., mag-c., mag-m., Merc., nat-c., nit-ac., petr., ph-ac., phos., Puls., rhus-t., sep., spong., sulph., tell.
Discharge	discharges, thick from eye	Alum., arg-n., calc-s., chel., euphr., hep., hydr., kali-bi., lyc., nat-m., puls., sep., sil., sulph., thuj.
Discharge	discharges, thin from eye	Graph.
Discharge	discharges, white from eye	Alum., hydr., lachn., petr., plb.
Discharge	discharges, yellow from eye	Agar., alum., arg-n., ars., aur., calc-s., calc., carb-s., carb-v., caust., chel., euphr., kali-bi., kali-c., kali-chl., kali-s., kreos., lyc., merc., nat-p., Puls., sep., Sil., sulph., thuj.
Discharge	erection, shortly after seminal discharge	Ph-ac., sulph.
Discharge	eruption, exuding	Crot-h., cupr., hell., kali-s., merc., nat-m., rhus-v., sol-n.
Discharge	eruption, exuding thin water	Crot-h., tarent-c.
Discharge	eruption, exuding yellow water	Cupr., hell., rhus-v., sol-n.
Discharge	eruption, moist with purulent discharge in upper limbs	Lyc., rhus-t.
Discharge	eruption, pimples exuding water in wrists	Hura., psor., rhus-v.
Discharge	eruption, pimples exuding water on pressure in wrists	Mag-c.
Discharge	eruption, pimples in palms hard itching, discharging stony concretion	Thuj.
Discharge	eruption, pimples oozing after scratching in forearm	Kali-n.
Discharge	eruption, pimples suppurating in hands	Anac., elaps.
Discharge	eruption, pustules suppurating in lower limbs	Con., thuj.
Discharge	eruption, with purulent discharge in forearm	Rhus-t.
Discharge	eruptions blotches itching & oozing	**Graph.**
Discharge	eruptions carbuncle discharging after scratching	Alum., ars., bar-c., bell., bov., bry., calc., carb-an., carb-v., caust., cic., con., dulc., **Graph.**, hell., hep., kali-c., kreos., **Lach.**, led., **Lyc.**, merc., mez., nat-c., nat-m., nit-ac., olnd., petr., **Rhus-t.**, ruta., sabin., sars., sel., sep., sil., squil., staph., sul-ac., sulph., tarax., thuj., viol-t.
Discharge	eruptions carbuncle discharging blood	Ant-c., calc., crot-h., lach., merc., nux-v.
Discharge	eruptions carbuncle discharging glutinous	Calc., carb-s., **Graph.**, nat-m., sulph.
Discharge	eruptions carbuncle discharging greenish	Ant-c., kali-chl., rhus-t.
Discharge	eruptions carbuncle discharging ichorous	Ant-t., clem., ran-s., *rhus-t.*
Discharge	eruptions carbuncle discharging moist	Alum., anac., anag., ant-c., ars-i., ars., bar-c., bell., bov., bry., bufo., cact., cadm., calc-s., calc., canth., caps., carb-an., **Carb-s.**, **Carb-v.**, caust., cham., cic., cist., clem., con., crot-h., crot-t., cupr., **Dulc**, **Graph.**, hell., hep., hydr., iod., jug-c., kali-ar., kali-br., kali-c., kali-p., kali-s., kreos., lach., led., **Lyc.**, manc., merc., **Mez.**, mur-ac., nat-a., nat-c., **Nat-m.**, nat-p., nat-s., nit-ac., olnd., petr., ph-ac., phos., phyt., psor., ran-b., **Rhus-t.**, rhus-v., ruta., sabin., sars., sel., **Sep.**, **Sil.**, **Sol-n.**, squil., staph., still., sul-ac., sul-i., sulph., tarax., tell., thuj., vinc., viol-t., zinc.

Body part/Disease	Symptom	Medicines
Discharge	eruptions carbuncle discharging pus	Clem., graph., hep., lyc., nat-m., nit-ac., sulph.
Discharge	eruptions carbuncle discharging thin	Cupr., dulc., hell., **Nat-m.**, rhus-t., rhus-v., sol-n.
Discharge	eruptions carbuncle discharging white	Bor., **Calc.**, carb-v., caust., dulc., graph., lyc., merc., nat-m., phos., **Puls.**, sep., **Sil.**
Discharge	eruptions carbuncle discharging yellow	Alum., anac., **Ant-c.**, ars., bar-c., calc., canth., carb-an., **Carb-s.**, **Carb-v.**, caust., clem., cupr., dulc., graph., hep., iod., kali-c., kali-s., lach., lyc., merc., nat-m., nat-p., **Nat-s.**, **Nit-ac.**, **Phos.**, **Puls.**, rhus-t., **Sep.**, **Sil.**, sol-n., **Sulph.**, thuj., viol-t.
Discharge	eruptions carbuncle oozing greenish bloody	Ant-c.
Discharge	eruptions carbuncle suppurating	Ars., plb., sil., sulph.
Discharge	eruptions, vesicles in first finger discharging water	Kali-c.
Discharge	even an emission of flatus causes easy discharge of prostatic fluid	Mag-c.
Discharge	excessive flow of blood in brain from suppressed discharges or suddenly ceasing pains	Cimic.
Discharge	excessive flow of blood in brain from suppressed lochia (the normal vaginal discharge of cell debris and blood after childbirth) from the vagina	Acon., bell., bry., cimic.
Discharge	excoriating bloody discharge	Ars-i., calc-p., carb-v., fl-ac., hep., lyc., merc., nat-m., puls., rhus-t., Sulph., syph., Tell.
Discharge	fetid discharge from urethra	Bar-c., benz-ac., carb-v., hep., psor., puls., sil., sulph., thuj.
Discharge	fistula lacrymalis discharging pus on pressure	Puls., sil., stann.
Discharge	flaky (thin dry flaking scales of skin) suppuration of foot	Sil.
Discharge	gelatinous discharge from urethra after urination	Nat-m.
Discharge	gleety discharge from urethra with impotency	Agn.
Discharge	gluey discharge from urethra	Graph.
Discharge	glutinous discharge from urethra	Agar., thuj.
Discharge	grayish discharge from urethra	Arg-m.
Discharge	greenish discharge from urethra	Bry., cinnb., cob., cop., hydr., kali-i., kali-s., merc-c., Merc., nat-m., nat-s., nit-ac., ter., thuj.
Discharge	ichorous (a watery or slightly bloody discharge from a wound or an ulcer) bloody discharge from ear	Am-c., Ars., calc-p., carb-an., carb-v., Lyc., nit-ac., Psor., sep., sil., tell.
Discharge	injuries with extravasations (leak, or cause blood or other fluid to leak, from a vessel into surrounding tissue as a result of injury, burns, or inflammation)	**Arn.**, bad., bry., cham., chin., cic., con., dulc., euphr., ferr., hep., iod., lach., laur., nux-v., par., plb., puls., rhus-t., ruta., sec., **Sul-ac.**, sulph.
Discharge	jelly like discharge from urethra	Kali-bi.
Discharge	large quantity of blood oozes on pressing the gums with fingers	Bapt., graph.
Discharge	milk like substance forcibly expelled from breast	Aeth., gamb.
Discharge	milky discharge from ears	Kali-chl.
Discharge	milky discharge from urethra	Cann-s., caps., cop., ferr., iod., kali-c., kali-chl., lach., merc., Nat-m., nux-v., petros., Sep.

Body part/Disease	Symptom	Medicines
Discharge	muco-pus discharge from bladder in old people	Alumn., carb-v., sulph., ter.
Discharge	nodules hard, painful, suppurating on penis,	Bov.
Discharge	obstruction in nose with watery discharge	Ars., arum-t., bov., brom., chin., cupr., graph., kali-i., merc-c., nux-v., sec., sin-n.
Discharge	odorless bloody discharge from ear	Lac-c.
Discharge	old cicatrices suppurating	Sil.
Discharge	oozing from oedematous legs	Graph., **Lyc.**, tarent-c.
Discharge	painful discharge from ear	Calc-s., ferr-p., Merc.
Discharge	painless gleety discharge from urethra	Agar., alum., arg-m., bar-c., cann-s., cop., ferr., hep., hydr., Kali-i., med., merc., mez., Nat-m., nat-s., petr., psor., puls., sang., Sep., sulph., thuj.
Discharge	phimosis with suppuration	Caps., cinnb., hep., merc., nit-ac.
Discharge	pimples oozing when scratched	Sulph.
Discharge	profuse discharge from urethra	Apis., arg-m., arg-n., ars-s-f., bufo., cann-i., chim., cop., cub., cur., ferr., hydr., kali-bi., med., petros., sep., Thuj.
Discharge	protracted discharge from urethra	Caps.
Discharge	purulent (consisting of pus) discharge from ear after abuse of mercury	Asaf., aur., Hep., Nit-ac., sil., sulph.
Discharge	purulent discharge from ear with eczema	Calc., hep., lyc., merc., sulph.
Discharge	purulent discharge from urethra	Agn., arg-n., arn., bar-c., bov., Calc-s., calc., cann-s., canth., caps., carb-v., chel., chim., clem., con., cop., cub., cupr-ar., ip., kali-i., kali-s., led., lyc., med., merc-c., merc., nat-m., Nit-ac., nux-v., ph-ac., phos., psor., puls., sabad., sabin., sars., sil., sulph., thuj.
Discharge	purulent discharge from urethra after abuse of sulphur	Calc., merc., puls.
Discharge	pus oozing from prostate gland	Hep., Sil.
Discharge	running oozing ulcer in lower limbs	Petr.
Discharge	scab behind ears exuding a glutinous moisture, sore on touch	Thuj.
Discharge	scabs (a hard crust of dried blood, serum, or pus that forms over a wound during healing) exuding a glutinous (sticky) in cervical region	Ant-t.
Discharge	scabs exuding a glutinous in coccyx	Bor., graph., sil.
Discharge	scabs exuding a glutinous in sacral region	Sil.
Discharge	scurfy scales, suppurating	Ars., bar-m., calc-s., cic., clem., graph., hep., lyc., mez., psor., rhus-t., sep., staph., Sulph., vinc.
Discharge	semen like discharge from urethra	Puls.
Discharge	seminal discharge (fluid ejaculated by male) failing during coition though the orgasm is present	Cann-i., graph.
Discharge	seminal discharge after urinating	Daph., kali-c.
Discharge	seminal discharge copious	Agar., bell., carb-s., carb-v., carl., iod., kali-c., merc-i-f., nat-m., par., petr., ph-ac., pic-ac., sep., sil., staph., sulph., zinc.
Discharge	seminal discharge copious with dream	Kali-c., pip-m., sars.

Body part/Disease	Symptom	Medicines
Discharge	seminal discharge during caresses	Arn., Con., gels., nat-c., nux-v., petr., phos., sars., sel., ust.
Discharge	seminal discharge during stool	Nat-m.
Discharge	seminal discharge every night	Nat-m., Nat-p., pic-ac., tarax.
Discharge	seminal discharge frequent in an old man	Bar-c., caust., nat-c.
Discharge	seminal discharge incomplete	Agar., aloe., anan., bar-c., berb., carb-s., dig., form., lyss., plb., zinc.
Discharge	seminal discharge larger and continues longer	Osm.
Discharge	seminal discharge painful	Agar., arg-n., berb., calc., canth., clem., con., kali-c., kali-i., kreos., merc., mosch., nat-ac., nit-ac., sars., sep., sul-ac., Sulph., thuj.
Discharge	seminal discharge too late	Agar., bor., Calc., eug., fl-ac., hydr., lach., lyc., lyss., merc-c., nat-m., petr., zinc.
Discharge	seminal discharge too late some time after the orgasm	Calc.
Discharge	seminal discharge too late, the orgasm subsides several times before it leads to ejaculation	Eug.
Discharge	seminal discharge too quick	Aloe., bar-c., berb., bor., brom., bufo., calad., calc., carb-s., carb-v., con., eug., gels., Graph., Ind., Lyc., nat-c., nat-m., onos., ph-ac., phos., pic-ac., plat., sel., sep., sulph., Zinc.
Discharge	seminal discharge while frolicking with a woman	Con., phos., sars.
Discharge	seminal discharge while unconscious	Caust., dios., ham., Ind., lach., merc-i-f., nat-p., plan., plb., sel., sep., uran.
Discharge	seminal discharge without dreams	Agar., anac., anan., ant-c., arg-m., arg-n., ars., bell., bism., camph., carb-v., cic., con., cor-r., dig., Dios., gels., graph., guai., ham., Ind., merc-i-f., nat-c., nat-p., phos., pic-ac., pip-m., sep., sin-a., stann., verb., vib., zinc.
Discharge	seminal discharge without erection	Absin., arg-m., bell., bism., calad., carb-an., chin., Cob., con., Dios., ery-a., fl-ac., gels., Graph., ham., kali-p., mosch., nat-c., nat-m., nat-p., nuph., nux-v., op., ph-ac., phos., sabad., sars., sel., spig., sulph.
Discharge	seminal discharge without excitement of fancy	Dios., phos.
Discharge	sensation of discharge hanging over eyes which must be wiped away	Croc., puls.
Discharge	sticky discharge from urethra	Nat-m., thuj.
Discharge	sticky discharge from urethra after stool	Iod.
Discharge	sticky discharge from urethra after urination	Cop., kali-c., lach., nat-m., petros., sep.
Discharge	sticky discharge from urethra before urination	Mez.
Discharge	stringy discharge from urethra	Kali-bi.
Discharge	suppurating (ooze pus) pimples	Chlor., kali-bi.
Discharge	suppurating pimples in cervical region	Calc-p., nat-c.
Discharge	suppuration around nails	Con., ph-ac.
Discharge	suppuration from bladder	Canth., sars., ter.
Discharge	suppuration from elbow	Dros., tep.
Discharge	suppuration from fingers	Bor., mang.

Body part/Disease	Symptom	Medicines
Discharge	suppuration from forearm	Lyc., plb.
Discharge	suppuration of ankle	Arn., hep.
Discharge	suppuration of foot	Rhus-v., sec., vip.
Discharge	suppuration of heel	Berb., bor., fago.
Discharge	suppuration of hip	Ars., asaf., asar., aur., calc-p., calc-s., calc-sil., calc., **Chin.**, graph., hep., merc., ph-ac., puls., rhus-t., sep., **Sil.**, staph., stram., sulph.
Discharge	suppuration of knee	Hippoz., iod.
Discharge	suppuration of left tonsil	Lach.
Discharge	suppuration of nails after vaccination	**Thuj.**
Discharge	suppuration of parotid (near ear) gland	Ars., Brom., bry., Calc., con., Hep., lach., Merc., nat-m., phos., Rhus-t., Sil., sul-ac.
Discharge	suppuration of right tonsil	Bar-c., lyc.
Discharge	suppuration of sole	Calc., kali-n., lyc., prun-s., spig.
Discharge	suppuration of tonsils	Aesc., alumn., am-m., anac., anan., apis., aur., bar-c., Bar-m., bell., calc-s., calc., canth., cham., cub., cupr., cur., daph., guai., Hep., ign., kali-bi., lac-c., lach., lyc., manc., merc-c., merc-i-f., merc-i-r., Merc., phyt., plb., sabad., sang., sep., Sil., sulph.
Discharge	suppuration under nail of great toe	Caust.
Discharge	suppuration under nails	Form.
Discharge	suppuration under nails of first finger	Calc., nat-s.
Discharge	suppurative kidneys	Ars., hep., hippoz., merc., sil.
Discharge	thick discharge from ears	Calc-s., Calc., carb-v., ery-a., Hydr., Kali-bi., kali-chl., lyc., nat-m., Puls., sep., Sil., tarent.
Discharge	thin discharge from ears	Ars., cham., elaps., graph., Kali-s., merc., petr., psor., sep., sil., sulph.
Discharge	tumours steatoma suppurating	Calc., carb-v.
Discharge	ulcer in gums discharging blood which tastes salty	Alum.
Discharge	ulcer in gums exuding blood on pressure	Bov.
Discharge	ulcer in skin suppurating	Acon., am-c., ambr., anac., ant-c., ant-t., arg-m., arn., ars-i., **Ars.**, **Asaf.**, aur., bar-c., bell., bov., bry., calc., canth., caps., carb-an., carb-s., carb-v., **Caust.**, cham., chel., chin., cic., clem., cocc., con., croc., dros., dulc., graph., hell., **Hep.**, hyos., ign., **Iod.**, ip., kali-ar., kali-c., kali-n., kali-s., kreos., lach., led., lyc., mang., **Merc.**, mez., mur-ac., nat-c., nat-m., nat-p., nit-ac., nux-v., petr., ph-ac., phos., plb., **Puls.**, ran-b., ran-s., **Rhus-t.**, ruta., sabad., sabin., sars., sec., sel., sep., **Sil.**, spig., spong., squil., staph., sul-ac., **Sulph.**, thuj., viol-t., zinc.
Discharge	ulcer in skin with corrosive (very strongly sarcastic or bitter) discharge	Agar., am-c., anac., **Ars-i.**, **Ars.**, bell., calc., carb-an., carb-v., **Caust.**, cham., chel., clem., con., crot-c., cupr., fl-ac., graph., hep., hippoz., ign., iod., **Kali-bi.**, kali-i., kreos., lach., lyc., **Merc.**, mez., nat-c., nat-m., nit-ac., nux-v., petr., phos., plb., puls., ran-b., ran-s., **Rhus-t.**, ruta., sep., **Sil.**, spig., squil., staph., sul-ac., sulph., zinc.

Body part/Disease	Symptom	Medicines
Discharge	ulcer in skin with tenacious (persisting for a long time) discharge	Ars., asaf., bov., cham., con., graph., hydr., merc., mez., ph-ac., phos., sep., sil., staph., viol-t.
Discharge	ulcer with albuminous discharge	Calc., puls.
Discharge	ulcer with blackish discharge	Anthr., bry., chin., lyc., sulph.
Discharge	ulcer with bloody discharge	Ant-t., anthr., arg-m., arn., ars-i., **Ars., Asaf.**, bell., calc-s., canth., carb-an., carb-s., carb-v., caust., com., con., croc., dros., graph., **Hep.**, hyos., iod., kali-ar., kali-c., kali-s., kreos., lach., lyc., **Merc.**, mez., nat-m., nit-ac., petr., ph-ac., phos., puls., pyrog., rhus-t., ruta., sabin., sars., sec., sep., sil., sul-ac., sulph., thuj., zinc.
Discharge	ulcer with cheesy discharge	Merc.
Discharge	ulcer with copious discharge	Acon., arg-n., ars., asaf., bry., calc., canth., carb-s., chin., cic., fl-ac., graph., **Iod.**, kali-c., kreos., lyc., mang., merc., mez., nat-c., ph-ac., phos., **Puls.**, rhus-t., ruta., sabin., **Sep.**, sil., squil., staph., sulph., thuj.
Discharge	ulcer with discharge of maggots (insect larva)	Ars., calc., merc., sabad., sil., sulph.
Discharge	ulcer with gelatinous discharge	Arg-m., arn., bar-c., cham., ferr., merc., sep., sil.
Discharge	ulcer with gray discharge	Ambr., ars., carb-ac., **Caust.**, chin., kali-chl., lyc., merc., sep., sil., thuj.
Discharge	ulcer with green disharge	Ars., asaf., aur., carb-v., caust., clem., com., kali-chl., kali-i., kreos., lyc., merc., naja., nat-c., nat-s., nux-v., par., phos., puls., rhus-t., sec., sep., sil., staph., sulph.
Discharge	ulcer with ichorous disharge	Am-c., ant-t., anthr., **Ars.**, asaf., aur., bov., calc., carb-an., carb-s., **Carb-v.**, caust., chin., cic., clem., con., dros., graph., hep., kali-ar., kali-c., kali-i., kali-p., kreos., lach., **Lyc.**, mang., **Merc.**, mez., mur-ac., **Nit-ac.**, nux-v., ph-ac., phos., plb., psor., ran-b., ran-s., **Rhus-t.**, sang., sec., sep., **Sil.**, squil., staph., sulph.
Discharge	ulcer with offensive discharge like herring brine (salt water for preserving fish)	Graph., tell.
Discharge	ulcer with old cheese like discharge	Hep., sulph.
Discharge	ulcer with putrid discharge	Am-c., anthr., **Ars., Asaf.**, bapt., bell., bor., calc-s., calc., **Chel.**, chin., cycl., graph., **Hep.**, lach., lyc., merc., **Mur-ac.**, nit-ac., ph-ac., phos., **Psor., Puls.**, rhus-t., sars., sep., **Sil.**, sulph.
Discharge	ulcer with sour smelling discharge	Calc., graph., **Hep.**, merc., nat-c., sep., sulph.
Discharge	ulcer with tallow like (substance made from vegetable matter) discharge	Merc-c., merc.
Discharge	ulcer with thin discharge	Ant-t., ars., **Asaf.**, carb-v., **Caust.**, dros., iod., kali-c., kali-i., lyc., **Merc.**, nit-ac., phos., plb., puls., pyrog., ran-b., ran-s., rhus-t., ruta., sil., staph., sulph., thuj.
Discharge	ulcer with watery discharge	Ant-t., ars-i., ars., asaf., calc., carb-v., **Caust.**, clem., con., dros., graph., iod., kali-c., lyc., **Merc.**, nit-ac., nux-v., petr., plb., puls., ran-b., ran-s., rhus-t., ruta., sil., squil., staph., sulph., thuj.
Discharge	ulcer with whitish discharge	Am-c., ars., calc., carb-v., hell., lyc., **Mez.**, puls., sep., sil., sulph.

Body part/Disease	Symptom	Medicines
Discharge	ulcer with yellow discharge	Acon., alum., am-c., ambr., anac., arg-m., ars., aur., bov., bry., calc-s., calc., caps., carb-s., carb-v., caust., cic., clem., con., croc., dulc., graph., hep., hydr., iod., **Kali-bi.**, kali-n., kali-p., kali-s., kreos., lyc., mang., merc., **Mez.**, nat-a., nat-c., nat-m., nat-p., nit-ac., nux-v., phos., **Puls.**, ran-b., rhus-t., ruta., sec., sel., sep., sil., spig., staph., sul-ac., sulph., thuj., viol-t.
Discharge	urticaria vesicular suppurating (oozing pus)	Am-m., aur., bov., calc., carb-v., graph., mag-c., nat-c., nit-ac., petr., phos., puls., ran-b., ran-s., rhus-t., sars., sulph., vip., zinc.
Discharge	vesicles discharging water from ears	Ptel.
Discharge	vesicles in mouth suppurating	Phos.
Discharge	vesicles on sides from ear discharge	Tell.
Discharge	vesicles on tongue suppurating	Mag-c.
Discharge	warts suppurating	Ars., bov., calc., caust., hep., nat-c., sil., thuj.
Discharge	watery discharge from ears	Calc., carb-v., cist., elaps., graph., Kali-s., merc., Sil., syph., Tell., thuj.
Discharge	watery discharge from urethra	Apoc., cann-s., canth., ferr-p., fl-ac., hydr., kali-s., lyc., merc-c., merc., mez., mur-ac., nat-m., ph-ac., phos., sumb., Thuj.
Discharge	watery discharge from urethra after injections of nitrate of silver	Nat-m.
Discharge	watery discharge from urethra with meatus glued up in morning with a watery drop	Phos.
Discharge	white discharge from ears	Ery-a., hep., kali-chl., Nat-m.
Discharge	white discharge from urethra in anæmic subjects	Calc-p.
Discharge	white discharge from urethra with impotence	Agn., calad., cob.
Discharge	yellow discharge from ears	Aeth., ars., calc-s., calc., crot-h., hydr., kali-ar., Kali-bi., kali-c., Kali-s., lyc., merc., nat-s., petr., phos., Puls., sil.
Discharge	yellowish discharge from urethra	Anan., arg-m., cinnb., cob., cub., cur., hydr., kali-i., kali-s., lith., lyc., Merc., Nat-s., nux-v., phyt., Puls., sep., ter., thuj.
Discharge	yellowish green discharge from ears	Cinnb., elaps., kali-chl., kali-s., merc., Puls.
Discoloration	discoloration between the toes bleached white	Bar-c., plb.
Discoloration	discoloration in legs with blotches	Lact-ac., nat-c., phos.
Discoloration	discoloration in thighs with blotches	Lact-ac.
Discoloration	discoloration like blood specks in legs	Phos.
Discoloration	discoloration of abdomen with redness	Anac., plb., rhus-t.
Discoloration	discoloration of ankle joints with redness	Lyc., mang., stann.
Discoloration	discoloration of ankle with redness	Agar., apis., calc., carb-s., carb-v., graph., hyos., lach., nat-c., phos., puls., rhus-t., sars., sep., sil., stann., thuj., vesp., vip., zinc.
Discoloration	discoloration of ankle with redness in evening	Apis.
Discoloration	discoloration of ankle with redness in spots	Apis., ars., bry., chin., elaps., lach., led., lyc., mang., phyt., thuj.

Body part/Disease	Symptom	Medicines
Discoloration	discoloration of ankle with white spots	Apis.
Discoloration	discoloration of ankle yellow grayish	Vip.
Discoloration	discoloration of back of ankle blue	Vip.
Discoloration	discoloration of back of ankle with red spots	Carb-o., puls., thuj.
Discoloration	discoloration of back of ankle with redness	Rhus-t., thuj.
Discoloration	discoloration of ball of ankle with redness	Rhus-t.
Discoloration	discoloration of fingers	Act-sp.
Discoloration	discoloration of fingers black	Sep., vip.
Discoloration	discoloration of fingers blue	Benz-n., caust., cocc., corn., crot-h., cupr., nat-m., nux-m., nux-v., op., petr., sil., vip.
Discoloration	discoloration of fingers blue in morning	Petr.
Discoloration	discoloration of fingers with brown spots	Ant-t.
Discoloration	discoloration of first finger with black spots	Apis., rhus-t.
Discoloration	discoloration of first finger with red blotches	Arg-n.
Discoloration	discoloration of hand black	Sol-n., sul-ac., tarent., vip.
Discoloration	discoloration of heel of legs purplish	Puls.
Discoloration	discoloration of heel of legs with redness	Ant-c., petr.
Discoloration	discoloration of joints with redness	Cocc., colch., kalm., merc., **Puls.**, **Rhus-t.**, verat-v.
Discoloration	discoloration of left leg during menses	Ambr.
Discoloration	discoloration of nail tip of first finger	Phos.
Discoloration	discoloration of nail tips white	Alum., der., fl-ac.
Discoloration	discoloration of nail tips yellow in spots	Elaps.
Discoloration	discoloration of nail tips, black	Sol-n.
Discoloration	discoloration of nail tips, blue	Agar., bor., colch., crot-c., op., phos.
Discoloration	discoloration of nail tips, blue in evening	Phos.
Discoloration	discoloration of nails	Ant-c., ars., graph., nit-ac., thuj.
Discoloration	discoloration of nails	Apis., ars., camph., dig., graph., nit-ac., ox-ac., sil.
Discoloration	discoloration of nails blue	Apis.
Discoloration	discoloration of nails red then black	Ars.
Discoloration	discoloration of palms with brown spots	Iod., nat-c., thuj.
Discoloration	discoloration of palms with red spots	Apis.
Discoloration	discoloration of palms with redness	Fl-ac.
Discoloration	discoloration of palms with yellowness	Chel.
Discoloration	discoloration of patella on going upstairs	Cann-s.
Discoloration	discoloration of second joint of second finger	Ars-h.
Discoloration	discoloration of skin after intermittent fever	Am-c., ars., chin-s., con., ferr., nat-c., nat-m., nux-v., sang., **Sep.**, tub.
Discoloration	discoloration of skin after vexation (anxiety/grief)	Cham., kali-c., nat-s.
Discoloration	discoloration of skin after washing	Kali-c.
Discoloration	discoloration of skin blackish	Acon., ant-c., apis., arg-n., **Ars.**, asaf., aur., carb-v., chel., crot-h., lach., nit-ac., ph-ac., phyt., **Plb.**, **Sec.**, spig.

Body part/Disease	Symptom	Medicines
Discoloration	discoloration of skin bluish	Acon., aeth., ail., am-c., ant-t., apis., arg-n., arn., ars., aur., bapt., bell., bism., brom., bry., bufo., cadm., calc., camph., carb-an., carb-s., **Carb-v.**, chin-a., chin., coca., cocc., con., cop., **Crot-c.**, crot-h., cupr., cur., **Dig.**, gels., hydr-ac., kali-bi., **Lach.**, laur., led., merc., mur-ac., naja., nat-m., nux-m., **Nux-v.**, **Op.**, ox-ac., ph-ac., phos., phyt., plb., puls., rhus-t., samb., sec., sil., spong., stram., syph., tarent., thuj., **Verat-v.**, **Verat.**, vip.
Discoloration	discoloration of skin dirty	Ars., bor., bry., bufo., ferr-i., ferr., iod., merc., nat-m., nit-ac., phos., plb., **Psor.**, sec., stram., **Sulph.**, tarent., thuj., tub.
Discoloration	discoloration of skin dirty gray	Iod.
Discoloration	discoloration of skin during pregnancy	Aur.
Discoloration	discoloration of skin every summer	Chin-a., chion.
Discoloration	discoloration of skin in new born children	Acon., bov., chin., nat-s., sep.
Discoloration	discoloration of skin like spots	Ambr., ant-t., **Arn.**, ars., canth., **Con.**, crot-c., elaps., **Ferr.**, hydrc., iod., kali-ar., kali-c., lach., lyc., nat-c., nat-p., **Petr.**, **Phos.**, psor., ruta., sabad., **Sep.**, stann., **Sulph.**, thuj., vip.
Discoloration	discoloration of skin red	Acon., **Agar.**, agn., am-c., ant-c., **Apis.**, arn., **Bell.**, bov., bry., calc., camph., canth., carb-v., chin., coc-c., cocc., coll., com., con., cop., crot-c., crot-h., crot-t., cur., cycl., dulc., eupho., ferr-p., **Graph.**, hyos., ign., kreos., lach., led., lyc., manc., **Merc.**, nat-m., nit-ac., nux-v., olnd., op., paeon., petr., ph-ac., phos., phyt., plb., puls., **Rhus-t.**, ruta., sabad., sec., sep., sil., spong., squil., stann., **Stram.**, sul-ac., sulph., tarax., tell., teucr., til., zinc.
Discoloration	discoloration of skin red after scratching	Agar., am-c., ant-c., arn., bell., bov., canth., chin., dulc., graph., kreos., lyc., merc., nat-m., nux-v., olnd., op., petr., ph-ac., puls., **Rhus-t.**, ruta., spong., tarax., teucr.
Discoloration	discoloration of skin white	**Apis.**, **Ars.**, calc., carb-v., fl-ac., **Kali-c.**, lac-c., sumb.
Discoloration	discoloration of skin with black spots	Aeth., ars., crot-h., ferr., lach., rhus-t., sec., vip.
Discoloration	discoloration of skin with blue spots	Aeth., anan., ant-c., anthr., apis., arg-n., **Arn.**, ars., bad., bar-c., bar-m., berb., bor., bry., calc., carb-an., carb-v., chlol., con., **Crot-h.**, dulc., euphr., ferr., hep., lac-c., **Lach.**, laur., led., lyc., merc., mosch., nit-ac., nux-m., nux-v., op., **Ph-ac.**, **Phos.**, plat., plb., puls., rhus-t., ruta., sars., **Sec.**, sil., **Sul-ac.**, sulph., tarent., ter.
Discoloration	discoloration of skin with bluish induration	Sars.
Discoloration	discoloration of skin with bluish recurring annually	Crot-h.
Discoloration	discoloration of skin with bluish red red spots	Anthr., apis., ars., bell., crot-h., elaps., lach., **Phos.**
Discoloration	discoloration of skin with brown liver spots	Am-c., ant-c., ant-t., arg-n., arn., ars-i., ars., aur., bad., bor., bry., cadm., calc-p., calc-s., calc., canth., carb-s., carb-v., caust., con., cop., cor-r., crot-h., **Cur.**, dros., dulc., ferr-i., ferr., graph., hyos., iod., kali-ar., kali-bi., kali-c., kali-p., **Lach.**, laur., **Lyc.**, merc-i-r., **Merc.**, mez., nat-a., nat-c., nat-p., **Nit-ac.**, nux-v., petr., phos., plb., puls., ruta., sabad., **Sep.**, sil., stann., sul-ac., **Sulph.**, tarent., thuj., tub.

Body part/Disease	Symptom	Medicines
Discoloration	discoloration of skin with brownish red red spots	Calc., cann-s., carb-v., **Nit-ac.**, phos., **Sep.**, thuj.
Discoloration	discoloration of skin with coppery red red spots	Alum., ars., calc., cann-s., **Carb-an.**, carb-v., cor-r., crot-t., kreos., **Lach.**, led., mez., nit-ac., phos., phyt., rhus-t., ruta., syph., ust., verat.
Discoloration	discoloration of skin with coppery red red spots after desquamation	Carb-an., fl-ac.
Discoloration	discoloration of skin with dark spots in old people	Ars., aur., bar-c., carb-an., con., lach., lyc., op., sec.
Discoloration	discoloration of skin with death spots in old people	Ars., aur., bar-c., con., lach., lyc., op., sec.
Discoloration	discoloration of skin with different colours	Ars., carb-v., chlol., cop., crot-h., **Lach.**, nux-m., nux-v., ox-ac., verat-v.
Discoloration	discoloration of skin with different colours during chill	Ars., crot-h., nux-v., rhus-t.
Discoloration	discoloration of skin with dirty spots	Berb., sabin., sec.
Discoloration	discoloration of skin with fiery (inflammed) red red spots	Acon., bell., ferr-ma., stram.
Discoloration	discoloration of skin with green spots	Arn., ars., bufo., carb-v., **Con.**, crot-h., lach., med., nit-ac., sep., sul-ac., verat., vip.
Discoloration	discoloration of skin with grey spots	Iod., nit-ac.
Discoloration	discoloration of skin with lense shaped spots	Calc., rhus-t., vip.
Discoloration	discoloration of skin with moist red spots	Crot-t.
Discoloration	discoloration of skin with moist spots	Ant-c., ars., carb-v., crot-t., hell., kali-c., lach., sel., **Sil.**, sulph., tarax.
Discoloration	discoloration of skin with pale spots	Lach.
Discoloration	discoloration of skin with pale red spots	Nat-c., phos., sil., teucr.
Discoloration	discoloration of skin with red rose coloured spots	Cann-s., carb-an., carb-v., cocc., cop., rhod., sars., sep., tep., teucr.
Discoloration	discoloration of skin with red spots after bathing	Am-c.
Discoloration	discoloration of skin with red spots in cold air	Sabad.
Discoloration	discoloration of skin with red wine spots	Cocc., **Sep.**
Discoloration	discoloration of skin with scarlet (bright red) spots	Acon., **Am-c.**, am-m., arn., ars., bar-c., **Bell.**, bry., carb-an., carb-v., caust., cham., coff., croc., dulc., eupho., hep., hyos., iod., ip., lach., **Merc.**, ph-ac., phos., rhus-t., stram., sulph.
Discoloration	discoloration of skin with shiny spots	Calc., phos.
Discoloration	discoloration of skin with small spots after scratching	Ant-t., bry., lach., led., lyc., merc., op., rat., squil., sul-ac., vip.
Discoloration	discoloration of skin with smarting spots	Bry., ferr., hep., led., nat-m., ph-ac., puls., sil., verat.
Discoloration	discoloration of skin with smooth indurated spots	Carb-an.
Discoloration	discoloration of skin with smooth spots	Carb-an., carb-v., cor-r., lach., mag-c., petr., sumb.
Discoloration	discoloration of skin with spots after scratching	Am-c., ant-c., bell., calc., cocc., cycl., graph., mag-c., mang., merc., nit-ac., ph-ac., phos., rhus-t., sabad., sep., sil., sul-ac., sulph., verat.
Discoloration	discoloration of skin with spots aggravated from warmth	Fl-ac.
Discoloration	discoloration of skin with spots burnt as if	Ant-c., ars., carb-v., caust., cycl., eupho., hyos., kreos., rhus-t., sec., stram.

Body part/Disease	Symptom	Medicines
Discoloration	discoloration of skin with spots like flea bites	Acon., pall.
Discoloration	discoloration of skin with spots returning yearly	Crot-h.
Discoloration	discoloration of skin with star shaped spots	Stram.
Discoloration	discoloration of skin with stinging spots	Canth., chel., lach., lyc., merc., nit-ac., puls., **Sil.**
Discoloration	discoloration of skin with violet (purplish blue) spots	Ferr., nit-ac., phos., verat.
Discoloration	discoloration of skin with white spots	Alum., am-c., **Ars.**, aur., berb., calc., carb-an., coca., merc., nat-c., nit-ac., phos., sep., **Sil.**, sulph.
Discoloration	discoloration of skin with white spots becoming bluish	Calc.
Discoloration	discoloration of skin with white spots with dark borders	Calc.
Discoloration	discoloration of skin yellow / jaundice after anger	Bry., cham., nat-s., **Nux-v.**
Discoloration	discoloration of skin yellow / jaundice after mortification (death and decay of living tissue	Bry., lyc.
Discoloration	discoloration of skin yellow / jaundice during heat	Ferr., lach., nux-v.
Discoloration	discoloration of skin yellow / jaundice with convulsion	Agar.
Discoloration	discoloration of sole of legs with blue spots	Kali-p.
Discoloration	discoloration of sole of legs with redness	Bry., kali-c., phos., puls.
Discoloration	discoloration of sole of legs with redness in spots	Ars.
Discoloration	discoloration of sole of legs with white spots	Nat-m.
Discoloration	discoloration of sole of legs with white spots as if bleached	Bar-c., plb.
Discoloration	discoloration of tibia with spots	Ambr., ant-c., caust., kali-n., lach., mag-c., phos., sil., sul-ac.
Discoloration	discoloration of tips of nails blue	Op.
Discoloration	discoloration of tips of nails red	Mur-ac., thuj.
Discoloration	discoloration of toes	Sec.
Discoloration	discoloration of toes violet	Stry.
Discoloration	discoloration of toes with blackness	Crot-h., phos., sec., sol-n.
Discoloration	discoloration of toes with redness	Agar., alum., am-c., apis., aster., aur-m., aur., berb., bor., carb-v., nat-m., nit-ac., nux-v., phos., sep., thuj., zinc.
Discoloration	discoloration of toes with redness shining	Thuj.
Discoloration	discoloration of upper limbs, black	Vesp.
Discoloration	discoloration of upper limbs, black in spots	Vip.
Discoloration	discoloration on abdomen in spots	Vip.
Discoloration	discoloration on back of hands with blotches	Apis., arg-n.
Discoloration	discoloration on back of hands with blotches and itching	Cit-v.
Discoloration	discoloration on back of hands with blotches and stinging	Apis.
Discoloration	discoloration on back of hands with blue spots	Sars., sec.
Discoloration	discoloration on back of hands with blueness	Carb-o., plb.
Discoloration	discoloration on back of hands with brown spots	Cop., lach., nat-m., petr., sulph.

Body part/Disease	Symptom	Medicines
Discoloration	discoloration on calf with blotches	Petr.
Discoloration	discoloration on calf with blue spots	Kali-p.
Discoloration	discoloration purple on ankle	Arn., lach.
Discoloration	discoloration purple on legs	Led., vesp.
Discoloration	discoloration purpura on legs	Kali-i., lach., **Phos.**, sec.
Discoloration	discoloration red of back of first finger	Arg-n.
Discoloration	discoloration white in spots in thigh	Calc.
Discoloration	discoloration with black dots on hand	Petr.
Discoloration	discoloration with blackness in hips	Crot-h.
Discoloration	discoloration with blotches on hand	Ars., sep.
Discoloration	discoloration with blotches on hand with itching	Sep.
Discoloration	discoloration with blue spots on ankles	Sul-ac.
Discoloration	discoloration with blue spots on hand	Nit-ac.
Discoloration	discoloration with blue spots on hand in old people	Bar-c.
Discoloration	discoloration with blueness on hand after waking at night	Samb.
Discoloration	discoloration with blueness on hand after washing in cold water	Am-c.
Discoloration	discoloration with blueness on hand at night	Phos., samb.
Discoloration	discoloration with blueness on hand during chill	Camph., nux-v., spong., stram., **Verat.**
Discoloration	discoloration with blueness on hand in morning	Spong.
Discoloration	discoloration with blueness on hand in winter	Cupr.
Discoloration	discoloration with blueness on hand when hanging down	Sep.
Discoloration	discoloration with blueness on hand with coldness	Nux-v., sep.
Discoloration	discoloration with blueness on hand with convulsion	Aesc.
Discoloration	discoloration with brown spots in legs	Petr., thuj.
Discoloration	discoloration with brownish back of hands	Iod., thuj.
Discoloration	discoloration with copper coloured spots on hands	Nit-ac.
Discoloration	discoloration with dark yellow spots on hands	Elaps., med.
Discoloration	discoloration with dark yellowness on hands	Aran.
Discoloration	discoloration with indurated spots in legs	Sars.
Discoloration	discoloration with purple hands	Apis., kali-p., lach., naja., op., phos., rhus-t., sec., thuj., vip.
Discoloration	discoloration with purple hands during chilliness	Thuj.
Discoloration	discoloration with purple spots on ankle	**Sul-ac.**
Discoloration	discoloration with purple spots on hands	Kali-c.
Discoloration	discoloration with purple spots on legs	**Apis.**, crot-h.
Discoloration	discoloration with red spots in knee	Lyc., petr.
Discoloration	discoloration with red spots in thigh	Bell., calc., caps., crot-t., cycl., graph., med., merc., petr., plan., rhod., rhus-t., sulph.

Body part/Disease	Symptom	Medicines
Discoloration	discoloration with red spots in thigh with burning	Ph-ac.
Discoloration	discoloration with red spots in thigh with itching	Nat-m.
Discoloration	discoloration with red spots in thigh with itching when scratched	Med.
Discoloration	discoloration with red spots on calf	Con., graph., kali-br., lach.
Discoloration	discoloration with red spots on hands	All-s., alum., bell., berb., cor-r., elaps., kali-i., lach., mag-m., mang., merc., nat-c., nat-m., ph-ac., sabad., sep., stann., tab., zinc.
Discoloration	discoloration with reddish spots on legs	Calc., con., dulc., graph., guare., kali-br., kali-n., lyc., merc., sars., sil., sul-ac., zinc.
Discoloration	discoloration with reddish spots on legs becomes covered with crusts	Zinc.
Discoloration	discoloration with redness in anterior part (in front) of knee	Merc., nat-m.
Discoloration	discoloration with redness in hips	Lact-ac., ph-ac., rhus-t., vip.
Discoloration	discoloration with redness in knee	Lachn., lact-ac., petr.
Discoloration	discoloration with redness in lower limbs	Petr., plb., ptel., sep., stram., vip.
Discoloration	discoloration with redness in nates	Cann-s., hyos.
Discoloration	discoloration with redness in posterior part (behind) of knee	Am-c., kreos.
Discoloration	discoloration with redness in spots in hips	Lact-ac., rhus-t.
Discoloration	discoloration with redness in spots in lower limbs	Ars., calc., caust., con., graph., kali-i., lach., lyc., merc., mez., petr., ph-ac., sil., sul-ac., sulph.
Discoloration	discoloration with redness in spots in nates	Cann-s., mag-c.
Discoloration	discoloration with redness in thigh	Anac., bell., kali-c., nat-m., puls., rhus-t., sil., thuj.
Discoloration	discoloration with redness in thigh at night	Rhus-v.
Discoloration	discoloration with redness on hands	**Agar.**, **Apis.**, bar-c., bell., berb., bry., carb-an., fl-ac., hep., mez., nat-s., nux-v., phos., plan., puls., rhus-t., seneg., staph., stram., sulph., sumb., vesp.
Discoloration	discoloration with redness on legs	Aeth., am-c., arn., arund., con., cop., elaps., hydr-ac., kali-bi., kali-br., lach., lyc., merc., nat-c., phos., puls., rhus-t., rhus-v., sulph., thuj.
Discoloration	discoloration with redness on legs in evening	Fago.
Discoloration	discoloration with redness on legs while walking	Nux-v.
Discoloration	discoloration with redness stripes in hips extending to umbilicus	Ph-ac.
Discoloration	discoloration with spots in legs	Sars., sul-ac.
Discoloration	discoloration with spots in lower limbs	Ant-c., bry., hyos., kali-br., kali-n., nat-c., sulph.
Discoloration	discoloration with spots in thigh	Am-c., ant-c., cann-i., cycl., graph., mur-ac., rhod.
Discoloration	discoloration with spots on calf	Con., graph., sars.
Discoloration	discoloration with spots on hand	Sol-n.
Discoloration	discoloration with spots on legs	Calc., chel., con., lyc., phos., stann., zinc.
Discoloration	discoloration with white spots on legs	Calc.
Discoloration	discoloration with yellow marks in thigh	Arn.

Body part/Disease	Symptom	Medicines
Discoloration	discoloration with yellow spots on legs	Carl., hydrc., stann., vip.
Discoloration	discoloration with yellow stripes in lower limbs	Vip.
Discoloration	discoloration with yellowness on hands	Canth., chel., cupr-ar., elaps., ign., lyc., sil., spig.
Discoloration	discoloration yellow in lower limbs	Kali-br, vip.
Discoloration	discoloration, black in spots in legs	Vip.
Discoloration	discoloration, black of legs	Iod., vip.
Discoloration	discoloration, black of nails	Ars., graph.
Discoloration	discoloration, blackness	Ars., tarent., vip.
Discoloration	discoloration, blackness in spots on shoulder	Vip.
Discoloration	discoloration, blackness on abdomen	Vip.
Discoloration	discoloration, blood settles under nails	Apis.
Discoloration	discoloration, blotches	Berb., cimx., cocc., hura.
Discoloration	discoloration, blotches (An irregularly shaped Reddish patch on the skin) on abdomen	Aloe., crot-t.
Discoloration	discoloration, blotches in lower limbs	Ant-c., crot-t., lach., nat-c., sulph.
Discoloration	discoloration, blotches on fingers	Arg-n.
Discoloration	discoloration, blotches on upper limbs	Chlol., rhus-v.
Discoloration	discoloration, blue in thigh	Anthr., bism., both., kreos.
Discoloration	discoloration, blue in legs	Ambr., anthr., arg-n., carb-an., carb-s., con., elaps., kali-br., lyc., mur-ac., **Nux-v.**, ox-ac., plb.
Discoloration	discoloration, blue marks on thigh	Arn.
Discoloration	discoloration, blue on forearm with blotches	Apis., arg-n., bism., plat., sep.
Discoloration	discoloration, blue on upper limbs	Apis., arg-n., bism., elaps., morph., sulph.
Discoloration	discoloration, blue on upper limbs with asthma	Kali-c.
Discoloration	discoloration, blue spots on abdomen	Ars., mosch.
Discoloration	discoloration, blue spots on thigh	Ant-c., arn., kreos., morph., mosch., vip.
Discoloration	discoloration, blue spots on upper arm	Plat.
Discoloration	discoloration, blue	Agar., apis., bism., bol., **Carb-v.**, crot-c., dig., kali-ar., lach., lyss., merc., op., rob.
Discoloration	discoloration, blueness of nails	Acon., aesc., agar., apis., apoc., arg-n., arn., ars., asaf., aur., cact., camph., carb-s., carb-v., chel., chin-a., chin-s., chin., chlf., cic., cocc., colch., con., cupr., dig., dros., eup-pur., ferr-ar., ferr-p., ferr., gels., gins., graph., ip., manc., merc-sul., merc., mez., mur-ac., nat-m., nit-ac., **Nux-v.**, op., ox-ac., petr., ph-ac., phos., plb., rhus-t., sang., sars., sep., sil., sulph., sumb., tarent., thuj., verat-v., **Verat.**
Discoloration	discoloration, blueness of nails during chill	Apis., arn., **Ars.**, asaf., carb-s., carb-v., chel., chin-s., chin., cocc., con., dros., eup-pur., ip., kali-ar., mez., **Nat-m.**, **Nux-v.**, petr., ph-ac., **Rhus-t.**, sulph., thuj., verat.
Discoloration	discoloration, blueness of nails during menses	Arg-n., thuj.
Discoloration	discoloration, bluish in lower limbs	Bism., cupr., ox-ac., sec., verat.
Discoloration	discoloration, bluish spots in lower limbs	Am-c., ant-c., con., lach., phos., **Sul-ac.**, sulph.
Discoloration	discoloration, bluish spots on forearm	**Sul-ac.**

Body part/Disease	Symptom	Medicines
Discoloration	discoloration, brown bluish in legs	Anthr., vip.
Discoloration	discoloration, brown spots in thigh	Cann-s., mez., nat-s.
Discoloration	discoloration, brown spots on abdomen	Ars., carb-v., cob., hydr-ac., kali-c., lach., Lyc., nit-ac., phos., sabad., Sep., thuj.
Discoloration	discoloration, brown spots on elbow	Cadm., lach., sep.
Discoloration	discoloration, brown spots on wrist	Petr.
Discoloration	discoloration, brownish in lower limbs	Arg-n.
Discoloration	discoloration, brownish inside thigh	Thuj.
Discoloration	discoloration, brownish on back of hands	Iod., thuj.
Discoloration	discoloration, copper coloured spots on upper arm	Nit-ac.
Discoloration	discoloration, cyanosis in thigh	Ars.
Discoloration	discoloration, cyanosis on legs	Con., elaps.
Discoloration	discoloration, dark of nails	Morph., ox-ac.
Discoloration	discoloration, dark on forearm	Acon., ant-c., ars., caust., com., sep.
Discoloration	discoloration, dark spreading up the limb	Naja.
Discoloration	discoloration, ecchymoses in lower limbs	Phos., sul-ac.
Discoloration	discoloration, ecchymoses of fingers	Coca.
Discoloration	discoloration, ecchymoses on legs	Crot-h.
Discoloration	discoloration, Ecchymosis	Merc-c., sec., **Sul-ac.**, tarent., vip.
Discoloration	discoloration, freckles	Ferr.
Discoloration	discoloration, greenish in lower limbs	Vip.
Discoloration	discoloration, greenish in thigh	Kali-n.
Discoloration	discoloration, greenish spots on abdomen	Rob.
Discoloration	discoloration, greenish yellow	Vip.
Discoloration	discoloration, grey of nails	Merc-c., sil.
Discoloration	discoloration, in joints of fingers	Cann-s., cham., chel., cinnb., lyc., pall., spong., sulph.
Discoloration	discoloration, inflammed spots on abdomen	Ars., bell., canth., kali-c., lach., led., lyc., nat-m., Phos., sabad., sep.
Discoloration	discoloration, mottled (irregular pattern of patches or spots of different colors)	Ars., **Lach.**
Discoloration	discoloration, of lower limbs black and painful spots	Nux-v.
Discoloration	discoloration, of thumb black	Vip.
Discoloration	discoloration, of thumb brownish	Sulph.
Discoloration	discoloration, of thumb dark	Cic.
Discoloration	discoloration, of thumb redness	Cimic., lach., vesp.
Discoloration	discoloration, of thumb white	Vip.
Discoloration	discoloration, of thumb white in spots	Sulph.
Discoloration	discoloration, of upper limb from ecchymoses	Vip.
Discoloration	discoloration, of upper limb from liver spots	Ant-c., guare., lyc., mez.
Discoloration	discoloration, of upper limb from liver spots becoming dark	Mez.
Discoloration	discoloration, of upper limb from liver spots with itching	Lyc.

Body part/Disease	Symptom	Medicines
Discoloration	discoloration, of upper limb from petechiæ	Berb., cop., cupr., phos., phys.
Discoloration	discoloration, of upper limbs having brown spots	Guare., lyc., petr., thuj.
Discoloration	discoloration, of upper limbs while hanging down	Sep.
Discoloration	discoloration, petechiæ (tiny red spot on skin) on back of hands	Berb.
Discoloration	discoloration, purple in spots in lower limbs	Bor., ptel.
Discoloration	discoloration, purple in spots of upper limb	Ars.
Discoloration	discoloration, purple in spots	Apis., lach.
Discoloration	discoloration, purple of nails	Apis., ars., op., samb., sec., stram.
Discoloration	discoloration, purple of upper limb	Naja., vesp.
Discoloration	discoloration, purple spots on forearm	Kali-c., kali-p.
Discoloration	discoloration, purple	Apis., verat-v., zinc.
Discoloration	discoloration, purpura haemorrhagica on back of hands	Lach., phos.
Discoloration	discoloration, purpura hemorrhagica in lower limbs	Lach., phos., sec., ter.
Discoloration	discoloration, red blotches	Lach., sulph.
Discoloration	discoloration, red of nails	Ars., crot-c., lith.
Discoloration	discoloration, red on forearm with blotches	Hura., kreos.
Discoloration	discoloration, red points on fingers	Lach.
Discoloration	discoloration, red spots on back of hands	Agar., bell., calc., cic., cop., hura., nat-c., osm., stann., sulph.
Discoloration	discoloration, red spots on back of hands with itching	Brom.
Discoloration	discoloration, red spots on elbow	Phos.
Discoloration	discoloration, red spots on fingers	Benz-ac., cor-r., plb., zinc.
Discoloration	discoloration, red streakes on back of hands with itching	Vip.
Discoloration	discoloration, red stripes on fingers	Apis.
Discoloration	discoloration, reddish of upper limbs while hanging down	Vip.
Discoloration	discoloration, redness after washing	Sulph.
Discoloration	discoloration, redness disappearing on pressure	Chin-s., kali-br., verat-v.
Discoloration	discoloration, redness in spots on forearm	Ars., berb., bor., chel., eupho., merc., olnd., rhus-v., sulph., tarent., tax., thuj., vesp.
Discoloration	discoloration, redness in spots with burning	Berb., sulph., tab.
Discoloration	discoloration, redness in spots	Cadm., elaps., lach., vip.
Discoloration	discoloration, redness of fingers	Agar., apis., apoc., arg-n., arum-i., benz-ac., berb., bor., cann-i., cit-v., fl-ac., graph., kali-bi., lach., lyc., nux-v., plb., sil., sulph., ther., zinc.
Discoloration	discoloration, redness of fingers in evening	Sulph.
Discoloration	discoloration, redness of fourth finger	Lyc.
Discoloration	discoloration, redness of nail tips	Berb., calc., fago., mur-ac.
Discoloration	discoloration, redness of nail tips after chilblains	Berb.

Body part/Disease	Symptom	Medicines
Discoloration	discoloration, redness on back of hands	Aur-s., berb., brom., cic., cimic., crot-h., ferr., mur-ac., sul-ac., sulph., sumb., vip.
Discoloration	discoloration, redness on back of hands as from nettles (plant with stinging leaves)	Nat-s.
Discoloration	discoloration, redness on back of hands in afternoon	Cimic.
Discoloration	discoloration, redness on back of hands in evening	Cimic., sulph.
Discoloration	discoloration, redness on back of hands in evening in open air	Dulc.
Discoloration	discoloration, redness on back of hands in morning	Sulph.
Discoloration	discoloration, redness on forearm	Anac., apis., arn., bell., colch., kreos., mang., rhus-t.
Discoloration	discoloration, redness on shoulder	Berb., chin-s., chin., lac-c., lach., ph-ac., puls-n., tab.
Discoloration	discoloration, redness on upper arm	Anac.
Discoloration	discoloration, redness with itching in spots	Berb., eupho., zinc.
Discoloration	discoloration, redness with swelling	Plb.
Discoloration	discoloration, redness	Bell., carb-o., merc-n., sep., stram., vip.
Discoloration	discoloration, spots on elbow	Calc., sep., vip.
Discoloration	discoloration, spots on fingers	Con., corn., lyc., mang., nat-m., ph-ac., plb.
Discoloration	discoloration, spots on forearm with blotches	Cimx., hura.
Discoloration	discoloration, spots on shoulder	Berb., ph-ac., sul-ac., tab.
Discoloration	discoloration, violet of fingers	Stry.
Discoloration	discoloration, white in spots of upper limb	Apis.
Discoloration	discoloration, white of fingers	Gins., lach., vip.
Discoloration	discoloration, white of fingers during coldness	Gins.
Discoloration	discoloration, white of nails	Cupr., nit-ac.
Discoloration	discoloration, white of upper limb	Berb.
Discoloration	discoloration, white spots on nails	Alum., ars., nit-ac., sep., **Sil.**, sulph.
Discoloration	discoloration, with red streaks on forearm	Anthr.
Discoloration	discoloration, with spots on forearm	Carb-o., mang., mill., nat-m.
Discoloration	discoloration, with white spots on forearm	Berb.
Discoloration	discoloration, with redness on wrist	Apis., cub.
Discoloration	discoloration, with spots on wrist	Dros., kali-c., merc., petr.
Discoloration	discoloration, yellow in spots of upper limb	Petr., vip.
Discoloration	discoloration, yellow of fingers	Ant-t., chel., con., elaps., ph-ac., sabad.
Discoloration	discoloration, yellow of fingers in spots	Ant-t., bism., con., elaps., sabad.
Discoloration	discoloration, yellow of nails	Am-c., ambr., aur., bell., bry., canth., carb-v., cham., chin., **Con.**, ferr., ign., lyc., merc., nit-ac., nux-v., op., plb., **Sep.**, **Sil.**, spig., sulph.
Discoloration	discoloration, yellow spots on shoulder	Ant-c.
Discoloration	discoloration, yellowish in spots	Vip.
Discoloration	discoloration, yellowish	Phos.
Discoloration	discolouration of cheeks	Cham.

Body part/Disease	Symptom	Medicines
Discoloration	discolouration of chin	Plat.
Discoloration	discolouration of external throat brown	Kali-s.
Discoloration	discolouration of external throat blue	Lach.
Discoloration	discolouration of external throat brown in spots	Kali-bi., sep.
Discoloration	discolouration of external throat purple	Tarent.
Discoloration	discolouration of external throat with redness	Am-caust., rhus-v.
Discoloration	discolouration of external throat with redness in spots	Bell., carb-v., iod., sep., stann., tarent.
Discoloration	discolouration of external throat yellow	Chel.
Discoloration	discolouration of external throat yellow in spots	Iod.
Discoloration	discolouration of face after anger	Con.
Discoloration	discolouration of face black	Camph., Chin., cor-r., crot-h., hydr-ac., lach., oena., op., stry., tarent.
Discoloration	discolouration of face blue during cough	Apis., bell., caust., coc-c., cor-r., Dros., Ip., mag-p., verat.
Discoloration	discolouration of face blue during headache	Cact., op.
Discoloration	discolouration of face blue in whooping cough	Ars., coc-c., cor-r., crot-h., dros., ip., nux-v.
Discoloration	discolouration of face blue in asthma	Stram., tab.
Discoloration	discolouration of face blue in cholera	Camph., Cupr., Verat.
Discoloration	discolouration of face blue in croup	Brom., carb-v.
Discoloration	discolouration of face blue in heart trouble	Apis., cact.
Discoloration	discolouration of face blue spots	Ail., apis., ars., aur., bapt., crot-h., ferr., hura., kali-br., kali-p., lach., led., mur-ac.
Discoloration	discolouration of face blue with convulsions	Cic., Cupr., hyos., ip., oena., phys., stry.
Discoloration	discolouration of face blue with dyspnœa (difficulty in breathing, often caused by heart or lung disease)	Bry., op., stram.
Discoloration	discolouration of face bronze	Ars-h.
Discoloration	discolouration of face brown when angry	Staph.
Discoloration	discolouration of face reddish	Bry., hyos., nit-ac., op., puls., samb., sep., stram., sulph.
Discoloration	discolouration of face, blue spots following eruptions	Ant-t., ferr., Lach., thuj.
Discoloration	discolouration of face, blue when angry	Staph.
Discoloration	discolouration of face, blue, during maniacal rage	Acon., ars., bell., con., hyos., lach., merc., op., puls., verat.
Discoloration	discolouration of face, changing colours	Acon., alum., ars., Bell., bor., bov., camph., caps., cham., chin., cina., croc., ferr., hyos., Ign., kali-c., laur., led., mag-c., mag-s., nux-v., olnd., op., ph-ac., Phos., Plat., puls., sec., spig., squil., sul-ac., verat., zinc.
Discoloration	discolouration of face, copper coloured	Alum., ars-h., ars., calc-p., calc., carb-an., cupr., kreos., led., rhus-t., ruta., stram., verat.
Discoloration	discolouration of face, copper coloured spots	Benz-ac., graph.
Discoloration	discolouration of face, dark coloured	Ail., apis., ars., Bapt., both., carb-s., carb-v., cupr., dub., elaps., gels., hura., hydr-ac., kali-i., lach., morph., Nit-ac., op., ox-ac., plb., sulph., verat.

Body part/Disease	Symptom	Medicines
Discoloration	discolouration of face, dirty looking	Apis., Arg-n., caps., card-m., chel., cupr., iod., kali-p., Lyc., mag-c., merc., phos., Psor., sanic., sec., Sulph., thuj.
Discoloration	discolouration of face, greenish	Ars., berb., Carb-v., Chel., crot-h., cupr., dig., ferr-ar., ferr., iod., kreos., med., merc-c., merc., nux-v., puls., verat.
Discoloration	discolouration of face, greenish spots	Ars.
Discoloration	discolouration of face, greenish spots about the eyes	Verat.
Discoloration	discolouration of face, mottled (patches or spots of different colors)	Ail., bapt., bell., cench., crot-h., dor., lach., rhus-t.
Discoloration	discolouration of face, pink spots	Ars., Carb-an., merc., nat-c.
Discoloration	discolouration of iris	Aur., coloc., euphr., kali-i., merc-i-f., nat-m., spig., syph.
Discoloration	discolouration of lips	Acet-ac., acon., agar., alum., alumn., am-c., amyg., Ant-t., apis., apoc., Arg-n., ars-i., ars., aur., bar-c., berb., cact., calc., Camph., caust., cedr., chin-s., chin., chlor., colch., con., crot-h., Cupr., cur., dig., dros., eup-pur., hep., Hydr-ac., iod., ip., kali-ar., kali-i., kreos., Lach., lachn., Lyc., merc-cy., merc., mosch., nat-m., Nux-v., op., phos., plan., prun-s., psor., samb., sec., stram., stry., verat., vip.
Discoloration	discolouration of pharynx	Acon., alumn., ant-t., Apis., ars., bell., bry., calc-p., calc-s., coc-c., cop., gent-c., iod., kali-n., merc-c., merc-i-f., merc., merl., nat-a., nat-m., ox-ac., phos., stram., sul-ac., ust., verat.
Discoloration	discolouration of throat, black	Merc-sul.
Discoloration	discolouration of throat, copper coloured	Kali-bi., Merc.
Discoloration	discolouration of throat, dark red	Acon., aesc., ail., Arg-n., Bapt., caps., Cham., crot-h., kali-bi., kali-i., kali-s., lach., merc-cy., merc-i-r., mez., naja., nat-a., phyt., puls., rhus-t.
Discoloration	discolouration of throat, purple	Ail., am-c., bapt., fl-ac., kali-bi., kali-chl., Lach., merc., nat-a., nit-ac., nux-v., ox-ac., puls., sulph., tarent.
Discoloration	discolouration of tonsils	Acon., apis., aur., bapt., Bell., cop., ferr-p., fl-ac., gymn., kali-bi., lach., merc-i-f., merc., phyt., puls., sulph.
Discoloration	discolouration of uvula	Acon., apis., Arg-n., ars., Bapt., Bar-m., Bell., calc-p., calc., caust., cimic., colch., crot-t., cupr., fl-ac., gent-c., kali-bi., kali-br., lach., merc-i-f., merc., nat-m., petr., sulph.
Discoloration	discolouration of uvula, dark red	Arg-n., Bapt., calc., caust., cupr-ac., lach.
Discoloration	discolouration of uvula, white spots	Mur-ac., nit-ac.
Discoloration	discolouration of uvula, yellow spots	Lac-c., lach., lyc., nit-ac.
Discoloration	discolouration, brown	Arg-n., ars-i., ars., bapt., bry., carb-ac., caust., con., crot-h., gels., hyos., iod., lyss., mag-m., nit-ac., op., puls., rhus-t., samb., sars., sep., staph., stram., sulph.
Discoloration	discolouration, cyanotic	Anan., Ars., aur., cact., cupr., hydr-ac., lyss., merc-cy., Nat-m., vesp.
Discoloration	discolouration, yellowish Face	Phos., vac.

Body part/Disease	Symptom	Medicines
Discoloration	discolouration, yellowish lip	Ant-t., ars-h., ars., bry., carb-v., chlor., hyos., olnd., op., phos., psor., squil., staph., sul-ac., verat.
Discoloration	discolouration, yellowish spots on lips	Caul., nat-c., sep.
Dislike	dislikes her own children	Glon., lyc., plat., verat.
Dislocation	dislocated feeling in ankle	Bry., calc-p., kali-bi., verat-v.
Dislocation	dislocated feeling in finger joints	Phos.
Dislocation	dislocated feeling in foot	Arum-t., bell.
Dislocation	dislocated feeling in hip	Agar., caust., ign., ip., laur., merc., mosch., pall., psor., **Puls.**, sulph., thuj.
Dislocation	dislocated feeling in hip from stepping	Caust., psor., sulph.
Dislocation	dislocated feeling in hip while sitting	Ip.
Dislocation	dislocated feeling in knee	Arg-m., arn., gels., ign., merc., pip-m., thuj.
Dislocation	dislocated feeling in left hip	Kreos., sulph.
Dislocation	dislocated feeling in lower limbs	Merc., sarr.
Dislocation	dislocated feeling in shoulder	Agar., ant-t., caust., ign., mag-c., mag-m., merc., sep., sulph.
Dislocation	dislocated feeling in thumb joints	Calc-p., cupr.
Dislocation	dislocated feeling in toes	Syph.
Dislocation	dislocated feeling in upper limbs	Ant-t., merc., rhus-t.
Dislocation	dislocated feeling in wrist on motion	Arn., bry., mez.
Dislocation	dislocation in last lower vertebra (a bone of spinal column)	Sanic.
Dislocation	dislocation of ankle	Bry., nat-c., nux-v., ruta., sulph.
Dislocation	dislocation of left ankle	Kali-bi.
Dislocation	dislocation of patella when going upstairs	Gels.
Dislocation	disposition to hawk (clear throat) during sleep	Calc-p.
Dislocation	disposition to hawk after sleep	Lach.
Dislocation	disposition to hawk from roughness	Alum.
Dislocation	disposition to hawk in open air	Carb-ac., nat-a.
Dislocation	disposition to hawk while talking	Calc-p.
Dislocation	disposition to masturbation after sexual excesses	Carb-v.
Dislocation	pain in first finger as of dislocation	Alum., ruta.
Dislocation	pain in shoulder as of dislocation	Ant-t., caps., cor-r., croc., fl-ac., ign., mag-c., mag-m., mez., myrt., nicc., olnd., **Rhus-t.**
Dislocation	pains from dislocation of hip	Carb-an., dros., kali-i., nit-ac.
Dislocation	pains from dislocation of hip on sitting down	Ip.
Dislocation	spontaneous (arising from internal cause) dislocation of hip	Bell., bry., calc., caust., coloc., lyc., puls., rhus-t., sulph., thuj., zinc.
Dissappointed love	ailments from disapointed love	Ant-c., aur., calc-p., caust., cimic., coff., hell., Hyos., Ign., kali-c., lach., Nat-m., nux-m., nux-v., Ph-ac., sep., staph., tarent.
Distension	distended as if uterus filled with wind	Ph-ac.

Body part/Disease	Symptom	Medicines
Distension	distension ameliorated by eructation (to expel stomach gases through the mouth)	Carb-v., sep., thuj.
Distension	distension of abdomen (to expand, swell, or inflate as if by pressure from within) after beer	Nat-m.
Distension	distension of abdomen after breakfast	Agar., chin-a., nat-m.
Distension	distension of abdomen after dinner	Alum., anac., calc., carb-an., Carb-v., euphr., grat., lyc., mag-c., mag-m., nat-m., nicc., nux-m., phos., sep., sulph., thuj., til.
Distension	distension of abdomen after drinking	Ambr., ars., carb-v., Chin., hep., nux-v., petr.
Distension	distension of abdomen after menses	Cham., kreos., lil-t., rat.
Distension	distension of abdomen after milk	Con.
Distension	distension of abdomen ameliorated by passing flatus	All-c., am-m., ant-t., bov., bry., carb-v., kali-i., Lyc., mag-c., mang., nat-c., nat-m., ph-ac., sulph.
Distension	distension of abdomen ameliorated by passing flatus (Intestinal gas, composed partly of swallowed air and partly of gas produced by bacterial fermentation of intestinal contents. It consists mainly of hydrogen, carbon dioxide, and methane in varying proportionsGas produced in the digestive system usually expelled from the body through the anus)	All-c., am-m., ant-t., bov., bry., carb-v., kali-i., Lyc., mag-c., mang., nat-c., nat-m., ph-ac., sulph.
Distension	distension of abdomen ameliorated from stool	Alum., am-m., asaf., calc-p., corn., hyper., nat-m.
Distension	distension of abdomen before dinner	All-c.
Distension	distension of abdomen before menses	Am-m., arn., berb., carb-an., carb-v., chin., cycl., hep., kreos., lach., lyc., mang., puls., zinc.
Distension	distension of abdomen before urination	Chin-s.
Distension	distension of abdomen before urination	Chin-s.
Distension	distension of abdomen during constipation	Bry., ery-a., graph., hyos., iod., lach., mag-m., nit-ac., phos., ter.
Distension	distension of abdomen during menses	Aloe., alum., berb., brom., carb-an., chin., Cocc., coff., croc., cycl., graph., ham., hep., ign., kali-c., kali-p., kreos., lac-c., lachn., lyc., mag-c., nat-c., nicc., nit-ac., nux-v., rat., Sulph., zinc.
Distension	distension of abdomen fasting while	Dulc.
Distension	distension of abdomen in children	Bar-c., Calc., Caust., cina., cupr., sil., staph., Sulph.
Distension	distension of abdomen in morning	Aloe., ars., asaf., cham., chin-a., chin., grat., nat-s., nit-ac., nux-v., ol-an., rhod., sulph.
Distension	distension of abdomen, after milk	Con.
Distension	distension of abdomen, after rising	Coc-c.
Distension	distension of abdomen, ameliorated by lying on abdomen	Con.
Distension	distension of abdomen, ameliorated from motion	Cedr.
Distension	distension of abdomen, ameliorated from stool	Corn.
Distension	distension of abdomen, ameliorated from walking	Calad., cedr.
Distension	distension of abdomen, before menses	Zinc.
Distension	distension of abdomen, from oysters	Bry., lyc.

Body part/Disease	Symptom	Medicines
Distension	distension of abdomen, painful	Acon., alum., ant-t., Ars., bar-c., bell., Bry., calad., canth., Caust., cham., hell., hyos., kali-i., Lach., merc-c., Merc., nat-c., nat-m., nux-v., Rhus-t., sulph., verat.
Distension	distension of abdomen, painful before stool	Ars., corn., fl-ac., phyt.
Distension	distension of blood vessels	Acon., agar., alum., am-c., arn., ars., bar-c., bar-m., **Bell.**, bry., calc-f., calc., camph., carb-s., carb-v., chel., chin-a., chin-s., **Chin.**, cic., coloc., con., croc., cycl., dig., ferr-ar., ferr-p., **Ferr.**, graph., ham., **Hyos.**, lach., led., lyc., meny., merl., mosch., nat-m., nux-v., olnd., op., ph-ac., phos., plb., podo., **Puls.**, rhod., rhus-t., sars., sec., sep., sil., spig., spong., staph., stront., sulph., **Thuj.**, vip., zinc.
Distension	distension of blood vessels during fever	Agar., bell., camph., chin-s., **Chin.**, **Hyos.**, **Led.**, **Puls.**
Distension	distension of blood vessels in evening	**Puls.**
Distension	distesion of abdomen, after contradiction	Nux-m.
Distension	distesion of abdomen, after dinner	Ant-c., dig., kalm., zinc.
Distension	distesion of abdomen, after drinking	Manc., tab.
Distension	distesion of abdomen, after pickled fish	Calad.
Distension	distesion of abdomen, ameliorated after eating	Cedr., rat.
Distension	distesion of abdomen, ameliorated after eructations	Arg-n., Carb-v., mag-c., nat-s.
Distension	distesion of abdomen, ameliorated after passing flatus	Rat.
Distension	distesion of abdomen, before dinner	Rat.
Distension	distesion of abdomen, during convulsion	Cic.
Distension	distesion of abdomen, in night, on waking	Asaf.
Distension	distesion of abdomen, in afternoon	Nat-m., petr., sulph.
Distension	distesion of abdomen, in evening	Dios., eupi., kali-bi., osm.
Distension	distesion of abdomen, in forenoon	Myric.
Distension	distesion of abdomen, in morning	Nux-v., phos.
Distension	distesion of abdomen, not ameliorated after eructations	Chin., echi., lyc.
Distension	distesion of abdomen, while eating	Con.
Distension	distesion, during chill	Cocc.
Distension	paralysis of bladder after over distension	Ars., canth., Caust., hell., hyos., nux-v., rhus-t., ruta., stry., sulph.
Distension	sensation of distension of oesophagus	Hyper., op., verat.
Dreads	dread of bathing	**Am-c.**, am-m., **Ant-c.**, bar-c., bar-m., bell., bor., bov., bry., calc., canth., carb-v., cham., **Clem.**, con., dulc., kali-c., kali-n., laur., lyc., mag-c., merc., mez., mur-ac., nat-c., nat-p., nit-ac., nux-m., nux-v., phos., **Psor.**, puls., **Rhus-t.**, sars., **Sep.**, sil., **Spig.**, stann., staph., stront., sul-ac., **Sulph.**, zinc.
Dreads	dreads being alone	Bufo., clem., con., elaps., kali-br., lyc., nat-c., sep.
Dream	after awaking falls to sleep again and continues same dream	Calad., nat-c.

Body part/Disease	Symptom	Medicines
Dream	breathing difficult after frightful dreams	Chel.
Dream	breathing difficult during dreams	Sang.
Dream	disturbed sleep by dreams	Acon., agar., ambr., arn., ars., atro., bell., benz-ac., bry., cact., calc-p., carb-s., carl., cham., cimic., coc-c., coloc., crot-t., cupr., cycl., dig., dulc., euphr., ferr-i., ferr., gamb., glon., graph., hell., ign., laur., lyc., lyss., mag-c., mag-s., merc., mur-ac., nat-m., nit-ac., nux-v., op., paeon., par., plb., psor., ptel., rhod., sin-n., sol-n., spig., spong., sulph., tab., valer.
Dream	dreams about children	Am-m., hura., kali-n., mag-c., merc.
Dream	dreams about disputes	Chin.
Dream	dreams about monsters	Aloe., hydr.
Dream	dreams absurd (meaningless)	Apis., chin., cina., coloc., ferr-m., glon., mygal., pip-m., rumx., sulph., thuj.
Dream	dreams accidents	Am-m., ant-c., arn., **Ars.**, bell., cham., chin., cinnb., con., **Graph.**, Ind., iod., iodof., jab., kali-c., kreos., lyc., nat-s., nux-v., puls., rumx., sars., sul-ac., sulph., thuj.
Dream	dreams amorous (feeling romantic love or sexual attraction) before menses	Calc., kali-c.
Dream	dreams amorous in morning	Aloe., colch., grat., lil-t., plb., sabin., sil., sumb.
Dream	dreams animals which bites	Daph., merc., phos., puls.
Dream	dreams animals	Aloe., am-c., am-m., **Arn.**, bell., bov., cham., daph., gran., hura., hydr., hyos., lyc., merc., nux-v., phos., phys., puls., ran-s., sil., sul-ac., sulph., tarent.
Dream	dreams another person lying with him in bed	Petr.
Dream	dreams before menses	Alum., calc., canth., caust., con., kali-c., sul-ac.
Dream	dreams being buried alive	Arn., chel., ign.
Dream	dreams black animals	Puls.
Dream	dreams burials (disposal of body)	Alum., hura.
Dream	dreams chased by bulls	Ind., tarent.
Dream	dreams continued after waking	All-s., arg-m., calc., chin., ign., lyc., nat-c., nat-m., psor., zinc.
Dream	dreams during menses	Alum., calc., cast., caust., con., kali-c., mag-c., nat-c., nat-m., thuj.
Dream	dreams during menses	Nat-m.
Dream	dreams he had a fit	Iris., mag-c., sil.
Dream	dreams he has committed crime	Cocc., nat-s., petr.
Dream	dreams he has committed rape	Petr.
Dream	dreams he is to die	Nit-ac., sil.
Dream	dreams he was a lion	Phys.
Dream	dreams he was blind	Phys.
Dream	dreams he was lost in a forest	Am-m., Ind., mag-c., mag-m., mag-s., sep.
Dream	dreams he was struck by lightning	Arn.
Dream	dreams he was strung by an insect	Phos.
Dream	dreams he was wrongfully accused	Clem.
Dream	dreams he would be crushed	Sulph.

Body part/Disease	Symptom	Medicines
Dream	dreams her mother had been drowned	Nicc.
Dream	dreams of a large dog following him	Sil.
Dream	dreams of a mad dog following him	Abrot., rumx.
Dream	dreams of battles	All-c., bell., bry., ferr., guai., plat., ran-s., sil., stann., thuj., verb.
Dream	dreams of beasts	Puls.
Dream	dreams of becoming emaciated	Kreos.
Dream	dreams of being accused of theft	Lach.
Dream	dreams of being at a banquet	Mag-s., ph-ac.
Dream	dreams of being bitten by dog	Calc., lyss., merc., sulph., verat.
Dream	dreams of being bitten by snakes	Bov.
Dream	dreams of being chased and had run backwards	Sep.
Dream	dreams of being cut with a knife	Guai.
Dream	dreams of being hung	Am-m.
Dream	dreams of being in underground room and walls falling	Bov.
Dream	dreams of being murdered	Am-m., chel., guai., ign., kali-i., lach., lact., lyc., merc., sil., zinc.
Dream	dreams of being poisoned	Kreos., nat-m., oci.
Dream	dreams of being stabbed	Chin., guai., nat-c., op.
Dream	dreams of being thirsty	Dros., mag-c., **Nat-m.**
Dream	dreams of being tightly encircled	Ruta.
Dream	dreams of being very tall	Ferr-i.
Dream	dreams of being wounded	Ant-c.
Dream	dreams of black cat	Daph.
Dream	dreams of black dog	Arn.
Dream	dreams of business	Anac., apis., asaf., bell., bry., bufo., calc., camph., canth., carb-v., carl., chel., cic., croc., cur., elaps., gels., hep., hura., kali-c., lach., lyc., merc., **Nux-v.**, phos., psor., puls., pyrog., **Rhus-t.**, sang., sars., sil., staph., tarent.
Dream	dreams of cats	Arn., ars., calc-p., daph., graph., hyos., lac-c., mez., nux-v., puls.
Dream	dreams of child had been beaten	Kali-n.
Dream	dreams of churches	Asc-t., coc-c., lyss., zing.
Dream	dreams of clairvoyant (psychic person)	Acon., ph-ac., phos., sulph.
Dream	dreams of coffins (long oblong container, usually made of wood, in which a dead body is placed for burial or cremation)	Brom., merc-i-f.
Dream	dreams of creeping worms	Am-c., mur-ac., nux-v., phos.
Dream	dreams of crimes	Hura., nat-ac., nat-m., nat-s., nit-ac., rumx.
Dream	dreams of cruelty	Nat-m., nux-v., sel., sil., stann.
Dream	dreams of dancing	Gamb., mag-c., mag-m., mag-s., zing.
Dream	dreams of death approaching	Kali-c., kali-chl., sil., sulph., tab.
Dream	dreams of desecting bodies	Iris., sang.

Body part/Disease	Symptom	Medicines
Dream	dreams of devils	Apis., arg-m., kali-c., lac-c., nat-c., nicc., sin-n.
Dream	dreams of difficulties	**Am-m.,** anac., ant-t., **Ars.,** cann-s., caps., croc., graph., mag-c., mag-m., mur-ac., phos., plat., rhus-t.
Dream	dreams of disappointments	Cann-s., ign., rumx., ust.
Dream	dreams of disaster	Sars.
Dream	dreams of dragons	Op.
Dream	dreams of driving of mule	Chin-b.
Dream	dreams of drowning	Alum., bov., ign., kali-c., lyc., merc-i-f., merc., nicc., ran-b., rumx., samb., sil., verat., zinc.
Dream	dreams of drowning in a sinking boat	Alum., lyc.
Dream	dreams of drowning man	Sol-t-ae.
Dream	dreams of dying	Am-c., arn., brom., camph., chel., dulc., fl-ac., sulph., thuj.
Dream	dreams of ears cut off	Nat-c.
Dream	dreams of earth quake	Rat., sil.
Dream	dreams of eating	Iod.
Dream	dreams of eating human flesh	Sol-t-ae.
Dream	dreams of enemies	Arg-m., con., ptel.
Dream	dreams of events not yet taken place	Mang., sulph.
Dream	dreams of explosion	Stann.
Dream	dreams of face covered with pustules	Anac.
Dream	dreams of falling from high places	Acon., alum., am-m., anan., aur., chin., dig., guai., hep., kali-c., kreos., merc., mez., nat-s., nicc., nux-m., op., phos., sep., sol-t-ae., sulph., sumb., **Thuj.,** zinc.
Dream	dreams of falling from high places into water	Am-m., dig., eupi., ferr., ign., iod., mag-m., mag-s., merc., nicc.
Dream	dreams of falling into water	Am-m., dig., eupi., ferr., ign., iod., mag-m., mag-s., merc., nicc.
Dream	dreams of farming	Mag-s., merc-i-r.
Dream	dreams of fighting with robbers	Ferr-i., mag-c., nat-c., sil.
Dream	dreams of fire	Alum., **Anac.,** ant-t., ars., bar-c., bell., calc-p., calc., carb-ac., carb-v., chin., clem., croc., cur., daph., euphr., fl-ac., graph., **Hep.,** iris., kali-ar., kali-c., kali-n., kreos., **Laur., Mag-c., Mag-m.,** mag-s., meph., merc-c., merc., naja., nat-c., nat-m., nat-p., nat-s., osm., phos., plat., rhod., rhus-t., sil., spig., spong., stann., stront., sul-ac., sulph., zinc., zing.
Dream	dreams of fishes swimming in water	Chin.
Dream	dreams of fishing	Arg-m., chin-b., mag-c., verat-v.
Dream	dreams of friend	Coff., con., fl-ac., kali-n., nicc.
Dream	dreams of friends long deceased	Arg-n., ferr., nat-c.
Dream	dreams of gold	Cycl., puls.
Dream	dreams of having committed theft	Alum., plb.
Dream	dreams of household affairs	Bell., bry.
Dream	dreams of humiliation	Alum., am-c., arn., asar., con., ign., led., mag-m., mosch., mur-ac., sil., staph.

Body part/Disease	Symptom	Medicines
Dream	dreams of hunting	Hura., hyper., merc-i-r., verat.
Dream	dreams of injuries	Am-m., ant-c., chin., nat-s., phos., sumb.
Dream	dreams of insects	Arg-n.
Dream	dreams of insults	Asar., nat-s., tarent.
Dream	dreams of journey	Am-c., am-m., anan., apis., brom., bufo., calc-f., calc-p., carb-ac., chel., chin., crot-h., elaps., hura., hydr., hyper., Ind., indg., **Kali-n.**, lac-c., lac-d., lach., mag-c., mag-m., mag-s., merc-i-r., merc., mez., nat-c., nat-m., op., psor., rhus-t., sang., sel., sil., ther.
Dream	dreams of journey by railroad	Apis.
Dream	dreams of journey on horse back	Nat-c., ther.
Dream	dreams of jumping	Verat.
Dream	dreams of jumping from window	Mag-m.
Dream	dreams of killing a mad dog	Rumx.
Dream	dreams of knives	Guai., lach., nat-c.
Dream	dreams of large meal (feast)	Anan., ant-c., asaf., hura., mag-s., nit-ac., ph-ac., tril., zinc.
Dream	dreams of laughing	Caust., coca., croc., kreos.
Dream	dreams of lice	Am-c., chel., gamb., mur-ac., nux-v., phos.
Dream	dreams of lightning	Arn., euphr., phel., spig.
Dream	dreams of living in tombs	Nicc.
Dream	dreams of long past	Am-c., calad., ferr-i., ferr., senec., **Sil.**, spig.
Dream	dreams of men	Nicc., puls.
Dream	dreams of men jumping into water	Mag-s.
Dream	dreams of mice	Colch., mag-s., sep.
Dream	dreams of misfortune	Alum., am-m., anac., ant-c., arn., ars., bar-c., bar-m., bell., cann-s., carb-an., cham., chin-a., chin., clem., cocc., croc., **Graph.**, guai., ign., kali-ar., kali-c., kali-n., kali-p., kali-s., laur., led., **Lyc.**, mag-c., mang., merc., mur-ac., **Nux-v.**, op., ph-ac., phos., **Puls.**, ran-b., rhus-t., sars., sel., spong., stann., staph., sul-ac., sulph., tarent., **Thuj.**, verat., verb., zinc.
Dream	dreams of money	Alum., cycl., mag-c., mag-m., phos., puls.
Dream	dreams of murder	Am-m., arn., bell., calad., calc., carb-an., cast., chel., guai., hura., ign., kali-i., kalm., kreos., lach., lact., led., lyc., mag-m., merc-c., merc., naja., nat-a., nat-c., nat-m., nicc., ol-an., petr., puls., rhus-t., rumx., sanic., sil., spong., staph., sulph., thuj., zinc.
Dream	dreams of music	Sarr.
Dream	dreams of naked men	Eupi., puls.
Dream	dreams of nausea	Arg-m.
Dream	dreams of nightmare	Acon., aloe., alum., alumn., am-c., am-m., ambr., ant-t., ars-i., ars., arum-t., bapt., bell., bor., bry., bufo., cadm., calc., camph., cann-i., canth., cham., chel., cina., cinnb., con., cycl., daph., dig., elaps., ferr-i., ferr-p., ferr., gels., guai., hep., ign., Ind., iod., iris., kali-ar., kali-bi., kali-c., kali-i., kali-n., led., lyc., mag-m., meph., merc., mez., nat-a., nat-c., nat-m., nat-p., nit-ac., nux-v., op., **Paeon.**, phos., plb., ptel., puls., rhus-t., ruta., sil., **Sulph.**, tab., tell., ter., thuj., valer., zinc.

Body part/Disease	Symptom	Medicines
Dream	dreams of nightmare (evil spirit) lying on back	Card-m., guai., **Sulph.**
Dream	dreams of people	Bell., calc-ar., merc.
Dream	dreams of people bathing in water	Chin-b.
Dream	dreams of persued for the purpose of rape	Kreos.
Dream	dreams of pins	Merc.
Dream	dreams of poison that he has taken	Kreos.
Dream	dreams of praying	Ars-h.
Dream	dreams of preaching	Anac., ant-t.
Dream	dreams of previous day events	Acon., arg-n., **Bry.**, calc-f., chel., cic., cur., ferr., fl-ac., graph., kali-c., kali-chl., lach., lyc., mag-c., merc., nux-v., puls., rhus-t., sars., sep., sil., stann.
Dream	dreams of previous events	Acon., aeth., am-c., anac., ant-t., arg-m., asaf., aster., bov., bry., calad., calc-p., carb-s., chel., chin., cic., coca., cocc., croc., crot-t., elaps., eupho., ferr-i., fl-ac., graph., Ind., jatr., kali-c., kali-chl., lach., nat-c., nat-p., nit-ac., nux-v., osm., ph-ac., phos., plan., rhus-t., sang., sars., sel., senec., sep., **Sil.**, sol-t-ae., spig., sulph., sumb., thuj.
Dream	dreams of quarrels	Alum., am-c., anan., ant-c., apis., arn., aur., bapt., bar-c., bell., brom., bry., calc., canth., carl., cast., caust., cham., con., crot-h., guai., guare., hep., kali-n., mag-c., mag-s., mosch., nat-c., nat-m., nat-s., nicc., **Nux-v.,** op., paeon., ph-ac., phos., plat., puls., sabin., sel., sep., sil., spig., stann., staph., tarax., verat., zinc.
Dream	dreams of rats	Sep.
Dream	dreams of relatives	Ferr., fl-ac., mag-c., mag-s., rheum., sars.
Dream	dreams of riots	Bry., con., guai., indg., kali-c., lyc., nat-c., nat-m., phos., puls., stann.
Dream	dreams of roaming over fields	**Rhus-t.**
Dream	dreams of robbers	**Alum.**, arn., aur., bell., calc-p., carb-v., cast., ferr-i., jac-c., kali-c., **Mag-c.**, mag-m., mag-s., merc., nat-c., **Nat-m.**, petr., phel., phos., psor., ptel., sanic., sil., sin-n., verat., zinc.
Dream	dreams of sailing in water	Chin., hura., nat-s., sang., senec., verat-v.
Dream	dreams of seeing a rape	Cench.
Dream	dreams of seeing a soldier shot	Am-m.
Dream	dreams of seeing murdered men	Rumx.
Dream	dreams of seeing persons hung	Merc-sul.
Dream	dreams of skelletons	Op.
Dream	dreams of smoking	Tell.
Dream	dreams of snakes	Alum., arg-n., bov., grat., iris., kali-c., lac-c., ptel., ran-s., rat., sep., sil., sol-n., spig., tab.
Dream	dreams of snow	Art-v., bapt., kreos.
Dream	dreams of snow storm	Kreos.
Dream	dreams of soldier	Chel.
Dream	dreams of spider	Cinnb., crot-c.
Dream	dreams of spider as large as an ox	Cinnb.
Dream	dreams of spiders	Cinnb., crot-c.
Dream	dreams of stars falling	Alum.

Body part/Disease	Symptom	Medicines
Dream	dreams of stealing fruit	Plb.
Dream	dreams of stone lying on him	Kali-c.
Dream	dreams of stool	Aloe., cast-v., psor., sars., zinc.
Dream	dreams of storms	All-s., ars., jac-c., mag-c., sil.
Dream	dreams of storms at sea	All-c., sil.
Dream	dreams of stream of water	Com.
Dream	dreams of suffocation	Arn., iris., kali-bi.
Dream	dreams of suicide	Naja.
Dream	dreams of swimming in water	Bell., hura., iod., lyc., merc-i-r., ran-b., rhus-t., sol-t-ae.
Dream	dreams of teeth breaking off	Kali-n., ther., thuj.
Dream	dreams of teeth falling out	Cocc., nicc., nux-v., tab.
Dream	dreams of teeth pulled out	Nat-m.
Dream	dreams of the evening	Ph-ac.
Dream	dreams of threats	Ars., sep.
Dream	dreams of threats of rape	Sep.
Dream	dreams of thunder storm	Arn., ars., euphr., nat-c.
Dream	dreams of tombs	Anac.
Dream	dreams of urinating	Ambr., kreos., lac-c., lyc., merc-i-f., seneg., sep., sulph.
Dream	dreams of violence	Led.
Dream	dreams of vomiting of worms	Chin.
Dream	dreams of vomiting of worms	Chin.
Dream	dreams of walking	Med., rhus-t.
Dream	dreams of walking in mud	Iod.
Dream	dreams of walking in water	Merc-i-r.
Dream	dreams of walking in water in which are serpants	Alum.
Dream	dreams of warts	Mez.
Dream	dreams of water	All-c., all-s., alum., **Am-m.**, arg-n., ars., bell., bov., carb-v., chin., com., dig., eupi., ferr., graph., hura., ign., iod., kali-c., kali-n., kalm., lyc., mag-c., mag-m., mag-s., meph., merc-i-r., merc., murx., nat-c., nat-m., nat-s., nicc., ox-ac., ran-b., rhus-t., sang., sil., sol-t-ae., sulph., tarent., valer., verat-v., verat., zinc.
Dream	dreams of wedding	Alum., chel., mag-c., mag-s., nat-c., nat-s.
Dream	dreams of weeping	Ang., elaps., glon., kali-c., kreos., mag-c., sil., spong.
Dream	dreams of working in snow	Bapt.
Dream	dreams of world on fire	Rhus-t.
Dream	dreams of writing	Senec.
Dream	dreams of yellow mice	Mag-s.
Dream	dreams only of a forest	Canth., mag-m., sep.
Dream	dreams only of fighting with ghosts	Sars., sep.
Dream	dreams only of fleeing	Zinc.
Dream	dreams only of floating	Hell.
Dream	dreams only of flowers	Mag-c., nat-s.
Dream	dreams only of flying	Apis., atro., indg., lyc., nat-s., xan.

Body part/Disease	Symptom	Medicines
Dream	dreams only of fruit	Cast-eq.
Dream	dreams only of funerals	Bart., brom., chel., form., mag-c., nicc., rat.
Dream	dreams only of ghosts	Aesc., alum., am-c., arg-n., asc-t., atro., bell., bov., camph., carb-s., carb-v., cham., crot-c., eupi., graph., ign., kali-c., kali-s., mag-c., manc., med., nat-c., nat-m., op., paeon., puls., sars., sep., sil., spig., sulph.
Dream	dreams only of giants	Bell., lyc.
Dream	dreams only of graves	Anac., arn., hura., iris., mag-c., ptel.
Dream	dreams only of high places	All-c., anac., brom., chin., laur., lyss.
Dream	dreams only of horses	Alum., am-m., asc-t., atro., crot-c., indg., mag-s., merc., phos., tarent., ther., zinc.
Dream	dreams only of horses changing into dogs	Zinc.
Dream	dreams only of horses riding	Nat-c., ther.
Dream	dreams only of horses running	Atro., indg.
Dream	dreams only of old friends	Ferr., rumx.
Dream	dreams only of stealing a horse	Rumx.
Dream	dreams smell of bodis	Calc.
Dream	dreams someone called	Ant-c., merc., sep.
Dream	dreams while awake	Acon., arn., bry., cham., chin., graph., hep., ign., merc., nux-v., op., petr., phos., rheum., sep., sil., stram., sulph.
Dream	dreams wild animals	Nux-v., sulph.
Dream	waking at midnight after dream	Fl-ac., zinc.
Dream	waking from dreams	Agar., arn., atro., aur., bad., bar-c., bell., bry., cham., coca., colch., coloc., gran., graph., hep., hyper., lyc., lyss., mag-s., merc., nat-m., nux-v., ph-ac., phos., plan., puls., sars., sil., stann., staph., **Sulph.**
Dream	weakness after a dream	Calc-s.
Dream	weakness on waking from a dream	Op., teucr.
Dropsy	dropsical hard swelling of penis	Arn., merc., nux-v., ph-ac., sabin., spong.
Dropsy	dropsical skin	Acon., **Ant-c.**, ars-i., **Ars.**, aur., bell., **Bry.**, canth., chel., chin-a., **Chin.**, colch., coloc., con., dig., dulc., eup-per., eupho., ferr-ar., ferr., guai., **Hell.**, hyos., iod., kali-ar., kali-c., kali-n., kali-s., lach., led., lyc., merc., mez., mur-ac., nat-c., nat-m., nat-p., nat-s., nit-ac., nux-m., olnd., op., phos., plb., **Puls.**, rhod., rhus-t., ruta., sabin., samb., sars., sec., seneg., sep., sil., **Squil.**, stram., **Sulph.**, **Tell.**, verat.
Dropsy	dropsical swelling of knee	Ant-t., apis., bry., calc., con., dig., fl-ac., hyper., iod., merc., **Rhus-t.**, sil., **Sulph.**
Dropsy	dropsy (a buildup of excess serous fluid between tissue cells) due to ascites (an accumulation of fluid serous fluid in the peritoneal cavity, causing abdominal swelling) with chronic diarrhoea	Apoc., oena.
Dropsy	Dropsy (watery state of the tissue of the body)	Arg.Phos
Dropsy	dropsy due to ascites (accumulation of fluid serous fluid in the peritoneal cavity, causing abdominal swelling) with induration (hardness in body tissue) of liver	Aur., lact.
Dropsy	dropsy external in morning	Chin., nat-c.

Body part/Disease	Symptom	Medicines
Dropsy	dropsy external	Acet-ac., agar., **Ant-c.**, *ant-t.*, **Apis.**, *apoc.*, ars-i., **Ars.**, *asc-c.*, *aur-m.*, aur., *bell.*, *bism.*, *bry.*, *cact.*, calad., *calc-ar.*, *calc.*, camph., *canth.*, *carb-s.*, *card-m.*, cedr., chel., *chin-a.*, **Chin.**, cinnb., coca., **Colch.**, *coll.*, coloc., *con.*, conv., cop., *crot-h.*, **Dig.**, *dulc.*, eup-pur., eupho., ferr-ar., *ferr-i.*, ferr-p., *ferr.*, **Graph.**, guai., **Hell.**, hyos., **Iod.**, kali-ar., *kali-c.*, *kali-i.*, kali-n., kali-p., kali-s., *lac-d.*, *lach.*, *led.*, *lyc.*, **Med.**, *merc.*, mez., mur-ac., nat-a., nat-c., *nit-ac.*, *nux-m.*, **Olnd.**, **Op.**, phos., pic-ac., plat., *plb.*, *puls.*, rhod., rhus-t., *ruta.*, *sabin.*, *samb.*, sars., sec., *seneg.*, *sep.*, sil., **Squil.**, stram., *sulph.*, **Ter.**, *teucr.*, *verat.*, *verb.*, zinc.
Dropsy	dropsy internal	Agn., am-c., ambr., ant-c., ant-t., **Apis.**, apoc., arg-m., arn., ars-i., **Ars.**, aur-m., aur., **Bell.**, bry., calc., camph., cann-s., canth., caps., carb-v., **Card-m.**, chin-a., **Chin.**, cina., **Colch.**, coloc., con., **Dig.**, dulc., eupho., ferr-ar., ferr-p., ferr., guai., **Hell.**, hep., hyos., iod., ip., kali-ar., kali-c., kali-p., kali-s., lach., lact., laur., led., lyc., merc., mez., mur-ac., nit-ac., ph-ac., phos., puls., rhus-t., sabad., samb., sars., seneg., sep., sil., spig., spong., squil., stann., stram., **Sulph.**, **Ter.**, teucr., verat., viol-t.
Dropsy	dropsy of chest can lie only on affected side	Ars.
Dropsy	dropsy of chest can lie only on right side with head low	Spig.
Dropsy	dropsy of chest with asthma	Psor.
Dropsy	dropsy of ovaries	Apis., arn., Ars., aur-m-n., bell., bry., Calc., carb-an., chin., coloc., con., ferr-i., graph., iod., kali-br., kali-c., kreos., lach., lil-t., Lyc., med., merc., nat-s., phos., plat., plb., podo., prun-s., rhod., rhus-t., sabin., ter., zinc.
Dropsy	dropsy of Pericardium (sac enclosing heart)	Apis., apoc., Ars., Colch., Dig., lach., Lyc., sulph., zinc.
Dropsy	dropsy of uterus	Aesc., apis., ars., bell., brom., bry., calc., camph., canth., chin., colch., con., dig., dulc., ferr., ham., Hell., iod., kali-c., lach., lact., led., lob., Lyc., merc., phos., puls., rhus-t., ruta., sabad., sep., sulph.
Drunkard	asthmatic in drunkards	Meph.
Drunkard	becoming heated in old drunkards	Bar-c.
Drunkard	convulsion in drunkards	Glon., nux-v., ran-b.
Drunkard	cough of drunkards	Ars., coc-c., lach., stram.
Drunkard	diarrhoea in old drunkards	Ant-t., apis., ars., chin., Lach., nux-v., phos.
Drunkard	eruption, pimples in drunkard	Kreos., lach., led.
Drunkard	haemorrhage from chest in drunkards	Ars., hyos., Nux-v., op.
Drunkard	heartburn in drunkards	Nux-v., sul-ac.
Drunkard	hiccough in drunkards	Ran-b.
Drunkard	inflammation of lungs in drunkards	Hyos., kali-br., nux-v., op.
Drunkard	nausea in drunkards	Ars., asar., Kali-bi., nux-v., sul-ac.
Drunkard	oedema (a buildup of excess serous fluid between tissue cells) affecting the lungs in drunkards	Crot-h.
Drunkard	pain in abdomen in drunkards	Calc., carb-v., lach., nux-v., sul-ac., sulph.
Drunkard	retching in drunkards	Ars., nux-v., op.

Body part/Disease	Symptom	Medicines
Drunkard	skin, crawling in drunkards	Carb-v., lach., nux-v., sulph.
Drunkard	trembling in drunkards	**Ars.**, bar-c., nux-v.
Drunkard	urine albuminous indication of kidney from abuse of alcohol	Ars., aur., bell., berb., calc-ar., Carb-v., chin., crot-t., cupr., ferr., lach., led., merc., nat-c., nux-v., sulph.
Drunkard	vision, dimness in drunkards	Nux-v.
Drunkard	vomiting blood in drunkards	Alumn., ars.
Drunkard	vomiting of drunkards	Alumn., Ars., cadm., calc., caps., carb-ac., crot-h., Kali-bi., kali-br., lach., nux-v., op., sang., sul-ac., sulph., zing.
Drunkard	Vomitting of Drunkards	Apomorphia
Dwarfishness	dwarfishness	**Bar-c.**, bar-m., **Calc-p.**, calc., carb-s., iod., lyc., med., merc., ol-j., sec., sil., **Sulph.**, zinc.
Dysentry	appetite, increased in dysentry	Nux-v.
Dysentry	Body aches during dysentery (a disease of the lower intestine caused by infection with bacteria, protozoans or parasites and marked by severe diarrhea, inflammation, and the passage of blood and mucus)	Arn.
Dysentry	eruptions herpetic alternating with chest affections and dysenteric stools	Rhus-t.
Dysentry	eruptions on skin alternating with dysentry	Rhus-t.
Dysentry	pain in sacral region with dysentry	Caps., nux-v.
Dysentry	retention of urine from dysentry	Ars., merc.
Dysmenorrhoea	dysuria during dysmenorrhoea (severe pain associated with menstruation)	Senec.
Dysmenorrhoea	perspiration in hand in dysmenorrhoea (severe pain associated with menstruation)	Tarent.
Dyspnoea	discolouration of face blue with dyspnœa	Bry., op., stram.
Dyspnoea	pain in back with dyspnoea	Lyc.
Dyspnoea	perspiration with dyspnoea	Anac., ant-t., apis., **Ars.**, arund., **Carb-v.**, lach., lyc., mang., sil., sulph., thuj., verat.
Dyspnoea	profuse perspiration with dyspnoea	Mang.
Dyspnoea	retching from dyspnoea	Am-c.
Dyspnoea	rheumatic pain in extremities alternating with dyspnoea	Guai.
Dyspnoea	swelling in ankle with dyspnoea	Hep.
Dysuria	dysuria (difficult or painful urination. This is usually associated with urgency and frequency of urination if due to cystitis or urethritis. The pain is burning in nature and is relieved by curing the underlying cause. A high fluid intake usually helps) with aching in back	Vesp.
Dysuria	dysuria alternating with bed wetting	Gels.
Dysuria	dysuria child cries at the close of urination	Sars.
Dysuria	dysuria during chill	Canth., cham., lyc., merc., nux-v., ph-ac., puls., sulph., thuj.
Dysuria	dysuria during dysmenorrhoea (severe pain associated with menstruation)	Senec.
Dysuria	dysuria during fever	Ant-c., cann-s., canth., cham., colch., dulc., nit-ac., nux-v., staph., sulph.

Body part/Disease	Symptom	Medicines
Dysuria	dysuria in newly married women	Cann-s., ery-a., Staph.
Dysuria	dysuria painful during perspiration	Canth., Cham., hep., lyc., merc., nit-ac., puls., sulph., thuj.
Dysuria	dysuria painful, after dinner and supper	Nux-m.
Dysuria	dysuria painful, aggravated after urination	Equis.
Dysuria	dysuria painful, aggravated from effort to urinate	Plb.
Dysuria	dysuria painful, aggravated from thinking of it	Hell., nux-v.
Dysuria	dysuria painful, child cries at close of urination	Sars.
Dysuria	dysuria painful, child cries before urine starts	Bor., lach., lyc., nux-v., Sars.
Dysuria	dysuria painful, from long retention of urine	Calc-p., caust., rhus-t., ruta., sulph.
Dysuria	dysuria painful, from spasm of bladder	Colch.
Dysuria	dysuria painful, so that he dances around the room in agony	Apis., cann-s., Canth., petros.
Dysuria	dysuria painful, with coldness, numbness and twitching down left leg	Agar.
Dysuria	dysuria painful, with difficulty in breathing and heart symptoms	Laur.
Dysuria	dysuria painful, with forcible stream	Agn., ant-c., carb-an., chel., cic., coc-c., cycl., nux-v., op., prun-s., spig., staph., sulph., verat-v.
Dysuria	dysuria painful, with forked stream	Arg-n., cann-s., canth., caust., chim., clem., Merc-c., merc., petr., prun-s., rhus-t., Thuj.
Dysuria	dysuria painful,spasmodic closure of the sphincter while finishing	Cann-s.
Dysuria	dysuria with aching in back	Vesp.
Dysuria	dysuria with suppressed menses and drawing pain in abdomen	Puls.
Dysuria	dysuria with violent pain in bladder	Calc-p.

E

Body part/Disease	Symptom	Medicines
Ear	abscess behind ear	Eup-per., rhus-t., tub.
Ear	abscess below ear	Nat-h.
Ear	abscess in meatus (the passage in the ear that leads to the eardrum)	Calc-s., crot-h., Hep., mag-c., puls., Sil.
Ear	abscess in meatus during menses	Puls.
Ear	air forced into ear when blowing nose	Sulph.
Ear	air rushing in ear	Lachn., mang., mez., staph.
Ear	air rushing in ear during eructation	Caust.
Ear	air rushing out as if from ear during eructation	Chel.
Ear	antitragus (a bump of cartilage just below the opening of the external ear)	Spong.
Ear	bald spot above ear	Phos.
Ear	blisters (a painful swelling on the skin containing fluid serum) of ears	Camph., kreos., meph.
Ear	bloody discharge from ear after measles	Bov., cact., carb-v., colch., crot-h., lyc., merc., nit-ac., Puls., sulph.
Ear	bloody discharge from ear after suppressed erruption	Cist., sulph.
Ear	bloody discharge from ear threatening caries	Asaf., Aur., calc-f., calc-s., calc., caps., nat-m., Sil., sulph.
Ear	bloody scabs (crust over healing wound) behind ears exuding a glutinous	Rhus-v.
Ear	blotches behind ears	Bry., calc., carb-an., caust., staph.
Ear	blowing sensation in right ear	Ail., rhus-t.
Ear	boils behind ears	Ang., bry., calc., con., nat-c., phyt., sulph., thuj.
Ear	boils below ears	Calc.
Ear	boils in front of ears	Bry., carb-v., laur., sulph.
Ear	boils in margins of ears	Bov., crot-h., Merc., Pic-ac., puls., rhus-t., Sulph.
Ear	boils in meatus	Bov., crot-h., Merc., Pic-ac., puls., rhus-t., Sulph.
Ear	boils on ears	Kali-c., sil., spong., sulph., syph.
Ear	boring fingers in ears	Agar., chel., mez., mill., phys., ruta., sal-ac., sil., thuj.
Ear	burning after scratching behind ears	Mag-m.
Ear	burning after scratching ears	Fl-ac.
Ear	burning in ear ameliorated by rubbing	Ol-an., phel.
Ear	burning in ear ameliorated by scratching	Caust., mag-c., nat-c.
Ear	burning in ear not ameliorated by rubbing	Zinc.

Body part/Disease	Symptom	Medicines
Ear	burning in ear not ameliorated by scratching	Am-m., arg-m., fl-ac., sars.
Ear	burning in ears aggravated by rubbing	Alum.
Ear	chilblains (red itchy swelling on the fingers, toes, or ears caused by exposure to cold and damp)	Agar.
Ear	child boring fingers in ears	Arund., cina., psor., sil.
Ear	constriction in ear	Thuj.
Ear	cracks behind ears	Chel., Graph., hep., hydr., lyc., petr., sep., sulph.
Ear	crusts below ears	Mur-ac., nat-p.
Ear	Deafnes	Bell.
Ear	discharge from ears after scarlet fever	Apis., asar., aur., bar-m., bov., brom., calc-s., Carb-v., crot-h., graph., hep., kali-bi., Lyc., merc., nit-ac., Psor., puls., sulph., tell., verb.
Ear	discharge of bloody wax from ear	Am-m., anac., hep., kali-c., lyc., merc., mosch., nat-m., nit-ac., phos., puls.
Ear	discharge of clear blood from ear	Bry.
Ear	discharge of copious blood from ear	Bar-m.
Ear	discharges from ear every seven days	Sulph.
Ear	discharges from ear in warm bed	Merc.
Ear	discharges from ear with putrid meat like smell	Kali-p., Psor., thuj.
Ear	discharges from left ear	Ferr., graph., psor.
Ear	discharges from right ear	Aeth., elaps., lyc., nit-ac., sil., thuj.
Ear	discharges of blood from ear	Am-c., arn., arund., asaf., bell., Both., bry., bufo., chin., cic., colch., con., Crot-h., elaps., ery-a., ham., merc., mosch., op., petr., Phos., puls., rhus-t., tell.
Ear	discharges of blood from ear instead of menses	Bry., phos.
Ear	discharges of blood from ear after prolonged suppuration (discharge of pus as a result of an injury or infection)	Chin.
Ear	discharges of blood from ear during cough	Bell.
Ear	eczema behind ears	Calc., Graph., Lyc., olnd., Psor., sulph., tell.
Ear	eczema in margins of ears	Nit-ac., psor.
Ear	eczema in meatus	Nit-ac., psor.
Ear	eczema of ear	Kali-bi., kali-s., psor.
Ear	eczema spreading from ear to face	Ars.
Ear	eruption, over margin of hair from ear to ear posteriorly	Nat-m., nit-ac., petr., Sulph.
Ear	excoriating bloody discharge	Ars-i., calc-p., carb-v., fl-ac., hep., lyc., merc., nat-m., puls., rhus-t., Sulph., syph., Tell.
Ear	excoriation of ears	Kali-bi., kali-c., kali-s., merc., petr., sulph.
Ear	formication in ear in morning	Zinc.
Ear	formication in ear while eating	Lachn.
Ear	fulness in ear from swallowing	Arum-d., mang.
Ear	fulness in ear when blowing nose	Mang., puls.

Body part/Disease	Symptom	Medicines
Ear	fulness in ear while eating	Nat-c.
Ear	fulness in ear, after stitching pains in ear	Iod.
Ear	fulness in ear, ameliorated by boring in ear	Mez.
Ear	fungus excrescence (a growth that sticks out from the body) in ear	Merc.
Ear	gangrenous vesicles on ears	Ars.
Ear	hard lump behind ear	Cinnb.
Ear	headache extending around the ears	Agar., lach., merc., nux-v., puls., rhus-t.
Ear	hearing impaired alternating with otorrhœa (discharge from ear)	Puls.
Ear	hearing impaired from paralysis of the auditory nerve (a nerve that conveys impulses relating to hearing and balance from the inner ear to the brain)	Bar-c., bell., calc., caust., chel., dulc., glon., graph., hyos., kali-p., lyc., merc., nit-ac., nux-v., op., petr., ph-ac., puls., sec., sil.
Ear	hearing impaired of left ear	Anac., arg-n., bor., bry., chel., coc-c., jac-c., mag-m., nat-c., op.
Ear	hearing impaired of left then right ear	Sulph.
Ear	hearing impaired of right ear	Arn., calc., cocc., cycl., ham., kali-s., led., merc., phys.
Ear	hearing impaired of right then left ear	Elaps.
Ear	ichorous (a watery or slightly bloody discharge from a wound or an ulcer) bloody discharge from ear	Am-c., Ars., calc-p., carb-an., carb-v., Lyc., nit-ac., Psor., sep., sil., tell.
Ear	inflamed and ulcerated wart-like growth behind ear	Calc.
Ear	inflammation of right parotid gland (salivary gland below ear)	
Ear	irritation extending to eustachian tube	Phyt.
Ear	itching behind ear ameliorated by scratching	Brom., mag-c., mag-m., ruta.
Ear	itching behind ear at night	Aur-m., mag-c., mag-m., merc-i-f., ruta.
Ear	itching behind ear followed by burning	Nat-m.
Ear	itching behind ear in evening while on bed	Merc-i-f., sulph.
Ear	itching behind ears with pimples	Rhus-t.
Ear	itching below ear ameliorated by scratching	Mag-c.
Ear	itching extended to eustachian tubes	Caust.
Ear	itching in concha (structure that resembles shell in shape) of the ear	Agar., arg-m., calc., chel., paeon., raph., spig., sulph.
Ear	itching in ear ameliorated by boring with finger	Aeth., agar., bov., coc-c., coloc., fl-ac., lachn., laur., mag-m., mill., ol-an., zinc.
Ear	itching in ear at night	Merc-i-r., sep., stry.
Ear	itching in ear at night alternating with anus	Sabad.
Ear	itching in ear compelling to swallow	Carb-v., Nux-v.
Ear	itching in ear in afternoon	Agar., laur., ol-an., puls.
Ear	itching in ear in evening	Acon., bor., calad., calc-p., elaps., graph., grat., mag-c., nat-m., psor., puls.
Ear	itching in ear in morning	Am-c., arg-m., kali-n., nat-c.
Ear	itching in ear not ameliorated by boring with finger	Agar., carb-v., laur., mang.

Body part/Disease	Symptom	Medicines
Ear	itching in ear while yawning	Acon.
Ear	itching in eustachian tubes (a bony passage extending from the middle ear to the naso pharynx that has a role in equalizing air pressure on both sides of the eardrum)	Agar., arg-m., calc., caust., coc-c., coloc., Nux-v., petr., Sil.
Ear	itching in eustachian tubes compelling swallowing	Nux-v.
Ear	itching in front of ear	Ol-an.
Ear	itching in left ear	Anag., benz-ac., calc., caust., cist., coc-c., form., ham., mang., mur-ac., nat-s., phel., rhus-t., sars., stann., sulph., tell., verat-v., zinc.
Ear	itching in right ear	Carb-ac., chel., cinnb., meny., merc-i-r., mez., nat-m., nat-p., psor., rat., rumx., tarent.
Ear	itching of ears	Kali-bi., mez., mosch., pall., psor., puls., sars., staph.
Ear	margins of ear moist	Sil.
Ear	meatus (the passage in the ear that leads to the eardrum) in margins	Kreos., nit-ac., psor.
Ear	meatus (the passage in the ear that leads to the eardrum) in margins	Kreos., nit-ac., psor.
Ear	milky discharge from ears	Kali-chl.
Ear	moist ears	Ant-c., bov., calc., Graph., kali-bi., kreos., lyc., merc., mez., petr., psor., ptel., staph.
Ear	moist on margins of ears	Sil.
Ear	must scratch ears until it bleeds	Alum., arg-m., nat-p.
Ear	noises in the ear of clock of bell	Mang.
Ear	noises in the ear on chewing	Aloe., alum., bar-c., bar-m., calc., carb-v., graph., iod., Kali-s., mang., meny., nat-m., Nit-ac., nux-v., petr., sil., sulph.
Ear	noises in the ear on moving the jaw	Graph.
Ear	noises in the ear when blowing nose	Bar-c., calc., carb-an., hep., kali-chl., lyc., mang., meny., ph-ac., stann., teucr.
Ear	noises in the ear when blowing nose ameliorated by boring into ear	Lach., meny., nicc.
Ear	noises in the ear when yawning,	Acon., cocc., mang., mez., verat.
Ear	odorless bloody discharge from ear	Lac-c.
Ear	pain behind left ear	Aur., kali-p., lach.
Ear	pain behind right ear	Aesc.
Ear	pain extending to other ear	Chel., hep., laur.
Ear	pain in back extending to ears	Gels.
Ear	pain in cervical region extending behind left ear	Apis.
Ear	pain in cervical region extending behind right ear	Elaps.
Ear	pain in cervical region extending to the ear	Bov., calc-p., cann-s., colch., elaps., lyss., thuj.
Ear	pain in ear after dinner	Agar., ant-c., bov., carb-an., plb.
Ear	pain in ear after suppression of ague (a feverish condition involving alternating hot, cold, and sweating stages, especially as a symptom of malaria)	Puls.

Body part/Disease	Symptom	Medicines
Ear	pain in ear at change of weather	Mang., rhod., rhus-t., sil.
Ear	pain in ear compelling to lie down	Cur.
Ear	pain in ear day and night	Hell.
Ear	pain in ear during chill	Acon., apis., calc., gamb., graph., nux-v., puls., sulph.
Ear	pain in ear during full moon	Sil.
Ear	pain in ear during headache	Ham., lach., merc., phos., psor., puls., ran-s., sang.
Ear	pain in ear extending from left to right	Calc-p.
Ear	pain in ear extending to left eye	Hura.
Ear	pain in ear extending to left face	Anac., bell., cann-s., merc., nux-v., stram., thea.
Ear	pain in ear extending to left forehead	Dig., nux-v., ptel.
Ear	pain in ear extending to left head	Sulph.
Ear	pain in ear extending to right eye	Glon., hura., puls., spig.
Ear	pain in ear extending to left shoulder	Nat-m.
Ear	pain in ear extending to malar bone (cheek bone)	Spig.
Ear	pain in ear extending to neck	Bell., lith., sil., tarax.
Ear	pain in ear extending to nose	Sil.
Ear	pain in ear extending to occiput	Ambr., fago.
Ear	pain in ear extending to parotid gland (salivary gland below ear) and mastoid process (bony part of ear)	Kali-bi., sep.
Ear	pain in ear from music	Ambr., cham., kreos., ph-ac., tab.
Ear	pain in ear from noises	Am-c., arn., bell., carb-v., Con., gad., mur-ac., op., phos., sang., sil., Sulph.
Ear	pain in ear from sound of hammer	Sang.
Ear	pain in ear from taking cold	Dulc., gels., kalm., merc., puls.,
Ear	pain in ear from taking cold in head	Bell., gels., led., puls.
Ear	pain in ear in cold wind	Ars-i., lac-c., sep., spong.
Ear	pain in ear in cold wind and rain	Nux-v.
Ear	pain in ear in damp weather	Calc-p., calc., dulc., nat-s., sil.
Ear	pain in ear on blowing nose	Act-sp., alum., bar-c., calc., caust., con., dios., hep., lyc., ph-ac., puls., sil., spig., stann., teucr., trom.
Ear	pain in ear when chewing	Aloe., anac., apis., arg-m., bell., cann-s., hep., lach., nux-m., nux-v., seneg., verb.
Ear	pain in ear when feet become cold	Stann.
Ear	pain in ear when laughing	Mang.
Ear	pain in ear while lying on bed	Caust., kali-i., kali-p., nux-v., sang., sulph., thuj.
Ear	pain in ear with face-ache	Bell., merc., ph-ac.
Ear	pain in ear with nausea	Dulc.
Ear	pain in ear with sore throat	Apis., bar-m., cham., Lach., merc., Nit-ac., par.
Ear	pain in ear with toothache	Glon., meph., merl., ph-ac., plan., Rhod., sep.
Ear	pain in external throat extending behind ear	Rhod.
Ear	pain in eye extending to ear	Fago., petr.

Body part/Disease	Symptom	Medicines
Ear	pain in face in left parotid gland	Coloc., rhus-t.
Ear	pain in face in right parotid gland	Bell., cocc., merc.
Ear	pain in left ear from swallowing	Carb-s., kali-bi., mang.
Ear	pain in nose extending to ears on swallowing	Elaps.
Ear	pain in right ear from swallowing	Brom.
Ear	pain in teeth alternating with itching in the ear	Agar.
Ear	pain in throat extending to ear	All-c., alum., ambr., bell., bry., calc., carb-ac., carb-an., cham., elaps., hep., ign., iris., kali-ma., kali-n., lac-c., lach., lith., lyc., merc-cy., merc., nat-m., nit-ac., nux-v., par., phyt., podo., sars., sec., sul-ac., tarent., tell.
Ear	pain in throat extending to ear on swallowing	Ail., brom., elaps., gels., kali-bi., kali-c., kali-ma., kali-n., lac-c., lach., merc., Nit-ac., Nux-v., par., phyt., tarent.
Ear	pain of ear aggravated from warmth of bed	Merc-i-f., Merc., nux-v., phos., puls.
Ear	pain of ear ameliorated from cold drinks	Bar-m.
Ear	pain of ear ameliorated from opening the mouth	Nat-c.
Ear	pain of ear ameliorated from pressure	Alum., bism., carb-an., caust., ham.
Ear	pain of ear ameliorated from sleep	Sep.
Ear	pain of ear ameliorated from swallowing	Rhus-t.
Ear	pain of ear ameliorated in open air	Am-m.
Ear	pain of ear ameliorated in warm room	Sep.
Ear	pain of ear extending to right shoulder	Cann-s., nat-m., rumx.
Ear	pain of ear extending to roof of mouth	Kali-bi.
Ear	pain of ear extending to side of neck	Carb-v., cocc., kali-bi., mag-p., meph., nat-m.
Ear	pain of ear extending to side of neck and clavicle and to last back teeth and side of occiput	Coc-c.
Ear	pain of ear extending to spine	Ptel.
Ear	pain of ear extending to teeth	Bell., chel., lyss., mosch., ol-an., spig., xan.
Ear	pain of ear extending to temples	Eupi., form., indg., lac-c., lach., nux-v., puls., sars., tarent.
Ear	pain of ear extending to throat	Carb-an., chel., fago., kali-bi., merc-i-f., spig.
Ear	pain of ear extending to vertex	Arn., chel.
Ear	pain of face extending to ears	Bell., calc., carb-an., caust., coloc., hep., Lach., lyc., mez., plan., Puls., sang., sep., spig., thuj.
Ear	painful discharge from ear	Calc-s., ferr-p., Merc.
Ear	periodical pain in ear	Arn., gels., nat-c., nat-m.
Ear	pimples above the ears	Cop., mur-ac.
Ear	pimples in meatus	Jug-r., kali-p.
Ear	pimples on ears	Agar., am-c., berb., calad., calc-p., cann-s., cic., coff., kali-c., kali-s., kreos., merc-c., merc., mur-ac., nat-m., petr., phos., psor., sabad., sel., spong., staph., sulph.
Ear	purulent (consisting of pus) discharge from ear after abuse of mercury	Asaf., aur., Hep., Nit-ac., sil., sulph.
Ear	purulent discharge from ear with eczema	Calc., hep., lyc., merc., sulph.

Body part/Disease	Symptom	Medicines
Ear	purulent vesicles on ears	Ptel.
Ear	pustules behind ears	Berb., cann-s., carb-v., cast-eq., crot-h., phyt., psor., ptel., Puls., spong., sumb.
Ear	pustules in front of ears	Mag-c.
Ear	pustules in margins of ears	Cast-eq.
Ear	pustules in meatus	Cast-eq.
Ear	rash in ears	Ant-c., nat-m.
Ear	scab behind ears exuding a glutinous moisture, sore on touch	Thuj.
Ear	scab behind ears	Aur-m., bar-c., Graph., kali-c., lach., Lyc., Sil., tell., thuj.
Ear	scaly ears	Cop., petr., psor., teucr.
Ear	scratching ears during sleep	Lyc.
Ear	scurfy in margins of ears	All-s., Lyc., psor.
Ear	scurfy of ears	Aur-m., bov., calc., com., graph., hep., iod., lach., Lyc., mur-ac., Psor., puls., sars., sil.
Ear	sensation as if Water in ear	Am-c., anan., asaf., bell., cina., dig., ferr., hep., mag-m.
Ear	sensation of air in ears	Graph., mez.
Ear	sensation of cold air in ears	Caust., dulc., mez., plat., staph., vinc.
Ear	sensation of fanning of air before ear	Calc., mang., nit-ac.
Ear	sensation of worms in ears	Acon., calc., coloc., guare., med., pic-ac., puls., rhod., ruta.
Ear	sensibility increased in ears	Kali-i., lach., merc., valer., zinc.
Ear	sleeplessness from pulsation in ear	Sil.
Ear	sore (painful or tender because of an injury, infection) behind ears	Graph., kali-c., nit-ac., Petr., Psor.
Ear	sounds seems distant	All-c., cann-i., cham., coca., eupi., Lac-c., nux-m., peti., sol-n.
Ear	stitching in ears	Lach.
Ear	stitching pain in larynx extending to ear when swallowing	Mang.
Ear	stitching pain in larynx extending to ear	Arg-m., nat-m.
Ear	suppuration of parotid (near ear) gland	Ars., Brom., bry., Calc., con., Hep., lach., Merc., nat-m., phos., Rhus-t., Sil., sul-ac.
Ear	swelling in left parotid gland	Brom., con., lach., Rhus-t., sul-ac.
Ear	swelling in left parotid gland after exanthemata (a disease characterized by the appearance of a skin rash, e.g. measles or scarlet fever)	Anthr., arn., bar-c., Brom., carb-v., dulc., iod., kali-bi., mag-c., sulph.
Ear	swelling in left parotid gland during menses	Kali-c.
Ear	swelling in right parotid gland	Am-c., Bar-c., bar-m., Bell., carb-an., graph., kali-bi., kali-c., merc., nit-ac., plb., sep., stram.
Ear	swelling in right then left parotid gland	Lyc.
Ear	thick discharge from ears	Calc-s., Calc., carb-v., ery-a., Hydr., Kali-bi., kali-chl., lyc., nat-m., Puls., sep., Sil., tarent.

Body part/Disease	Symptom	Medicines
Ear	thin discharge from ears	Ars., cham., elaps., graph., Kali-s., merc., petr., psor., sep., sil., sulph.
Ear	typhus fever with swelled parotid, and sensitive bones	Mang.
Ear	vesicles below ears	Ptel.
Ear	vesicles discharging water from ears	Ptel.
Ear	vesicles in front of ears	Cic.
Ear	vesicles in margins of ears	Nicc.
Ear	vesicles in meatus	Nicc.
Ear	vesicles on ears	Alum., ars., meph., olnd., phos., ptel., rhus-v., sep., tell.
Ear	vesicles on ears extending to face	Graph., sep.
Ear	vesicles on ears extending to scalp	Hep.
Ear	vesicles on ears filled with serum (liquid part of blood)	Rhus-v.
Ear	vesicles on ears surrounded by inflamed base	Ars.
Ear	vesicles on sides from ear discharge	Tell.
Ear	watery discharge from ears	Calc., carb-v., cist., elaps., graph., Kali-s., merc., Sil., syph., Tell., thuj.
Ear	wax of ears black	Elaps., Puls.
Ear	wax of ears brown	Calc-s.
Ear	wax of ears dry	Elaps., lac-c., lach., mur-ac., petr.
Ear	wax of ears hardened	All-s., con., elaps., lach., Puls., sel.
Ear	wax of ears increased	Agar., am-m., anan., bell., calc., Caust., con., cycl., dios., elaps., hep., kali-c., lyc., merc-i-r., merl., mosch., mur-ac., petr., sel., sep., sil., sulph., tarent., thuj., zinc.
Ear	wax of ears peeling off in scales	Mur-ac.
Ear	wax of ears red or dark	Mur-ac.
Ear	wax of ears soft	Sil.
Ear	wax of ears thick	Chel., petr.
Ear	wax of ears thin	Am-m., con., hep., iod., kali-c., lach., merc., mosch., petr., sel., sil., sulph., tell.
Ear	white discharge from ears	Ery-a., hep., kali-chl., Nat-m.
Ear	yellow discharge from ears	Aeth., ars., calc-s., calc., crot-h., hydr., kali-ar., Kali-bi., kali-c., Kali-s., lyc., merc., nat-s., petr., phos., Puls., sil.
Ear	yellowish green discharge from ears	Cinnb., elaps., kali-chl., kali-s., merc., Puls.
Ebola	haemorrhagic fever including Ebola (a virus transmitted by blood and body fluids that causes the linings of bodily organs and vessels to leak blood and fluids, usually resulting in death) & Dengue (a tropical disease caused by a virus that is transmitted by mosquitoes and marked by high fever and severe muscle and joint pains)	Carb-v., **Crot-h.**, lach., mill., **Phos.**, sul-ac.
Ecchymoses	discoloration, ecchymoses on legs	Crot-h.
Ecchymoses	ecchymoses (bleeding from broken blood vessels into surrounding tissue) on upper arm	Vip.

Body part/Disease	Symptom	Medicines
Ecchymoses	ecchymosis from lids	Arn., led.
Ecchymoses	ecchymosis in chest	Lach., phos., sul-ac.
Ecchymoses	ecchymosis in eye	Acon., aeth., am-c., arg-n., Arn., bell., Cact., cham., chlol., con., crot-h., cupr-ac., erig., glon., ham., kali-bi., kali-chl., kreos., lach., Led., lyc., lyss., nux-v., phos., plb., ruta., sul-ac., ter.
Ecchymoses	ecchymosis in eye from coughing	Arn., bell.
Ecchymoses	ecchymosis in skin	Anth., arg-n., **Arn.**, bad., bar-c., bar-m., bry., calc., carb-v., cham., chin., chlol., coca., con., crot-h., dulc., euphr., ferr., hep., lach., laur., **Led.**, nux-v., par., **Ph-ac.**, **Phos.**, plb., puls., rhus-t., ruta., **Sec.**, **Sul-ac.**, sulph., tarent., ter.
Ecchymoses	ecchymosis of lumbar region	Merc-c., vip.
Ecchymoses	ecchymosis on right Eyelids	Con.
Ecchymoses	ecchymosis on skin returning yearly	Crot-h.
Eczema	asthmatic with face ache and disappearance of tetter (eruption) on face	Dulc.
Eczema	bleeding eczema on face	Alum., ars., dulc., hep., lyc., merc., petr., psor., sep., sulph.
Eczema	burning eczema on face	Cic., viol-t.
Eczema	burning pain in hand in eczema	Merc.
Eczema	eczema around mouth	Mez., mur-ac., nat-m.
Eczema	eczema at corner of mouth	Arund., graph., hep., lyc., rhus-t., sil.
Eczema	eczema at margins of hair	Sulph.
Eczema	eczema behind ears	Calc., Graph., Lyc., olnd., Psor., sulph., tell.
Eczema	eczema in axilla	Hep., jug-r., merc., nat-m., petr., Psor., sep.
Eczema	eczema in cervical region	Anac., lyc., psor., sil.
Eczema	eczema in coccyx	Arn., merc., sil.
Eczema	eczema in margins of ears	Nit-ac., psor.
Eczema	eczema in meatus	Nit-ac., psor.
Eczema	eczema of chin	Bor., cic., graph., merc-i-r., phos., rhus-t., sep.
Eczema	eczema of ear	Kali-bi., kali-s., psor.
Eczema	eczema on chest	Anac., calc-s., calc., carb-v., cycl., Graph., hep., kali-s., petr., Psor., Sulph.
Eczema	eczema on eyelids	Clem., Graph., hep., mez., tell., Thuj.
Eczema	eczema on face like dried honey	Ant-c., Cic., mez.
Eczema	eczema on male genitalia	Arg-n., ars., chel., crot-t., graph., hep., lyc., nat-m., nit-ac., petr., rhus-t., sep., sulph., thuj.
Eczema	eczema on mammae	Anac.
Eczema	eczema on nipples	Graph.
Eczema	eczema scrotum	Crot-t.
Eczema	eczema spreading from ear to face	Ars.
Eczema	eczema spreading from occiput	Lyc., sil.
Eczema	eruption, eczema	Anil., arn., ars., kali-br., merc., psor.

Body part/Disease	Symptom	Medicines
Eczema	eruption, eczema in ankle	Chel., nat-p., psor.
Eczema	eruption, eczema in back of foot	Merc., psor.
Eczema	eruption, eczema in back of hands	Graph., jug-c., merc., **Mez.**, nat-c., phos., sep.
Eczema	eruption, eczema in bend of elbow	Cupr., graph., mez., **Psor.**
Eczema	eruption, eczema in bends of joints	Am-c., **Graph.**, led., merc., sep., sulph.
Eczema	eruption, eczema in calf	Graph.
Eczema	eruption, eczema in elbow	Brom.
Eczema	eruption, eczema in forearm	Graph., merc., mez., sil., thuj.
Eczema	eruption, eczema in hands	Ars., canth., clem., **Graph.**, jug-c., lyc., merc., mez., nit-ac., phos., sil.
Eczema	eruption, eczema in hollow of knee	Graph.
Eczema	eruption, eczema in joints	Led., phos.
Eczema	eruption, eczema in legs	Apis., **Ars.**, carb-v., **Graph.**, kali-br., lach., led., lyc., merc., nat-m., **Petr.**, rhus-t., sars., **Sulph.**
Eczema	eruption, eczema in shoulder	Petr.
Eczema	eruption, eczema in thighs	Petr., rhus-t.
Eczema	eruption, eczema in upper limbs	Canth., graph., merc., mez., phos., psor., sil.
Eczema	eruption, eczema in wrists	Jug-c., mez., psor.
Eczema	eruption, eczema rubrum in knee	Anil., arn., rhus-t.
Eczema	eruption, herpes like ringworm in elbow	Cupr.
Eczema	eruptions eczema	Alum., am-c., am-m., anac., ant-c., arg-n., **Ars-i.**, **Ars.**, astac., aur-m., aur., **Bar-m.**, bell., bor., brom., bry., calad., **Calc-s.**, **Calc.**, canth., carb-ac., carb-s., carb-v., caust., **Cic.**, clem., cop., **Crot-t.**, cycl., **Dulc.**, fl-ac., **Graph.**, **Hep.**, hydr., iris., **Jug-c.**, **Jug-r.**, kali-ar., kali-bi., kali-c., kali-chl., kali-s., lach., **Lappa-m.**, led., lith., lyc., merc., **Mez.**, nat-m., nat-p., nat-s., nit-ac., **Olnd.**, **Petr.**, phos., phyt., **Psor.**, ran-b., **Rhus-t.**, rhus-v., sars., sep., sil., staph., **Sul-i.**, **Sulph.**, thuj., viol-t.
Eczema	eruptions eczema alternating with internal affections	Graph.
Eczema	eruptions eczema elevated	Anac., ars., asaf., bry., calc., carb-v., caust., cop., crot-h., cupr-ar., dulc., graph., lach., merc., mez., op., phos., sulph., tab., tarax., valer.
Eczema	eruptions eczema excoriated	Alum., arg-m., aur., bry., calc., colch., dros., graph., hep., **Merc.**, **Nat-m.**, nit-ac., par., **Petr.**, ph-ac., puls., rhus-t., sep., **Sulph.**, viol-t.
Eczema	eruptions eczema fetid	Ars., graph., hep., kali-p., lach., lyc., merc., mez., nit-ac., **Psor.**, rhus-t., sep., sil., staph., **Sulph.**, vinc.
Eczema	eruptions eczema flat	Am-c., ant-c., ant-t., ars., asaf., **Bell.**, carb-an., eupho., **Lach.**, lyc., merc., nat-c., nit-ac., petr., ph-ac., phos., puls., ran-b., sel., sep., sil., staph., sulph., thuj.
Eczema	eruptions eczema granular	Agar., am-c., ars., carb-v., cocc., graph., hep., kreos., led., nat-m., nux-v., par., phos., valer., vinc.
Eczema	eruptions eczema grape shaped	Agar., **Calc.**, rhus-t., staph., verat.
Eczema	eruptions eczema gritty	Am-c., graph., hep., nat-m., phos., zinc.

Body part/Disease	Symptom	Medicines
Eczema	eruptions eczema hard	Agar., ant-c., aur., caust., mez., ran-b., rhus-t., spig., valer.
Eczema	eruptions eczema on hairy parts	Agar., calc., kali-i., lach., lith., lyc., merc., nat-m., nit-ac., ph-ac., **Rhus-t.**, sil.
Eczema	eruptions, eczema in fingers	Lyc., sil., staph.
Eczema	eruptions, eczema in lower limbs	Anil., apis., ars., bov., chel., jug-r., kali-br., merc., petr., psor., rhus-t.
Eczema	eruptions, painful eczema in fingers	Arn.
Eczema	fetid (having a rotten or offensive smell) eczema on face	Lyc.
Eczema	moist eczema on face	Cic., Graph., Lyc., petr., psor., rhus-t.
Eczema	purulent discharge from ear with eczema	Calc., hep., lyc., merc., sulph.
Elbow	ankylosis of elbow	Sil.
Elbow	arthritic nodosities on condyles above elbow	Mag-c.
Elbow	arthritic nodosities on condyles above elbow with stiffness	Lyc.
Elbow	arthritic nodosities on olecranon	Still.
Elbow	bubbling sensation in elbow	Kreos., mang., rheum., spong.
Elbow	burning pain in elbow	Agar., alum., arg-m., arund., asaf., bell., berb., calc-p., carb-an., carb-v., coc-c., colch., coloc., kali-n., merc., mur-ac., ph-ac., phos., plat., sep., sulph., ter.
Elbow	burning pain in elbow at night	Sep.
Elbow	burning pain in elbow in evening	Arg-m., carb-an.
Elbow	burning pain in elbow in forenoon	Sulph.
Elbow	burning pain in olecranon	Chel., ph-ac.
Elbow	caries of elbow	Sil.
Elbow	coldness in elbow	Agar., cedr., gins., graph., ir-f.
Elbow	coldness in elbow extending to hands towards noon	Cedr.
Elbow	coldness in olecranon (elbow bone)	Agar.
Elbow	compression of elbow	Chlor., nat-s.
Elbow	compression of elbow in evening	Nat-s.
Elbow	constrictions in bend of elbow	Elaps., rat.
Elbow	constrictions in elbow	Agar., caust., lach., mang., petr., rat., sep.
Elbow	constrictions in elbow as with a cord	Rat.
Elbow	constrictions in elbow in morning	Petr.
Elbow	constrictions in elbow on bending	Rat.
Elbow	constrictions in left elbow	Agar.
Elbow	constrictions in right upper arm above the elbow	Phys.
Elbow	contraction of muscles & tendons of bend of elbow	Caust., elaps., puls., sars., sulph.
Elbow	contraction of muscles & tendons of elbow	Ars., glon., lyc., nux-v., tep.
Elbow	convulsion ameliorated by bending elbow	Nux-v.
Elbow	cracking in elbow	Am-c., ant-c., brom., cinnb., con., dios., kalm., merc., mur-ac., nat-m., sulph., tep., thuj., zinc., zing.

Body part/Disease	Symptom	Medicines
Elbow	cracking in elbow from stretching	Thuj.
Elbow	cracking in elbow in afternoon	Kalm.
Elbow	cramp in third finger from extending to elbow	Sep., sulph.
Elbow	discoloration, brown spots on elbow	Cadm., lach., sep.
Elbow	discoloration, red spots on elbow	Phos.
Elbow	discoloration, spots on elbow	Calc., sep., vip.
Elbow	elbow hot	Alum., arg-m., arund., berb., sep.
Elbow	eruption, black blister in elbow	Ars.
Elbow	eruption, black vesicles in elbow	Ars.
Elbow	eruption, blister (painful swelling on skin) in elbow	Crot-h.
Elbow	eruption, crusts (a dry hardened outer layer of blood, pus, or other bodily secretion that forms over a cut or sore) in bend of elbow	Cupr., mez., **Psor.**
Elbow	eruption, desquamation in elbow	Sulph.
Elbow	eruption, dry in bend of elbow	Mez.
Elbow	eruption, dry, furfuraceous in olecranon	Aster., sep.
Elbow	eruption, eczema in bend of elbow	Cupr., graph., mez., **Psor.**
Elbow	eruption, eczema in elbow	Brom.
Elbow	eruption, elevations in elbow	Merc.
Elbow	eruption, elevations itchy & scaly in elbow	Merc.
Elbow	eruption, fissures (a break in the skin lining the anal canal, usually causing pain during bowel movements and sometimes bleeding. Anal fissures occur as a consequence of constipation or sometimes of diarrhoea) in bend of elbow	Kali-ar.
Elbow	eruption, herpes in bend of elbow	Cupr., graph., kreos., **Nat-m.**, sep., thuj.
Elbow	eruption, herpes in elbow	Bor., cact., **Cupr.**, hep., kreos., phos., psor., sep., staph., thuj.
Elbow	eruption, herpes like ringworm in elbow	Cupr.
Elbow	eruption, in bend of elbow	Am-m., bry., calad., calc., cupr., graph., hep., merc., mez., nat-c., nat-m., psor., sep., staph., sulph.
Elbow	eruption, in elbow	Aster., berb., brom., cact., cupr., hep., iris., kali-s., kreos., lach., merc., phos., psor., sabin., sep., staph., sulph., tep., thuj., zinc.
Elbow	eruption, itching in elbow	Merc., sep.
Elbow	eruption, nodules in elbow	Eupi., mur-ac.
Elbow	eruption, painful in bend of elbow	Am-m., ant-c., dros., dulc., hura., lachn., nat-c., ol-an., phos., rhus-t., sep.
Elbow	eruption, painful in elbow	Merc.
Elbow	eruption, pimples biting in elbow	Kali-n.
Elbow	eruption, pimples in elbow	Ant-c., asc-t., berb., bry., dulc., hyos., kali-n., lach., merc., nat-c., ol-an., sabin., sep., staph., sulph., tarax., thuj.
Elbow	eruption, pimples burning in elbow	Kali-n.

Body part/Disease	Symptom	Medicines
Elbow	eruption, pimples in bend of elbow	Ant-c., hura., hyos., ol-an., phos., sep., thuj.
Elbow	eruption, pimples on inflamed base in elbow	Tarax.
Elbow	eruption, pustules in bend of elbow	Sulph.
Elbow	eruption, pustules in elbow	Eup-per., hep., jug-c., lach.
Elbow	eruption, pustules itchy in elbow	Hep.
Elbow	eruption, pustules yellowish in elbow	Jug-c.
Elbow	eruption, rash in bend of elbow	Calad., hep., sep., zinc.
Elbow	eruption, rash in elbow	Calad., mez., sulph.
Elbow	eruption, red in bend of elbow	Cor-r., rhus-t.
Elbow	eruption, red in elbow	Cinnb., rhus-t.
Elbow	eruption, red vesicles in bend of elbow	Nat-c.
Elbow	eruption, scabies in bend of elbow	Bry., merc.
Elbow	eruption, scaly in elbow	Calc., jug-r., kali-s., merc., sep., staph., sulph.
Elbow	eruption, suppurating (Oozing pus) in elbow	Sulph.
Elbow	eruption, suppurating vesicles in elbow	Sulph.
Elbow	eruption, tubercle in elbow	Am-c., caust., mag-c., mur-ac.
Elbow	eruption, urticaria in elbow	Aran.
Elbow	eruption, vesicles in bend of elbow	Calc., nat-c., rhus-v., sulph.
Elbow	eruption, vesicles in elbow	Ars., calad., nat-p., sulph.
Elbow	eruption, white vesicles in elbow	Sulph.
Elbow	eruption, yellowish vesicles in elbow	Sulph.
Elbow	erysipelatous inflammation in elbow	Ars., lach., sulph.
Elbow	extremities flexed at elbow	Lyc.
Elbow	heaviness in elbow	Chin-a., con., samb.
Elbow	hot & red swelling of elbow	**Merc.**
Elbow	inflammation in elbow	Ant-c., lach., lact-ac., sil.
Elbow	itching in bend of elbow	Canth., carb-s., cupr., hep., laur., nat-c., nit-ac., ol-an., petr., psor., rumx., **Sep.**, sulph., ter.
Elbow	itching in bend of elbow in afternoon	Sulph.
Elbow	itching in bend of elbow in evening	Cupr.
Elbow	itching in elbow	Agar., alum., arg-m., berb., calc-i., caust., crot-h., cycl., fago., ign., indg., kali-n., lachn., laur., mang., med., merc-i-f., merc., mur-ac., **Nat-c.**, nat-p., ol-an., pall., petr., phos., psor., rhus-v., sep., sulph.
Elbow	itching in elbow aggravated in evening	Sulph.
Elbow	itching in elbow ameliorated by rubbing	Ol-an.
Elbow	itching in elbow ameliorated by scratching	Ol-an.
Elbow	itching in olecranon of elbow	Agar., ars-m., mag-m., nit-ac., olnd., phos.
Elbow	jerking of elbow	Nat-m., stram., zinc.
Elbow	lameness in elbow	All-c., dios., dulc., hydr., iris., merc-i-f., mez., petr.
Elbow	lameness in elbow in morning	Dios.
Elbow	lupus (disease of connective tissue) in one elbow	Hep.

Body part/Disease	Symptom	Medicines
Elbow	numbness in bend of elbow	Hura., plb., sulph.
Elbow	numbness in elbow	All-c., cinnb., dig., dios., jatr., kali-n., phos., pip-m.
Elbow	numbness in elbow aggravated on motion	All-c.
Elbow	numbness in elbow extending to tips of fingers	Jatr.
Elbow	numbness in elbow in evening when lying down	Phos.
Elbow	pain in elbow after carrying a weight	Cham.
Elbow	pain in elbow after going to bed	Dios.
Elbow	pain in elbow after riding	Verat.
Elbow	pain in elbow after walking	Valer.
Elbow	pain in elbow aggravated from warmth	Guai.
Elbow	pain in elbow aggravated on motion	Agn., **Bry.**, carb-s., guai., kali-bi., led., plb., sulph., ust.
Elbow	pain in elbow alternating with pain in knees	Dios.
Elbow	pain in elbow alternating with pain in shoulder	Kalm.
Elbow	pain in elbow ameliorated from warmth	Caust., **Rhus-t.**
Elbow	pain in elbow ameliorated on motion	Arg-m., aur-m-n., bism., dulc., lyc., mez., **Rhus-t.**
Elbow	pain in elbow at night	Dig., gels., kali-n., merc-i-f., phos., ter.
Elbow	pain in elbow during chill	Ang., **Podo.**
Elbow	pain in elbow extending to hand	Kali-bi., lach., nicc., tarent.
Elbow	pain in elbow extending to little finger	Aesc., arund., jatr., lyc., phyt., puls., seneg.
Elbow	pain in elbow extending to shoulder	Cycl., phos., still.
Elbow	pain in elbow extending to wrist	Ars., guai., kali-n., phyt., prun-s., rhus-t.
Elbow	pain in elbow in afternoon	Sulph.
Elbow	pain in elbow in evening	Cast-eq., cop., dios., dulc., fl-ac., jac-c.
Elbow	pain in elbow in forenoon	Abrot., dios., plan.
Elbow	pain in elbow in morning	Brach., dios., lyc., ran-b., sep., sumb., thuj.
Elbow	pain in elbow in noon	Arg-m., cedr.
Elbow	pain in elbow when bending arm	All-s., chel., dulc., mag-c., mur-ac., puls.
Elbow	pain in elbow when stretching arm	Hep., kali-c., puls., ruta.
Elbow	pain in elbow when touched	Ambr., calc-p., dulc., hyos., ph-ac.
Elbow	pain in elbow while leaning on it	Carb-an., kreos., nat-s., phos.
Elbow	pain in elbow while leaning on opposite side	Nux-v.
Elbow	pain in elbow while lying	Nat-c., phos.
Elbow	pain in elbow while sitting	Phos.
Elbow	pain in fingers extending to elbow	Nat-m., plat., plb.
Elbow	pain in forearm extending to elbow	Spig.
Elbow	pain in knee alternating with pain in elbow	Dios.
Elbow	pain in olecranon	Alum., am-c., carb-an., caust., chin-a., hep., kali-n., rhod., spong., verat.
Elbow	pain in olecranon on motion	Hep.
Elbow	pain in shoulder extending to elbow	Abrot., cupr-ar., ferr., fl-ac., Ind., petr., phos., plb.
Elbow	pain in thumb extending to elbow	Calc-s.

Body part/Disease	Symptom	Medicines
Elbow	paralysis in elbow	Fago., petr., sabin.
Elbow	rheumatic swelling of elbow	Agar., **Bry.**, chel., coloc., com., lyc.
Elbow	sensation as if cold water were dripping from elbow	Stry.
Elbow	sensation as if cold water were through elbow	Graph.
Elbow	sensation as if elbow bandaged	Caust.
Elbow	sensation of paralysis in elbow	Ambr., arg-m., mez., samb., stront., sulph., valer.
Elbow	sensation of paralysis in elbow at night	Stront.
Elbow	sensation of paralysis in elbow during motion	Arg-m.
Elbow	sensation of paralysis in elbow from raising the arm	Mez.
Elbow	sensation of paralysis in elbow in afternoon	Sulph.
Elbow	sensation of paralysis in right wrist extending to elbow	Euphr.
Elbow	shocks in elbow	Agar., nat-m., verat.
Elbow	shocks in elbow to head	Agar.
Elbow	stiffness in elbow	Acon., aeth., alum., am-c., anac., ang., asaf., bell., **Bry.**, calc., chel., ham., kali-c., lach., lact-ac., led., lyc., phos., pip-m., puls., sep., spig., stann., sulph., thuj., zinc.
Elbow	stiffness in elbow in evening	Com., sep., valer.
Elbow	stiffness in elbow in morning	Dios.
Elbow	stitching pain in chest extending to elbow	Sil.
Elbow	suppuration from elbow	Dros., tep.
Elbow	swelling in condyles of elbow	**Calc-p.**, mez.
Elbow	swelling in elbow	Acon., agar., benz-ac., bry., calc-f., chel., cic., colch., coloc., con., dios., hydr., lac-c., lact-ac., **Merc.**, petr., puls., sil., spig., tep., ter.
Elbow	swelling in forearm near elbow	Lyc.
Elbow	swelling in hand extending to elbow	Crot-c., crot-h., ruta.
Elbow	tingling in elbow	Meny., verat.
Elbow	tumours on elbow point	Hep.
Elbow	twitching in band of elbow	Arg-n., bar-c.
Elbow	twitching in elbow ameliorated from motion	Agn., arg-m.
Elbow	twitching in elbow ameliorated from sretching arm	Nat-m.
Elbow	twitching in elbow in afternoon	Nat-m.
Elbow	twitching in elbow in afternoon at 3.00 p.m.	Arg-m.
Elbow	twitching in elbow in morning	Nat-m.
Elbow	twitching in elbow in noon while lying	Zinc.
Elbow	ulcer in elbow	Calc., hydr., lach., nat-s.
Elbow	wandering pain in elbow	Cact.
Elbow	wandering pain in fingers	Ars-h., iris., nat-a.
Elbow	warts on bend of elbow	Calc-f.
Elbow	weakness in bend of elbow at 5.00 a.m.	Cann-i.
Elbow	weakness in elbow	Ang., chin-s., coloc., dios., fago., glon., hyper., led., nat-s., op., plb., raph., sarr., staph., sulph., thuj., valer.

Body part/Disease	Symptom	Medicines
Elbow	weakness in elbow at 5.00 a.m.	Valer.
Elephantiasis	elephantiasis (a chronic disease in which parasitic worms obstruct the lymphatic system, causing enlargement of parts of the body, e.g. the legs and scrotum, and hardening of the surrounding skin. It is transmitted by mosquitoes) of scrotum	Sil.
Emaciation	appetite, increased with emaciation	Abrot., Calc., Iod., Nat-m., Petr., phos., psor., sulph., tub.
Emaciation	appetite, increased with marasmus .	Abrot., ars-i., bar-c., bar-i., calc-p., Calc., caust., chin., Cina., Iod., lyc., mag-c., Nat-m., nux-v., petr., sil., sulph.
Emaciation	dry cough in emaciated boys	Lyc.
Emaciation	emaciation	Ars., calc., carb-s., clem., nit-ac., phyt., **Plb.**, sec., stront., **Sulph.**
Emaciation	emaciation (become thin) of the muscles of abdomen	Plb.
Emaciation	emaciation after grief	Petr., ph-ac.
Emaciation	emaciation after vaccination	Maland., thuj.
Emaciation	emaciation from loss of animal fluids	**Chin., Lyc., Sel.**
Emaciation	emaciation in old people	Ambr., **Bar-c., Iod., Lyc.**, sec., sel.
Emaciation	emaciation in paralyzed	Kali-p., nux-v., **Plb.**, sec., sep.
Emaciation	emaciation in right upper limb	Carb-an., cupr., plb., thuj.
Emaciation	emaciation of affected parts	Ars., bry., carb-v., dulc., **Graph., Led.**, lyc., mez., nat-m., nit-ac., nux-v., ph-ac., phos., plb., **Puls., Sec.**, sel., sep., sil.
Emaciation	emaciation of back	Tab.
Emaciation	emaciation of buttocks (either of the two fleshy mounds above the legs and below the hollow of the back)	Bar-m., lach., nat-m., sacc.
Emaciation	emaciation of calf	Sel.
Emaciation	emaciation of certain parts	Bry., calc., caps., carb-v., con., dulc., graph., iod., led., mez., nat-m., nit-ac., ph-ac., sel., sil.
Emaciation	emaciation of cervical region	Calc., iod., lyc., Nat-m., sanic., sars.
Emaciation	emaciation of chest	Kali-i.
Emaciation	emaciation of diseased limb	Ars., bry., carb-v., dulc., graph., **Led.**, mez., nat-m., nit-ac., ph-ac., phos., **Plb., Puls.**, sec., sel., sep., sil.
Emaciation	emaciation of dorsal region	Plb.
Emaciation	emaciation of face	Acet-ac., agar., anac., ars-i., ars., bar-c., calc., chin-s., cupr., guai., hura., iod., kali-bi., kali-i., lac-d., merc-c., mez., naja., nat-c., nat-p., nux-m., plb., psor., sel., sep., sil., sulph., sumb., tab.
Emaciation	emaciation of face after neuralgia	Plb.
Emaciation	emaciation of face and hands	Grat., sel.
Emaciation	emaciation of fingers	Lach., sil., thuj.
Emaciation	emaciation of foot	Ars., **Caust.**, chin., nat-m., plb.
Emaciation	emaciation of forearm	Phos., **Plb.**

Body part/Disease	Symptom	Medicines
Emaciation	emaciation of gluteal muscle	Lath., plb.
Emaciation	emaciation of hand	Ars., chin., cupr., graph., phos., **Plb.**, **Sel.**
Emaciation	emaciation of hips (the area on each side of the body between the waist and the thigh)	Calc.
Emaciation	emaciation of index finger	Lach., thuj.
Emaciation	emaciation of leg	Abrot., apis., benz-ac., berb., bov., calc., caps., chin., nit-ac., **Nux-v.**, **Rhus-v.**, sarr., sel., syph., thuj.
Emaciation	emaciation of lower limbs	Abrot., am-m., apis., arg-m., arg-n., ars., berb., calc., chin., dulc., lath., nat-m., nit-ac., ph-ac., plb., sanic., sel.
Emaciation	emaciation of lumbar region	Plb., sel.
Emaciation	emaciation of mammae	Coff., nux-m.
Emaciation	emaciation of painful lower limb	Ol-j., plb.
Emaciation	emaciation of shoulder	Plb., sumb.
Emaciation	emaciation of thighs	Bar-m., calc., nit-ac., plb., sacc., sel.
Emaciation	emaciation of thumb	Thuj.
Emaciation	emaciation of tips of fingers	Ars.
Emaciation	emaciation of upper arm	Nit-ac., plb.
Emaciation	emaciation of wrist	**Plb.**
Emaciation	emaciation upwards	Abrot., arg-n.
Emaciation	emaciation with downward spreads	Lyc., nat-m., sars.
Emaciation	emaciation with insanity	Arn., ars., calc., chin., graph., lach., lyc., nat-m., nit-ac., nux-v., phos., puls., sil., sulph., verat.
Emaciation	enlarged abdomen of children with marasmus (a gradual wasting away of the body, generally associated with severe malnutrition or inadequate absorption of food and occurring mainly in young children)	Calc., sanic., sars.
Emaciation	marasmus (gradual wasting away of the body) of children	Abrot., alum., ant-c., arg-n., **Ars-i.**, **Ars.**, bar-c., **Calc-p.**, **Calc.**, carb-v., caust., chin., cina., hydr., **Iod.**, kali-c., kreos., lyc., mag-c., **Nat-m.**, nux-m., nux-v., ol-j., op., petr., phos., plb., psor., puls., sars., sep., **Sil.**, sulph.
Emaciation	tabes mesentrica (progressive wasting of the body, usually as a result of a chronic disease)	Ars-i., ars., aur-m., aur., bar-c., bar-i., bar-m., calc-p., calc-s., **Calc.**, carb-an., carb-s., caust., con., hep., iod., kreos., lyc., merc-i-f., merc., nat-s., ol-j., sulph., tub.
Emission	Aching in lumbar region after emissions	Ham.
Emission	anxiety after emissions	Carb-an., petr.
Emission	breathing difficult after emission	Phos., Staph.
Emission	burning pain in back after emission	Merc., phos.
Emission	burning pain in urethra after emission	Carb-an., carb-v., caust., cob., dig., merc., sep., sulph., thuj.
Emission	burning pain in urethra during emission	Ant-c., bor., clem., sars., sep., Sulph., thuj.
Emission	burning pain in urethra on waking after emission	Carb-an.
Emission	chill in morning after nightly emissions	Merc.
Emission	coldness in foot after emission	Aloe., nux-v.

Body part/Disease	Symptom	Medicines
Emission	coldness in hands after emission	Merc.
Emission	convulsion during emission of semen	Art-v., grat., nat-p.
Emission	emission of prostatic fluid after stool	Am-c., anac., calc., caust., cur., hep., iod., kali-c., lyss., nat-c., nit-ac., phos., sel., sep., sil., Sulph., zinc.
Emission	emission of prostatic fluid after urination	Anac., calc., cur., daph., hep., hipp., kali-c., lyc., lyss., nat-c., nat-m., sel., sep., sil., Sulph.
Emission	emission of prostatic fluid before urination	Psor.
Emission	emission of prostatic fluid during lascivious thoughts	Con., lyc., nat-m., Nit-ac., ph-ac., phos., pic-ac.
Emission	emission of prostatic fluid during urination	Anac., hep., nat-c., nit-ac., sep., sulph.
Emission	emission of prostatic fluid in drops	Phos., Sel.
Emission	emission of prostatic fluid while fondling women	Agn., Con.
Emission	emission of prostatic fluid while passing flatus	Con., mag-c.
Emission	emission of prostatic fluid while talking to young lady	Nat-m., phos.
Emission	emission of prostatic fluid while walking	Agn., Sel., sil.
Emission	emission of prostatic fluid with every emotion	Con., hep., puls., sel., zinc.
Emission	emission of prostatic fluid with stool	Agar., agn., alum., am-c., anac., ars., aur-m., calc., carb-v., carl., caust., Con., cor-r., elaps., hep., ign., iod., kali-bi., nat-c., nat-m., nat-p., nit-ac., Nux-v., petr., Ph-ac., phos., Sel., Sep., sil., staph., sulph., zinc.
Emission	emission of prostatic fluid without erection	Aur., bell., cann-s., con., eupho., lyc., lyss., nat-m., phos., Sel., thuj.
Emission	emmission of prostatic fluid after stool	Am-c., anac., calc., caust., cur., hep., iod., kali-c., lyss., nat-c., nit-ac., phos., sel., sep., sil., Sulph., zinc.
Emission	emmission of prostatic fluid after urination	Anac., calc., cur., daph., hep., hipp., kali-c., lyc., lyss., nat-c., nat-m., sel., sep., sil., Sulph.
Emission	emmission of prostatic fluid before urination	Psor.
Emission	emmission of prostatic fluid during erection	Nit-ac., Ph-ac., puls.
Emission	emmission of prostatic fluid during lascivious (showing a desire for, or unseemly interest in,sex) thoughts	Con., lyc., nat-m., Nit-ac., ph-ac., phos., pic-ac.
Emission	emmission of prostatic fluid during urination	Anac., hep., nat-c., nit-ac., sep., sulph.
Emission	emmission of prostatic fluid while passing flatus	Con., mag-c.
Emission	emmission of prostatic fluid while sitting	Sel.
Emission	emmission of prostatic fluid while talking to a young lady	Nat-m., phos.
Emission	emmission of prostatic fluid while thinking of a young lady	Nat-m.
Emission	emmission of prostatic fluid while walking	Agn., Sel., sil.
Emission	emmission of prostatic fluid with difficult stool	Agn., alum., am-c., anac., arn., cann-i., carb-v., con., gels., hep., nat-c., Nit-ac., Ph-ac., phos., psor., sep., Sil., staph., Sulph., zinc.
Emission	emmission of prostatic fluid with every emotion	Con., hep., puls., sel., zinc.
Emission	emmission of prostatic fluid with soft stool	Anac., sel.

Body part/Disease	Symptom	Medicines
Emission	emmission of prostatic fluid with stool	Agar., agn., alum., am-c., anac., ars., aur-m., calc., carb-v., carl., caust., Con., cor-r., elaps., hep., ign., iod., kali-bi., nat-c., nat-m., nat-p., nit-ac., Nux-v., petr., Ph-ac., phos., Sel., Sep., sil., staph., sulph., zinc.
Emission	emmission of prostatic fluid without erection	Aur., bell., cann-s., con., eupho., lyc., lyss., nat-m., phos., Sel., thuj.
Emission	faintness after emission	**Asaf.**, ph-ac.
Emission	feeling of insects crawling on skin after emission	Ph-ac.
Emission	formication after emission	Ph-ac.
Emission	heaviness in extremities after emission	Ph-ac., puls.
Emission	heaviness in left upper limbs after emission	Staph.
Emission	interrupted sleep after midnight after emissions	Petr.
Emission	itching in male genitalia all over the genital especially after emission	Ph-ac.
Emission	pain in back descends after emissions (a bodily discharge, especially of semen)	Ant-c., cob., kali-br., ph-ac., sars., staph.
Emission	pain in lumbar region down the spermatic cords (a cord by which a testis is suspended in the scrotum) after emission	Sars.
Emission	pain in sacral region after emission	Graph.
Emission	pain in thigh after emission	Agar.
Emission	pain in urethra from emissions	Cob., pip-m., sars.
Emission	palpitation of heart after emission	Asaf.
Emission	Paralytic sensation after emission	Sil.
Emission	perspiration after emissions	Calc., puls., sep., sulph.
Emission	perspiration on back after emission	Sil.
Emission	restless sleep after emission	Aloe.
Emission	trembling after emissions	**Nat-p.**
Emission	trembling in knee after emissions	Nat-p.
Emission	vision, blurred after emission	Calc., chin., lil-t., Phos.
Emission	weakness after emissions	Acet-ac., agar., aur., bar-c., calc., canth., carb-an., carl., chin., con., cupr., dig., gels., hydr., iod., kali-c., **Lyc.**, naja, nat-m., nat-p., **Nux-v.**, **Ph-ac.**, **Phos.**, pic-ac., plb., puls., sars., sel., sep., **Sil.**, stann., **Staph.**, ust.
Emission	weakness in back from emissions	Sel.
Emission	weakness in lumbar region after emissions	Ham., nat-p., phos.
Emission	weakness in thigh after emission	Agar., calc.
Emission	weakness in upper limbs after emissions	Staph.
Emphysema	emphysema (a chronic medical disorder of the lungs in which the air sacs are dilated or enlarged and lack flexibility, so that breathing is impaired and infection sometimes occurs) of chest	Am-c., Ant-a., Ant-t., ars., bell., brom., camph., carb-s., carb-v., chlor., cupr., cur., dig., dros., Hep., ip., lac-d., Lach., Lob., merc., nat-m., nit-ac., op., phel., phos., sars., seneg., sep., sulph., ter.
Emphysema	emptyness of abdomen, after breakfast	Am-m., coca., colch., dig., lyc., puls.
Emphysema	emptyness of abdomen, after dinner	Lyc., ptel., thea., zinc.

Body part/Disease	Symptom	Medicines
Emphysema	emptyness of abdomen, after nursing	Carb-an., olnd.
Emphysema	emptyness of abdomen, after siesta (afternoon rest)	Ang.
Emphysema	emptyness of abdomen, after stool	Aloe., ambr., dios., fl-ac., Petr., ph-ac., puls., sep., sulph.
Emphysema	emptyness of abdomen, after vomitting	Ther.
Emphysema	emptyness of abdomen, aggravated from inspiration	Calad.
Emphysema	emptyness of abdomen, ameliorated from eructations	Sep.
Emphysema	emptyness of abdomen, before sleep	Dig.
Emphysema	emptyness of abdomen, during fever	Zinc.
Emphysema	emptyness of abdomen, during headache	Cocc., nat-m., phos., ptel., sang., Sep.
Emphysema	emptyness of abdomen, during menses	Kali-p., spong., tab.
Emphysema	emptyness of abdomen, when thinking of food	Sep.
Emphysema	emptyness of abdomen, with aversion to food	Bar-c., carb-s., carb-v., chin., cocc., coff., dulc., grat., hell., hydr., nat-m., nux-v., rhus-t., sil., stann., sulph., verb.
Emphysema	emptyness of abdomen, with diarrhoea	Fl-ac., lyc., petr., stram., sulph.
Emphysema	emptyness of abdomen, without hunger	Act-sp., agar., alum., am-m., ars., bar-c., berb., bry., chin-s., chin., cocc., dulc., hell., kali-n., Lach., mur-ac., nat-m., nicc., olnd., op., phos., psor., rhus-t., sil., sul-ac., sulph., tax.
Encephalitis	encephalitis (Inflammation of brain)	Acon., apis., Bell., bry., cadm., camph., canth., cham., cina., con., crot-h., cupr., glon., hell., hyos., lach., merc., nux-v., op., par., phos., phys., plb., puls., rhus-t., stram., sulph., verat-v.
Encephalitis	encephalitis of meninges (protective spine or brain mebranes)	Acon., apis., arg-n., arn., Bell., bry., calc-p., calc., canth., cina., cocc., cupr., gels., glon., Hell., hippoz., hyos., kali-br., lach., merc., nat-m., op., phos., plb., rhus-t., sil., Stram., sulph., Zinc.
Encephalitis	encephalitis of meninges (protective spine or brain mebranes)	Acon., apis., arg-n., arn., Bell., bry., calc-p., calc., canth., cina., cocc., cupr., gels., glon., Hell., hippoz., hyos., kali-br., lach., merc., nat-m., op., phos., plb., rhus-t., sil., Stram., sulph., Zinc.
Encephalitis	encephalitis of periosteum (the sheath of connective tissue that surrounds all bones except those at joints)	Aur-m., aur., Fl-ac., kali-i., led., mang., merc-c., merc., Mez., nit-ac., Ph-ac., phos., puls., rhod., rhus-t., ruta., sil., staph.
Encephalitis	encephalitis with deep sleep or unconsciousness	Bor.
Encephalitis	tubercular (affected by tuberculosis) encephalitis	Calc., iod., lyc., merc., nat-m., sil., sulph., tub., zinc.
Endocardium	inflammation of endocardium (the thin membranous lining of the heart's cavities) rheumatic	Ars., aur-m., Aur., cact., dig., hyos., kali-n., Kalm., Lach., phos., plat., spig., spong., sumb., verat.
Endocardium	inflammation of endocardium with pain and great anxiety	Aur., kalm.
Endocardium	inflammation of endocardium with scanty menses	Nat-m.
Epilepsy	chill after epilepsy	Calc., **Cupr.**, sulph.

Body part/Disease	Symptom	Medicines
Epilepsy	chill left sided before epilepsy	Sil.
Epilepsy	clenching from epileptic covulsion	Lach., mag-p., oena.
Epilepsy	clenching thumbs in epilepsy	Bufo., caust., cic., lach., stann., staph., sulph.
Epilepsy	coldness in shoulder in epilepsy	Caust.
Epilepsy	coldness in shoulder in epilepsy extending to small of back	Kreos.
Epilepsy	coldness of skin on left side before epilepsy	Sil.
Epilepsy	constriction in heart before epilepsy	Calc-ar., lach.
Epilepsy	contraction of muscles & tendons of fingers in epilepsy	Lach., mag-p., merc.
Epilepsy	convulsion before epilepsy with sensation of expansion of body	Arg-n.
Epilepsy	convulsion epileptic from heart	**Calc-ar.**, lach., naja.
Epilepsy	convulsion epileptic from right heel to occiput	Stram.
Epilepsy	convulsion epileptic from solar plexus (a point on the upper abdomen just below where the ribs separate)	Art-v., bell., bufo., calc., caust., **Cic.**, cupr., indg., **Nux-v.**, sil., **Sulph.**
Epilepsy	convulsion epileptic in uterus to throat	Lach.
Epilepsy	convulsion epileptic in uterus	Bufo.
Epilepsy	convulsion epileptic knees	Cupr.
Epilepsy	convulsion epileptic like a mouse running	**Bell.**, **Calc.**, ign., nit-ac., *sil.*, *sulph.*
Epilepsy	convulsion epileptic with aura (warning sensation before epileptic episode) abdomen to head	Indg.
Epilepsy	convulsion epileptic with coldness running down spine	Ars.
Epilepsy	convulsion epileptic with drawing in limbs	Ars.
Epilepsy	convulsion epileptic with jerk in nape	Bufo.
Epilepsy	convulsion epileptic with nervous feeling	Arg-n., nat-m.
Epilepsy	convulsion epileptic with numbness of brain	Bufo.
Epilepsy	convulsion epileptic with sensation of cold air over spine and body	Agar.
Epilepsy	convulsion epileptic with shocks	Ars., laur.
Epilepsy	convulsion epileptic with warm air streaming up spine	Ars.
Epilepsy	convulsion epileptic with waving sensation in brain	Cimic.
Epilepsy	convulsion of upper limbs from epileptic starting	Sulph.
Epilepsy	convulsion on left side before epilepsy	Sil.
Epilepsy	convulsion with aura	Calc., lach., sulph.
Epilepsy	delirium after epilepsy	Arg-m., plb.
Epilepsy	delirium during epilepsy	Op.
Epilepsy	epileptic (periodic sudden loss or impairment of consciousness, often accompanied by convulsions) warning / force creeping down spine	Lach.
Epilepsy	epileptic aura (warning sensation before epileptic episode) from heel to occiput	Stram.

Body part/Disease	Symptom	Medicines
Epilepsy	epileptic in arm	Calc., lach., sulph.
Epilepsy	icy coldness running down back before epilepsy	Ars.
Epilepsy	jerking of fingers in epilepsy	**Cic.**
Epilepsy	numbness before epilepsy	Bufo.
Epilepsy	numbness in fingers during epileptic	Cupr.
Epilepsy	numbness in upper arm between attacks of epilepsy	Cupr.
Epilepsy	pain in heart at before epilepsy	Calc-ar., lyc.
Epilepsy	pain in left upper limb before epilepsy	Calc-ar.
Epilepsy	pain in upper limb before epilepsy	Calc-ar.
Epilepsy	palpitation of heart before epilepsy	Ars., calc-ar., calc., cupr., lach.
Epilepsy	retching before epilepsy	Cupr.
Epilepsy	sensation of mouse running up upper limbs before epilepsy	**Bell., Sulph.**
Epilepsy	shocks like electric before epilepsy	Ars.
Epilepsy	stiffness before epilepsy	Bufo.
Epilepsy	stiffness in lower limbs before epilepsy	Bufo.
Epilepsy	stiffness in right upper limbs before epilepsy	Bufo.
Epilepsy	sweating of scalp before epilepsy	Caust.
Epilepsy	trembling in upper limbs before epilepsy	Sil.
Epilepsy	urine copious with amenorrhoea after epilepsy	Cupr.
Epilepsy	weakness after epileptic convulsions	Camph.
Epistaxis	excessive flow of blood in brain at night with epistaxis	Ant-c., bell., bry., carb-v., croc., lach., lil-t., meli., nux-v., pic-ac., psor.
Epistaxis	inflammation in leg with epistaxis (Nose bleed)	Bor.
Epistaxis	pain in vagina after epistaxis	Calc-p.
Epistaxis	palpitation of heart with epistaxis	Graph.
Epistaxis	Stream of blood from chest to head like a gust of wind with epistaxis (bleeding from nose)	Mill.
Erection	Aching in lumbar region after violant erections	Mag-m.
Erection	burning pain in urethra after erection	Anag., cahin., calc-p., canth., carb-s., ferr-i., mag-m., mosch., nat-m., nit-ac.
Erection	chronic want of erection	Lyc.
Erection	contraction of urethra during erection	Canth.
Erection	emission of prostatic fluid during erection	Nit-ac., Ph-ac., puls.
Erection	emission of prostatic fluid without erection	Aur., bell., cann-s., con., eupho., lyc., lyss., nat-m., phos., Sel., thuj.
Erection	emmission of prostatic fluid during erection	Nit-ac., Ph-ac., puls.
Erection	erection after urinating	Aloe., form., lil-t., lith., nat-c., rhus-t.
Erection	erection during sleep	Aster., fl-ac., merc-c., nat-c., nux-v., op., rhod.
Erection	erection seldom during sleep	Aster., fl-ac., merc-c., nat-c., nux-v., op., rhod.
Erection	erection seldom during stool	Carl., ign., samb., thuj.

Body part/Disease	Symptom	Medicines
Erection	erection strong	Ars-i., Canth., cedr., cham., clem., corn., Fl-ac., graph., helon., lach., mag-m., merc-c., mez., nux-v., Phos., Pic-ac., puls., sabin., sep., tarax., zinc.
Erection	erection strong with pain in abdomen	Zinc.
Erection	erection without sexual desire	Agn., am-c., ambr., anac., arn., asc-t., bry., bufo., calad., calc-p., cann-i., cann-s., canth., carb-v., eug., eupho., fl-ac., graph., ham., hyos., iod., kali-c., kali-p., kalm., lyss., mag-s., nat-c., nat-m., nat-p., nit-ac., nux-v., ph-ac., phos., pic-ac., sel., sil., spig., sulph., tab., tarent.
Erection	erection, shortly after seminal discharge	Ph-ac., sulph.
Erection	expectoration bloody after violent erection	Nat-m.
Erection	formication during erection	Tarent.
Erection	haemorrhage from urethra during erection	Canth.
Erection	hemorrhage from urethra during erection	Canth.
Erection	itching in urethra during erections	Nux-v., sel.
Erection	pain in prostate gland during erection	Alum.
Erection	pain in spermatic cord after erection	Mag-m., nux-m., sars.
Erection	pain in urethra after erection	Cann-s.
Erection	pain in urethra during erection	Nit-ac.
Erection	seminal discharge without erection	Absin., arg-m., bell., bism., calad., carb-an., chin., Cob., con., Dios., ery-a., fl-ac., gels., Graph., ham., kali-p., mosch., nat-c., nat-m., nat-p., nuph., nux-v., op., ph-ac., phos., sabad., sars., sel., spig., sulph.
Erection	sleeplessness from erections	Sep.
Erection	want of erection after gonorrhoea	Agn., cob., cub., hydr., med., sulph., thuj.
Erection	weakness from erections	Aur., carb-s.
Eructation	air rushing in ear during eructation	Caust.
Eructation	air rushing out as if from ear during eructation	Chel.
Eructation	anxiety ameliorated after eructations	Kali-c., mag-m.
Eructation	asthmatic ameliorated from eructations	Carb-v., nux-v.
Eructation	breathing difficult ameliorated from eructations	Aur., Carb-v., nux-v.
Eructation	constriction in stomach in forenoon before eructations	Thuj.
Eructation	convulsion ameliorated from eructations	Kali-c.
Eructation	cough ameliorated from eructations	Sang.
Eructation	cough excited from eructations	Ambr., bar-c., lact-ac., sol-t-ae., staph.
Eructation	cramps in chest with eructations	Dig.
Eructation	diarrhoea ameliorated after eructations	Arg-n., carb-v., grat., hep., lyc.
Eructation	distension ameliorated by eructation (to expel stomach gases through the mouth)	Carb-v., sep., thuj.
Eructation	distesion of abdomen, ameliorated after eructations	Arg-n., Carb-v., mag-c., nat-s.
Eructation	distesion of abdomen, not ameliorated after eructations	Chin., echi., lyc.
Eructation	emptyness of abdomen, ameliorated from eructations	Sep.

Body part/Disease	Symptom	Medicines
Eructation	eructations on stooping	Cic., ip., phos.
Eructation	eructations after acids	Ph-ac., staph.
Eructation	eructations after beer	Ferr.
Eructation	eructations after bread	Bry., chin., crot-h., merc., nat-m.
Eructation	eructations after bread and milk	Zinc.
Eructation	eructations after breakfast	Ars., calc-p., carb-ac., cham., con., cycl., grat., hell., hyper., kali-br., phos., pic-ac., plat., sars., sep., sulph., verat.
Eructation	eructations after butter	Carb-v., Puls.
Eructation	eructations after cabbage	Mag-c.
Eructation	eructations after dinner	Agar., aloe., am-c., ang., apis., ars., bar-c., carl., coca., cycl., dig., fl-ac., ham., kreos., lach., lyc., mag-m., merc., nat-m., nicc., petr., rat., sars., sul-ac., sulph., zinc.
Eructation	eructations after fatty foods	Caust., ferr-m., ferr., Puls., Sep., thuj.
Eructation	eructations after meat	Ruta.
Eructation	eructations after milk	Alum., am-c., ant-t., calc., carb-ac., carb-s., carb-v., chin., cupr., iris., lyc., mag-c., nat-m., nat-s., petr., phos., sulph., zinc.
Eructation	eructations after pork	Psor.
Eructation	eructations after potato	Alum., gran.
Eructation	eructations after rich food	Bry., Carb-v., ferr., nat-m., Puls., sep., staph., thuj.
Eructation	eructations after soup	Alum., anac., carb-v., mag-c.
Eructation	eructations after starchy foods	Nat-c., sulph.
Eructation	eructations after stool	Aesc., anac., ars., bar-c., calc-s., cob., coloc., merc., sil.
Eructation	eructations after super	Alum., carb-v., chin-s., ferr., ham., lyc., sars., sep., sil., zinc.
Eructation	eructations after sweets	Arg-n., caust., raph., zinc.
Eructation	eructations after tiny oceon fish	Eupi.
Eructation	eructations after wine	Lyc.
Eructation	eructations alternates with hiccough	Agar., sep., wye.
Eructation	eructations alternates with yawning	Berb., lyc.
Eructation	eructations ameliorated after sleep	Chel., chin.
Eructation	eructations ameliorated on lying	Aeth., rhus-t.
Eructation	eructations ameliorated while walking	Lyc.
Eructation	eructations at daytime	Bry., Iod., petr.
Eructation	eructations at night	Ant-t., calc-s., calc., canth., carb-v., chel., crot-h., ham., kali-c., lyc., mang., merc., mur-ac., nux-v., ox-ac., phos., pip-m., Puls., sulph., tanac., ther.
Eructation	eructations before breakfast	Bov., ran-s.
Eructation	eructations before stool	Sumb.
Eructation	eructations bitter food comes up	Lyc., nat-s.
Eructation	eructations bloody	Merc-c., nux-v., phos., raph., sep.
Eructation	eructations burning	Caust., coff., crot-t., ferr., iod., lyc.

Body part/Disease	Symptom	Medicines
Eructation	eructations constant	Chel., con., cupr., nit-ac., sars., sulph.
Eructation	eructations during apyrexia	Am-c.
Eructation	eructations during breakfast	Ox-ac., zinc.
Eructation	eructations during stool	Cham., con., dulc., kali-c., merc., puls., ruta.
Eructation	eructations followed by pain in stomach	Con.
Eructation	eructations in evening	Abrot., alum., am-c., ambr., bell., calc., carb-v., caust., coc-c., con., crot-h., cupr., cycl., dros., eupi., fl-ac., gels., grat., ham., hyper., kali-bi., mag-c., mez., phos., Puls., ran-s., rhus-t., rumx., sars., sep., sil., sin-n., sol-t-ae., stram., sulph., verat., zinc., zing.
Eructation	eructations like spoiled eggs	Acon., agar., ant-t., Arn., brom., bufo., coff., dios., elaps., kali-c., mag-m., mag-s., petr., phos., podo., psor., ptel., rhus-t., sep., stann., sulph., valer.
Eructation	eructations on vomiting	Phyt.
Eructation	eructations painful	Anan., bry., carb-an., caust., Cham., con., nat-c., nux-v., ox-ac., par., phos., plb., sabad., sep.
Eructation	eructations tasting bitter after fatty foods	Ferr-m., ferr.
Eructation	eructations tasting bitter after potatoes	Alum.
Eructation	eructations tasting bitter after rich food	Ferr-m., ferr.
Eructation	eructations tasting bitter after sour food	Ph-ac.
Eructation	eructations tasting bitter after supper	Zinc.
Eructation	eructations tasting bitter during stool	Cham.
Eructation	eructations tasting bitter when stooping	Cast.
Eructation	eructations tasting bitter while fasting	Nux-v.
Eructation	eructations tasting like almond	Caust., laur.
Eructation	eructations tasting like apples	Agar.
Eructation	eructations while fasting	Acon., bov., cina., croc., nit-ac., nux-v., plat., valer.
Eructation	faintness after eructation	Nux-v.
Eructation	faintness ameliorated after eructation	Mag-m.
Eructation	fullness of stomach, ameliorated by eructation	Carb-v., euphr., iris., mag-c., nux-v., phos., sil.
Eructation	headache ameliorated by eructations	Bry., cinnb., gent-c., lach., sang.
Eructation	hiccough after eructations	Bry., cycl., til.
Eructation	nausea ameliorated during eructations	Agar., all-c., am-m., ant-t., camph., carb-s., caust., chel., cinnb., fago., glon., grat., kali-p., lac-c., lyc., mag-m., nicc., ol-an., osm., phos., rhod., rumx., sabad., sul-ac., verat-v.
Eructation	nausea during eructations	Coloc., crot-t., grat., kali-c., ptel.
Eructation	pain in abdomen aggravated by eructations	Cham., cocc., phos.
Eructation	pain in abdomen from suppressed eructations	Bar-c., con.
Eructation	pain in back ameliorated from erructation	Sep.
Eructation	pain in chest ameliorated from eructations	Bar-c., kali-c., lyc.
Eructation	pain in chest from eructations	Cocc., phos., staph.
Eructation	pain in region of heart ameliorated from eructations	Lyc.

Body part/Disease	Symptom	Medicines
Eructation	pain in uvula after eructations	Alum., sulph.
Eructation	palpitation of heart ameliorated from eructations	Aur., bar-c., carb-v.
Eructation	sensation of lump in abdomen ameliorated after eructation	Bar-c.
Eruption	anaesthesia in skin after suppressed eruption	Zinc.
Eruption	asthma alternating with eruptions	Calad., crot-t., hep., kalm., lach., mez., rhus-t., sulph.
Eruption	asthmatic after suppressed eruptions	Apis., ars., carb-v., dulc., ferr., hep., ip., psor., Puls., sec., sulph.
Eruption	asthmatic with face ache and disappearance of tetter (eruption) on face	Dulc.
Eruption	blueness of scrotum after eruption	Tep.
Eruption	breathing difficult from suppressed eruptions	Apis.
Eruption	breathing difficult with eruptive disease	Apis.
Eruption	burning eruption on head	Ars., bar-c., cic., graph., kali-bi., nit-ac., petr., sars., Sulph.
Eruption	catarrh go back from eruption	Sep.
Eruption	chorea from suppressed eruptions	Caust., **Sulph.**, zinc.
Eruption	comatose (coma) sleep after suppressed eruption	Zinc.
Eruption	convulsion from suppressed eruption	Agar., bry., calc., caust., cupr., stram., sulph., zinc.
Eruption	convulsion when eruptions fail to break out	Ant-t., **Cupr., Zinc.**
Eruption	convulsion when skin rash repelled or do not appear	Ant-t., bry., camph., cupr., gels., ip., stram., sulph., **Zinc.**
Eruption	copper colored eruptions	Calc.
Eruption	copper coloured eruption on clavicle (bone at front of human shoulder)	Stram.
Eruption	copper coloured eruption on head	Carb-an., lyc., sulph.
Eruption	coppery patches in chest	Stram.
Eruption	cough alternating with eruptions	Ars., crot-t., mez., psor., sulph.
Eruption	cough ameliorated by developing eruptions of measles	Cupr.
Eruption	cough from suppressed eruptions	Dulc.
Eruption	crusty, scabby , bloody eruption on head	Calc.
Eruption	desquamating (remove layer of skin) eruption on head	Calc., lach., merc-c., merc., mez., nat-m., Olnd., phos., staph.
Eruption	diarrhoea after suppressed eruptions	Bry., dulc., hep., lyc., mez., psor., Sulph., urt-u.
Eruption	diarrhoea alternating with erruptions	Calc-p., crot-t.
Eruption	dirty eruption on head	Psor., sulph., thuj.
Eruption	discolouration of face, blue spots following eruptions	Ant-t., ferr., Lach., thuj.
Eruption	dry eruption on head	Ars., calc., fl-ac., kali-ar., merc., mez., Psor., sep., sil., Sulph.
Eruption	eruption (rash or blemish on skin) with scales	Arn., kali-c.
Eruption	eruption between toes	Alum., petr.

Body part/Disease	Symptom	Medicines
Eruption	eruption crusty black on face	Ars.
Eruption	eruption crusty greenish yellow on face	Merc., petr.
Eruption	eruption crusty offensive on face	Merc., petr., Psor.
Eruption	eruption crusty serpiginous on face	Sulph.
Eruption	eruption crusty white on face	Mez.
Eruption	eruption crusty yellow on face	Ant-c., calc., cic., Dulc., hyper., merc., mez., ph-ac., sulph., viol-t.
Eruption	eruption desquamating on face	Apis., ars., bell., canth., chin-s., hydr., kali-ar., lach., merc., ol-an., phos., psor., puls., rhus-t., rhus-v., sulph., thuj.
Eruption	eruption in back of foot	Aster., bov., carb-o., caust., lach., led., med., merc., petr., psor., puls., sars., tarax., thuj., zinc.
Eruption	eruption in fingers	Arn., ars., bor., canth., caust., cist., cupr., cycl., fl-ac., graph., hep., kali-s., lach., mez., mur-ac., ph-ac., ran-b., rhus-t., rhus-v., sars., sep., sil., spig., sulph., tab., tarax., thuj.
Eruption	eruption in foot	Anan., ars., aster., bar-c., bov., calc., carb-o., caust., chin-s., con., croc., crot-c., elaps., genist., lach., med., mez., phos., rhus-t., rhus-v., sec., sep., stram., sulph.
Eruption	eruption in forearm aggravated from scratching	Mang., mez.
Eruption	eruption in hands	Alum., am-m., anag., ant-t., ars., bar-m., **Carb-v.**, cic., cist., clem., cocc., com., con., cop., dulc., **Graph.**, hep., kali-s., kalm., kreos., lach., **Lyc.**, med., merc., mez., mur-ac., nat-c., nat-m., nat-s., nit-ac., oena., petr., phos., psor., puls., rhus-t., rhus-v., ruta., sanic., sars., sel., sep., staph., still., sul-ac., sulph., zinc.
Eruption	eruption in knee	Anac., ant-c., arn., canth., carb-v., dulc., iod., lac-c., lach., merc., nat-m., nat-p., nux-v., ph-ac., phos., psor., rhus-t., sabad., samb., sars., sep., thuj.
Eruption	eruption in legs	Agar., alum., am-m., ars., arund., bov., bry., calc., caust., chin-s., chlor., cupr-ar., cupr., daph., fago., kali-ar., kali-bi., kali-br., kali-c., lach., merc., mez., murx., nat-c., nat-m., nit-ac., petr., ph-ac., podo., puls., rhus-t., rumx., sec., sep., staph., stram., sulph., thuj., zinc.
Eruption	eruption in legs bleeding after scratching	Cupr-ar.
Eruption	eruption in nates	Ant-c., bor., canth., caust., graph., mez., nat-c., nat-m., nux-v., sel., thuj., til.
Eruption	eruption in palm	Anag., arn., aur., crot-h., graph., kali-c., nat-s., sep., sulph.
Eruption	eruption in sole of foot	Anan., ars., bell., bry., bufo., chin-s., con., elaps., kali-bi., manc., nat-m., pip-m., sulph.
Eruption	eruption like fish scales in coccyx	Ars-i., mez.
Eruption	eruption on female gentialia with vesicles	Graph., lyc., nat-s., Rhus-t., sep., staph., sulph.
Eruption	eruption on head with cracks	Graph., petr.
Eruption	eruption on head with thick white pus beneath	Mez.
Eruption	Eruption on head, bleeding after scratching	Alum., ars., bov., calc., cupr-ar., dulc., lach., lyc., merc., nat-a., petr., psor., staph., Sulph.

Body part/Disease	Symptom	Medicines
Eruption	Eruption over margin of hair	Calc., nat-m., nit-ac., petr., sep., Sulph., tell.
Eruption	eruption over occiput	Caust., clem., lyc., nat-m., sil.
Eruption	eruption over temples	Dulc., mur-ac.
Eruption	eruption, burning in upper limbs	Con., merc., nat-c., **Rhus-t.**, spig.
Eruption	eruption, small red vesicles in upper limbs	Nat-m.
Eruption	eruption, urticaria after scratching in lower limbs	Clem., zinc.
Eruption	eruption, urticaria in lower limbs	Apis., calc., **Chlol.**, clem., kali-i., merc., plan., sulph., zinc.
Eruption	eruption, vesicles between second and third fingers	Sulph.
Eruption	eruption, vesicles yellow in back of hands	Arg-n.
Eruption	eruption, areola (dark area around nipple) red	Nat-m.
Eruption	eruption, between first and second fingers	Cic.
Eruption	eruption, between nates	Olnd.
Eruption	eruption, between second and third fingers	Sulph.
Eruption	eruption, between third and fourth fingers	Mag-c.
Eruption	eruption, black	Ars., sec.
Eruption	eruption, black blister in elbow	Ars.
Eruption	eruption, black blisters in legs	Ars.
Eruption	eruption, black blisters in thighs	Anthr.
Eruption	eruption, black in foot	Ars., sec.
Eruption	eruption, black in hands	Sec.
Eruption	eruption, black in upper limbs	Sec.
Eruption	eruption, black pustules in upper limbs	Anthr., ars., lach., sec.
Eruption	eruption, black vesicles discharging acrid serum in upper limbs	Rhus-t.
Eruption	eruption, black vesicles in elbow	Ars.
Eruption	eruption, black vesicles in foot	**Ars.**, nat-m.
Eruption	eruption, black vesicles in hands	Sec.
Eruption	eruption, black vesicles in thighs	Anthr.
Eruption	eruption, black vesicles in upper limbs	Ars.
Eruption	eruption, black vesicles periodical every 4 to 6 weeks in upper limbs	Sulph.
Eruption	eruption, black vesicles with itching in upper limbs	Daph.
Eruption	eruption, blebs (bubble like blister) in knee	Anthr.
Eruption	eruption, bleeding	Calc.
Eruption	eruption, bleeding after scratching	Cupr-ar.
Eruption	eruption, bleeding after scratching on upper limbs	Cupr-ar.
Eruption	eruption, bleeding in foot	Calc.
Eruption	eruption, bleeding in hands	Alum., lyc., merc., petr.
Eruption	eruption, blister (painful swelling on skin) in elbow	Crot-h.
Eruption	eruption, blisters	Ars.

Body part/Disease	Symptom	Medicines
Eruption	eruption, blisters after scratching in thighs	Lach.
Eruption	eruption, blisters forming scabs in wrists	Am-m.
Eruption	eruption, blisters in heels	Calc., caust., graph., lach., led., nat-c., nat-m., petr., phos., sep., sil.
Eruption	eruption, blisters in palm	Bufo., ran-b.
Eruption	eruption, blisters in sole of foot	Ars., calc.
Eruption	eruption, blisters in toes	Ars., nit-ac., ph-ac.
Eruption	eruption, blood blisters becoming gangrenous	Sec.
Eruption	eruption, blood boils in legs	Mag-c.
Eruption	eruption, blood boils in nates	Aur-m.
Eruption	eruption, blotches	Ant-c., aur., berb., carb-v., cimx., cocc., hura., lach., merc., mur-ac., nat-c., nat-m., sars., sulph., zinc.
Eruption	eruption, blotches in calf	Aur., carb-v., lach., merc., petr., phos., thuj.
Eruption	eruption, blotches in fingers	Ant-c., arg-n., ars., berb., caust., cocc., con., lach., led., nat-c., rhus-t., verat.
Eruption	eruption, blotches in foot	Ant-c., jug-r., kreos., lyc., sep., sulph.
Eruption	eruption, blotches in hands	Arg-n., ars., carb-an., indg., kali-chl., merc., rhus-t., rhus-v., sep., spig., stann., sulph., urt-u.
Eruption	eruption, blotches in knee	Ant-c., sulph.
Eruption	eruption, blotches in legs	Ant-c., arg-n., aur., carb-v., cocc., hura., jug-r., kreos., lact-ac., merc., nat-c., petr., phos., rhod., thuj.
Eruption	eruption, blotches in nates	Ant-c., bry., sars.
Eruption	eruption, blotches in thighs	Aur., carb-v., crot-h., merc., rhod., zinc.
Eruption	eruption, blotches in toes	Ant-c., lach., sulph., zinc.
Eruption	eruption, blotches in upper limbs	Cimx., hura., mur-ac., nat-m.
Eruption	eruption, blotches in wrists	Aur-m., carb-v., cocc.
Eruption	eruption, blue spots in thighs	Arn.
Eruption	eruption, bluish hard lump oozing with scabs in upper limbs	Calc-p.
Eruption	eruption, boils	All-c., am-c., apoc., ars., aur-m., bell., brom., calc., carb-s., clem., cob., elaps., graph., guare., **Hep.**, hyos., iris., kali-bi., kali-n., lyc., merc., mez., nat-m., nit-ac., nux-v., petr., ph-ac., psor., rat., rhus-t., rhus-v., sec., sep., stram., **Sulph.**, thuj.
Eruption	eruption, boils in ankle	Merc.
Eruption	eruption, boils in back of hands	Calc.
Eruption	eruption, boils in calf	Bell., **Sil.**
Eruption	eruption, boils in foot	Anan., calc., led., sars., sil., **Stram.**
Eruption	eruption, boils in forearm	Calc., carb-v., cob., iod., lach., lyc., mag-m., nat-s., petr., sil.
Eruption	eruption, boils in hands	Calc., coloc., iris., lach., led., lyc., psor.
Eruption	eruption, boils in heels	Calc., lach.
Eruption	eruption, boils in hips	Alum., am-c., bar-c., graph., hep., jug-r., lyc., nit-ac., ph-ac., rat., sabin.

Body part/Disease	Symptom	Medicines
Eruption	eruption, boils in knee	Am-c., calc., nat-m., nux-v.
Eruption	eruption, boils in legs	Anan., anthr., ars., calc., cast-eq., mag-c., nit-ac., nux-v., **Petr.**, **Rhus-t.**, sil.
Eruption	eruption, boils in nates	Agar., alum., am-c., aur-m., bar-c., bart., cadm., calad., graph., hep., indg., lyc., nit-ac., ph-ac., phos., plb., psor., rat., sabin., sars., sec., sep., sil., sulph., thuj.
Eruption	eruption, boils in right thigh	Calc., hell., kali-bi., kali-c., rhus-v.
Eruption	eruption, boils in shoulder	Am-c., am-m., bell., hydr., kali-n., nit-ac., ph-ac., sulph.
Eruption	eruption, boils in sole of foot	Rat.
Eruption	eruption, boils in thighs	Agar., all-s., alum., am-c., apoc., aur-m., bell., calc., carb-s., clem., cocc., hep., hyos., ign., kali-bi., lach., lyc., mag-c., nit-ac., nux-v., petr., ph-ac., phos., plb., rhus-v., sep., **Sil.**, thuj.
Eruption	eruption, boils in upper limbs	Aloe., am-c., ars., bar-c., bell., brom., calc., carb-an., carb-v., cob., coloc., elaps., graph., guare., iod., iris., kali-n., lyc., mag-m., mez., **Petr.**, ph-ac., **Rhus-t.**, sil., sulph., syph., zinc.
Eruption	eruption, boils in wrists	Iod., sanic.
Eruption	eruption, boils on ulnar side of palms	Coloc.
Eruption	eruption, bran (husks of cereal grain) like in upper limbs	Bor.
Eruption	eruption, brown in hands	Nat-m.
Eruption	eruption, brownish rash in thighs	Mez.
Eruption	eruption, burning after scratching in hands	Mez., **Staph.**
Eruption	eruption, burning after scratching in thighs	Til.
Eruption	eruption, burning after scratching	Staph., til.
Eruption	eruption, burning in foot	Bov., mez.
Eruption	eruption, burning in hands	Bufo., rhus-t.
Eruption	eruption, burning in hollow of knee	Merc.
Eruption	eruption, burning in knee	Nux-v.
Eruption	eruption, burning in legs	Lact-ac., rhus-t.
Eruption	eruption, burning in pimples when scratched in thighs	Staph., til.
Eruption	eruption, burning in thighs	Fago., til.
Eruption	eruption, burning on touch in hands	Canth., **Cic.**
Eruption	eruption, burning pimples in hands	Bov., rhus-t.
Eruption	eruption, burning pimples in thighs	Mang.
Eruption	eruption, burning vesicles between the fingers	Canth.
Eruption	eruption, burning vesicles in back of hands	Mez.
Eruption	eruption, burning vesicles in forearm	Sil.
Eruption	eruption, burning vesicles in hands	Canth., rhus-v.
Eruption	eruption, burning vesicles in lower limbs	Verat.
Eruption	eruption, burning vesicles in thighs	Verat.
Eruption	eruption, burning vesicles in wrists	Am-m., bufo., mez.

Body part/Disease	Symptom	Medicines
Eruption	eruption, burning	**Ars.**, bov., fago., lact-ac., **Merc.**, nux-v., **Rhus-t.**, til.
Eruption	eruption, chronic psoriasis in back of hands	Ars., aur., bar-c., **Graph.**, hep., lyc., maland., **Petr.**, phos., phyt., rhus-t., sars., sulph.
Eruption	eruption, confluent (place where two or more things meet)	Cop., phos., rhus-v.
Eruption	eruption, confluent in foot	Cop., rhus-v.
Eruption	eruption, confluent in upper limbs	Cop., phos.
Eruption	eruption, confluent in upper limbs	Cop., phos.
Eruption	eruption, copper coloured in back of hands	Psor.
Eruption	eruption, copper coloured in knee	Stram.
Eruption	eruption, copper coloured spot in palm	Cor-r.
Eruption	eruption, copper coloured spot in thighs	Mez.
Eruption	eruption, copper coloured spots in legs	Graph.
Eruption	eruption, coppery spots in foot	Graph.
Eruption	eruption, corroding (destroy progressively by chemical action) vesicles in sole of foot	Ars., sulph.
Eruption	eruption, corroding vesicles in nates	Bor.
Eruption	eruption, cracked in hands	Alum., lyc., merc., petr.
Eruption	eruption, cracked in upper limbs	Phos.
Eruption	eruption, cracked	Phos.
Eruption	eruption, cracks in back of hands	Merc.
Eruption	eruption, crusts (a dry hardened outer layer of blood, pus, or other bodily secretion that forms over a cut or sore) in bend of elbow	Cupr., mez., **Psor.**
Eruption	eruption, crusts in forearm	Mez.
Eruption	eruption, crusts in thighs	Anac., clem., graph., ph-ac.
Eruption	eruption, crusty & full of cracks in hands	Anthr., **Graph.**, petr., sanic.
Eruption	eruption, crusty in hollow of knee	Bov.
Eruption	eruption, crusty in knee	Psor., sil.
Eruption	eruption, denuded (remove covering) spots in legs	Calc.
Eruption	eruption, desquamating (remove a thin layer of skin, especially as a treatment for acne)	Agar., am-c., am-m., arn., ars., bar-c., calc., chin-s., crot-t., elaps., ferr., hydr., kreos., merc., **Mez.**, rhus-v., sep., sulph., thuj.
Eruption	eruption, desquamating dry on face	Ars., kali-i., led., lyc., psor., sep.
Eruption	eruption, desquamating in back of hands	Am-m., bar-c., calc., graph., merc.
Eruption	eruption, desquamating in heels	Elaps.
Eruption	eruption, desquamating in legs	Agar., carb-an., merc., sulph., thuj.
Eruption	eruption, desquamating in sole of foot	Ars., chin-s., elaps., manc., sulph.
Eruption	eruption, desquamating in upper limbs	Agar., am-c., am-m., arn., bar-c., calc., chin-s., crot-t., ferr., hydr., led., merc., **Mez.**, **Rhus-t.**, rhus-v., sep., sulph.
Eruption	eruption, desquamating in wrists	Rhus-v.
Eruption	eruption, desquamating thick whitish scales in upper limbs	Crot-t.

Body part/Disease	Symptom	Medicines
Eruption	eruption, desquamation between index finger and thumb	Am-m.
Eruption	eruption, desquamation between the fingers	Am-m.
Eruption	eruption, desquamation in calf	Mag-c.
Eruption	eruption, desquamation in elbow	Sulph.
Eruption	eruption, desquamation in foot	Chin-s., dulc., **Mez.**
Eruption	eruption, desquamation in joints	Phos.
Eruption	eruption, desquamation in shoulder	Ferr., merc.
Eruption	eruption, desquamation in thighs	Chin-s., crot-t., kreos., sulph.
Eruption	eruption, desquamation of palm	Am-c., arn., chin-s., hydr., sabad., sep., sulph.
Eruption	eruption, dry in ankle	Cact.
Eruption	eruption, dry in bend of elbow	Mez.
Eruption	eruption, dry in foot	Mez.
Eruption	eruption, dry in hands	Anag., bov., lyc., merc., psor.
Eruption	eruption, dry in hollow of knee	Bry., psor.
Eruption	eruption, dry in legs	Calc-p., clem., dol.
Eruption	eruption, dry in upper limbs	Dol., hyper., merc., **Psor.**
Eruption	eruption, dry in wrists	Merc., psor.
Eruption	eruption, dry tetter in palms	Caust., nat-s., sel., sulph.
Eruption	eruption, dry	Bry., merc.
Eruption	eruption, dry, furfuraceous in olecranon (Elbow bone)	Aster., sep.
Eruption	eruption, elevated & shiny in upper limbs	Crot-t.
Eruption	eruption, elevated bleeding after scratching in upper limbs	Cupr-ar.
Eruption	eruption, elevated in upper limbs	Alumn., anac., carb-v., cic., crot-h., crot-t., dros., graph., hep., kali-br., kreos., merc., nat-m., nit-ac., plb., sul-ac., urt-u.
Eruption	eruption, elevated in upper limbs exuding thin water	Crot-h.
Eruption	eruption, elevated in upper limbs exuding yellow water	Cupr., hell., rhus-t., sol-n.
Eruption	eruption, elevated red blotches in palms	Fl-ac.
Eruption	eruption, elevated spots in calf	Mag-c.
Eruption	eruption, elevated spots in legs	Syph.
Eruption	eruption, elevated white scabs in lower limbs	Mez.
Eruption	eruption, elevated with excoriation (tear somebody's skin off) in upper limbs	Arn., ruta., sul-ac.
Eruption	eruption, elevated with excrescences (growth that sticks out from the body) in upper limbs	Ars., lach., thuj.
Eruption	eruption, elevated with spots in upper limbs	Syph.
Eruption	eruption, elevated with whitish tips in upper limbs	Crot-t.
Eruption	eruption, elevations in back of foot	Petr., puls., thuj.

Body part/Disease	Symptom	Medicines
Eruption	eruption, elevations in elbow	Merc.
Eruption	eruption, elevations in foot	Cop.
Eruption	eruption, elevations in shoulder	Alumn.
Eruption	eruption, elevations itchy & scaly in elbow	Merc.
Eruption	eruption, erysipelatous vesicles in wrists	Rhus-t., rhus-v.
Eruption	eruption, erythematous (Redness of skin)	Ars., thuj.
Eruption	eruption, excoriation in nates	Rhus-t., thuj.
Eruption	eruption, excoriations in legs	Graph., tarent-c.
Eruption	eruption, excrescences	Ars., thuj.
Eruption	eruption, excrescences, wart-like in back of hands	**Thuj.**
Eruption	eruption, exuding	Crot-h., cupr., hell., kali-s., merc., nat-m., rhus-v., sol-n.
Eruption	eruption, exuding thin water	Crot-h., tarent-c.
Eruption	eruption, exuding yellow water	Cupr., hell., rhus-v., sol-n.
Eruption	eruption, fissures (a break in the skin lining the anal canal, usually causing pain during bowel movements and sometimes bleeding. Anal fissures occur as a consequence of constipation or sometimes of diarrhoea) in bend of elbow	Kali-ar.
Eruption	eruption, fissures in wrists	Kali-ar.
Eruption	eruption, flat pimples in thighs	Ant-c., plan.
Eruption	eruption, forearm moist	Alum., merc., mez., rhus-t.
Eruption	eruption, furfuraceous in hands	Alum.
Eruption	eruption, gradually reducing rash in thighs after scratching	Mez.
Eruption	eruption, greenish vesicles in knee	Iod.
Eruption	eruption, gritty (small pieces of sand or stone)	Nat-m.
Eruption	eruption, gritty in knee	Nat-m.
Eruption	eruption, hard in upper limbs	Caust., mez., sep., sil.
Eruption	eruption, hard pustules in wrists	Cocc.
Eruption	eruption, hard	Bov.
Eruption	eruption, herped in nates	Bor., caust., kreos., nat-c., nicc.
Eruption	eruption, herpes	Alum., bor., caust., com., con., cupr., dulc., graph., led., lyc., manc., mang., merc., mur-ac., nat-m., nicc., nux-v., petr., psor., sars., sec., sep., staph., thuj., zinc.
Eruption	eruption, herpes between index finger and thumb	Ambr.
Eruption	eruption, herpes between the fingers	Ambr., graph., merc., nit-ac.
Eruption	eruption, herpes between toes	Alum., graph.
Eruption	eruption, herpes in ankle	Cact., cycl., kreos., nat-c., nat-m., petr., sulph.
Eruption	eruption, herpes in back of hands	Carb-s., graph., lyc., nat-c., petr., sep., thuj.
Eruption	eruption, herpes in bend of elbow	Cupr., graph., kreos., **Nat-m.**, sep., thuj.
Eruption	eruption, herpes in calf	Cycl., lyc., sars.
Eruption	eruption, herpes in elbow	Bor., cact., **Cupr.**, hep., kreos., phos., psor., sep., staph., thuj.

Body part/Disease	Symptom	Medicines
Eruption	eruption, herpes in foot	**Alum.**, mez., nat-m., petr., **Sulph.**
Eruption	eruption, herpes in forearm	Alum., con., mag-s., mang., **Merc.**, nat-m., sulph.
Eruption	eruption, herpes in hands	Bor., bov., calc., cist., con., **Dulc.**, graph., kreos., merc., mez., nat-c., nat-m., ran-b., sars., sep., staph., verat., **Zinc.**
Eruption	eruption, herpes in hips	Nat-c., nicc., sep.
Eruption	eruption, herpes in hollow of knee	**Ars.**, calc., con., **Graph.**, kreos., led., nat-c., **Nat-m.**, petr., phos., psor., sulph.
Eruption	eruption, herpes in joints	Dulc., kreos., staph.
Eruption	eruption, herpes in knee	Ars., carb-v., dulc., graph., kreos., merc., nat-c., **Nat-m.**, petr., phos., sulph.
Eruption	eruption, herpes in legs	Ars., calc-p., calc., com., graph., kali-c., lach., lyc., lyss., mag-c., merc., nat-m., petr., sars., sep., staph., zinc.
Eruption	eruption, herpes in palms	Aur., kreos., psor., ran-b., sep.
Eruption	eruption, herpes in shoulder	Kali-ar.
Eruption	eruption, herpes in thighs	Clem., graph., kali-c., lyc., **Merc.**, mur-ac., **Nat-m.**, nit-ac., petr., sars., sep., staph., zinc.
Eruption	eruption, herpes in toes	Alum.
Eruption	eruption, herpes in upper limbs	Alum., bor., **Bov.**, calc., caust., con., cupr., dol., dulc., graph., kali-c., kreos., lyc., mag-s., manc., mang., **Merc.**, nat-c., nat-m., nux-v., phos., psor., sars., sec., sep., sil.
Eruption	eruption, herpes in wrists	Ip., merc., psor.
Eruption	eruption, herpes like ringworm in elbow	Cupr.
Eruption	eruption, herpes, crusty in upper limbs	Con., thuj.
Eruption	eruption, herpes, furfuraceous	Merc., phos.
Eruption	eruption, herpes, in the joints of upper limbs	Calc., merc.
Eruption	eruption, hot herpes in thighs	Fago.
Eruption	eruption, hot reddish knots in thighs	Kali-bi.
Eruption	eruption, hot	Fago.
Eruption	eruption, impetigo (contagious infection of the skin characterized by blisters that form yellow-brown scabs) in back of foot	Carb-s.
Eruption	eruption, in ankle	Cact., calc-p., calc., chel., osm., psor., puls., rhus-v., sel., sep., stront., tep.
Eruption	eruption, in back of hands	Berb., bov., chel., cupr., jug-r., kali-chl., kali-s., kreos., merc., mez., mur-ac., nat-c., phos., sanic., sep., **Sulph.**
Eruption	eruption, in back of hands in cold weather	Sep.
Eruption	eruption, in bend of elbow	Am-m., bry., calad., calc., cupr., graph., hep., merc., mez., nat-c., nat-m., psor., sep., staph., sulph.
Eruption	eruption, in calf	Apis., bell., caust., kali-ar., mag-c., petr., phyt., sars., sep., sil., thuj.
Eruption	eruption, in cluster (bunch) in upper limbs	Rhus-t.
Eruption	eruption, in elbow	Aster., berb., brom., cact., cupr., hep., iris., kali-s., kreos., lach., merc., phos., psor., sabin., sep., staph., sulph., tep., thuj., zinc.

Body part/Disease	Symptom	Medicines
Eruption	eruption, in forearm	Alum., ant-t., ars., bry., calad., carb-an., caust., cinnb., con., cupr., graph., mag-s., mang., merc., mez., phos., rhus-t., sel., spong., tarax., zinc.
Eruption	eruption, in group, in legs	Nat-m.
Eruption	eruption, in hands in cold weather	Sep.
Eruption	eruption, in hips	Nat-c., nicc., osm.
Eruption	eruption, in olecranon	Berb.
Eruption	eruption, in shoulder	Alumn., ars., nux-v., sep.
Eruption	eruption, in shoulder with black pores	Dros.
Eruption	eruption, in thighs	Agar., ars., aster., bar-m., calc., chin-s., crot-t., fago., graph., kali-ar., kali-bi., kali-c., kreos., merc., nat-c., nat-m., nit-ac., nux-v., osm., petr., phos., plan., psor., rhus-t., rhus-v., sil., staph., sulph., thuj., til.
Eruption	eruption, in toes	Am-c., crot-c., cupr-ar., cupr., graph., kali-bi., lach., med., nat-c., nit-ac., ph-ac., rhus-v., ruta., sil., sulph., zinc.
Eruption	eruption, in upper parts between nates	Hep.
Eruption	eruption, in wrists	Am-m., ant-c., ant-t., apis., ars-i., ars., calc., caust., cimic., crot-h., dros., eupho., hep., led., merc., mez., olnd., psor., rhus-t., sulph., tarax.
Eruption	eruption, inside thighs during menses	Sil.
Eruption	eruption, itching between the fingers	Canth., lyc., **Psor.**, **Sulph.**
Eruption	eruption, itching biting in foot	Calc.
Eruption	eruption, itching burning in foot	Bov., mez.
Eruption	eruption, itching burning rash in thighs during menses	Rhus-v.
Eruption	eruption, itching in back of foot	Aster., calc., lach., psor., tarax.
Eruption	eruption, itching in back of hands	Am-m., merc., mez., sanic., **Sulph.**
Eruption	eruption, itching in back of hands at night	Merc.
Eruption	eruption, itching in calf	Sil.
Eruption	eruption, itching in elbow	Merc., sep.
Eruption	eruption, itching in foot	Aster., bov., calc., con., mez., sep., sil.
Eruption	eruption, itching in forearm	Mez.
Eruption	eruption, itching in hands	**Carb-v.**, daph., graph., jug-r., mez., phos., psor., sanic., staph., urt-u., zinc.
Eruption	eruption, itching in hollow of knee	Agar., **Ars.**, bry., led., psor., zinc.
Eruption	eruption, itching in joints	Phos.
Eruption	eruption, itching in knee	Nat-m., nux-v.
Eruption	eruption, itching in legs	Arund., calc., carb-v., lact-ac., psor., puls., rhus-t., rumx.
Eruption	eruption, itching in nates	Calc-p., caust., graph., thuj., til.
Eruption	eruption, itching in thighs	Agar., carb-v., fago., merc., nat-m., sep., til.
Eruption	eruption, itching in upper limbs	Agar., anag., ant-c., ant-t., berb., bov., calad., carb-an., carb-v., caust., cupr., dulc., jug-c., kali-c., kali-chl., kali-i., kreos., lach., laur., led., lyc., mag-c., mag-s., mang., merc., mez., nat-m., nat-s., nux-v., phos., psor., puls., **Rhus-t.**, **Sep.**, spig., sulph., tab., til., urt-u., zinc.

Body part/Disease	Symptom	Medicines
Eruption	eruption, itching in wrists	Merc., mez., psor., rhus-t.
Eruption	eruption, itching like in upper limbs	Alum., berb., graph., lach., merc., nit-ac., phos., rhus-t., sars., sel., sep., sulph.
Eruption	eruption, itching pimples between index finger and thumb	Ars., sulph.
Eruption	eruption, itching pimples in back of hands	Am-m., zinc.
Eruption	eruption, itching pimples in hands	Acon., am-c., bov., kreos., lyc., sel., sulph.
Eruption	eruption, itching pimples in hands when becoming warm in bed	Mur-ac.
Eruption	eruption, itching pimples in legs	Asc-t., bell., elaps., kali-bi., sep., stront., ziz.
Eruption	eruption, itching pimples in nates	Kali-n., lyc., til.
Eruption	eruption, itching pimples in thighs	Asc-t., stann., staph., sulph., zinc.
Eruption	eruption, itching pustules in legs	Arg-n., asc-t.
Eruption	eruption, itching pustules in wrists	Cocc.
Eruption	eruption, itching rash in thighs worse after scratching	Mez.
Eruption	eruption, itching rash in wrists	Calad., led.
Eruption	eruption, itching vesicles between the fingers	Canth., psor., **Sulph.**
Eruption	eruption, itching vesicles in back of foot	Aster.
Eruption	eruption, itching vesicles in back of hands	Cic., kali-chl., **Mez.**, phos.
Eruption	eruption, itching vesicles in hands	**Carb-ac.**
Eruption	eruption, itching vesicles in knee	Carb-v.
Eruption	eruption, itching vesicles in lower limbs	Calc., carb-v.
Eruption	eruption, itching vesicles in palms	Kali-c., rhus-t.
Eruption	eruption, itching vesicles in thighs	Aster., clem.
Eruption	eruption, itching vesicles in wrists	Am-m., bufo., calc-p., kali-i., nat-m.
Eruption	eruption, itching	Agar., arg-n., bov., bry., calc., fago., gent., lach., lact-ac., led., mag-s., merc., nat-m., nux-v., phos., puls., rhus-t., rumx., sep., sulph., tarax., til., urt-u.
Eruption	eruption, knots in nates	Ther.
Eruption	eruption, large blood boils in shoulder	Calc., jug-r., lyc., zinc.
Eruption	eruption, large patches in legs	Caust.
Eruption	eruption, large pustules in upper limbs	Sep.
Eruption	eruption, large vesicles in palms	Anthr.
Eruption	eruption, leprous (affecting the skin and nerves that can cause tissue change and, in severe cases, loss of sensation and disfigurement. Leprosy is transmitted following close personal contact and has an incubation period of 1-30 years. It can now be cured if treated with a combination of drugs) in upper limbs	Meph., phos.
Eruption	eruption, leprous spots annular (shaped like ring) in nates	Graph.
Eruption	eruption, leprous spots in legs	Graph., nat-c.

Body part/Disease	Symptom	Medicines
Eruption	eruption, like chicken pox in upper limbs	Led.
Eruption	eruption, like flea (small wingless insect that sucks blood and lives as a parasite on warm-blooded animals) bite	Sec.
Eruption	eruption, like flee (small wingless insect that sucks blood and lives as a parasite on warm-blooded animals)bite in foot	Sec.
Eruption	eruption, like measles	Cop., rhus-t.
Eruption	eruption, like nodules in upper limbs	Hippoz., petr., sep.
Eruption	eruption, like varicella (chicken pox) in lower limbs	Ant-t.
Eruption	eruption, like varicella in legs	Ant-t.
Eruption	eruption, lumps in calf	Nit-ac.
Eruption	eruption, lumps in upper limbs	Phos.
Eruption	eruption, lumps, hard , bluish, oozing & scabbing in upper limbs	Calc-p.
Eruption	eruption, malleolus (either of the hammer-shaped bony protuberances at the sides of the ankle joint) in ankle	Cact.
Eruption	eruption, measles like in upper limbs	Cop., rhus-v.
Eruption	eruption, measles-like in back of hands	Cop.
Eruption	eruption, miliary in foot	Ars.
Eruption	eruption, miliary in foot	Ars.
Eruption	eruption, miliary in upper limbs	Alum., ant-t., bry., cop., merc., nux-v., rhus-v., sel., sulph.
Eruption	eruption, miliary in upper limbs	Alum., ant-t., bry., cop., merc., nux-v., rhus-v., sel., sulph.
Eruption	eruption, millet seed-like in hands	Bar-m.
Eruption	eruption, moist	Bry., merc., nat-m.
Eruption	eruption, moist between the fingers	Graph.
Eruption	eruption, moist in back of hands	Bov., kreos., mez.
Eruption	eruption, moist in hands	Clem., kali-c., kali-s., mang., merc., mez., petr., ran-s., rhus-t.
Eruption	eruption, moist in upper limbs	Alum., bov., con., kreos., rhus-t.
Eruption	eruption, moist pimples in legs	Puls.
Eruption	eruption, moist vesicles in back of hands	Mez.
Eruption	eruption, moist with purulent discharge in upper limbs	Lyc., rhus-t.
Eruption	eruption, moistness in ankle	Chel.
Eruption	eruption, moistness in hollow of knee	Graph., **Merc.**, **Sep.**
Eruption	eruption, moistness in legs	Apis., bry., calc., graph., merc., petr., rhus-t., tarent-c.
Eruption	eruption, moistness in thighs	Crot-t., merc., nat-m.
Eruption	eruption, moisture between nates	Arum-t., thuj.
Eruption	eruption, nodes in foot	Ang.

Body part/Disease	Symptom	Medicines
Eruption	eruption, nodules (Cell or tissue mass) in back of foot	Petr.
Eruption	eruption, nodules in elbow	Eupi., mur-ac.
Eruption	eruption, nodules in forearm	Hippoz.
Eruption	eruption, nodules in hands	Petr., sep.
Eruption	eruption, nodules in legs	Agar., merc.
Eruption	eruption, over margin of hair from ear to ear posteriorly	Nat-m., nit-ac., petr., Sulph.
Eruption	eruption, painful	**Arn.,** bov., hep., merc.
Eruption	eruption, painful in back of foot	Bov., psor.
Eruption	eruption, painful in bend of elbow	Am-m., ant-c., dros., dulc., hura., lachn., nat-c., ol-an., phos., rhus-t., sep.
Eruption	eruption, painful in elbow	Merc.
Eruption	eruption, painful in foot	Lyc., phos., spig., sulph.
Eruption	eruption, painful in knee	Arn.
Eruption	eruption, painful in nates	Graph.
Eruption	eruption, painful in upper limbs	Ars., kali-c., lyc., merc., petr.
Eruption	eruption, patches in ankle	Calc.
Eruption	eruption, pemphigus (an autoimmune disease characterized by large blisters on the skin and mucous membranes, often accompanied by itching or burning sensations) in upper limbs	Sep., ter.
Eruption	eruption, pemphigus in back of hands	Sep.
Eruption	eruption, pemphigus in wrists	Sep.
Eruption	eruption, petechia (a tiny purplish red spot on the skin caused by the release into the skin of a very small quantity of blood from a capillary) in back of hands	Berb.
Eruption	eruption, petechia in legs	Am-m., phos.
Eruption	eruption, petechia in thighs	Ars.
Eruption	eruption, petechiæ in upper limbs	Berb.
Eruption	eruption, pimples in upper limbs during menses	Sulph.
Eruption	eruption, pimples itching after scratching in thighs	Mag-c.
Eruption	eruption, purple in hands	Petr.
Eruption	eruption, rash in upper limbs	Alum., ant-t., bell., berb., bry., calad., chlol., cupr., daph., dig., elaps., form., kali-ar., led., mag-p., merc., mez., nux-v., phyt., puls., rheum., rhus-t., sec., sep., sil., stram., sul-i., sulph., tep.
Eruption	eruption, raw in forearm	Petr., rhus-t.
Eruption	eruption, rawness in hands	Petr., sulph.
Eruption	eruption, red areola in thighs	Nat-m.
Eruption	eruption, red in ankle	Calc., chel., sars.
Eruption	eruption, red in back of hands	Jug-r.
Eruption	eruption, red in bend of elbow	Cor-r., rhus-t.

Body part/Disease	Symptom	Medicines
Eruption	eruption, red in calf	Mag-c.
Eruption	eruption, red in elbow	Cinnb., rhus-t.
Eruption	eruption, red in foot	Bov., crot-c.
Eruption	eruption, red in forearm	Petr.
Eruption	eruption, red in hands	Bell., berb., bov., canth., carb-an., cic., cycl., jug-r., lyc., merc., ran-s., spig., spong., sul-ac., sulph., verat.
Eruption	eruption, red in hollow of knee	Merc., nat-m.
Eruption	eruption, red in legs	Bell., kali-bi., merc., sulph.
Eruption	eruption, red in lower limbs	Bell., bov., chel., crot-c., kali-bi., mag-c., merc., nat-m., rhus-v.
Eruption	eruption, red in thighs	Merc., rhus-v.
Eruption	eruption, red patches in back of hands	Calc.
Eruption	eruption, red patches in legs	Calc., sil., sul-ac.
Eruption	eruption, red patches in thighs	Calc.
Eruption	eruption, red pimples in hands	Acon., anac., ars., bov., sulph., til.
Eruption	eruption, red pimples in legs	Ir-f., kali-chl., rumx.
Eruption	eruption, red pimples in thighs	Asc-t., chel., clem., graph., kali-c., sars., sulph., thea., til.
Eruption	eruption, red pustules in lower limbs	Lyc., mez.
Eruption	eruption, red spots in calf	Con., lyc., phyt.
Eruption	eruption, red spots in palms	Apis.
Eruption	eruption, red	Bell., bov., chlol., crot-c., gins., jug-r., kali-bi., mag-s., merc., nat-m., rhus-v., valer.
Eruption	eruption, roseola (red rash on the skin, seen in diseases such as measles, scarlet fever, and syphilis) after abuse of mercury	Kali-i.
Eruption	eruption, rough	Rhus-v.
Eruption	eruption, rough in lower limbs	Rhus-v.
Eruption	eruption, rough in thighs	Kreos., rhus-v.
Eruption	eruption, scales (thin flat piece or flake of something such as dead skin)	Arn., ars-i., kali-s., merc., mez., phos., pip-m., rhus-t., rhus-v., sec., sulph., zinc.
Eruption	eruption, scales fall off on scratching in upper limbs	Sulph.
Eruption	eruption, scales in hands	Anac., anthr., arn., clem., graph., hep., merc., mur-ac., petr., psor., sars., sec., sep.
Eruption	eruption, scales in hands worse in winter	Petr., sep.
Eruption	eruption, scales in lower limbs	Calc-p., clem., kali-ar., kali-s., pip-m., rhus-v.
Eruption	eruption, scales in palms	Hep., lyc., nat-s., petr., pip-m., rhus-t., sabad., sars., sel., sep., sulph.
Eruption	eruption, scales in sole of foot	Pip-m.
Eruption	eruption, scales in spots in lower limbs	Merc., zinc.
Eruption	eruption, scales in spots in upper limbs	Merc.
Eruption	eruption, scales in upper limbs	Agar., anthr., arn., **Ars.**, berb., cupr., fl-ac., iris., kali-s., merc., phos., pip-m., puls., rhus-t., sec., sil., sulph.

Body part/Disease	Symptom	Medicines
Eruption	eruption, scaly between the fingers	Laur.
Eruption	eruption, scaly in back of foot	Psor.
Eruption	eruption, scaly in back of hands	Lyc., sars., sep., sulph.
Eruption	eruption, scaly in elbow	Calc., jug-r., kali-s., merc., sep., staph., sulph.
Eruption	eruption, scaly in foot	Rhus-v.
Eruption	eruption, scaly in forearm	Alum., merc., petr.
Eruption	eruption, scaly in knee	Hydr.
Eruption	eruption, scaly in thighs	Mez.
Eruption	eruption, scaly in wrists	Ars-i., merc., rhus-t.
Eruption	eruption, scurfy (thin dry flaking scales of skin, usually as a result of a skin condition such as dandruff) brownish in upper limbs	Am-m., cinnb.
Eruption	eruption, scurfy brownish	Am-m., bar-m., cinnb., merc.
Eruption	eruption, scurfy in foot	Sil.
Eruption	eruption, scurfy in hands	Sars., sep.
Eruption	eruption, scurfy in legs	Ars., calc., kali-bi., sabin., sep., staph., zinc.
Eruption	eruption, scurfy in lower limbs	Bar-m., merc., petr.
Eruption	eruption, scurfy in nates	Calc-p.
Eruption	eruption, scurfy in spots in lower limbs	Merc.
Eruption	eruption, scurfy in spots in thighs	Merc.
Eruption	eruption, scurfy in thighs	Bar-m., merc., mez.
Eruption	eruption, scurfy tetters in palms	Cinnb., lyc., nat-s., sulph.
Eruption	eruption, smarting (stinging) in upper limbs	Anag., hyper., urt-u.,Mag-c., puls.
Eruption	eruption, smooth spots in palms	Cor-r.
Eruption	eruption, sore in hollow of knee	Merc.
Eruption	eruption, sore in lower limbs	Merc.
Eruption	eruption, soreness between toes	Berb., carb-an., graph., lyc., merc-i-r., mez., nat-c., ph-ac., ran-b.
Eruption	eruption, spots in ankle	Puls.
Eruption	eruption, spots in hollow of knee	Petr.
Eruption	eruption, spots in wrists	Apis., calc., dros., jac-c., merc.
Eruption	eruption, spots like a burn in lower limbs	Lach.
Eruption	eruption, spreading vesicles in sole of foot	**Ars.**, calc.
Eruption	eruption, spreading vesicles in toes	Graph., nit-ac.
Eruption	eruption, stinging in lower limbs	Ant-c., nux-v., petr., sabin.
Eruption	eruption, stinging vesicles in forearm	Rhus-t.
Eruption	eruption, stinging vesicles in knee	Rhus-t.
Eruption	eruption, suppurating (Oozing pus) in elbow	Sulph.
Eruption	eruption, suppurating vesicles in elbow	Sulph.
Eruption	eruption, suppurating vesicles in foot	Con., graph., nat-c., sel.
Eruption	eruption, syphilitic psoriasis in back of hands	Ars., aur., merc., phos.

Body part/Disease	Symptom	Medicines
Eruption	eruption, syphilitic psoriasis in palms	Ars-i., ars., aur., merc., phos., sel.
Eruption	eruption, transparent vesicles in forearm	Rhus-t.
Eruption	eruption, transparent vesicles in palms	Merc.
Eruption	eruption, tubercle (small rounded swelling on the skin or on a mucous membrane) in elbow	Am-c., caust., mag-c., mur-ac.
Eruption	eruption, tubercles	Ant-c., caust., crot-h., nat-c.
Eruption	eruption, tubercles in calf	Petr.
Eruption	eruption, tubercles in foot	Carb-an., rhus-t.
Eruption	eruption, tubercles in forearm	Agar., am-c., jug-r., kali-n., lach., mur-ac., ph-ac.
Eruption	eruption, tubercles in hands	Ars., carb-an., hydrc., kali-chl., merc., nit-ac., rhus-t., rhus-v., sep., spig., stram.
Eruption	eruption, tubercles in hips	Rat., rhus-t.
Eruption	eruption, tubercles in legs	Ant-c., caust., crot-h., nat-c., petr.
Eruption	eruption, tubercles in nates	Hep., mang., phos.
Eruption	eruption, tubercles in shoulder	Crot-h., kali-chl., phos., rhus-t.
Eruption	eruption, tubercles in thighs	Nat-c.
Eruption	eruption, tubercles in upper limbs	Ars., crot-h., nat-c., phyt., rhus-t.
Eruption	eruption, tubercles in wrists	Am-c., crot-h., mag-c.
Eruption	eruption, tubercles painful in upper limbs	Ars.
Eruption	eruption, tubercles ulcerating in upper limbs	Nat-c.
Eruption	eruption, ulcerated in heels	Nat-c.
Eruption	eruption, ulcerating in lower limbs	Ph-ac.
Eruption	eruption, ulcerating vesicles in sole of foot	**Ars.**, calc., psor., sulph.
Eruption	eruption, ulcerative tubercles in legs	Nat-c.
Eruption	eruption, ulcerative vesicles in back of foot	Zinc.
Eruption	eruption, watery in hands	Rhus-t.
Eruption	eruption, white in legs	Agar.
Eruption	eruption, white nodes in calf	Thuj.
Eruption	eruption, white pimples in legs	Staph.
Eruption	eruption, white pimples in thighs	Plan.
Eruption	eruption, white scales in hands	Graph., sep.
Eruption	eruption, white spots in legs	Calc.
Eruption	eruption, with brownish scurfs in wrists	Am-m.
Eruption	eruption, with burning in wrists	Merc.
Eruption	eruption, with crusts in wrists	Mez.
Eruption	eruption, with desquamation in hands	All-s., alum., am-c., am-m., bar-c., ferr., graph., laur., merc., mez., nat-m., ph-ac., phos., rhus-t., sep., sulph.
Eruption	eruption, with exudation in bend of elbow	Sulph.
Eruption	eruption, with hard reddish knots	Kali-bi.
Eruption	eruption, with nodules	Petr., sep.
Eruption	eruption, with patches	Carb-v., iris., jug-c., phos., puls., sars., thuj., viol-t.

Body part/Disease	Symptom	Medicines
Eruption	eruption, with petechiæ (a small red or purple spot on the skin caused by minor bleed from tiny blood vessels	Ars., aur-m., berb.
Eruption	eruption, with purulent discharge in forearm	Rhus-t.
Eruption	eruption, with white scales in forearm	Merc.
Eruption	eruption, with white scales in forearm smelling like cheese	Calc.
Eruption	eruption, with yellow exudation in hands	Rhus-v.
Eruption	eruption, with yellow scales in forearm	Rhus-t.
Eruption	eruption, yellow crusts in back of hands	Merc., mez.
Eruption	eruption, yellow vesicles in palms	Anthr., bufo., rhus-t., rhus-v.
Eruption	eruption, yellowish vesicles in elbow	Sulph.
Eruption	eruptions pimples itching when warm	Caust., sars., tell., til.
Eruption	eruptions (rash or blemish) burning at night	Ars., caust., merc., **Rhus-t.**, staph., til.
Eruption	eruptions (rash or blemish) carbuncle stinging	**Apis.**, carb-an., nit-ac.
Eruption	eruptions (rash or blemish) from rhus poisoning	Agar., am-c., **Anan.**, arn., bry., **Crot-t.**, cupr., graph., grin., kali-s., led., lob., nuph., plan., sang., sep., sulph.
Eruption	eruptions after scratching	Agar., alum., **Am-c.**, am-m., ant-c., arn., ars., bar-c., bell., bov., bry., calc., canth., carb-an., carb-s., carb-v., **Caust.**, chin., cic., con., cycl., dulc., eupho., graph., hell., hep., ip., kali-c., kali-s., kreos., lach., laur., **Lyc.**, mag-c., merc., mez., nat-c., nat-m., nit-ac., nux-v., olnd., petr., ph-ac., phos., plb., puls., rhod., **Rhus-t.**, sabin., sars., sep., sil., spong., squil., staph., stront., sul-ac., **Sulph.**, thuj., verat., viol-t., zinc.
Eruption	eruptions around cervical region	Agar., ant-c., ant-s., ars., bar-m., bell., berb., bry., caust., cham., chel., clem., graph., hep., kali-bi., lyc., mang., nat-a., nat-m., petr., psor., rhus-t., sec., sep., Sil., staph., stram., sulph., thuj.
Eruption	eruptions around cervical region in margins of hair	Nat-m., petr.
Eruption	eruptions around coccyx	Bor., graph., merc.
Eruption	eruptions around lumbar region	Arund., rhus-t.
Eruption	eruptions around mouth	Agar., am-c., anac., Ant-t., Ars., bell., bor., bov., cadm., calc-f., calc., carb-s., carb-v., caust., cham., chel., chin-s., Graph., hell., hep., hydr., hyper., ign., kali-ar., kali-bi., kali-c., Kali-chl., kali-i., Kreos., lach., laur., led., lyc., mag-c., mag-m., mang., merc-c., merc., mez., mur-ac., Nat-a., Nat-c., Nat-m., nat-p., nat-s., Nit-ac., nux-v., par., petr., phos., Rhus-t., rhus-v., Sep., sil., Staph., Sulph., tarax., zinc.
Eruption	eruptions around nose	Alum., am-c., ant-c., bar-c., calc., caust., dulc., elaps., mag-m., nat-c., par., Rhus-t., sep., sil., sul-ac., sulph., tarax., zinc.
Eruption	eruptions black pimples	Carb-v., spig.
Eruption	eruptions blackish	Ant-c., **Ars.**, asaf., bell., bry., chin., con., crot-h., hyos., lach., mur-ac., nit-ac., ran-b., rhus-t., sec., sep., sil., spig., still., vip.

Body part/Disease	Symptom	Medicines
Eruption	eruptions bleeding	Alum., ant-t., apis., ars., calc., dulc., eupho., hep., kali-ar., kali-c., kali-n., lach., lyc., med., merc-c., **Merc.**, nit-ac., olnd., par., petr., psor., sep., **Sulph.**
Eruption	eruptions bleeding after scratching	Alum., ars., bov., calc., chin., cocc., cupr-ar., dulc., lach., lyc., nux-v., petr., psor., **Sulph.**, til.
Eruption	eruptions blisters (छाला) as from a burn	Ambr., aur., bell., canth., carb-an., clem., lyc., nat-c., phos., sep., sulph.
Eruption	eruptions blotches (छाला)	Anac., ant-c., arn., ars., asaf., bar-c., bell., berb., bry., calc., caps., chel., chlol., cocc., coff., con., croc., crot-h., crot-t., dulc., fl-ac., hell., hep., hyos., ign., kali-c., kreos., lach., led., lyc., mag-c., mang., merc., nat-c., nat-m., nit-ac., nux-v., op., petr., ph-ac., phos., puls., rhus-t., rhus-v., ruta., sabin., sars., sec., sel., sep., sil., spig., squil., staph., stram., sul-ac., sulph., valer., verat., vip.
Eruption	eruptions blotches after scratching	Kali-c., lach., lyc., merc., nat-c., nit-ac., op., rhus-t., spig., verat., zinc.
Eruption	eruptions blotches indurated	Am-m., phos., sars.
Eruption	eruptions blotches inflammed	Hep., mang., merc., phos., sil.
Eruption	eruptions blotches itching & oozing	**Graph.**
Eruption	eruptions blotches red	Arg-n., carb-v., crot-t., fl-ac., merc., mur-ac., op., phos., urt-u.
Eruption	eruptions blotches red & desquamating	Fl-ac.
Eruption	eruptions blotches red & elevated	Fl-ac., rhus-t.
Eruption	eruptions blotches stinging	Petr., sars., stram., zinc.
Eruption	eruptions blotches watey	Graph., mag-c.
Eruption	eruptions blotches yellow	Ant-c., sulph.
Eruption	eruptions blue dark	Ail., arg-n., crot-h., lach., ran-b., sars., sulph.
Eruption	eruptions boils at injured places	Dulc.
Eruption	eruptions boils in the spring	Bell., crot-h., lach.
Eruption	eruptions boils maturing slowly	Hep., sil., sulph.
Eruption	eruptions boils stinging when touched	Mur-ac., sil.
Eruption	eruptions boils with greenish pus	Sec.
Eruption	eruptions brownish	Anag., dulc., nit-ac., ph-ac., phos.
Eruption	eruptions burning	Agar., alum., am-c., am-m., ambr., anac., ant-c., ant-t., **Apis.**, arg-m., **Ars.**, aur., bar-c., bell., berb., bov., bry., bufo., calad., calc-s., calc., cann-s., canth., caps., **Carb-ac.**, carb-an., carb-s., carb-v., **Caust.**, chin-a., chin., **Cic.**, clem., cocc., coff., colch., com., con., crot-t., cub., dig., dulc., eupho., **Graph.**, guai., hell., hep., ign., kali-ar., kali-bi., kali-c., kali-i., kali-n., kali-s., kreos., lach., laur., led., lyc., mang., **Merc.**, mez., nat-a., nat-c., nat-m., nat-p., nit-ac., nux-v., olnd., par., petr., ph-ac., phos., plat., plb., psor., puls., ran-b., **Rhus-t.**, sabad., sars., seneg., sep., sil., spig., spong., squil., stann., staph., stram., stront., sulph., teucr., thuj., urt-u., verat., viol-o., viol-t., zinc.
Eruption	eruptions burning aggravated from touch	Cann-s., canth., merc.

Body part/Disease	Symptom	Medicines
Eruption	eruptions burning ameliorated after scratching	Kali-n.
Eruption	eruptions burning in open air	Led.
Eruption	eruptions burning pocks	**Ars.**, lach., merc.
Eruption	eruptions burning when washing	Merc.
Eruption	eruptions burning when washing in cold water	Clem., thuj.
Eruption	eruptions carbuncle	Agar., ant-t., anthr., apis., arn., **Ars.**, **Bell.**, bufo., caps., carb-an., coloc., crot-c., crot-h., echi., hep., hyos., lach., mur-ac., nit-ac., phyt., pic-ac., rhus-t., sec., **Sil.**, sulph., tarent-c.
Eruption	eruptions carbuncle after abuse of mercury	**Kali-i.**
Eruption	eruptions carbuncle after scratching	Alum., am-c., am-m., ant-c., ars., bar-c., bell., bov., bry., calc., caps., carb-an., carb-s., carb-v., cic., con., dulc., graph., hep., kali-ar., kali-c., kali-s., kreos., led., **Lyc.**, merc., mez., nat-m., petr., phos., puls., ran-b., **Rhus-t.**, sabad., sabin., sars., sep., sil., staph., **Sulph.**, thuj., verat., viol-t., zinc.
Eruption	eruptions carbuncle burning	Anthr., apis., ars., coloc., crot-c., crot-h., hep., **Tarent-c.**
Eruption	eruptions carbuncle clustered	Agar., calc., ph-ac., ran-b., rhus-t., staph., verat.
Eruption	eruptions carbuncle confluent	Agar., ant-t., caps., chlol., cic., hyos., ph-ac., phos., rhus-v., valer.
Eruption	eruptions carbuncle like chicken pox	Acon., **Ant-c.**, ant-t., ars., asaf., bell., canth., carb-v., caust., coff., con., cycl., hyos., ip., led., merc., nat-c., nat-m., **Puls.**, rhus-t., sep., sil., **Sulph.**, thuj.
Eruption	eruptions carbuncle serpiginous	Clem., psor., sulph.
Eruption	eruptions during lactation	Sep.
Eruption	eruptions during leprosy	Alum., anac., ant-t., ars., bar-c., calc., carb-ac., carb-an., carb-s., carb-v., caust., com., con., crot-h., form., graph., hell., hydrc., iod., iris., kali-c., kali-i., lach., mag-c., mang., meph., nat-c., nat-m., nit-ac., nuph., petr., phos., psor., **Sec.**, sep., sil., **Sulph.**, tub., zinc.
Eruption	eruptions during menses	Dulc., graph., nux-m.
Eruption	eruptions from being over heated	Bov., carb-v., con., **Nat-m.**, psor., puls.
Eruption	eruptions horny	Ant-c., ran-b.
Eruption	eruptions impetigo	Alum., am-c., ant-c., ars-i., ars., bar-c., calc., carb-ac., carb-v., caust., cic., clem., con., crot-t., dulc., graph., hep., iris., jug-c., kali-bi., kreos., lact., lyc., merc., nat-c., nat-m., nit-ac., olnd., ph-ac., phos., rhus-t., sars., sep., sil., staph., sulph., viol-t.
Eruption	eruptions in corners of mouth	Ant-c., bell., bov., calc-f., Calc., carb-v., cic., cund., Graph., hep., ign., iris., kreos., lyc., mang., Merc., mez., nat-c., nat-m., Nit-ac., nux-v., petr., ph-ac., phos., psor., rhus-t., seneg., sep., sil., tab., verat.
Eruption	eruptions in left nose	Bell., bor., calc., cob., sars.
Eruption	eruptions in lower lips	Bor., Bry., calc., nat-c., nat-m., ph-ac., phos., Sep., sulph.
Eruption	eruptions in nails of fingers	Eug., merc., sel.

Body part/Disease	Symptom	Medicines
Eruption	eruptions in right nose	Calc., carb-an., dulc., gamb., kali-n., lach.
Eruption	eruptions in septum (a thin partition or membrane dividing something into two or more cavities. Examples include the tissue separating the nostrils)	Bar-c., bov., calad., caps., crot-t., ol-an., psor., teucr., thuj., vinc.
Eruption	eruptions in spring	*Nat-s., rhus-t., sars., sep.*
Eruption	eruptions in summer	Kali-bi., led.
Eruption	eruptions in upper lips	Ars., bar-c., bell., carb-v., cic., cinnb., graph., Kali-c., Kreos., lyc., mag-c., mag-m., mang., nat-c., nat-m., nit-ac., par., phyt., rhus-t., sep., sil., squil., Staph., Sulph., thuj., viol-t.
Eruption	eruptions inflamed	Ars., calc., lyc.
Eruption	eruptions inside nose	Am-m., mag-c., phel., podo., sars., sel., sil.
Eruption	eruptions itching aggravated from fire	Mez.
Eruption	eruptions itching aggravated from touch	Mez.
Eruption	eruptions itching aggravated from warmth	Alum., bov., caust., clem., led., lyc., **Merc.**, mez., nat-a., psor., puls., sulph.
Eruption	eruptions itching aggravated from warmth of bed	Aeth., alum., anac., ant-c., caust., clem., cocc., kali-a., kreos., mag-m., merc., mur-ac., **Psor.**, puls., rhus-t., sars., staph., **Sulph.**, til., verat.
Eruption	eruptions itching aggravated from washing	Mez., sulph.
Eruption	eruptions itching aggravated in cold water	Clem.
Eruption	eruptions itching aggravated in warm room	Sep.
Eruption	eruptions itching ameliorated from heat of stove	Rumx., tub.
Eruption	eruptions itching ameliorated in cold air	Kali-bi.
Eruption	eruptions itching at night	Ant-c., ant-t., ars-i., ars., clem., crot-t., graph., iris., kali-bi., kreos., **Merc.**, mez., olnd., rhus-t., staph., ust., verat., viol-t.
Eruption	eruptions itching before storm	Graph.
Eruption	eruptions itching during menses	Carb-v., kali-c.
Eruption	eruptions itching in cold air	Kali-ar., psor., rumx.
Eruption	eruptions itching in evening	Alum., bor., graph., kreos., mag-m., staph.
Eruption	eruptions itching in open air	Led., nit-ac.
Eruption	eruptions itching patches bleeding after scratches	**Sulph.**
Eruption	eruptions itching when undressing	Ars-i., kali-ar., nat-s., **Rumx.**
Eruption	eruptions mealy	Am-c., **Ars.**, aur., bov., bry., bufo., **Calc.**, cic., *dulc.*, graph., kreos., led., *lyc.*, merc., mur-ac., nit-ac., **Phos.**, *sep.*, **Sil.**, sulph., thuj., verat.
Eruption	eruptions mealy white	Ars., calc., dulc., **Kali-chl.**, lyc., sep., sil., thuj.
Eruption	eruptions moist after scratching	Kali-c., sars.
Eruption	eruptions of nose painful when touched	Chin., clem., kali-c., petr., ph-ac.
Eruption	eruptions of nose red	Aur., bell., carb-s., crot-t., lach., ph-ac., syph., thuj.
Eruption	eruptions of nose stinging	Apis., squil.
Eruption	eruptions on abdomen	Agar., anac., apis., ars., bar-m., bry., calc., graph., kali-ar., kali-bi., kali-c., merc-c., merc., nat-c., nat-m., phos., rhus-t., sulph.

Body part/Disease	Symptom	Medicines
Eruption	eruptions on abdomen, itching	Agar., calc., merc., rhus-t., sulph.
Eruption	eruptions on abdomen, moist	Merc.
Eruption	eruptions on face aggravated at night	Ars., mag-m.
Eruption	eruptions on face aggravated at night in warm room	Mag-m.
Eruption	eruptions on face aggravated by cold air	Ars., dulc.
Eruption	eruptions on face aggravated from warmth	Euphr., mez., psor., sulph., teucr.
Eruption	eruptions on face aggravated from washing	Nux-v., sulph.
Eruption	eruptions on face ameliorated from warmth	Ars.
Eruption	eruptions on face before menses	Mag-m., sars.
Eruption	eruptions on face during menses	Calc., dulc., eug., graph., psor., sang.
Eruption	eruptions on face painful	Alum., apis., bell., berb., calc., cic., clem., eug., led., phos., plat., sep., staph., Sulph.
Eruption	eruptions on face painful at night	Viol-t.
Eruption	eruptions on face painful when touched	Ant-c., bell., hep., lach., led., nit-ac., par., sabad., stann., valer.
Eruption	eruptions on face red	Ant-c., aur., calc-p., calc., carb-s., caust., cham., cic., euphr., fago., hyper., lac-c., led., nit-ac., par., petr., phos., psor., sep., sulph.
Eruption	eruptions on female genitalia moist	Sep.
Eruption	eruptions on female gentialia, erysipelatous	Rhus-t.
Eruption	eruptions on nose moist	Aur-m-n., carb-v., Graph., nat-c., thuj.
Eruption	eruptions on skin alternating with asthma	Calad., mez., rhus-t., sulph.
Eruption	eruptions on skin alternating with diarrhoae	Calc-p.
Eruption	eruptions on skin alternating with dysentry	Rhus-t.
Eruption	eruptions on skin alternating with internal affections	Graph.
Eruption	eruptions on skin alternating with respiratory symptoms	Crot-t., lach.
Eruption	eruptions on skin alternating with tightness of chest	Calad., kalm., rhus-t.
Eruption	eruptions on skin of chest in every spring	Nat-s.
Eruption	eruptions on skin painful	Agar., alum., ambr., ant-c., apis., arg-m., **Arn.**, *ars.*, *asaf.*, aur., bar-c., **Bell.**, berb., bov., calc., cann-s., canth., caps., chel., *chin.*, cic., *clem.*, *con.*, *cupr.*, *dulc.*, guai., *hep.*, kali-ar., *kali-c.*, kali-s., *lach.*, led., *lyc.*, *mag-m.*, *mag-m.*, merc., nat-a., nat-c., nat-p., **Nux-v.**, par., petr., **Ph-ac.**, phos., *puls.*, ran-b., ran-s., rhus-t., ruta., sel., seneg., *sep.*, **Sil.**, *spig.*, spong., squil., **Sulph.**, thuj., valer., *verat.*, verb.
Eruption	eruptions on skin painful as from splinters when touched	Hep., nit-ac.
Eruption	eruption, blisters	Alum., am-c., anac., **Ant-c.**, ars., aur., bor., bry., bufo., canth., carb-an., carb-s., **Caust.**, cham., clem., crot-h., dulc., graph., hep., kali-ar., kali-c., kali-s., lach., mag-c., merc., nat-a., nat-c., nat-m., nat-p., nit-ac., petr., phos., ran-b., ran-s., **Rhus-t.**, rhus-v., sep., sil., sulph., verat., vip., zinc.

Body part/Disease	Symptom	Medicines
Eruption	eruption, painless	Ambr., anac., ant-c., ant-t., bell., cham., cocc., con., cycl., dros., hell., hyos., lach., laur., **Lyc.**, olnd., ph-ac., phos., puls., rhus-t., samb., sec., spig., staph., stram., sulph.
Eruption	eruption, pamphigus (large blisters)	Acon., anac., ars., bell., bufo., calc., canth., caust., chin., crot-h., dulc., hep., hydrc., jug-c., **Lach.**, lyc., merc., nat-m., nat-s., nit-ac., ph-ac., phos., psor., ran-b., ran-s., rhus-t., sars., sep., sil., sul-ac., sulph., thuj.
Eruption	eruption, papular	Aur., calc., caust., cham., cycl., gels., grin., hippoz., hydrc., iod., kali-bi., kali-c., **Kali-i.**, kali-s., lyc., merc., petr., phos., pic-ac., sep., sil., sulph., syph., zinc.
Eruption	eruption, patches (cover for wound)	Agar., ail., ars., berb., calc., carb-v., graph., iris., jug-c., kali-bi., kali-c., lith., mang., phos., puls., sars., sep., thuj., viol-t.
Eruption	eruption, petechiae (tiny red spot on skin)	Apoc., arn., **Ars.**, aur-m., bapt., bell., berb., **Bry.**, camph., canth., con., crot-h., cupr., dulc., eup-per., hyos., lach., led., nat-m., nux-v., ph-ac., phel., **Phos.**, **Rhus-t.**, ruta., sec., sil., squil., stram., sul-ac., ter.
Eruption	eruption, petechiae in old people	Con.
Eruption	eruption, pustular (a small round raised area of inflamed skin filled with pus) on abdomen	Crot-c., crot-t., kali-bi., merc., puls., squil.
Eruption	eruption, pustular (a small round raised area of inflamed skin filled with pus) on abdomen	Crot-c., crot-t., kali-bi., merc., puls., squil.
Eruption	eruption, pustules	Agar., am-c., am-m., anac., *ant-c.*, *ant-s.*, **Ant-t.**, arn., ars-i., **Ars.**, *aur.*, *bell.*, bry., bufo., calad., calc-p., *calc-s.*, *calc.*, carb-ac., carb-s., carb-v., caust., cham., *chel.*, *cic.*, cina., *clem.*, cocc., *con.*, cop., *crot-h.*, crot-t., cupr-ar., cycl., *dulc.*, eupho., fl-ac., gnaph., *hep.*, hippoz., *hydrc.*, hyos., iod., *iris.*, jug-c., jug-r., kali-ar., *kali-bi.*, *kali-br.*, kali-c., *kali-i.*, kali-s., *kreos.*, lach., *merc.*, *mez.*, nat-m., *nit-ac.*, nux-v., *petr.*, ph-ac., phos., *psor.*, *puls.*, **Rhus-t.**, rhus-v., *sars.*, sec., *sep.*, *sil.*, squil., **Staph.**, **Sulph.**, tab., tell., thuj., viol-t., zinc.
Eruption	eruption, pustules after scratching	Am-m., ant-c., ars., bell., bry., cycl., hyos., merc., puls., **Rhus-t.**, sil., staph., sulph.
Eruption	eruption, pustules aggravated from bathing	Dulc.
Eruption	eruption, pustules black	Ant-t., **Anthr.**, bry., **Lach.**, mur-ac., nat-c., rhus-t.
Eruption	eruption, pustules bleeding	Ant-t.
Eruption	eruption, pustules brown	Ant-t.
Eruption	eruption, pustules burning	Am-c., jug-r., petr.
Eruption	eruption, pustules containing water	Kali-i., rhus-t., stram.
Eruption	eruption, pustules covered with spots	Jug-r., lyc.
Eruption	eruption, pustules cracked	Rhus-t.
Eruption	eruption, pustules dry	Merc.
Eruption	eruption, pustules fetid	Anthr., ars., bufo., viol-t.
Eruption	eruption, pustules green	Jug-r., sec., viol-t.
Eruption	eruption, pustules greesy	Kreos.
Eruption	eruption, pustules hard	Anac., ant-c., crot-h., nit-ac.
Eruption	eruption, pustules humid (with a relatively high level of moisture in the air)	Bell.

Body part/Disease	Symptom	Medicines
Eruption	eruption, pustules indolent	Kali-br., psor.
Eruption	eruption, pustules inflamed	Anac., crot-t., kali-bi., rhus-t., sep., stram.
Eruption	eruption, pustules itching at night	Kali-bi.
Eruption	eruption, pustules itching	Ant-t., anthro., berb., crot-t., dulc., graph., hydr-ac., kali-bi., merc., nux-v., petr., rhus-t., sars., sulph.
Eruption	eruption, pustules lumpy	Anthro., cham.
Eruption	eruption, pustules malignant	**Anthr.**, apis., **Ars.**, bell., bufo., canth., carb-v., cench., crot-h., **Lach.**, ran-b., rhus-t., sec., sil., tarent-c.
Eruption	eruption, pustules mixed with vesicles	Ant-t.
Eruption	eruption, pustules painful	Ant-t., ars., berb., kali-br., stram., viol-t.
Eruption	eruption, pustules red areola	Anac., ant-t., bor., calad., lach., nit-ac., par., thuj.
Eruption	eruption, pustules red	Anac., ant-t., ars., berb., caust., **Cic.**, cimic., crot-h., crot-t., graph., hydr-ac., hydrc., kali-c., mez., nit-ac.
Eruption	eruption, pustules rose coloured	Ars., dulc.
Eruption	eruption, pustules scaly	Merc.
Eruption	eruption, pustules scurfy (thin dry flaking scales of skin, usually as a result of a skin condition such as dandruff)	Anac., ant-c., ant-t., bov., crot-t., dulc., kali-chl., merc.
Eruption	eruption, pustules small	Ant-t., hydrc., kali-i., kali-n., puls.
Eruption	eruption, pustules sore	Calad., merc.
Eruption	eruption, pustules stinging	Am-c., berb., dros., rhus-t., sep.
Eruption	eruption, pustules syphilitic	Kali-bi.
Eruption	eruption, pustules tensive	Ant-t., crot-h., kali-n., mag-s.
Eruption	eruption, pustules thin which break and send out ichorous pus, which corrodes the skin and spreads	Ant-t.
Eruption	eruption, pustules titillating	Mez.
Eruption	eruption, pustules ulcerated	Ant-t., ars., crot-t., cupr-ar., dulc., mag-m., merc., nat-c., sars., sil.
Eruption	eruption, pustules white	Calad., cimic., cop., cycl.
Eruption	eruption, pustules with white tips	Ant-c., ant-t., puls.
Eruption	eruption, pustules yellow	Anac., carb-v., hyos., merc., staph., viol-t.
Eruption	eruption, rash (outbreak on the surface of the skin that is often reddish and itchy) after abuse of belladona	Hyos.
Eruption	eruption, rash after scratching	Am-c., am-m., ant-c., bov., bry., calc., carb-s., caust., dulc., graph., ip., lach., led., merc., mez., ph-ac., phos., puls., rhus-t., sars., sel., sil., spong., staph., sulph., verat., viol-t., zinc.
Eruption	eruption, rash at night	Chlol.
Eruption	eruption, rash black	Lach.
Eruption	eruption, rash blotches	Agar., lyc.
Eruption	eruption, rash bluish	**Acon.**, ail., am-c., bell., coff., **Lach.**, phos., sep., stram., sulph.
Eruption	eruption, rash brownish	Mez.

Body part/Disease	Symptom	Medicines
Eruption	eruption, rash chronic	Am-c., clem., mez., staph.
Eruption	eruption, rash fiery & moist	Carb-v.
Eruption	eruption, rash fiery (inflamed) before menses	Dulc.
Eruption	eruption, rash fiery during menses	Con.
Eruption	eruption, rash fiery in lying in (time around childbirth) women	Bry., cupr., ip.
Eruption	eruption, rash fiery receding in eruptive fevers	**Bry.**
Eruption	eruption, rash fiery red	**Acon., Bell.,** stram., sulph.
Eruption	eruption, rash fiery scarlet (bright red color)	**Acon., Am-c.,** ars., **Bell., Bry.,** calc., carb-v., caust., chlol., coff., com., dulc., hyos., iod., ip., kali-bi., lach., merc., ph-ac., phos., rhus-t., sulph., zinc.
Eruption	eruption, rash fiery when overheated	Apis., lyc.
Eruption	eruption, rash fiery with patches	Ail.
Eruption	eruption, rash from changing air	Apis.
Eruption	eruption, rash from tightness of chest alternating with asthma	Calad.
Eruption	eruption, rash in children	Acon., bry., cham., ip., sulph.
Eruption	eruption, rash in cold air	Apis., dulc., sars., sep.
Eruption	eruption, rash on coming into warm room from open air	Apis., ars.
Eruption	eruption, rash stinging	Nat-m., viol-t.
Eruption	eruption, rash suppressed	Ip.
Eruption	eruption, rash white	Agar., apis., **Ars.,** bov., bry., calad., ip., nux-v., phos., rhus-v., sulph., **Valer.**
Eruption	eruption, rash white in open air	Sars.
Eruption	eruption, rash white in room	Calc.
Eruption	eruption, rash with burning & itching	Agar., bry., calad., clem., sulph., teucr.
Eruption	eruption, rash with burning	Agar., bry., nux-v.
Eruption	eruption, rash with excoriated skin	Sulph.
Eruption	eruption, red	Acon., agar., **Am-c.,** anac., anan., ant-c., apis., arn., ars., aur., berb., calc., cham., chel., chin-s., chlol., cic., clem., cocc., com., con., cop., crot-t., cycl., dulc., fl-ac., graph., kali-bi., **Kali-c.,** kali-s., lach., lyc., mag-c., **Merc.,** mez., nit-ac., ox-ac., petr., ph-ac., **Phos.,** rhus-t., sabad., sars., sep., sil., spig., staph., stram., **Sul-ac., Sulph.,** thuj., til., valer., vip.
Eruption	eruption, roseola (red rash on the skin, seen in diseases such as measles, scarlet fever, and syphilis)	**Acon.,** bell., **Bry.,** carb-v., coff., hyos., ip., merc., nux-v., phos., **Puls.,** rhus-t., sars., sulph.
Eruption	eruption, scabies (contagious skin disease marked by intense itching, inflammation, and red papules)	Ambr., ant-c., ant-t., **Ars.,** aster., bar-m., bry., calc., canth., carb-ac., carb-an., **Carb-s., Carb-v., Caust.,** clem., coloc., con., cop., crot-t., cupr., dulc., graph., guai., hep., **Kali-s.,** kreos., lach., led., lyc., mang., merc-i-f., merc., mez., nat-c., olnd., petr., ph-ac., **Psor.,** puls., sabad., **Sel., Sep.,** sil., squil., staph., sul-ac., **Sulph.,** tarax., valer., verat., zinc.
Eruption	eruption, scabies bleeding	Calc., dulc., merc., sulph.

Body part/Disease	Symptom	Medicines
Eruption	eruption, scabies dry	Ars., calc., carb-v., caust., cham., cupr., dulc., graph., hep., kreos., led., lyc., merc-i-f., merc., nat-c., petr., ph-ac., psor., **Sep., Sil.,** staph., sulph., valer., verat., zinc.
Eruption	eruption, scabies fatty	Ant-c., caust., clem., cupr., kreos., **Merc.,** sel., sep., squil., sulph.
Eruption	eruption, scabies moist	Calc., carb-v., caust., clem., con., dulc., graph., kreos., lyc., merc., petr., sep., sil., squil., staph., sulph.
Eruption	eruption, scabies suppressed	Alum., ambr., ant-c., ant-t., ars., carb-v., **Caust.,** dulc., graph., kreos., lach., nat-c., nat-m., ph-ac., sel., sep., sil., **Sulph.,** verat., zinc.
Eruption	eruption, scabies suppressed with mercury & sulphur	Agn., ars., bell., calc., carb-v., **Caust.,** chin., dulc., hep., iod., nit-ac., **Psor.,** puls., rhus-t., sars., sel., **Sep.,** sil., staph., thuj., valer.
Eruption	eruption, scaly	Agar., am-m., anac., ant-c., ars-i., **Ars.,** aur., bar-m., bell., bor., bufo., cact., cadm., calad., calc-s., calc., canth., cic., **Clem.,** com., cupr., cycl., dulc., fl-ac., hep., hydrc., hyos., iod., kali-ar., kali-bi., kali-c., kali-s., led., mag-c., merc., mez., nat-a., nat-m., nit-ac., olnd., petr., **Phos., Phyt.,** plb., psor., rhus-t., sang., sars., **Sep.,** sil., staph., sulph., teucr., thuj.
Eruption	eruption, scaly ichthyosis (skin to become dry, thick, and scaly)	Anag., ars-i., ars., aur., calc., chin., clem., coloc., graph., hep., lac-c., lyc., mez., ol-j., petr., **Phos.,** plb., sep., sil., sulph., thuj.
Eruption	eruption, scaly like bran (husks of cereal grain)	Agar., alum., am-c., anac., arg-m., ars-i., **Ars.,** aur., bor., bry., **Calc.,** canth., carb-ac., carb-an., carb-v., chlor., cic., clem., dulc., graph., iod., kali-ar., **Kali-chl.,** kali-i., **Kreos.,** lach., led., lyc., mag-c., mang., merc., mez., nat-a., nat-m., nit-ac., olnd., petr., phos., **Phyt.,** ran-b., rhus-t., sep., **Sil.,** staph., sulph., thuj.
Eruption	eruption, scaly spots	Hydrc., kali-c., merc., **Nit-ac.,** puls., sabin., sil., thuj., zinc.
Eruption	eruption, scaly white	Anac., ars., graph., **Kali-chl.,** lyc., thuj., zinc.
Eruption	eruption, scaly yellow	**Kali-s.**
Eruption	eruption, scarlatina gangrenous	Ail., **Am-c.,** ars., **Carb-ac.,** lach., phos.
Eruption	eruption, scarlatina in patches	Ail.
Eruption	eruption, scarlatina receding	Am-c., phos., sulph., **Zinc.**
Eruption	eruption, scarlatina scorbutic spots	Anan., merc-c., merc.
Eruption	eruption, scarlatina smooth	Am-c., **Bell.,** euphr., hyos., merc.
Eruption	eruption, scarlet	Anan., cop.
Eruption	eruption, serpiginous	Clem., hep., psor., sars., sulph.
Eruption	eruption, shining through	Merc.
Eruption	eruption, small boils	**Arn.,** bar-c., dulc., fl-ac., **Kali-i.,** lyc., mag-c., mag-m., nat-m., nux-v., sulph., tarent., viol-t., zinc.
Eruption	eruption, smarting	Acon., agar., alum., ambr., ant-c., apis., **Arg-m.,** ars., aur., bar-c., bry., calc., cann-s., canth., caps., carb-an., carb-s., chel., chin., cic., coff., colch., dol., dros., ferr., **Graph.,** hell., **Hep.,** ign., kali-c., kali-s., lach., led., lyc., mag-c., mang., merc., mez., nat-c., nat-m., nit-ac., nux-v., olnd., par., petr., ph-ac., phos., plat., puls., ran-b., rhus-t., ruta., sabin., sars., sel., **Sep.,** sil., spig., spong., squil., staph., sulph., teucr., valer., verat., zinc.

Body part/Disease	Symptom	Medicines
Eruption	eruption, spotted	Merc., verat.
Eruption	eruption, suppressed	Acon., alum., am-c., ambr., ars-i., ars., bell., **Bry.**, calad., calc., carb-an., carb-v., caust., cham., con., cupr., **Dulc.**, gels., graph., hep., **Ip.**, kali-c., kali-s., lach., lyc., merc., mez., nat-c., nit-ac., nux-m., op., **Petr.**, **Ph-ac.**, phos., **Psor.**, puls., rhus-t., sars., sel., sep., sil., staph., **Stram.**, sul-ac., **Sulph.**, thuj., tub., verat., viol-t., **Zinc.**
Eruption	eruption, suppurating pocks	Bell., merc., sulph.
Eruption	eruption, suppurating	Alum., am-c., **Ant-c.**, ant-t., apis., ars., bar-c., bell., bor., cadm., calc-s., calc., carb-s., carb-v., caust., **Cham.**, chel., cic., clem., cocc., con., croc., cycl., dulc., euphr., **Graph.**, hell., hep., jug-c., kali-c., kali-s., lach., led., **Lyc.**, mag-c., mang., **Merc.**, mur-ac., nat-a., nat-c., nat-m., nat-p., **Nit-ac.**, nux-v., olnd., par., **Petr.**, ph-ac., phos., plb., psor., puls., **Rhus-t.**, samb., sars., sec., **Sep., Sil.**, spig., squil., staph., sulph., tarax., thuj., verat., viol-o., viol-t., zinc.
Eruption	eruption, syphilitic roseola	**Kali-i.**, phos.
Eruption	eruption, syphilitic	Arg-n., **Ars-i.**, ars., aur., bad., dulc., fl-ac., guai., hep., kali-bi., kali-chl., **Kali-i.**, kreos., lach., lyc., **Merc-c.**, **Merc-i-f.**, **Merc-i-r.**, **Merc.**, **Nit-ac.**, petr., phyt., plat., rhus-t., rumx., sang., sars., sep., sil., staph., still., **Syph.**, thuj.
Eruption	eruption, tubercles	Agar., alum., am-c., am-m., anac., ang., ant-c., apis., aran., ars., aur., bar-c., bar-m., bry., calc-p., calc-s., **Calc.**, carb-an., carb-s., carb-v., **Caust.**, cic., cocc., con., crot-h., dulc., fl-ac., graph., hell., hep., hydrc., kali-ar., kali-bi., kali-br., kali-c., kali-i., kali-n., kali-s., **Lach.**, **Led.**, lyc., mag-c., mag-m., mag-s., mang., merc-c., merc., mez., mur-ac., nat-a., nat-c., nat-m., nit-ac., nux-v., olnd., petr., ph-ac., phos., rhus-t., sec., sel., sep., sil., stann., staph., sul-ac., sulph., tarax., thuj., valer., verat., zinc.
Eruption	eruption, tubercles erysipelatous (severe skin rash accompanied by fever and vomiting)	Nat-c., phos., sil.
Eruption	eruption, tubercles gnawing (uncomfortable)	Rhus-t.
Eruption	eruption, tubercles hard	Am-c., am-m., ant-c., bar-c., bov., bry., con., lach., mag-c., mag-s., nat-m., phos., rhus-t., valer.
Eruption	eruption, tubercles humid	Kali-n., sel.
Eruption	eruption, tubercles in summer	Kali-bi.
Eruption	eruption, tubercles in winter	Kali-br.
Eruption	eruption, tubercles inflamed	Am-m., rhus-t.
Eruption	eruption, tubercles itching	Aur., canth., carb-an., cham., cocc., dulc., graph., kali-c., kali-n., lach., lyc., mag-c., mag-s., mur-ac., nat-m., nit-ac., op., rhus-t., staph., stram., stront., tub., zinc.
Eruption	eruption, tubercles leprous	Nat-c., phos., sil.
Eruption	eruption, tubercles malignant	Ars.
Eruption	eruption, tubercles miliary (small nodules or lesions resembling millet seeds)	Nat-m.

Body part/Disease	Symptom	Medicines
Eruption	eruption, tubercles mucous	Fl-ac., nit-ac., thuj.
Eruption	eruption, tubercles painful as if sore	Ant-c., caust., ph-ac.
Eruption	eruption, tubercles painful	Am-c., ars., bell., bov., lach., lyc., ph-ac., zinc.
Eruption	eruption, tubercles painless	Arn., bell., graph., ign., led., olnd., squil., verat.
Eruption	eruption, tubercles raised	Olnd., rhus-v., valer.
Eruption	eruption, tubercles red	Am-c., berb., bov., carb-an., carb-v., dig., hep., kali-chl., kali-i., lach., led., mag-c., mag-m., merc., mur-ac., nat-m., nit-ac., op., ph-ac., puls., sep., spig., sulph., thuj., verat.
Eruption	eruption, tubercles scurfy	Sulph.
Eruption	eruption, tubercles smooth	Ph-ac.
Eruption	eruption, tubercles soft	Bell., crot-h., lach.
Eruption	eruption, tubercles sore	Sep
Eruption	eruption, tubercles stinging	Calc., caust., dulc., kali-i., led., mag-c., phos., rhus-t., squil., stram.
Eruption	eruption, tubercles suppurating	Am-c., bov., caust., fl-ac., kali-bi., nat-c., nit-ac., sil.
Eruption	eruption, tubercles syphilitic	Ars-i., ars., dulc., fl-ac., hep., kali-bi., kali-i., merc., nit-ac., phyt., sil., thuj.
Eruption	eruption, tubercles tearing	Cham., con.
Eruption	eruption, tubercles ulcerative	Am-c., bov., caust., fl-ac., nat-c., sec.
Eruption	eruption, tubercles umbilicated (Navel Shaped)	Kali-bi., kali-br.
Eruption	eruption, tubercles wart shaped	Lyc., thuj.
Eruption	eruption, tubercles watery	Graph., mag-c.
Eruption	eruption, tubercles white	Ant-c., dulc., sep., sulph., valer.
Eruption	eruption, tubercles yellow	Ant-c., rhus-t.
Eruption	eruption, white pimples after scratching	Agar., ars., bov., bry., ip., sulph.
Eruption	eruption, with biting	Agn., alum., am-c., am-m., ant-c., arn., ars., bell., bor., bov., bry., calc., camph., canth., caps., carb-an., carb-s., carb-v., caust., cham., chel., chin., cocc., colch., coloc., con., dros., **Eupho.**, hell., ip., lach., **Led.**, lyc., mag-c., mang., merc., mez., mur-ac., nat-c., nat-m., nux-v., olnd., op., petr., ph-ac., phos., plat., **Puls.**, ran-b., ran-s., rhod., rhus-t., sel., sil., spig., spong., still., stront., sulph., thuj., verat., viol-t.
Eruption	eruption, with biting	Agn., alum., am-c., am-m., ant-c., arn., ars., bell., bor., bov., bry., calc., camph., canth., caps., carb-an., carb-s., carb-v., caust., cham., chel., chin., cocc., colch., coloc., con., dros., **Eupho.**, hell., ip., lach., **Led.**, lyc., mag-c., mang., merc., mez., mur-ac., nat-c., nat-m., nux-v., olnd., op., petr., ph-ac., phos., plat., **Puls.**, ran-b., ran-s., rhod., rhus-t., sel., sil., spig., spong., still., stront., sulph., thuj., verat., viol-t.
Eruption	eruption, with black pocks(a small indentation, pit, or hole)	Ars., bell., hyos., lach., mur-ac., rhus-t., sec.
Eruption	eruption, with black pocks	Ars., bell., hyos., lach., mur-ac., rhus-t., sec.
Eruption	eruption, with jerking pain	Asar., calc., caust., cham., chin., cupr., lyc., puls., **Rhus-t.**, sep., sil., staph.

Body part/Disease	Symptom	Medicines
Eruption	eruption, with pocks (small hole)	Ant-c., ant-t., arn., ars., bell., bry., caust., clem., cocc., euon., hyos., kali-bi., kreos., merc., mill., psor., puls., rhus-t., sil., sulph., thuj.
Eruption	eruption, with pocks (small hole)	Ant-c., ant-t., arn., ars., bell., bry., caust., clem., cocc., euon., hyos., kali-bi., kreos., merc., mill., psor., puls., rhus-t., sil., sulph., thuj.
Eruption	eruption, with red areola	Anac., ant-t., bor., cocc., tab.
Eruption	eruptions on tip of nose	Acon., aeth., am-c., anan., asaf., carb-an., carb-v., caust., clem., lyc., nit-ac., pall., ph-ac., sep., sil., spong.
Eruption	eruptions over temples	Alum., ant-c., arg-m., bell., bry., calc., carb-v., caust., dulc., lach., lyc., mur-ac., nat-m., nit-ac., sabin., spig., sulph., thuj.
Eruption	eruptions tubercles red areola	Cocc., dulc., ph-ac.
Eruption	eruptions under nose	Arn., bor., bov., sars., squil.
Eruption	eruptions with swelling	Acon., am-c., arn., ars., bell., bry., calc., canth., carb-v., caust., chin., cic., con., eupho., hep., kali-c., lyc., mag-c., **Merc.**, nat-c., nat-m., nit-ac., petr., ph-ac., phos., puls., **Rhus-t.**, ruta., samb., sars., sep., sil., sulph., thuj.
Eruption	eruptions with tearing pain	Acon., arn., ars., bry., calc., canth., carb-v., caust., clem., cocc., dulc., graph., kali-c., **Lyc.**, merc., mez., nat-c., nit-ac., phos., puls., rhus-t., sep., sil., staph., sulph., zinc.
Eruption	eruptions with ulcerative pain	Am-c., am-m., ant-c., ars., bar-c., caps., caust., con., graph., kali-c., laur., mang., merc., phos., puls., rhus-t., sep., **Sil.**, staph., sulph., tarax., zinc.
Eruption	eruptions with whitish pocks	Iod., lyc.
Eruption	eruptions with whitish pocks	Iod., lyc.
Eruption	eruptions, black in lower limbs	Sec.
Eruption	eruptions, black pustules in lower limbs	Ars., nat-c., sec.
Eruption	eruptions, bleeding after scratching in lower limbs	Calc., cupr.
Eruption	eruptions, bleeding pimples in lower limbs	Agar., thea.
Eruption	eruptions, blisters in thumb	Hep.
Eruption	eruptions, blisters in tips of fingers	Alum., cupr.
Eruption	eruptions, blotches in lower limbs	Ant-c., lach., nat-c., sulph.
Eruption	eruptions, bluish vesicles in fingers	Ran-b.
Eruption	eruptions, burning after scratching in lower limbs	Til.
Eruption	eruptions, burning in fingers	Ran-b.
Eruption	eruptions, burning in lower limbs	Bov., fago., lact-ac., merc., nux-v., til.
Eruption	eruptions, burning pustules (small round raised area of inflamed skin filled with pus) in lower limbs	Mez.
Eruption	eruptions, burning vesicles in fingers	Ran-b.
Eruption	eruptions, copper coloured spots in fingers	Cor-r.
Eruption	eruptions, crusts in nails of fingers	Ars.
Eruption	eruptions, desquamation in fingers	Agar., bar-c., elaps., graph., merc., mez., rhus-v., sabad., sep., still., sulph.

Body part/Disease	Symptom	Medicines
Eruption	eruptions, desquamation in lower limbs	Agar., ars., calc-p., chin-s., crot-t., elaps., kreos., mag-c., merc., sulph., thuj.
Eruption	eruptions, desquamation in nails of fingers	Chlol.
Eruption	eruptions, desquamation in tips of fingers	Bar-c., elaps., ph-ac., phos.
Eruption	eruptions, dry in fingers	Anag., psor.
Eruption	eruptions, dry in joints of fingers	**Psor.**
Eruption	eruptions, dry in lower limbs	Bry.
Eruption	eruptions, elevated spots in fingers	Syph.
Eruption	eruptions, excrescences in fingers	Ars., thuj.
Eruption	eruptions, flat pimples in lower limbs	Ant-c., plan.
Eruption	eruptions, from flee bites in lower limbs	Sec.
Eruption	eruptions, gangrenous in lower limbs	Hyos.
Eruption	eruptions, greenish excrescences in fingers	Ars.
Eruption	eruptions, hot in lower limbs	Chel., fago.
Eruption	eruptions, hot reddish like knots in lower limbs	Kali-bi.
Eruption	eruptions, in first finger	Agar., calc., kali-c., mag-c., nat-c., sil.
Eruption	eruptions, in fourth finger	Cycl.
Eruption	eruptions, in groups in lower limbs	Nat-m.
Eruption	eruptions, in joints of fingers	Cycl., hydr., mez., **Psor.**
Eruption	eruptions, in lower limbs ameliorated from cold bathing	Lyc.
Eruption	eruptions, in sides of fingers	Mez., sabad., tax.
Eruption	eruptions, in third finger	Cycl.
Eruption	eruptions, in thumb	Hep., sanic.
Eruption	eruptions, in tip of thumb	Ail.
Eruption	eruptions, in tips of fingers	Ars., bar-c., cist., cupr., elaps., nat-c., psor.
Eruption	eruptions, itching in fingers	Ran-b.
Eruption	eruptions, itching in lower limbs	Agar., anac., arg-n., bov., bry., calc., caust., daph., dulc., fago., jug-r., kali-c., lach., lact-ac., led., mang., merc., mur-ac., nat-c., **Nat-m.**, nat-p., nicc., nux-v., petr., puls., rhus-t., rumx., sel., **Sep.**, sil., **Staph.**, sulph., tarax., til.
Eruption	eruptions, itch-like in lower limbs	Ars., bry., chel., sulph.
Eruption	eruptions, lumpy in lower limbs	Petr., ther., thuj.
Eruption	eruptions, miliary in lower limbs	Alum., ars., bov., daph., merc., nux-v., sil., sulph.
Eruption	eruptions, moist in lower limbs	Bov., bry., chel., kreos., merc., nat-m.
Eruption	eruptions, nodules in lower limbs	Petr., ther., thuj.
Eruption	eruptions, painful in lower limbs	Arn., bov.
Eruption	eruptions, painful nodules in fingers	Calc.
Eruption	eruptions, papule in lower limbs	Lach., lachn., merc., nux-v., ph-ac., rhus-t., sel., sep., thuj.
Eruption	eruptions, pemohigus (large blisters on the skin and mucous membranes, often accompanied by itching or burning sensations) in fingers	Lyc.

Body part/Disease	Symptom	Medicines
Eruption	eruptions, pemohigus (large blisters on the skin and mucous membranes, often accompanied by itching or burning sensations) in fingers	Lyc.
Eruption	eruptions, pemphigus in thumb	Lyc.
Eruption	eruptions, pemphigus in thumb	Lyc.
Eruption	eruptions, petechia in lower limbs	Am-m., ars., kali-i.
Eruption	eruptions, phagedenic (rapidly spreading) blisters in fingers	Calc., graph., hep., kali-c., mag-c., nit-ac., ran-b., sil., sulph.
Eruption	eruptions, phagedenic in first finger after washing with cold water	Nat-c.
Eruption	eruptions, phagedenic in first finger discharging water	Calc.
Eruption	eruptions, phagedenic in lower limbs	Ars., nux-v., sulph.
Eruption	eruptionson skin, scarlatina (contagious bacterial infection marked by fever, a sore throat, and a red rash, mainly affecting children)	Acon., **Ail.**, **Am-c.**, **Apis.**, arn., ars., arum-t., bar-c., **Bell.**, bry., calc., carb-ac., carb-v., cham., crot-h., cupr., gels., hep., hyos., **Lach.**, **Lyc.**, **Merc.**, **Nit-ac.**, ph-ac., phos., phyt., **Rhus-t.**, stram., sulph., zinc.
Eruption	excoriated eruptions during menses	All-c., am-c., bov., carb-v., caust., graph., hep., kali-c., nat-s., sars., sil., sulph.
Eruption	excoriated eruptions in aged women	Merc.
Eruption	excoriating eruption on head	Calc., graph., hep., Merc., nat-m., nit-ac., Petr., ph-ac., psor., rhus-t., sep., Sulph., viol-t.
Eruption	excoriating with perspiration in foot	Bar-c., calc., carb-v., coff., **Fl-ac.**, graph., hell., iod., lyc., nit-ac., ran-b., sanic., sec., sep., sil., squil., zinc.
Eruption	excoriation	Cham., Hep., podo., rhod., sulph.
Eruption	excoriation between nates	Arg-m., arum-t., bufo., carb-s., **Graph.**, nat-m., nit-ac., puls., sep., sulph.
Eruption	excoriation between sides of both the thighs	Berb., sumb., thuj.
Eruption	excoriation between thighs	Aeth., am-c., ambr., anan., ars., bar-c., bufo., calc., carb-s., **Caust.**, chin-a., chin., goss., graph., **Hep.**, kali-ar., **Kali-c.**, **Kreos.**, lyc., **Merc.**, nat-c., nat-m., nit-ac., petr., rhod., **Sep.**, squil., sul-ac., **Sulph.**, zinc.
Eruption	excoriation between thighs from walking	**Graph.**, ruta., sul-ac., sulph.
Eruption	excoriation between toes	Aur-m., berb., carb-an., clem., fl-ac., graph., lach., lyc., mang., merc-i-f., mez., nat-c., nat-m., nit-ac., ran-b., sep., **Sil.**, syph., zinc.
Eruption	excoriation in bend of knee	Ambr., **Sep.**
Eruption	excoriation in bends of joints	Bell., caust., **Graph.**, lyc., mang., ol-an., petr., sep., squil., sulph.
Eruption	excoriation in leg	Lach.
Eruption	excoriation of axilla	Ars., aur., carb-v., con., graph., mez., sanic., sep., sulph., zinc.
Eruption	excoriation of ears	Kali-bi., kali-c., kali-s., merc., petr., sulph.
Eruption	excoriation of eyelids	Apis., Arg-n., Ars., calc., graph., hep., med., merc-c., Merc., nat-m., sulph.
Eruption	excoriation of glans	Anan., cor-r., merc-i-r., Merc., nat-c., nat-m., nit-ac., sep., sulph., Thuj.

Body part/Disease	Symptom	Medicines
Eruption	excoriation of nipples	Alumn., anan., arg-n., arn., calc-p., calc., cast-eq., Caust., cham., crot-t., dulc., Fl-ac., graph., ham., hell., hyper., ign., lyc., merc., nit-ac., phos., Phyt., puls., sang., sep., sil., sulph., zinc.
Eruption	excoriation of penis	Cop., kali-i., Nit-ac.
Eruption	excoriation of prepuce (the loose fold of skin that covers the tip of penis)	Anan., carb-v., hep., ign., Merc., mez., mur-ac., nit-ac., psor., sep., thuj.
Eruption	Felon (a pus-filled infection on the skin at the side of a fingernail or toenail) ameliorated from cold application	Apis., fl-ac., led., **Nat-s., Puls.**
Eruption	Felon at root of nail	Caust., graph.
Eruption	Felon beginning in nail	Par., petr., phyt., plb., puls., rhus-t., sep., **Sil.**, sulph.
Eruption	felon in palm	Lach., sil., sulph.,Hep.
Eruption	felon in thumb	All-c., am-m., bor., bufo., eug., fl-ac., gran., hep., kali-c., kali-i., nux-v., op., sep., sil., sul-ac., sulph.
Eruption	felon under nail	Alum., caust., coc-c., sulph.
Eruption	felon with caries of bone	Asaf., aur., fl-ac., lach., lyc., merc., mez., ph-ac., **Sil.**, sulph.
Eruption	felon with caries of bone and deep seated pain aggravated from warmth of bed	Sep.
Eruption	felon, bone caries with offensive pus	Fl-ac.
Eruption	felon, burning panaritium	**Anthr.**
Eruption	felon, deep seated panaritium	Bry., hep., lyc., rhus-t.
Eruption	felon, from hangnails	Lyc., nat-m., sulph.
Eruption	felon, from injury	Led.
Eruption	felon, gangrenous	Ars., lach.
Eruption	felon, itching	**Apis.**
Eruption	felon, lymphatic (a network of vessels that transport fluid, fats, proteins, and lymphocytes to the bloodstream) inflamed	All-c., bufo., hep., lach., rhus-t.
Eruption	felon, malignant (likely to spread or cause death) with burning	Anthr., ars., **Tarent-c.**
Eruption	felon, maltreated (treat somebody or something badly)	Hep., phos., sil., stram., sulph.
Eruption	felon, panaritium	All-c., alum., **Am-c.**, am-m., anac., **Anthr., Apis.**, arn., asaf., bar-c., benz-ac., berb., bov., bufo., calc., caust., chin., cist., con., cur., **Dios.**, eug., ferr., **Fl-ac.**, gins., **Hep.**, hyper., iod., iris., kali-c., kalm., lach., led., lyc., merc., nat-c., nat-h., nat-m., nat-s., **Nit-ac.**, par., petr., phyt., plb., puls., rhus-t., sang., sep., **Sil.**, sulph., **Tarent-c.**, teucr.
Eruption	felon, periosteum (tissue around bone)	Am-c., asaf., calc-p., calc., canth., dios., fl-ac., mez., phos., sep., **Sil.**, sulph.
Eruption	gangrenous upper limbs due to abscess	Anan.
Eruption	hard eruption on head	Ant-c., carb-an., nat-m.
Eruption	headache from suppressed eruptions	Ant-c., bry., lyc., mez., nux-m., psor., sulph.

Body part/Disease	Symptom	Medicines
Eruption	hydrocele (an accumulation of watery liquid in a body cavity, especially in the sac around the testes) After suppressed eruptions	Abrot., calc., hell.
Eruption	indurations (becoming hard) after eruptions	Kali-br.
Eruption	insanity after suppressed erruption	Bell., caust., stram., sulph., zinc.
Eruption	itching in eruptions in female genitalia during menses	Agar., aur-m., bry., calc., caust., con., dulc., graph., kali-c., merc., nux-v., petr., sep., staph.
Eruption	itching in eruptions in female genitalia	Ambr., graph., lach., nit-ac., nux-v., sep., sil., sulph., urt-u.
Eruption	itching in eruptions in female genitalia before menses	Aur-m., dulc., verat.
Eruption	itching in eruptions in female Genitalia when warm	Aeth.
Eruption	itching in upper limbs after suppressed eruption	Hep.
Eruption	malignant eruption on head	Brom., phos.
Eruption	measly (like measles) spots in cervical region	Ars., cop., morph.
Eruption	moist eruption on head	Anan., bar-c., calc., graph., Psor., ruta., staph.
Eruption	moist eruptions	Carb-v., Graph., Hep., merc., nat-m., petr., ph-ac., Rhus-t., sars., sep., sil.
Eruption	moist eruptions around cervical region	Caust., clem.
Eruption	offensive eruption on head	Merc., sep., sulph.
Eruption	pain in knee after suppressed eruption	Sep.
Eruption	pain of face after suppressed ereuption	Dulc., kalm., mez., thuj.
Eruption	painful eruptions	Sil., viol-t.
Eruption	palpitation of heart after suppressed eruptions	Ars., calc.
Eruption	paralysis agitans after suppression of eruption	Caust., hep.
Eruption	paralysis from suppressed eruption	Caust., dulc., hep., psor., sulph.
Eruption	paralysis of left upper limb from suppressed eruption	Hep.
Eruption	paralysis of lower limb from suppressed eruption	Psor.
Eruption	perspiration at night with miliary itching eruption	Rhus-t.
Eruption	perspiration with eruption	Dulc.
Eruption	petechia on chest	Ars., cop., stram.
Eruption	petechia on chest , purple	Ars.
Eruption	petechial (tiny purplish red spot on the skin caused by the release into the skin of a very small quantity of blood from a capillary) fever with fetid stool intestinal hæmorrhage, sopor so weak that he settles down in bed into a heap	**Mur-ac.**
Eruption	petechial fever with foul smell	**Arn.**
Eruption	petechial fever with foul smell, putrid, foul, cadaverous smell to stool, brown, dry, leathery-looking tongue, extreme prostration	**Ars.**
Eruption	petechial fever	Anthr., arn., ars., bapt., camph., caps., carb-v., chin., **Chlor.**, lach., **Mur-ac.**, nit-ac., phos., rhus-t., sec., sulph.
Eruption	respiration arressted from suppressed eruptions	Ars., sulph.

Body part/Disease	Symptom	Medicines
Eruption	rheumatic pain in extremities after acute eruptions	Dulc.
Eruption	rheumatic pain in extremities alternating with eruptions	Crot-t., staph.
Eruption	sensation of crawling in eruption in upper limbs	Lach.
Eruption	serpiginous eruption on head	Psor., sars.
Eruption	skin, crawling without eruption	**Alum., Ars.,** cist., dol., gels., lach., med., merc., **Mez.,** petr., psor., sulph.
Eruption	skin, itching suppressed eruptions after	Ars.
Eruption	skin, moisture (wetness) on spots	Ant-c., carb-v., hell., kali-c., lach., led., petr., sabin., sel., **Sil.,** sulph., tarax., vinc.
Eruption	skin, moisture (wetness)	Alum., ars., bar-c., bell., bov., bry., calc., carb-an., **Carb-v.,** caust., cic., clem., con., dulc., **Graph.,** hell., hep., kali-ar., kali-c., kreos., lach., led., **Lyc.,** merc., mez., nat-c., nat-m., nit-ac., olnd., petr., ph-ac., phos., **Rhus-t.,** ruta., sabin., sel., sep., sil., squil., staph., sul-ac., sulph., tarax., thuj., viol-t.
Eruption	skin, moisture after scratching	Alum., ars., bar-c., bell., bov., bry., calc., carb-an., carb-v., caust., cic., con., dulc., **Graph.,** hell., hep., kali-ar., kali-c., kali-s., kreos., **Lach.,** led., **Lyc.,** merc., mez., nat-c., nat-m., nit-ac., olnd., petr., **Rhus-t.,** ruta., sabin., sars., sel., sep., sil., squil., staph., sul-ac., sulph., tarax., thuj., viol-t.
Eruption	smarting (sharp stinging localized pain) with eruption on back	Bry., spig.
Eruption	sudden weakness after the eruption, comes out	Ars.
Eruption	swelling in fingers with eruptions	Psor.
Eruption	swelling in left parotid gland after exanthemata (a disease characterized by the appearance of a skin rash, e.g. measles or scarlet fever)	Anthr., arn., bar-c., Brom., carb-v., dulc., iod., kali-bi., mag-c., sulph.
Eruption	syphilitic rash	Ars-i., merc., Nit-ac.
Eruption	unconsciousness after suppression of eruptions	Zinc.
Eruption	vertigo after suppressed erruption	Bell., bry., calc., carb-v., cham., hep., ip., lach., phos., rhus-t., sulph.
Eruption	white eruption on head	Alum., calc., mez., Nat-m., tell., thuj.
Eruption	yellow eruption on head	Calc-s., calc., dulc., kali-bi., Kali-s., merc., nat-p., petr., psor., spong., staph., sulph., viol-t.
Eryrhema	erythema (redness of the skin as a result of a widening of the small blood vessels near its surface) in cervical region	Apis.
Eryrhema	erythematous discolouration iof clavicle	Apis.
Eryrhema	erythematous penis	Petr., samb.
Erysipelas	eruptions on female gentialia, erysipelatous	Rhus-t.
Erysipelas	eruption, tubercles erysipelatous (severe skin rash accompanied by fever and vomiting)	Nat-c., phos., sil.
Erysipelas	erysipela	Apis., graph., kali-i., merc., ph-ac., rhus-t.
Erysipelas	erysipela (a severe skin rash accompanied by fever and vomiting and caused by a streptococcal bacterium) extending to face	Apis.

Body part/Disease	Symptom	Medicines
Erysipelas	erysipela (skin rash accompanied by fever and vomiting) across the shoulders	Apis.
Erysipelas	erysipela extending to forehead	Apis., kali-i., ruta., sulph.
Erysipelas	erysipela extending to occiput	Ph-ac., rhus-t.
Erysipelas	erysipela in cervical region	Graph., kali-i., ph-ac.
Erysipelas	erysipela in cervical region extending to face	Rhus-t.
Erysipelas	erysipela in lumbar region	Merc.
Erysipelas	erysipelas aggravated after scratching	Am-c., ant-c., arn., ars., bell., bor., bry., calc., canth., carb-an., carb-v., graph., hep., hyos., lach., lyc., mag-c., **Merc.**, nat-a., nat-c., nit-ac., petr., phos., puls., ran-b., **Rhus-t.**, samb., sil., spong., sulph., thuj.
Erysipelas	erysipelas of mammae	Anan., Apis., arn., bell., cadm., carb-an., carb-s., carb-v., cham., coll., graph., phos., plan., sulph.
Erysipelas	erysipelas on abdomen	Graph.
Erysipelas	erysipelas on face from bites of insects	Led.
Erysipelas	erysipelas on face	Ars., camph., Carb-v., chin., hippoz., Lach., mur-ac., rhus-t., Sec., sil.
Erysipelas	erysipelas on face, oedematous	Apis., ars., chin., crot-t., hell., lyc., merc., rhus-t., sulph., thuj.
Erysipelas	erysipelas on left face	Agn., bor., cham., lach.
Erysipelas	erysipelas on left to right face	Lach., Rhus-t.
Erysipelas	erysipelas on right face	Arund., bell., stram.
Erysipelas	erysipelas on right to left face	Apis., arund., Graph., lyc., sulph.
Erysipelas	erysipelas on skin, chronic	Graph., ter.
Erysipelas	erysipelas on skin, during menses	Graph.
Erysipelas	erysipelas on skin, erratic (often changing direction)	Arn., bell., mang., mur-ac., puls., rhus-t., sabin., sulph.
Erysipelas	erysipelas on skin, gangrenous	Acon., anthr., apis., **Ars.**, bell., camph., **Carb-v.**, chin., com., **Crot-c.**, hippoz., hyos., **Lach.**, mur-ac., rhus-t., sabin., **Sec.**, sil., ter.
Erysipelas	erysipelas on skin, in old people	Am-c.
Erysipelas	erysipelas on skin, left to right	Lach., rhus-t.
Erysipelas	erysipelas on skin, recurrent	Apis., crot-h.
Erysipelas	erysipelas on skin, right to left	Apis., arund., graph., lyc., sulph.
Erysipelas	erysipelas on skin, running in streakes (linear growth of bacteria)	Graph.
Erysipelas	erysipelas on skin, smooth	Apis., **Bell.**
Erysipelas	erysipelas on skin, vesicular (fluid-filled cyst/blister)	Am-c., anac., ars., astac., bar-c., bell., bry., canth., carb-an., carb-s., com., crot-t., **Eupho.**, graph., hep., kali-chl., kali-s., lach., mez., petr., phos., puls., ran-b., **Rhus-t.**, rhus-v., sabad., sep., staph., stram., sulph., urt-u.
Erysipelas	erysipelas on skin, with swelling	Acon., am-c., **Apis.**, arn., ars., **Bell.**, bry., calc., canth., carb-s., carb-v., caust., chin., **Crot-c.**, eupho., graph., hep., kali-c., lach., lyc., mag-c., **Merc.**, nat-a., nat-c., nat-m., nit-ac., petr., ph-ac., phos., puls., **Rhus-t.**, rhus-v., ruta., samb., sars., sep., sil., sulph., thuj., verat-v., zinc.

Body part/Disease	Symptom	Medicines
Erysipelas	erysipelatous inflammation in ankle	Lach., rhus-t., tep.
Erysipelas	erysipelatous inflammation in elbow	Ars., lach., sulph.
Erysipelas	erysipelatous inflammation in fingers	Rhod., rhus-t., sulph., thuj.
Erysipelas	erysipelatous inflammation in foot	Apis., arn., bry., dulc., nux-v., puls., rhus-t., sil., sulph.
Erysipelas	erysipelatous inflammation in foot after dancing	Berb.
Erysipelas	erysipelatous inflammation in forearm	Anan., ant-c., apis., bufo., kali-c., **Lach.**, merc., petr.
Erysipelas	erysipelatous inflammation in hand	Graph., lach., rhus-t.
Erysipelas	erysipelatous inflammation in knee	Nux-v, Rhus-t., sulph.
Erysipelas	erysipelatous inflammation in leg	Anan., **Apis.**, arn., ars., bor., bufo., calc., hep., hydr., **Lach.**, lyc., merc., nat-c., puls., rhus-t., sil., sulph., ter., zinc.
Erysipelas	erysipelatous inflammation in psoas (loin muscle)	Sulph.
Erysipelas	erysipelatous inflammation in toes	**Apis.**
Erysipelas	erysipelatous inflammation in upper arm	Bell., petr.
Erysipelas	erysipelatous inflammation of upper limbs	Am-c., apis., arn., ars., bell., bufo., carb-ac., form., hippoz., kali-c., kalm., **Lach.**, petr., ph-ac., **Rhus-t.**, rhus-v.
Erysipelas	erysipelatous infllamation on skin	Anan., **Lach.**, vip.
Erysipelas	erysipelatous rash in cervical region	Hydr.
Erysipelas	erysipelatous spots in foot	Apis.
Erysipelas	inflammation erysipelatous of throat	Apis., bapt., bell., crot-c., lach., lyc., merc., phyt., rhus-t.
Erysipelas	Inflammation of eye erysipelatous	Acon., anac., Apis., bell., com., graph., hep., led., merc-c., merc., Rhus-t., vesp.
Erysipelas	swelling in hand with erysipelatous	**Rhus-t.**, rhus-v.
Expectoration	asthma ameliorated from expectorations	Hyper.
Expectoration	breathing difficult ameliorated from expectoration	Ail., Ant-t., grin., guai., ip., manc., nit-ac., sep., zinc.
Expectoration	breathing difficult ameliorated from expectoration in morning	Sep.
Expectoration	constriction in chest ameliorated from expectoration	Calc., manc.
Expectoration	coryza with cough and expectoration	Euphr.
Expectoration	cough ameliorated by expectoration	Ail., alum., alumn., bell., calc., carb-an., caust., guai., hep., iod., ip., kali-n., kreos., lach., lob., meli., mez., phos., phyt., plan., sang., sep., sulph., zinc.
Expectoration	cough with copious greenish salty expectorations aggravated in morning	Stann.
Expectoration	cough with expectoration	Dulc., sil.
Expectoration	dry cough at night followed by profuse salty expectoration with pain as if something were torn loose from larynx	Calc.
Expectoration	dry cough with expectoration only in morning	Alum., am-c., bell., bry., calc., carb-v., coc-c., eupho., ferr., hep., kali-c., led., lyc., mag-c., mang., mur-ac., nat-c., nat-m., nit-ac., nux-v., ph-ac., phos., Puls., sep., sil., Squil., stann., sul-ac.

Body part/Disease	Symptom	Medicines
Expectoration	dry cough with expectoration only in morning on hawking later copious green sputum	Carb-v.
Expectoration	expectoration acrid (unpleasantly strong and bitter in smell or taste)	Alum., am-c., am-m., anac., ars., carb-v., caust., cham., coc-c., con., ferr., ign., iod., kreos., lach., lyc., mag-m., merc., mez., nat-m., nit-ac., nux-v., phos., puls., rhus-t., sep., sil., spig., squil., sul-ac., sulph.
Expectoration	expectoration after bath	Calc-s.
Expectoration	expectoration after breakfast	Sep.
Expectoration	expectoration after dinner	Alumn.
Expectoration	expectoration after rising	Chin-s., coca., mag-m., puls., sep., sulph.
Expectoration	expectoration after scrub skin	Chin-s.
Expectoration	expectoration after sea bathing	Mag-m.
Expectoration	expectoration after waking	Agar., aur., carb-v., lyc., psor., sulph., thuj.
Expectoration	expectoration aggravated from air	Chin-s., cob., merc., nux-v., plan., sacc., sep.
Expectoration	expectoration ameliorated from drinking	Am-c.
Expectoration	expectoration ameliorated in cold air	Calc-s.
Expectoration	expectoration ameliorated in open air	Arg-n., calc-s.
Expectoration	expectoration as if mixed with dust	Phos.
Expectoration	expectoration at night in bed	Sulph.
Expectoration	expectoration before midnight on getting into bed	Sep.
Expectoration	expectoration blackish	Arn., aster., bell., chin., cur., elaps., hydr-ac., kali-bi., lyc., nux-v., ox-ac., puls., rhus-t.
Expectoration	expectoration blackish yellow	Hydr-ac.
Expectoration	expectoration bloody after a fall	Ferr-p., mill.
Expectoration	expectoration bloody after drinking	Calc.
Expectoration	expectoration bloody after eating	Sep.
Expectoration	expectoration bloody after exertion	Ip., mill.
Expectoration	expectoration bloody after violent erection	Nat-m.
Expectoration	expectoration bloody at night	Arn., ars., ferr., mez., puls., rhus-t., sulph.
Expectoration	expectoration bloody at night acrid	Am-c., ars., canth., carb-v., hep., Kali-c., kali-n., rhus-t., Sil., sul-ac., sulph., zinc.
Expectoration	expectoration bloody before menses	Zinc.
Expectoration	expectoration bloody black at night	Arn., bism., canth., chin., croc., crot-c., dig., dros., Elaps., kali-bi., nit-ac., nux-v., ph-ac., puls., zinc.
Expectoration	expectoration bloody during lactation (the production of milk by the mammary glands. the period during which milk is produced by the mammary glands)	Ferr.
Expectoration	expectoration bloody during menses	Iod., nat-m., phos., sep., Zinc.
Expectoration	expectoration bloody during suppressed menses	Acon., carb-v., dig., led., lyc., Nux-v., phos., puls., sulph.
Expectoration	expectoration bloody in afternoon	Alum., clem., lyc., mag-c., mez., mill., nux-v.
Expectoration	expectoration bloody in evening	Cub., nat-c., sep.
Expectoration	expectoration bloody in evening after lying down	Sep.

Body part/Disease	Symptom	Medicines
Expectoration	expectoration bloody in evening when coughing	Nat-c.
Expectoration	expectoration bloody in morning during menses	Zinc.
Expectoration	expectoration bloody in morning on bed	Nit-ac., Nux-v.
Expectoration	expectoration bloody in morning on rising	Aesc., ferr.
Expectoration	expectoration bloody in noon	Sil.
Expectoration	expectoration bloody on coughing	Bell., sep.
Expectoration	expectoration bloody on hawking	Cham., ferr., hyper., kali-n., nit-ac.
Expectoration	expectoration bloody when clearing the throat	Am-c.
Expectoration	expectoration bloody while lying down in morning	Merc.
Expectoration	expectoration bloody while walking	Cham., merc., sul-ac., zinc.
Expectoration	expectoration bloody while working	Merc.
Expectoration	expectoration blue & white alternately	Arund.
Expectoration	expectoration bluish	Arund., brom., kali-bi., nat-a., sulph.
Expectoration	expectoration bluish gray	Coc-c.
Expectoration	expectoration brick dust coloured	Bry., phos., rhus-t.
Expectoration	expectoration bright red at night	Acal., Acon., am-c., arn., ars., Bell., bry., calc., canth., carb-an., carb-v., cench., chin., cob., dig., dros., Dulc., ferr-p., ferr., Hyos., ip., kali-bi., kali-n., laur., led., merc., mill., nux-m., nux-v., phos., puls., rhus-t., sabad., Sabin., sec., sep., sil., zinc.
Expectoration	expectoration brown at night	Bry., calc., Carb-v., con., puls., rhus-t., sil.
Expectoration	expectoration brownish	Agar., ars., bry., caps., carb-an., carb-v., hyos., lyc., mag-c., phos., puls., sil.
Expectoration	expectoration brownish lumps	Agar., phos.
Expectoration	expectoration brownish yellow	Lyc.
Expectoration	expectoration chronic	Sul-ac.
Expectoration	expectoration constant almost day and evening	Arg-m., Squil.
Expectoration	expectoration containing blood and mucus	Op.
Expectoration	expectoration copious after each paroxysmal cough	Agar., alumn., anan., arg-n., Coc-c., kali-bi., sulph.
Expectoration	expectoration copious after meals	Sanic.
Expectoration	expectoration copious at day time	Cic., sil.
Expectoration	expectoration copious at night	Carb-v., kali-bi.
Expectoration	expectoration copious in evening	Carb-v., graph.
Expectoration	expectoration copious in evening on lying down	Graph.
Expectoration	expectoration copious in morning	Agar., alum., calc-s., calc., carb-v., cob., coc-c., dig., eupho., euphr., kali-bi., ph-ac., phos., psor., sanic., squil., stann.
Expectoration	expectoration copious in old people	Ammc., ant-t., ars., Bar-c., kreos.
Expectoration	expectoration copious in warm room	Kali-c.
Expectoration	expectoration copious mouthful at a time	Euphr., lyc., phos., rumx.
Expectoration	expectoration copious while moving	Ferr.
Expectoration	expectoration copious, bitter	Iod.

Body part/Disease	Symptom	Medicines
Expectoration	expectoration cream like yellowish white	Ambr.
Expectoration	expectoration dark	Ars., bism., carb-an., cupr., kali-bi., med., naja., nux-m., oena.
Expectoration	expectoration difficult in afternoon	Chin-s., chin.
Expectoration	expectoration difficult in aged people	Ammc.
Expectoration	expectoration easier after each cough	Aspar.
Expectoration	expectoration easier after eating	Bell., lyc., nux-m., phos., sanic., sil., staph., thuj.
Expectoration	expectoration easy at day time	Ail., arg-m., coc-c., dig., sil., staph.
Expectoration	expectoration easy at night	Meli.
Expectoration	expectoration easy in evening	Arg-m., dig.
Expectoration	expectoration easy in morning	Arund., mang.
Expectoration	expectoration easy on motion	Ip.
Expectoration	expectoration easy on waking	Meli.
Expectoration	expectoration flies forcibly out of mouth	Bad., chel., kali-c.
Expectoration	expectoration from cold wind	Lycps.
Expectoration	expectoration frothy (full of foam) in morning	Cub., dios., sulph., thuj.
Expectoration	expectoration gelatinous (semi solid)	Agar., alumn., Arg-m., arg-n., arn., bar-c., bry., cact., chin-s., chin., cupr., cur., dig., ferr., kreos., laur., med., Samb., sil., sulph., viol-o.
Expectoration	expectoration glairy (like egg white)	Arn., carb-h., Nat-m., nat-s.
Expectoration	expectoration globular (consisting of globules)	Agar., alumn., calad., cinch-b., coc-c., sel., sil., Stann., thuj.
Expectoration	expectoration granular (made up of grains or particles)	Agar., bad., calc., chin., hyper., kali-bi., lach., lyc., mang., mez., phos., sel., sep., sil., spong., thuj.
Expectoration	expectoration granular in morning	Lyc.
Expectoration	expectoration granular offensive	Sil.
Expectoration	expectoration granular while sneezing	Mez.
Expectoration	expectoration greenish in evening while lying down	Psor.
Expectoration	expectoration greenish in morning	Ars., crot-c., ferr., lyc., mang., nat-m., nit-ac., par., psor., sil., stann.
Expectoration	expectoration greenish on waking	Ferr., psor.
Expectoration	expectoration in afternoon	Alum., am-m., anac., ars., bad., caust., chin-s., chin., clem., coc-c., eucal., hydr., lyc., mag-c., mill., naja., nux-v., op., phos.
Expectoration	expectoration in bed	Calc., nit-ac.
Expectoration	expectoration in bed	Am-c., calc., ferr., phos., sep.
Expectoration	expectoration in bed in evening	Calc., nux-m., sep.
Expectoration	expectoration in bed in evening on getting warm	Nux-m.
Expectoration	expectoration in cold air	Lach., plan.
Expectoration	expectoration in forenoon	Bry., calc-s., chin-s., coc-c., iris., lyc., oena., sil., Stann., sulph., zinc.
Expectoration	expectoration in masses	Ars., coc-c., kali-n., sin-n.
Expectoration	expectoration in noon	Bell., calc-s., sil.
Expectoration	expectoration in open air	Chin-s., cob., lach., merc., nux-v., sacc., sep.

Body part/Disease	Symptom	Medicines
Expectoration	expectoration in pieces	Alum., nit-ac., rhus-t., sep.
Expectoration	expectoration in shape of balls	Agar., arg-n., coc-c., lyc., med., ph-ac., sil., squil., Stann., sulph.
Expectoration	expectoration in shape of little albuminous balls	Ph-ac.
Expectoration	expectoration like bile	Bar-c., dig., puls., samb.
Expectoration	expectoration like cheese	Chin., fago., lyc., puls., sal-ac., sanic.
Expectoration	expectoration like oil	Petr.
Expectoration	expectoration like starch	Agar., arg-m., bar-c., cact., coca., dig., laur., nat-a., phyt., sel., sulph.
Expectoration	expectoration looking dirty	Calc.
Expectoration	expectoration milky	Am-c., ars., aur., carb-v., ferr., Kali-chl., phos., plb., puls., sep., sil., sulph., zinc.
Expectoration	expectoration on rising	Calc., ferr., phos., Puls.
Expectoration	expectoration painful	Ars., cub., elaps., merc-c.
Expectoration	expectoration painful as if from heart	Elaps.
Expectoration	expectoration pasty	Kali-bi.
Expectoration	expectoration purulent	Arg-n., chin., sulph.
Expectoration	expectoration ropy	All-s., alumn., apis., coc-c., hydr., ip., Kali-bi., lach., lob., med., merc., nat-s., seneg., stict., viol-o.
Expectoration	expectoration stringy	Croc.
Expectoration	expectoration stringy	Aesc., agar., alum., Alumn., arg-m., ars-i., arum-i., asaf., calc-s., caust., chin-s., cimic., coc-c., ery-a., ferr., hydr., iber., Kali-bi., lach., lob., phos., rumx., ruta., sang., sanic., seneg., stict.
Expectoration	expectoration thick	Cupr.
Expectoration	expectoration thin	Ferr., nux-m., sabin.
Expectoration	expectoration viscid (thick and sticky)	Croc., cupr., mag-c., sec.
Expectoration	expectoration when dry on the floor looks as if burned	Phos.
Expectoration	expectoration while walking in open air	Merc., nux-v., sacc.
Expectoration	expectoration with blackish grains	Chin.
Expectoration	expectoration with threads of blood mixed with white sputa	Aur-m.
Expectoration	Expectoration, can raise sputa only on to tongue whence it must be removed by wiping	Apis.
Expectoration	fullness in chest ameliorated after expectoration	Ail.
Expectoration	gagging (restraint of speech) during expectoration	Arg-n., coc-c., par.
Expectoration	loose cough without expectoration	Am-c., arn., arum-t., brom., caust., con., crot-t., dros., kali-s., lach., phos., sep., stann., sulph.
Expectoration	pain in chest ameliorated from expectoration (to cough up and spit out phlegm, thus clearing the bronchial passages)	Chel., euon., mag-s.
Expectoration	pain in region of heart from expectorations	Asaf.
Expectoration	pain in throat aggravated on expectoration	Bell.

Body part/Disease	Symptom	Medicines
Expectoration	sensation of emptyness in chest after expectoration	Calad., stann., zinc.
Expectoration	weakness from cough & expectoration	Nux-v.
Expectoration	weakness in chest after expectoration	Stann.
Expectoration	wheezing breath ameliorated on expectoration	Ip.
Extension	extension of fingers difficult	Arn., ars., camph., carb-s., coloc., cupr-ar., cupr., hyos., merc., mosch., plat., plb., stram., syph., tab.
Extension	extension of legs difficult	Carb-o., pic-ac., stry.
Extension	extension of legs impossible	Con., plb.
Extension	extension of legs impossible while sitting	Lath.
Extension	extension of legs necessary	Sul-ac.
External Throat	pustules in external throat	Chel., psor.
External Throat	rash in external throat	Am-c.
External Throat	recurrent fibroid (benign growth composed of fibrous and muscle tissue, especially one that develops in the wall of the womb and is associated with painful and excessive menstrual flow) tumours in external throat	Sil.
Extremity	acute pain in extremities	**Acon.**, ant-c., ars., asc-c., bell., **Bry.**, calc-s., caul., cham., chel., chin-s., chin., cimic., **Colch.**, dulc., glon., ign., kali-bi., kalm., lac-c., lach., **Merc.**, nux-v., puls., rhod., **Rhus-t.**, sal-ac., sang., verat.
Extremity	extremities flexed (bend)	Acon., ars., carb-h., carb-o., colch., sec.
Extremity	extremities flexed and extended alternately	Carb-o., cic., cupr., hyos., lyc., nux-v., plb., sec., tab.
Extremity	extremities flexed at elbow	Lyc.
Extremity	extremities flexed backward	Acon., lyc.
Extremity	extremities flexed during convulsion	Colch., hydr-ac., hyos., phos., plb.
Extremity	extremities flexed in sleep	Ant-t.
Extremity	extremities flexed over chest	Morph., olnd., tab.
Extremity	extremities flexed spasmodically	Caust., hydr-ac., nux-m., nux-v., plb., stry.
Extremity	extremities flexed, extended while sitting	Nit-ac.
Extremity	heaviness in extremities after breakfast	Verat., Ther.
Extremity	heaviness in extremities after coition	Bufo.
Extremity	heaviness in extremities after dinner	Ant-c., sulph.
Extremity	heaviness in extremities after during storm	Phos.
Extremity	heaviness in extremities after emission	Ph-ac., puls.
Extremity	heaviness in extremities after exertion	Lach.
Extremity	heaviness in extremities after sexual excesses	Puls.
Extremity	heaviness in extremities after waking	Cham., tep.
Extremity	heaviness in extremities after while walking	Acon., calc., paeon., **Pic-ac.**
Extremity	heaviness in extremities after while walking in open air	Lyc., sil., zinc.
Extremity	heaviness in extremities ameliorated after rising	Lyc., nat-m.
Extremity	heaviness in extremities ameliorated after while walking in open air	Carb-v.

Body part/Disease	Symptom	Medicines
Extremity	heaviness in extremities ameliorated on motion	Caps., cham.
Extremity	heaviness in extremities ameliorated on rising after sittiing	Merc., nat-m.
Extremity	heaviness in extremities at night	Carb-v., caust., petr., sep.
Extremity	heaviness in extremities before chill	Ther.
Extremity	heaviness in extremities before menses	Bar-c., com., lyc., merc., nit-ac., zinc.
Extremity	heaviness in extremities during chill	Coc-c.
Extremity	heaviness in extremities during day time	Sulph.
Extremity	heaviness in extremities during fever	**Calc., Gels., Nux-v., Rhus-t.,** sulph.
Extremity	heaviness in extremities during menses	Cocc., nat-m.
Extremity	heaviness in extremities during pregnancy	Calc-p.
Extremity	heaviness in extremities from mental exertion	Ph-ac.
Extremity	heaviness in extremities in afternoon	Mag-m.
Extremity	heaviness in extremities in evening	Am-c., ammc., par., phos., sabad.
Extremity	heaviness in extremities in forenoon	Caust., cham., grat., sabad., stront.
Extremity	heaviness in extremities in morning	Calad., carb-an., caust., nat-m., nit-ac., pall., zinc.
Extremity	heaviness in extremities in morning in bed	Nat-m., nit-ac., phos., zinc.
Extremity	heaviness in extremities in noon after eating	Lyc.
Extremity	heaviness in extremities in noon while walking	Dig.
Extremity	heaviness in extremities on motion	Lach., mez.
Extremity	heaviness in extremities on rising	Phos.
Extremity	heaviness in extremities on rising after sittiing	Carb-v.
Extremity	heaviness in extremities on waking	Bar-c., clem., lyc., nat-m., phos., sulph., verat., zinc.
Extremity	heaviness in extremities on walking	Nux-v., pic-ac.
Extremity	heaviness in extremities while ascending stairs	Clem., lyc.
Extremity	heaviness in extremities while lying on left side	Merc-i-f.
Extremity	heavyness in extremities after breakfast and dinner	Agar.
Extremity	heavyness in extremities after drinking	Asaf.
Extremity	heavyness in extremities after stool	Agar., mur-ac., sep.
Extremity	heavyness in extremities before menses	Puls.
Extremity	heavyness in extremities during menses	Apis., graph., nat-m., puls.
Extremity	inflamation of extremities	Lach., merc-n., vip.
Extremity	itching in extremities after coition	Agar.
Extremity	itching in extremities after menses	Calc-s., calc., colch., con., cur., elaps., ferr., graph., kali-br., kali-c., kreos., lyc., mag-c., nat-m., Nit-ac., ph-ac., sil., sulph., Tarent., zinc.
Extremity	itching in extremities aggravated after scratching	Alum., ars., bism., corn., ham., led., petr., ph-ac., rhus-v., stront., **Sulph.**
Extremity	itching in extremities ameliorated after scratching	Alum., ant-t., bov., camph., cann-i., chel., chin., coloc., graph., jug-c., kali-c., laur., led., mag-c., mag-m., mang., merc., mill., **Nat-c.,** nat-s., nicc., ol-an., olnd., pall., ph-ac., tarax., thuj.

Body part/Disease	Symptom	Medicines
Extremity	itching in extremities in afternoon	Fago.
Extremity	itching in extremities in bed	Fago., lyc., nux-v., rumx.
Extremity	itching in extremities in bed at night	Rumx.
Extremity	itching in extremities when undressing	Nat-s., rumx.
Extremity	jerking of extremities painful	Sec.
Extremity	jerking of extremities while falling asleep	Agar., alum., arg-m., **Ars.**, cob., gels., hyper., **Ign.**, **Kali-c.**, nat-a., nat-m., phys., sel., sil., sulph., thuj.
Extremity	jerking of extremities, periodical	Bar-m.
Extremity	numbness in upper half of body	Bar-c.
Extremity	numbness of left half of body	Caust.
Extremity	numbness of whole body	Arg-n., bar-m., cedr., **Kali-br.**, lyss., ox-ac.
Extremity	numbness on one side the other side paralyzed	Cocc.
Extremity	pain in extremities after coition	**Sil.**, tub.
Extremity	pain in extremities after convulsions	Plb.
Extremity	pain in extremities after eating	Bry., indg., kali-bi., sep.
Extremity	pain in extremities after giving birth	Rhod.
Extremity	pain in extremities after midnight	**Ars.**, gels., merc., sars., sulph., thuj.
Extremity	pain in extremities after slight exertion	Agar., alum., bar-c., berb., calc., **Caust.**, cimic., con., gels., ign., kali-c., kali-n., mag-c., nat-c., nat-m., phos., rhus-t., ruta., sabin., sep., sil., stann., sul-ac., sulph., zinc.
Extremity	pain in extremities after walking	Raph., rhod., rhus-t., ruta.
Extremity	pain in extremities aggravated after sleep	Agar., lach., merc-c., op.
Extremity	pain in extremities aggravated from cold water	Ant-c., ars., phos., rhus-t., tarent.
Extremity	pain in extremities aggravated from drinking	**Crot-c.**
Extremity	pain in extremities aggravated from pressure	Cina., cocc., merc., plb.
Extremity	pain in extremities aggravated from thinking about the pain	Ox-ac.
Extremity	pain in extremities aggravated from thunderstorm	**Med.**, nat-c., **Rhod.**
Extremity	pain in extremities aggravated from touch during thunderstorm	**Chel.**, chin., cocc., vip.
Extremity	pain in extremities aggravated from warmth	Ant-t., apis, bry., guai., iod., kali-i., ptel., puls., **Sec.**, sep., stel., sulph., thuj.
Extremity	pain in extremities aggravated from warmth of bed	Apis., lac-c., led., **Merc.**, phyt., stel., sulph., verat.
Extremity	pain in extremities alternating sides	**Lac-c.**
Extremity	pain in extremities alternating with chill and heat	Brom.
Extremity	pain in extremities ameliorated after eating	Nat-c.
Extremity	pain in extremities ameliorated from applying cold	Apis., guai., lac-c., **Led.**, **Puls.**, **Sec.**, thuj.
Extremity	pain in extremities ameliorated from coffee	Arg-m.
Extremity	pain in extremities ameliorated from cold water	Puls.
Extremity	pain in extremities ameliorated from perspiration	Ars., bry., nux-v., thuj.
Extremity	pain in extremities ameliorated from pressure	Ars., bry., mag-p., plb.

Body part/Disease	Symptom	Medicines
Extremity	pain in extremities ameliorated from warmth	Aesc., agar., am-c., ant-c., arg-m., **Ars.**, bry., cact., caust., cham., chin., colch., coloc., graph., **Kali-bi.**, kali-c., **Kali-p.**, kalm., lyc., **Mag-p.**, merc., nux-v., ph-ac., pyrog., **Rhus-t.**, **Sil.**, sulph.
Extremity	pain in extremities ameliorated from warmth of bed	**Ars.**, kali-bi., nux-v., ph-ac., pyrog., **Rhus-t.**
Extremity	pain in extremities ameliorated in open air	**Kali-s.**, **Puls.**, sabin.
Extremity	pain in extremities ameliorated on continued motion	Agar., **Cham.**, **Rhus-t.**
Extremity	pain in extremities ameliorated on motion	Agar., arg-m., aur., cham., chin., con., dig., dulc., ferr., kali-c., kali-p., **Kali-s.**, lach., lyc., med., merc., mur-ac., nat-s., psor., **Puls.**, **Pyrog.**, rat., **Rhod.**, **Rhus-t.**, ruta., sep., thuj., tub., valer., zinc.
Extremity	pain in extremities ameliorated on walking	Agar., arg-m., ars., cham., chin., ferr., kali-i., kali-s., lyc., merc., nat-a., phos., puls., rhod., **Rhus-t.**, ruta., seneg., valer., verat.
Extremity	pain in extremities appear and disappear gradually	Stann.
Extremity	pain in extremities as after violent exercise	Aesc.
Extremity	pain in extremities at 2.00 to 3.00 a.m.	**Kali-c.**
Extremity	pain in extremities at 4.00 a.m.	Gels.
Extremity	pain in extremities at midnight	Sulph.
Extremity	pain in extremities at night	Acon., agar., alum., am-c., arn., ars., asaf., aur., bry., calc., carb-v., **Cham.**, cinnb., dulc., ferr., fl-ac., gels., graph., hep., kali-bi., kali-c., kali-i., kalm., lach., lyc., merc-i-f., merc-sul., **Merc.**, mez., nat-m., nit-ac., nux-v., phos., phyt., **Plb.**, podo., puls., rhod., rhus-t., sabin., sars., sulph., syph., thuj.
Extremity	pain in extremities at night drives out of bed	**Cham.**, ferr., **Merc.**
Extremity	pain in extremities before chill	**Arn.**, calc., carb-v., cina., **Eup-pur.**, lyc., nux-v., rhus-t.
Extremity	pain in extremities before midnight	Bry.
Extremity	pain in extremities during chill	Ang., aran., arn., **Ars.**, asaf., aur., bar-c., **Bov.**, bry., calc-s., calc., caps., carb-s., caust., chin-s., cimx., cina., cocc., **Coloc.**, cycl., **Dulc.**, **Eup-per.**, eup-pur., eupho., ferr., form., gels., graph., hell., hep., ign., **Ip.**, kali-ar., kali-c., **Kali-n.**, kali-s., lach., led., **Lyc.**, **Mez.**, mur-ac., nat-a., nat-c., nat-m., **Nux-v.**, op., petr., ph-ac., plb., psor., **Puls.**, **Pyrog.**, ran-b., **Rhus-t.**, sabad., **Sep.**, sil., squil., stram., sulph., **Tub.**, xan.
Extremity	pain in extremities during fever	Arn., ars., bell., **Bry.**, calc., chin., **Eup-per.**, ferr., merc., nat-m., **Nux-v.**, phos., ptel., puls., pyrog., rhod., rhus-t., sec., sep., sulph., tub., valer.
Extremity	pain in extremities during influenza	Acon., **Bry.**, caust., chel., **Eup-per.**, eupho., gels., naja.
Extremity	pain in extremities during menses	Bell., berb., bry., cast., cimic., con., graph., kali-n., kalm., nit-ac., nux-m., nux-v., phos., sep., spong., stram., verat.
Extremity	pain in extremities during sleep	Ars.
Extremity	pain in extremities even from draft of warm air	Sel.

Body part/Disease	Symptom	Medicines
Extremity	pain in extremities from becoming cold	**Ars.**, bry., calc., graph., kalm., **Nux-v.**, ph-ac., phos., puls., ran-b., **Rhus-t.**, tarent.
Extremity	pain in extremities from changes of the weather	Calc-p., **Rhod.**, sil.
Extremity	pain in extremities from cold air	**Ars.**, daph., kali-ar., kalm., sel., tarent.
Extremity	pain in extremities from fright	Merc.
Extremity	pain in extremities from jerking	Am-m., **Carb-s.**, puls.
Extremity	pain in extremities from lying on	Ars., bry., iod., lyc., merc., nux-v., rhus-t., verat.
Extremity	pain in extremities from mental exertion	Colch.
Extremity	pain in extremities from noise	Cocc., **Coff.**, nux-v.
Extremity	pain in extremities from sour wine	Ant-c.
Extremity	pain in extremities from wine	Led., mez., zinc.
Extremity	pain in extremities in afternoon	Calc., cina., glon., kali-c., lyc., lycps., nit-ac., ptel., staph., thuj.
Extremity	pain in extremities in afternoon	Calc., cina., glon., kali-c., lyc., lycps., nit-ac., ptel., staph., thuj.
Extremity	pain in extremities in evening	Am-c., apoc., ars., bell., cact., calc-p., calc., colch., kali-s., kalm., led., mag-s., petr., ph-ac., plan., **Plb.**, puls., rhus-t., sol-n., sulph.
Extremity	pain in extremities in evening after lying down	Ars.
Extremity	pain in extremities in forenoon	Am-c., mag-m., merc., nat-a., plan.
Extremity	pain in extremities in morning	Arg-n., calc-p., cinnb., clem., kali-bi., lyc., phos., sulph.
Extremity	pain in extremities in morning in bed	Nux-v., **Puls.**, rhus-t.
Extremity	pain in extremities in noon	Bry., sulph.
Extremity	pain in extremities in noon until midnight	Bell., mag-s., rhus-t.
Extremity	pain in extremities in wet weather	Am-c., ant-c., arg-m., bell., bor., bry., **Calc.**, carb-v., caust., **Colch.**, con., dulc., hep., lyc., **Merc.**, nat-s., nit-ac., nux-m., phyt., **Puls.**, **Rhod.**, **Rhus-t.**, ruta., sars., sep., sil., sulph., tub., **Verat.**
Extremity	pain in extremities on beginning to move	Agar., caps., carb-v., caust., **Ferr.**, fl-ac., graph., kali-p., lach., led., **Lyc.**, med., nit-ac., petr., ph-ac., **Phos.**, plb., psor., **Puls.**, pyrog., rhod., **Rhus-t.**, ruta., sil., valer.
Extremity	pain in extremities on changing place	Sang.
Extremity	pain in extremities on going to sleep	Kali-c.
Extremity	pain in extremities on motion	Aesc., berb., **Bry.**, calc-p., caps., chin., cocc., **Colch.**, coloc., dulc., euphr., guai., kalm., led., merc-c., naja., nat-m., nux-m., nux-v., ox-ac., phyt., plb., ran-b., sil., squil., zinc.
Extremity	pain in extremities on part lain on	Dros., graph., Kali-c., Nux-m., nux-v., sep.
Extremity	pain in extremities on walking	Coff., lyc., merc., op., ruta.
Extremity	pain in extremities towards morning	Ars., bov., kali-c., nux-v., rhus-t., thuj.
Extremity	pain in extremities towards morning on waking	Aesc., aur., hep., op., puls., sulph., tell., zinc.
Extremity	pain in extremities while ascending stairs	Calc., phos.
Extremity	pain in extremities while riding	Bry.
Extremity	pain in extremities while sitting	Pyrog., **Valer.**

Body part/Disease	Symptom	Medicines
Extremity	paralytic pain in extremities	Aur., fl-ac., mag-m., merc-c., nux-v., rhus-t., sabad., thuj.
Extremity	paroxysmal pain in extremities	**Carb-s.**, caul., caust., cocc., mag-p., **Nux-v.**, phos., **Plb.**, **Puls.**, sec.
Extremity	rheumatic pain in extremities after a cold	Acon., arn., bry., calc-p., calc., coloc., dulc., gels., guai., merc., nit-ac., ph-ac., rhus-t., sulph.
Extremity	rheumatic pain in extremities after becoming cold	Ph-ac., **Rhus-t.**
Extremity	rheumatic pain in extremities alternating with chest affection	Led.
Extremity	rheumatic pain in extremities alternating with diarrhoea	Cimic., dulc., kali-bi.
Extremity	rheumatic pain in extremities alternating with dyspnoea	Guai.
Extremity	rheumatic pain in extremities alternating with eruptions	Crot-t., staph.
Extremity	rheumatic pain in extremities alternating with gastric symptoms	**Kali-bi.**
Extremity	rheumatic pain in extremities alternating with haemorrhoids	Abrot.
Extremity	rheumatic pain in extremities alternating with pain in heart	Benz-ac.
Extremity	rheumatic pain in extremities alternating with pulmonary troubles	**Kali-bi.**
Extremity	rheumatic pain in extremities ameliorated after a cold	Guai., lac-c., **Led.**, **Puls.**, **Sec.**
Extremity	rheumatic pain in extremities drive him out of bed	**Cham.**, ferr., lac-c., led., **Merc.**, sulph., verat.
Extremity	rheumatic pain in extremities extending to lower limbs	Kali-c.
Extremity	rheumatic pain in extremities extending upward	Kalm., **Led.**
Extremity	rheumatic pain in extremities following diarrhoea	Kali-bi.
Extremity	rheumatic pain in extremities from abuse of mercury	Arg-m., arn., asaf., bell., calc., carb-v., cham., **Chin.**, **Guai.**, **Hep.**, kali-i., lach., lyc., mez., nit-ac., ph-ac., phyt., podo., puls., rhod., **Sars.**, sulph., valer.
Extremity	rheumatic pain in extremities from checked diarrhoea	Abrot.
Extremity	rheumatic pain in extremities from left to right	**Lach.**, naja., rhus-t.
Extremity	rheumatic pain in extremities from overheated and exertion	Zinc.
Extremity	rheumatic pain in extremities from right to left	**Lyc.**
Extremity	rheumatic pain in extremities from suppressed haemorrhoids	Abrot.
Extremity	rheumatic pain in extremities in chronic diarrhoea	Nat-s.
Extremity	rheumatic pain in extremities in cold weather	Ars., **Bry.**, **Calc-p.**, carb-v., colch., dulc., kali-bi., kalm., nit-ac., nux-v., ph-ac., phos., puls., rhod., **Rhus-t.**, sul-ac., tub.
Extremity	rheumatic pain in extremities in first warm days	Bry.

Body part/Disease	Symptom	Medicines
Extremity	rheumatic pain in extremities in injured parts	Caust.
Extremity	rheumatic pain in extremities in places least covered by flesh	Sang.
Extremity	rheumatic pain in extremities in spring	Colch.
Extremity	rheumatic pain in extremities in warm weather	**Colch.**, kali-bi.
Extremity	rheumatic pain in extremities with perspiration	**Form.**, **Merc.**, sulph., til.
Extremity	rheumatic syphilitic pain in extremities	Benz-ac., fl-ac., kali-bi., **Kali-i.**, kalm., merc., nit-ac., phyt.
Extremity	shaking of extremities	Kali-br., op.
Extremity	shaking of extremities after faintness	Arn., asaf., colch., kali-br., kreos., lyc., merc-c., sec., stry.
Extremity	shaking of extremities at night	Stram.
Extremity	shaking of extremities in evening	Nux-v.
Extremity	shaking of extremities in noon after eating	Graph.
Extremity	shaking of extremities when sleeping after dinner	Nux-v.
Extremity	ulcerative pain in extremities	Agar.
Extremity	walking difficult	Aur., chin., olnd., ter.
Eye	after cataract operation	Arn., seneg.
Eye	after operation for cataract	Guare., phyt.
Eye	alter shape of iris	Apis., merc., rhus-t.
Eye	amaurosis (partial or complete vision impairment, especially when there is no obvious damage to the eye) of the right optic nerve (either of the second pair of cranial nerves whose nerve fibers transmit visual light signals from the eye to the brain) then the left	Chin.
Eye	amaurosis of the right optic nerve	Bov.
Eye	Ameliorated from closing eyes	Kali-c., zinc.
Eye	Anaemia of cojunctiva (a delicate mucous membrane that covers the internal part of the eyelid and is attached to the cornea)	Dig., plb.
Eye	Anaemia of retina (a light-sensitive membrane in the back of the eye containing rods and cones that receive an image from the lens and send it to the brain through the optic nerve)	Agar., chin., dig., lith.
Eye	anxiety from exertion of eyes	Sep.
Eye	anxiety on closing eyes	Calc., Carb-v., mag-m.
Eye	atrophy of optic nerve	Nux-v., Phos., tab.
Eye	atrophy of optic nerve from tobacco	Ars.
Eye	bleeding from eyes	Acon., aloe., am-c., am-caust., arn., bell., Both., calc., camph., carb-v., cham., cor-r., Crot-h., dig., elaps., euphr., kali-chl., Lach., nit-ac., Nux-v., Phos., plb., raph., ruta., sulph.
Eye	bleeding from eyes, from blowing nose	Nit-ac.
Eye	blindness, after injury to eye	Arn.
Eye	blindness, after pain in head and eyes	Con.

Body part/Disease	Symptom	Medicines
Eye	blinking	Chel., kalm., mez., nux-v.
Eye	bluish black vesicles (fluid-filled cyst) above the eyes	Ran-b.
Eye	boils, about the eyes	Sil.
Eye	breathing difficult on closing eyes	Carb-an., carb-v.
Eye	burning, back of the eyes	Form.
Eye	cancer,epithelioma of lachrymal glands (relating to tears)	Carb-an.
Eye	carbuncles on eye	Agar., Arg-n., cann-i., kali-c., zinc.
Eye	cataract (an eye disease in which the lens becomes covered in an opaque film that affects sight, eventually causing total loss of sight)	Sulph.
Eye	cataract of right eye	Am-c., kali-c., nit-ac., sil.
Eye	cataract, beginning	Caust., puls., sec., sep.
Eye	cataract, from contusion (an injury in which skin and bone are not broken but damage is done to tissues under the skin, causing a bruise)	Arn., con.
Eye	cataract, senile (after the age of 65 years)	Carb-an., sec.
Eye	cataract, in women	Sep.
Eye	chemosis (swelling of eye whites) of cornea	Hep.
Eye	chemosis of left eye	Bell.
Eye	chemosis of right eye	Syph., vesp.
Eye	chest symptoms alternating with eye symptoms	Ars.
Eye	Chill on closing the eyes	Mag-m.
Eye	Condylomata at corner of eye	Calc., nit-ac.
Eye	Condylomata in iris (the colored part of the eye that consists of a muscular diaphragm surrounding the pupil and regulates the light entering the eye by expanding and contracting the pupil)	Cinnb., Merc., staph., thuj.
Eye	Condylomata on eye bleeding when touched	Nit-ac.
Eye	Conical (cone shaped transparent convex membrane that covers the pupil and iris of the eye) cornea	Euphr., puls.
Eye	conjunctiva	Apis., arg-n., ars., bell., bry., cadm., cedr., cham., chel., chlol., eupho., graph., ip., led., nat-a., nat-c., nat-m., nux-v., sep.
Eye	constant movements of eyeballs	Agar., bell., benz-n., iod., sil., stram.
Eye	constant movements of eyeballs under closed eyelids	Benz-n.
Eye	Constriction in brain extending to eyes and nose	Nit-ac.
Eye	cornea become worse or useless	Ars.
Eye	cough excited from closing eyes at night	Hep.
Eye	cracks in corner of eye	Alum., Graph., iod., Lyc., merc., nat-m., nit-ac., petr., phos., plat., sep., sil., sulph., zinc.
Eye	crawling in corner of eye	Plat.

Body part/Disease	Symptom	Medicines
Eye	crawling in eye	Agar., asar., bell., chin., cina., colch., nat-c., nat-s., seneg., sep., spig., sulph., verat.
Eye	dermoid (a benign tumor that contains skin or skin derivatives, found in the ovaries or on the face, especially around the eyes) around the eyes	Calc., nat-c., nat-m., thuj.
Eye	desire to close eyes	Agar., ant-t., bell., calc., caust., chel., con., dios., elaps., gels., lact-ac., med., ox-ac., sil.
Eye	desire to rub eye	All-c., apis., bor., carb-ac., caust., con., croc., fl-ac., gymn., kali-bi., mez., morph., nat-c., op., plb., puls., rat., squil., sulph.
Eye	discharges of mucous or pus from eye at night	Alum.
Eye	discharges of mucous or pus from eye in evening	Kali-p.
Eye	discharges of mucous or pus from eye in morning	Arg-n., ars., cinnb., kali-bi., mag-c., plb., sep., sil., staph., sulph.
Eye	discharges, acrid from eye	Am-c., ars-i., ars., calc., carb-s., cham., coloc., euphr., fl-ac., graph., hep., kali-ar., merc., nit-ac., sulph.
Eye	discharges, bloody from eye	Ars., asaf., carb-s., carb-v., caust., cham., hep., kali-c., kreos., lach., lyc., merc., mez., nat-m., petr., ph-ac., phos., puls., rhus-t., sep., sil., sulph., thuj.
Eye	discharges, from corner of eye	Ant-c., bell., berb., bism., dig., eupho., kali-bi., nat-c., nat-m., nux-v., pic-ac., psor.
Eye	discharges, from lachrymal sac (bone of eye socket)	Ars., arum-t., con., hep., iod., merc., nat-m., Petr., puls., sil., stann., sulph.
Eye	discharges, like acrid water from eye	Clem.
Eye	discharges, milky-white from eye	Kali-chl.
Eye	discharges, of pus from corner of eye	Cham., graph., kali-bi., kali-c., kali-i., led., Nux-v., ph-ac., ran-b., zinc.
Eye	discharges, purulent from eye	Ail., alumn., arg-m., Arg-n., Calc., carb-s., carb-v., caust., cham., chlor., ery-a., eupho., ferr-i., graph., grin., Hep., kali-i., lach., led., Lyc., lyss., mag-c., mag-m., Merc., nat-c., nit-ac., petr., ph-ac., phos., Puls., rhus-t., sep., spong., sulph., tell.
Eye	discharges, thick from eye	Alum., arg-n., calc-s., chel., euphr., hep., hydr., kali-bi., lyc., nat-m., puls., sep., sil., sulph., thuj.
Eye	discharges, thin from eye	Graph.
Eye	discharges, white from eye	Alum., hydr., lachn., petr., plb.
Eye	discharges, yellow from eye	Agar., alum., arg-n., ars., aur., calc-s., calc., carb-s., carb-v., caust., chel., euphr., kali-bi., kali-c., kali-chl., kali-s., kreos., lyc., merc., nat-p., Puls., sep., Sil., sulph., thuj.
Eye	discolouration of iris	Aur., coloc., euphr., kali-i., merc-i-f., nat-m., spig., syph.
Eye	ecchymosis in eye	Acon., aeth., am-c., arg-n., Arn., bell., Cact., cham., chlol., con., crot-h., cupr-ac., erig., glon., ham., kali-bi., kali-chl., kreos., lach., Led., lyc., lyss., nux-v., phos., plb., ruta., sul-ac., ter.
Eye	ecchymosis in eye from coughing	Arn., bell.
Eye	excoriation (tear somebody's skin off) of canthi (corner of eye)	Alum., apis., Ars., bor., eupho.

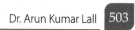

Body part/Disease	Symptom	Medicines
Eye	eye symptoms ameliorated from moon light	Aur.
Eye	eyeballs, floating	Kali-c.
Eye	fistula (an anal fistula may develop after an abscess in the rectum has burst , creating an opening between the anal canal and the surface of the skin) in eye	Sil.
Eye	fistula lacrymalis	Agar., apis., arg-n., aur-m., brom., Calc., chel., Fl-ac., hep., lach., lyc., mill., nat-c., nat-m., nit-ac., Petr., phyt., Puls., Sil., stann., sulph.
Eye	fistula lacrymalis discharging pus on pressure	Puls., sil., stann.
Eye	fungus growth in eye	Bell., Calc., lyc., Phos., sep., sil., thuj.
Eye	glaucoma (an eye disorder marked by unusually high pressure within the eyeball that leads to damage of the optic disk)	Areca 3,6., Phos., prun-s., spig., sulph.
Eye	green colour around eyes	Canth., cupr-ac.
Eye	headache extending around the eyes	Arg-n., asaf., brom., calc., caust., croc., crot-h., ign., kali-c., kali-s., lach., lyss., mag-m., merc., nat-m., nicc., Nit-ac., Puls., rhus-t., seneg., spig., Sulph.
Eye	headache on closing eyes	All-c., aloe., alumn., ant-t., apis., ars., chin., ferr-p., ferr., grat., hep., ip., lac-c., lach., nux-v., op., ph-ac., sabin., sil., ther., thuj.
Eye	hearing impaired alternating with eye symptoms	Guare.
Eye	heaviness of Head from motion of eyes	Bry., chin., nux-v., rhus-t.
Eye	heaviness of Head on exertion of eyes	Mur-ac.
Eye	herpes in eye	Alum., bry., caust., con., kreos., lach., olnd., spong., sulph.
Eye	herpes of cornea	Graph., hep., ign.
Eye	hyperesthesis of the retina	Con., crot-h., ign., lact-ac., Nat-m., nux-v.
Eye	Impossible to walk with closed eyes	Alumina
Eye	inclination to wipe eye	Agar., alum., arg-n., calc., carb-an., croc., kreos., lac-c., lyc., nat-c., plb., puls., rat., sep.
Eye	inflammation , after adhesions of iris	Calc., clem., merc-c., nit-ac., sil., spig., staph., sulph., ter.
Eye	Inflammation of eye after injuries	Acon., Arn., calc., puls., Sil., sulph.
Eye	Inflammation of eye after measles	Arg-m., carb-v., crot-h., euphr., puls.
Eye	Inflammation of eye aggravated from becoming wet	Calc., dulc., rhus-t.
Eye	Inflammation of eye aggravated from cold	Ars., sil.
Eye	Inflammation of eye aggravated from dry cold wind	Acon.
Eye	Inflammation of eye aggravated from warmth of bed	Merc.
Eye	Inflammation of eye aggravated from washing	Sulph.
Eye	Inflammation of eye alternating with sore throat	Par.
Eye	Inflammation of eye ameliorated from cold	Apis., Arg-n., asar., bry., caust., Puls., sep.
Eye	inflammation of eye ameliorated from cold applications	Apis., asar., puls.

Body part/Disease	Symptom	Medicines
Eye	Inflammation of eye ameliorated from warm covering	Hep.
Eye	inflammation of eye due to choroid (a brownish membrane between the retina and the white of the eye that contains blood vessels and large pigmented cells)	Ars., aur., bell., Bry., cedr., coloc., gels., ip., jab., kali-chl., kali-i., merc-c., merc-d., merc., nux-v., phos., phyt., prun-s., psor., puls., ruta., sil., spig., sulph., thuj.
Eye	Inflammation of eye erysipelatous	Acon., anac., Apis., bell., com., graph., hep., led., merc-c., merc., Rhus-t., vesp.
Eye	Inflammation of eye from wounds	Arn., calad., Staph.
Eye	Inflammation of eye from bites of insects	Led.
Eye	Inflammation of eye from burns	Canth.
Eye	inflammation of eye from carbuncles (Inflammed swelling)	Bell., berb., cann-i.
Eye	Inflammation of eye from foreign bodies	Acon., Arn., calc., puls., Sil., sulph.
Eye	Inflammation of eye from heat	Apis., Bad., Bell., bry., Glon., kali-i., med., merc., still.
Eye	Inflammation of eye from sand and dust	Sulph.
Eye	Inflammation of eye from wounds in canthi (corner of eye)	Am-c., apis., Arg-n., bor., bufo., calc-s., calc., clem., graph., kali-c., mag-c., merc., nat-c., sulph., zinc.
Eye	Inflammation of eye from wounds in canthi (corner of eye)	Am-c., apis., Arg-n., bor., bufo., calc-s., calc., clem., graph., kali-c., mag-c., merc., nat-c., sulph., zinc.
Eye	Inflammation of eye gonorrhœal	Ant-t., chin., cor-r., cub., med., merc., Nit-ac., Puls., spig., sulph., thuj.
Eye	Inflammation of eye in infants	Acon., alumn., Apis., arg-m., Arg-n., arn., Ars., arund., bell., bor., bry., Calc., cham., dulc., euphr., hep., ign., lyc., merc-c., merc., Nit-ac., nux-v., Puls., rhus-t., sulph., Thuj., zinc.
Eye	Inflammation of eye in summer	Sep.
Eye	Inflammation of eye in wet weather	Dulc., Rhus-t., sil.
Eye	inflammation of eye meibomian (Swelling)	Cham., colch., dig., euphr., hep., indg., kreos., phos., puls., staph., stram., sulph.
Eye	inflammation of eye of sclerotics (white of the eye)	Acon., cocc., hura., kalm., merc., psor., rhus-t., spig., thuj.
Eye	Inflammation of eye recurrent	Ars., bry., Calc., sulph.
Eye	Inflammation of eye syphilitic	Arg-m., arg-n., ars., Asaf., aur-m-n., aur-m., aur., cinnb., clem., graph., hep., Kali-i., Merc-c., merc-cy., merc-i-f., Merc., Nit-ac., Phyt., staph., syph., thuj.
Eye	inflammation of eye tubercular	Bar-i., tub.
Eye	Inflammation of eye with headache	Apis., led., verat.
Eye	Inflammation of eye with swelling of feet	Ars.
Eye	inflammation of eye with ulceration	Apis., bufo., kali-c., zinc.
Eye	inflammation of iris aggravated at night	Ars., dulc., Kali-i., Merc-c., Merc., nit-ac., rhus-t., staph., sulph., zinc.
Eye	inflammation of iris with bursting pain in eyeball, temple and side of face	Staph.
Eye	inflammation of iris, syphilitic	Arg-n., ars., asaf., aur-m., aur., cinnb., hep., Kali-i., Merc-c., merc-i-f., merc., Nit-ac., petr., staph., syph., thuj., zinc.
Eye	inflammation of optic nerve	Bell., phos., plb., puls., tab.

Body part/Disease	Symptom	Medicines
Eye	inflammation of retina	Ars., asaf., aur., calc., crot-h., gels., kalm., lach., merc-c., merc., phos., prun-s., puls., sec., sulph.
Eye	inflammation of sclerotics (relating to the dense outer coating of the eyeball that forms the white of the eye sclera) with stitches and aversion to sunlight	Nux-v.
Eye	inflammation of throat alternating with sore eyes	Par.
Eye	Inflammation, of eye after vaccination	Thuj.
Eye	inversion of eye lids	Anan., bor., calc., graph., merc., nat-m., nit-ac., sulph., zinc.
Eye	irritation in eye	Apis., ars., caust., con., fago., ign., iod., lyc., merc-i-f., nat-a., puls., ran-s., rhus-t., ruta., sang.
Eye	itching in eye after dinner	Mag-c.
Eye	itching in eye aggravated from rubbing	Mag-c.
Eye	itching in eye ameliorated from cold application	Puls.
Eye	itching in eye ameliorated from rubbing	Agar., caust., euphr., mag-c., nat-c., nux-v., ol-an., spong., stram., sulph., zinc.
Eye	itching in eye ameliorated in open air	Puls.
Eye	itching in eye at night	Ars., sulph.
Eye	itching in eye during coryza	Caps.
Eye	itching in eye from exertion of vision	Rhus-t.
Eye	itching in eye from light	Anan.
Eye	itching in eye from warm bathing	Mez.
Eye	itching in eye in evening	Acon., calc-p., calc., cupr., dios., erig., eug., eupho., ferr., gamb., mag-c., meph., merc-c., pall., phos., Puls., sil., Sulph., vesp.
Eye	itching in eye in forenoon	Sulph.
Eye	itching in eye in morning	Agar., am-c., dios., fago., meph., nat-m., nat-s., sulph.
Eye	itching in eye after rising in morning	Nat-m.
Eye	itching in eyelids	Sars.
Eye	itching of canthi (borner of eye) aggravated in open air	Staph.
Eye	itching of canthi ameliorated in open air	Gamb.
Eye	itching of canthi in evening	Mag-c., puls.
Eye	itching under eyes	Apis., con.
Eye	lachrymation (the production of tears in the eyes, especially excessive production as in crying or in reaction to a foreign body) aggravated from looking upward steadily	Ars., bell., carb-v., chel., colch., sulph.
Eye	lachrymation at day time only	Alum., lyc., sars., zinc.
Eye	lachrymation at night	Acon., all-s., apis., Zinc.
Eye	lachrymation during chill	Elat.
Eye	lachrymation during coryza	agar., All-c., alum., anac., anan., arg-n., ars-i., ars., carb-ac., Carb-v., chin., dulc., Euphr., iod., jab., kali-c., lach., lyc., Nux-v., phos., phyt., puls., ran-s., sabad., sang., sin-n., spig., staph., Tell., verb.

Body part/Disease	Symptom	Medicines
Eye	lachrymation during headache	Agar., arg-n., asar., bell., bov., carb-an., carb-v., chel., com., con., eug., hep., ign., Ind., kali-i., lac-c., lil-t., merc., osm., plat., puls., rhus-r., spong., stram., tax.
Eye	lachrymation from bright light	Ail., chel., chin-s., kreos., mag-m., sabad., spong.
Eye	lachrymation from light	Dig., kreos., puls., spong.
Eye	lachrymation from light of sun	Bry., graph., ign., staph.
Eye	lachrymation from looking steadily	Agar., Apis., cadm., caust., chel., cinnb., croc., echi., eupho., ign., kali-c., merc., nat-a., osm., ruta., seneg., spong., tab., thuj.
Eye	lachrymation from right eye	Brom., calc., hyos., verb., vesp.
Eye	lachrymation in cold air	Cob., dig., echi., euphr., kreos., lyc., phos., Puls., sep., sil., thuj.
Eye	lachrymation in damp weather	Crot-h., graph.
Eye	lachrymation in evening	Acon., all-c., asar., calc., eug., mag-m., merc., nicc., phos., rhus-t., ruta., sep., ter., Zinc.
Eye	lachrymation in fornoon	Nat-c., squil.
Eye	lachrymation in left eye	Carb-ac., clem., coloc., dios., ign., sin-n., uran.
Eye	lachrymation in morning	Alum., calc., carb-an., kali-n., kreos., lachn., mag-c., merc., nat-c., nat-m., nicc., phel., phos., Puls., rat., rhus-t., sep., staph., Sulph., zinc.
Eye	lachrymation in wind	Euphr., lyc., nat-m., phos., Puls., rhus-t., sanic., sil., sulph., thuj.
Eye	lachrymation when laughing	Nat-m.
Eye	lachrymation when yawning	when : Ant-t., calc-p., ign., kali-c., kreos., meph., nux-v., rhus-t., sabad., sars., staph., viol-o.
Eye	lachrymation while looking at the fire	Ant-c., chel., mag-m., merc., sabad.
Eye	lachrymation while reading	Am-c., carb-s., croc., grat., ign., nat-a., nit-ac., olnd., phos., ruta., seneg., sep., still., sul-ac.
Eye	lachrymation while writing	Calc., ol-an.
Eye	lachrymation with cough	Acon., agar., aloe., brom., bry., calc., carb-ac., carb-v., cench., chel., cina., cycl., eup-per., eupho., Euphr., graph., hep., ip., kali-c., kali-ma., kreos., merc., Nat-m., op., phyt., Puls., rhus-t., sabad., sil., Squil., staph., sulph.
Eye	lachrymation with pain in the eye	Calc., chel., coloc., ferr.
Eye	left pupil (the dark circular opening at the center of the iris in the eye, where light enters the eye) dilated more than right	Nat-a., urt-u.
Eye	left pupils contracted	Arg-m., tarent.
Eye	left pupils contracted with right pupil dilated	Colch., lyss., rhod., tarent.
Eye	lens of eye enlarged	Colch.
Eye	movements of eye up and down	Benz-ac., sulph.
Eye	must close eyes	Agar., arn., calc., canth., carb-v., chel., eupho., kali-c., lyc., mez., sil., spig.
Eye	must keep the eyes open and look into the light	Puls.

Body part/Disease	Symptom	Medicines
Eye	myopia (a common condition in which light entering the eye is focused in front of the retina and distant objects cannot be seen sharply)	Agar., am-c., anac., apis., arg-n., ars., calc., carb-s., carb-v., chin., cimic., coff-t., con., cycl., dig., euphr., gels., graph., grat., hyos., jab., lach., lyc., mang., meph., mez., nat-a., nat-c., nat-m., nat-p., nit-ac., petr., ph-ac., Phos., Phys., pic-ac., plb., psor., Puls., raph., ruta., sel., spong., stram., sul-ac., sulph., syph., thuj., tub., valer., verb., viol-o., viol-t.
Eye	nausea aggravated from motion of eyes	Con., graph., jab., puls., sep.
Eye	nausea ameliorated from closing the eyes	Con.
Eye	nausea from using the eyes	Con., graph., jab., sep., ther.
Eye	nausea on closing the eyes	Lach., sabad., ther.
Eye	numbness around eyes	Asaf.
Eye	opacity (material through which light cannot pass) of left cornea with arcus senilis (an opaque circle around the cornea of the eye that can develop late in life)	Acon., ars., cocc., coloc., kali-bi., merc-c., merc., mosch., Puls., Sulph., zinc.
Eye	opacity of left cornea	Hep., sulph.
Eye	operation for cataract, after evening, while at work	Mez.
Eye	operation for cataract, after evening, while at work	Mez.
Eye	ovaries painful with pain in eye	Sulph.
Eye	pain around the eyes	Cinnb., gels., ign., Mag-m., merc-c., merc., nit-ac., pall., phyt., puls., Spig., sulph., ter.
Eye	pain in cervical region extending to eye	Gels., sel., Sil., sulph., thea.
Eye	pain in ear extending to left eye	Hura.
Eye	pain in ear extending to right eye	Glon., hura., puls., spig.
Eye	pain in external throat extending to eye	Sel.
Eye	pain in eye after coition (sexual intercourse)	Bart.
Eye	pain in eye aggravated by closing	Bell., canth., carb-v., cimic., clem., con., fago., lact-ac., sil., staph., sumb.
Eye	pain in eye aggravated from dim light	Am-m., apis., sars., stram.
Eye	pain in eye aggravated from pressure	Brom., dros., ham., plan., sars.
Eye	pain in eye aggravated from rest	Coloc., dros., dulc., merc-i-f., mur-ac., thuj.
Eye	pain in eye aggravated from sun light	Aml-n., calc., clem., hep., kali-p., mang., nat-a., nat-m., sulph.
Eye	pain in eye aggravated from thinking of the pain	Lach., spig.
Eye	pain in eye aggravated from warmth	Arn., chel., merc., mez., nat-m., puls.
Eye	pain in eye aggravated from wet weather	Calc., dulc., merc., rhus-t., spig.
Eye	pain in eye alternates with pain in abdomen	Euphr.
Eye	pain in eye alternates with pain in left arm	Plb.
Eye	pain in eye alternates with pain in ovary	Sulph.
Eye	pain in eye amelioratd from warmth	Ars., aur-m., dulc., ery-a., Hep., kali-ar., lac-d., mag-p., nat-a., nat-c., seneg., sil., spig., thuj.
Eye	pain in eye ameliorated by closing	Chel., lac-d., nit-ac., ph-ac., pic-ac., plat., sin-n.
Eye	pain in eye ameliorated by covering eyes with hand	Aur-m., thuj.

Body part/Disease	Symptom	Medicines
Eye	pain in eye ameliorated by dark	chin., euphr., nux-m., staph.
Eye	pain in eye ameliorated from lying on left side	Nat-a.
Eye	pain in eye ameliorated from lying on painful side	Lach., zinc.
Eye	pain in eye ameliorated from motion of eyes	Dulc., op.
Eye	pain in eye ameliorated from pressure	Asaf., bapt., bry., calc., caust., chel., chin-s., cimic., coloc., con., ham., mag-m., mag-p., mur-ac., pic-ac.
Eye	pain in eye ameliorated from rest	Berb., pic-ac.
Eye	pain in eye ameliorated when lying on	Chel., cimic.
Eye	pain in eye at each beat of heart	Atro.
Eye	pain in eye at each step	Hep.
Eye	pain in eye during menses	Carb-an., coloc., croc.
Eye	pain in eye extending to arm	Rumx.
Eye	pain in eye extending to ear	Fago., petr.
Eye	pain in eye extending to forehead	Agar., croc., hura., kalm., ran-b.
Eye	pain in eye extending to frontal sinus (a cavity filled with air in the bones of the face and skull, especially one opening into the nasal passages)	Spig.
Eye	pain in eye extending to occiput (back part of the head)	Bry., coc-c., colch., com., crot-t., dios., kali-p., lach., nat-a., pic-ac., sil.
Eye	pain in eye extending to over side of face	Lyc., op.
Eye	pain in eye extending to temples	Anac., bad., chel., coc-c., ip., phys.
Eye	pain in eye extending to vertex	Cimic., croc., lach., phyt.
Eye	pain in eye from artificial light	Calc-p., calc., carb-an., chel., cina., croc., ip., lith., lyc., mang., nat-a., nat-m., nux-v., petr., pic-ac., plat., sars., seneg., sep., staph.
Eye	pain in eye from day light	Am-c., hell., hep., lact-ac., merc., sars., sil.
Eye	pain in eye from glaring at fire	Merc.
Eye	pain in eye from sunrise until sunset	Kalm.
Eye	pain in eye in glaucoma	Mez., phos.
Eye	pain in eye on reading and writing	Nat-a.
Eye	pain in eye when looking at near objects	Echi., mang.
Eye	pain in eye when looking at strong light	Acon., anac., apis., caust., Nat-m., ph-ac., phos., rheum., ruta., sars., sulph., tab.
Eye	pain in eye when swallowing	Tarent.
Eye	pain in eye while reading	Calc., mill., nat-s., phys., Ruta.
Eye	pain in eye while sewing	Apis., ars-m., cina., dig., mez.,Ruta.
Eye	pain in eye with nausea	Thuj.
Eye	pain in left eye	Agar.
Eye	pain in lower limb alternating with eye symptoms	Kreos.
Eye	pain in nose extending to eyes	Hep., lyc.
Eye	pain of eyes ameliorated by cold water	Acon., apis., asar., aur., form., lac-d., nat-a., nit-ac., phos., pic-ac., puls.
Eye	pain of eyes ameliorated from profuse urination	Acon., ferr-p., gels., ign., kalm., sang., sil., ter., verat.

Body part/Disease	Symptom	Medicines
Eye	pain of face below eye	Acon., arg-n., ars., aur-m-n., bell., chin., coloc., gels., hydrc., iris., mag-p., mez., nux-v., plat., sil., spig., sulph., verb., zinc.
Eye	pain of face on closing eyes	Cimic., med.
Eye	painin eye from fine work	Carb-v., coloc., con., jab., merc., mur-ac., nat-m., Ruta., seneg., sulph.
Eye	palpitation of heart in morning must lie still with closed eyes	Carb-an.
Eye	palpitation of heart upon opening eyes	Carb-an.
Eye	paralysis of iris (the colored part of the eye that consists of a muscular diaphragm surrounding the pupil and regulates the light entering the eye by expanding and contracting the pupil)	Ars., kali-bi., par.
Eye	paralysis of lower limb with jerking of eyes	Alum-m., arg-n.
Eye	perspiration at day time when closing the eyes	**Con.**
Eye	perspiration in hand with ophthalmia (inflammation of eyes)	Brom., cadm., calc., con., dulc., **Fl-ac.**, gymn., Ind., iod., led., petr., **Sulph.**
Eye	perspiration on closing the eyes	Bry., calc., carb-an., **Con.**, lach., thuj.
Eye	photophobia (very low tolerance of the eye for light) at night	Con., gels.
Eye	photophobia, chronic	Aeth., nat-s., sil.
Eye	photophobia, desires lamp light	Stram.
Eye	photophobia, from artificial light	Agar., arg-n., aster., bor., calc-p., calc., cast., chel., coff., con., crot-h., cupr., dros., euphr., gels., ip., lac-d., lith., merc., nat-m., phos., puls., stram., sulph.
Eye	photophobia, from blue light	Tab.
Eye	photophobia, from sunlight	Acon., ars., asar., berb., bry., calc., camph., cast., Chin., cic., clem., euphr., Graph., hep., ign., kali-ar., lac-c., lith., merc-c., merc-sul., merc., petr., ph-ac., phos., Sulph., zinc.
Eye	photophobia, in afternoon	Zing.
Eye	photophobia, in evening	bor., Calc., carb-an., caust., eug., euphr., lyc., merc., ph-ac., sil., stram., sumb., zinc., zing.
Eye	photophobia, in morning	Am-c., am-m., ant-c., calc., kali-n., nat-s., Nux-v., phyt., sil., verat.
Eye	protrusion (eye sticks out from its surroundings) of right eye more than left	Com.
Eye	protrusion, exophthalmus (bulge in artery)	Aml-n., ars., aur., bad., bar-c., bell., cact., calc., con., crot-h., dig., Ferr-i., Ferr., ign., Iod., lycps., nat-m., phos., Sec., spong.
Eye	pterygium	Am-br., arg-n., ars-m., ars., calc., chim., euphr., form., lach., nux-m., psor., rat., spig., sulph., tell., zinc.
Eye	pterygium (a triangular patch of tissue that obstructs vision by growing over usually the inner side of the eye that results from degeneration of the cornea and is associated with prolonged exposure to sun and wind) of pink colour	Arg-n.

Body part/Disease	Symptom	Medicines
Eye	pulsation in head aggravated from closing eyes	Sep.
Eye	quivering of eye	Alum., am-m., apis., aran., carb-v., con., fl-ac., glon., hyos., petr., phos., rat., rhus-t., sars., seneg., stann., zinc.
Eye	quivering of left eye	Alum.
Eye	quivering of right eye	Sars.
Eye	rash above the eyes	Ran-b.
Eye	rash at canthi	Lact., syph.
Eye	rash below eyes	Dulc., guai., sel., thuj.
Eye	rash on eyes	Sulph.
Eye	redness of eyes after injuries	Acon., arn., euphr., hep., sil.
Eye	redness of eyes after sexual excesses	Staph.
Eye	redness of eyes ameliorated in open air	Arg-n.
Eye	redness of eyes at daytime	Sulph.
Eye	redness of eyes during headache	Bell., cimic., glon., sulph.
Eye	redness of eyes during menses	Acon., bell., cham., euphr., glon., hep., ign., merc., nux-v., puls., zinc.
Eye	redness of eyes in evening	Apoc., dig., hyos., kali-chl., lyc.
Eye	redness of eyes in morning	Ambr., apoc., bry., caps., dios., fago., mez., nat-a., raph., rhus-t., sang., sep., Sulph., valer.
Eye	redness of eyes while reading	Ammc., Arg-n., lact., merl., nat-m.
Eye	redness of eyes while sewing	Arg-n., Nat-m., ruta.
Eye	redness of veins of eyes	Acon., aeth., all-c., alumn., ambr., ant-t., apis., arg-n., ars., bar-m., bell., calc-p., camph., carb-s., caust., clem., con., crot-t., elaps., euphr., graph., hep., ign., kali-ar., kali-bi., kali-c., kali-i., kali-s., lach., lyc., meph., merc-c., merc., Nat-a., Nat-m., nat-p., onos., ph-ac., phos., sang., sil., spig., stram., sulph., ter.
Eye	restless eyes	Bell., chin-s., kali-p., lyss., stram., stry., valer., verat.
Eye	retinal hæmorrhage of eyes	Arn., bell., crot-h., glon., ham., Lach., merc-c., phos., prun-s., sulph.
Eye	sarcoma of eyes	Iod., phos.
Eye	sensation of discharge hanging over eyes which must be wiped away	Croc., puls.
Eye	sensation of eye lashes in eye	Plan., puls., sang., tab.
Eye	separation (detachment) of retina	Apis., aur., dig., gels., phos.
Eye	stiffness in muscles about the eyes	Agar., Kalm., nat-m.
Eye	Stinging pain in eye	Asarumeuropium
Eye	stitching pain in eye at midnight	Ars.
Eye	stitching pain in eye from lying on left side	Lac-f.
Eye	stitching pain in left eye	Chim., chin., cimic., cist., croc., lac-f., mur-ac., spig., thuj., zinc.
Eye	stitching pain in right eye	Dios., nat-m., phys., rhus-t.
Eye	styes, at canthi (corner of eye)	Bar-c., nat-m., stann.

Body part/Disease	Symptom	Medicines
Eye	swelling about the eyes	Apis., ars., colch., elaps., ferr., merc., nit-ac., phos., rhus-t.
Eye	swelling above eyes	Kali-c., lyc., nat-a., ruta., sep.
Eye	swelling around eyes	All-c., Apis., ars., chin., colch., cupr., elaps., ferr., Kali-c., merc., nit-ac., phos., Rhus-t., sang., stram.
Eye	swelling over the eyes	Ruta., sep.
Eye	swelling under eyes	Apis., apoc., Ars., aur., bry., calc-ar., cinnb., fl-ac., Kali-c., kali-i., med., merc., nit-ac., nux-v., olnd., phos., puls.
Eye	swollen in left eye	Coloc.
Eye	swollen right eye	Lyc.
Eye	thickening of cornea	Apis., arg-n., asar., bell., nit-ac., sil.
Eye	tired sensation in eyes	Am-m., ars., graph., iod., jab., nat-a., nat-m., phos., psor., ruta., sep., stann., stram., sulph., zinc.
Eye	unconsciousness cannot open eyes	Gels.
Eye	unconsciousness with fixed eyes	Aeth., ars., bov., camph., canth., caust., cupr., stram.
Eye	vertigo ameliorated from closing eyes	Alum., con., dig., ferr., gels., graph., phel., pip-m., sel., sulph., tab., verat-v.
Eye	vertigo ameliorated from rubbing the eyes	Alum.
Eye	vertigo ameliorated on wiping eyes	Alum.
Eye	vertigo from looking with eyes turned	Spig.
Eye	vision blurred ameliorated on closing eyes	Calc-f.
Eye	vision, a sea of fire on closing eyes	Phos., spig.
Eye	vision, blurred on turning eyes	Gels.
Eye	vision, dimness after exertion of eyes	Calc., mang., nat-m., nit-ac., petr.
Eye	vision, dimness after exertion of eyes, on fine work	Agar., calc., nat-m., Ruta.
Eye	vision, dimness ameliorated from wiping eyes	Alum., arg-n., carl., cina., croc., euphr., lyc., nat-a., nat-c., puls., sil.
Eye	vision, dimness by straining eyes	Agar., calc., Ruta.
Eye	vision, foggy in incipient (beginning to appear or develop) cataract	Caust.
Eye	vision, golden chain dangling (to swing or hang loosely) before eyes	Chin.
Eye	vision, objects move in a circle on closing eyes	
Eye	vision, red circles floating before the eye	Cact.
Eye	vision, red masses floating before the eye	Spig.
Eye	vision, red sparks floating before the eye	Fl-ac., stry.
Eye	vision, red spots floating before the eye	Elaps., hyos., lac-c., lyc.
Eye	vision, red stripes floating before the eye	Am-c., bell., Con., nat-m., puls., sep., thuj.
Eye	vision, round objects pass before eyes while lying	Caust.
Eye	vision, serpent-like waves floating before the eye	Phys.
Eye	vision, serpents floating before the eyes	Cund.
Eye	vision, sparks floating before the eyes	Stry.

Body part/Disease	Symptom	Medicines
Eye	vision, spots floating before the eyes	Con., elaps.
Eye	vision, spots floating before the eyes after reading	Cocc., cur.
Eye	vision, spots floating before the eyes on rising from seat	Verat.
Eye	vision, spots floating before the eyes sewing while	Am-c.
Eye	vision, stars floating before the eye	Psor.
Eye	vision, stripes floating before the eyes while reading	Kali-c., sol-n.
Eye	vision, stripes floating before the right eyes while reading	Phos.
Eye	vision, yellow colour spots floating before eyes	Agar., am-c., am-m., plb.
Eye	vision, yellow colour spots floating before left eyes	Agar.
Eye	vomitting ameliorated from closing eyes	Tab.
Eye	weakness ameliorated from resting head on something and closing eyes	Anac.
Eye	white spots in canthi	Colch.
Eye	winking (to close one eye briefly, usually as a friendly greeting or to show that something just done or said is a joke or a secret)	Agar., am-c., anan., apis., arg-n., aster., Bell., caust., chel., chin., con., croc., cycl., Euphr., fl-ac., glon., ign., mez., nit-ac., nux-v., op., petr., plat., spig., sulph., sumb.
Eye	winking looking at bright objects	Acon., apis.
Eye Lash	eye lashes (hair at edge of eyelid), white	Ars-h.
Eye Lash	falling of eye lashes	Alum., apis., ars., aur., bufo., calc-s., chel., chlol., euphr., med., merc., ph-ac., psor., Rhus-t., sel., sep., sil., staph., sulph.
Eyeball	involuntary movements of eyeballs	Agar., calc., canth., cupr., mag-p., nux-v., sulph.
Eyeball	paralysis of ciliary (the tissue and muscle that surrounds the lens of the eye) muscles of eyeball	Acon., arg-n., con., dub., gels., graph., kali-br., nat-m., nux-v., par., phys., Ruta., seneg.
Eyeball	paralysis of muscles of eyeball	Caust., con., euphr., Gels., kali-i., merc-i-f., nat-m., Nux-v., rhus-t., seneg.
Eyeball	pendulum like movements of eye balls from side to side	Agar., amyg., ars., benz-n., carb-h., cic., cupr., gels., sabad., sulph.
Eyeball	stiffness in eyeballs	Agar., ars., bar-m., calc-p., calc., camph., caust., crot-c., cupr-s., hep., Kalm., nat-a., Nat-m., onos., phos., seneg., spig., stry.
Eyebrow	Condylomata in eyebrows	Anan., caust., thuj.
Eyebrow	Condylomata in left eyebrows	Caust., cinnb., nit-ac., sulph., Thuj.
Eyebrow	Condylomata in right lower eyebrows	Nit-ac.
Eyebrow	hair falling of eye brows (hair above eye socket)	Agar., ail., alum., anan., aur-m., hell., Kali-c., mill., plb., sel., sil., sulph.
Eyebrow	itching in eyebrows	Nat-m.
Eyebrow	itching of eyebrows	Agar., agn., all-c., alum., ars., arund., berb., bry., caust., com., con., ferr., fl-ac., laur., manc., mez., nat-m., pall., par., rhod., sel., sil., spig., Sulph., verat., viol-t.
Eyebrow	pain in nose extending to eyebrows	Inul.
Eyebrow	pimples in eyebrows	Kali-c.

Body part/Disease	Symptom	Medicines
Eyebrow	psoriasis in eyebrows	Phos.
Eyebrow	swelling between lids and eyebrows	Cench., Kali-c.
Eyebrow	swollen glands on Glabella ((just above the nose and between the eyebrows),	Kali-c.
Eyelash	sensation of eye lashes in eye	Plan., puls., sang., tab.
Eyelid	blotches on eyelids	Aur., bry., calc., ran-s., staph., thuj.
Eyelid	constant movements of eyeballs under closed eyelids	Benz-n.
Eyelid	convulsion while touching eyelids	Coc-c.
Eyelid	ecchymosis from lids	Arn., led.
Eyelid	ecchymosis on right Eyelids	Con.
Eyelid	eczema on eyelids	Clem., Graph., hep., mez., tell., Thuj.
Eyelid	eversion (turning inside out) of eyelids	Alum., apis., Arg-m., Arg-n., bell., calc., graph., ham., hep., lyc., merc-c., merc., mez., nat-m., nit-ac., psor., staph., sulph., zinc.
Eyelid	eversion of lower eyelids	Apis
Eyelid	excoriation of eyelids	Apis., Arg-n., Ars., calc., graph., hep., med., merc-c., Merc., nat-m., sulph.
Eyelid	hardness of meibomian glands (a sebaceous gland in the eyelid)	Bad., lith., staph.
Eyelid	herpes on eyelids	Bry., corn., graph., kreos., psor., rhus-t., sep., sulph., tarent.
Eyelid	hypertrophy of conjunctiva (membrane under eyelid)	Apis.
Eyelid	itching of eyelids	Alum., ambr., anag., apis., Arg-m., asaf., asc-t., aur-m., aur., bell., berb., bry., bufo., calc., carb-s., caust., con., croc., crot-t., cycl., dros., eupho., euphr., graph., hep., kali-ar., kali-bi., lob., mez., nat-p., nux-v., paeon., pall., petr., ph-ac., phos., Puls., Rhus-t., sep., sin-n., spong., Sulph., tarent., Tell., vesp., vinc., zinc.
Eyelid	nodules on eye lids	Staph., sulph., thuj.
Eyelid	nodules on the eye lid	Con., sil., Staph., thuj.
Eyelid	Oedema of lower left lid	Calc., merc.
Eyelid	Oedema of lower lid	Aur., cahin., crot-c., dig., Kali-ar., op., phos., raph.
Eyelid	Oedema of upper left lid	Asar., cahin., tell.
Eyelid	Oedema of upper lid	Apis., bry., con., cycl., ign., Kali-c., kali-i., med., nat-c., petr., squil., syph., teucr.
Eyelid	Oedema of upper right lid	Caust., nat-c., phos.
Eyelid	pain in eye lids	Caust., chel., chin., ign., lyc., mez., sep., sulph., vesp., xan.
Eyelid	paralysis of eye lids	Alum., ars., bapt., bar-m., bell., cadm., cocc., con., graph., guare., hydr-ac., merc-i-f., nat-a., nit-ac., op., plb., puls., Sep., Spig., stram., verat., vip., zinc.
Eyelid	paralysis of eye lids after injury	Led.
Eyelid	paralysis of left eyelids	Nux-v., plb.

Body part/Disease	Symptom	Medicines
Eyelid	paralysis of right eye lids	Alum., apis., cur., mag-p., phys., rhus-t., sulph.
Eyelid	paralysis of upper eye lids	Alum., apis., arn., ars., bufo., cadm., Caust., chlol., cina., cocc., con., crot-c., crot-h., cur., dulc., eupho., Gels., graph., led., lyss., mag-p., med., merl., morph., naja., nat-a., nat-c., Nit-ac., nux-m., op., phos., plb., Rhus-t., sec., Sep., Spig., stann., syph., verat., zinc.
Eyelid	pimples on eyelids	Alum., chel., guai., Hep., lyc., merc-c., nat-m., rhus-t., sel., seneg.
Eyelid	pustules on eyelids	Ant-t., arg-m., carb-s., lyc., merc., sep., sil., sulph., Tell.
Eyelid	rash on eyelids	Sulph.
Eyelid	scales on eyelids	Ars., psor., Sep.
Eyelid	scaly herpes on eyelids	Chel., kreos., nat-m., Psor., sep.
Eyelid	scurfy on eyelids	Mez., Petr., Sep., tub.
Eyelid	sleepiness from contraction of eyelids	Ant-t., con., croc., kali-c.
Eyelid	spasm (involuntary muscle contraction) of eyelids	Agar., alum., bell., calc-p., calc., camph., chin-a., croc., cupr., euphr., mag-p., merc-c., nat-m., nux-v., plat., plb., puls., ruta., sep., sil.
Eyelid	stiffness in eyelids	Apis., arum-d., camph., gels., Kalm., nat-a., nux-m., rhus-t., sep., spig., verat.
Eyelid	sty (a temporary swelling on an eyelid at the base of an eyelash) on right eye	Am-c., cupr., ferr-p., nat-m.
Eyelid	sty on left eye	Bar-c., colch., elaps., hydr., hyper., staph.
Eyelid	styes on lower lid	Colch., cupr., elaps., ferr-p., graph., hyper., kali-p., phos., puls., rhus-t., seneg.
Eyelid	styes on upper lid	Am-c., bell., ferr., merc., ph-ac., Puls., staph.
Eyelid	swelling between lids and eyebrows	Cench., Kali-c.
Eyelid	tubercles on eyelids	Aur., bry., calc., ran-s., staph., thuj.
Eyelid	tumours on right lower eyelid	Zinc.
Eyelid	tumours on right upper lid	Zinc.
Eyelid	ulcer in conjunctiva	Alum., Caust., coloc., crot-t., hydr., lyss., nit-ac.
Eyelid	vesicles on eyelids	Berb., cimic., crot-t., mez., pall., psor., rhus-t., rhus-v., sars., sel.

Body part/Disease	Symptom	Medicines
Face	abscess on face	Anan., bell., Hep., kali-i., Merc., phos., sil. antrum : Kali-i., lyc., merc., mez., Sil.
Face	acne on face aggravated on becoming heated	Caust.
Face	acne on face	Ant-c., ars-i., ars., Aur., bar-c., bell., calc-s., Calc-sil., calc., Carb-an., Carb-s., Carb-v., Caust., chel., con., cop., crot-h., eug., Hep., iod., Kali-br., kreos., lach., led., med., nat-m., nit-ac., Nux-v., ph-ac., psor., puls., sabin., sanic., sel., Sep., Sil., sul-i., sulph., thuj., tub., uran.
Face	ameliorated from bathing face	Asar., calc-s., mez., sabad.
Face	asthmatic with face ache and disappearance of tetter (eruption) on face	Dulc.
Face	bleeding eczema on face	Alum., ars., dulc., hep., lyc., merc., petr., psor., sep., sulph.
Face	bleeding from face when scratched	Merc., mez., par., petr., rhus-t., sulph.
Face	blotches of face aggravated at night	Mag-m.
Face	blotches of face aggravated before menses	Mag-m.
Face	blotches of face aggravated by washing	Am-c., phyt.
Face	blotches of face aggravated from warmth of bed	Mag-m.
Face	blotches of face itching	Graph.
Face	boils on face burning	Alum., am-m., anac., ant-c., apis, ars., calc., caust., chin-s., cic., euphr., graph., kali-c., led., mag-m., merc., nat-m., phos., rat., rhus-t., sars., seneg., sep., staph., sulph.
Face	boils on face burning when scratched	Nat-s., sars.
Face	boils on face burning when wet	Euphr.
Face	boils on face burning, cannot sleep without cold applications	Am-m.
Face	boils on face painful	Hep.
Face	burning eczema on face	Cic., viol-t.
Face	cancer of face	aur., carb-an., con., kali-ar., kali-c., kali-i., lach., nit-ac., phos., sil., sulph., zinc.
Face	chapped face	Arum-t., graph., lach., petr., sil.
Face	chill beginning in and extending from face	Acon., arn., bar-c., berb., bor., calc., carb-ac., caust., cham., ign., kreos., laur., merc., petr., phos., puls., rhod., ruta., staph., stram.
Face	chill in afternoon with violent chill with thirst and red face	**Ferr.**
Face	chill in fever followed by heat with sweat of the face	Alum.

Body part/Disease	Symptom	Medicines
Face	chilliness in evening with flashes of heat in the face	Nit-ac., petr.
Face	cobwebs (spider web) sensation on face	Alum., bar-c., bor., brom., bry., calad., calc., carb-s., carl., con., Graph., laur., mag-c., mez., morph., ph-ac., plb., ran-s., sul-ac., sulph., sumb.
Face	coldness in foot in afternoon with hot face	Hura.
Face	coldness in foot in noon during heat and redness of the face	Sep.
Face	coldness in foot with heat of face	Acon., asaf., cocc., gels., ign., ruta., samb., sep., Stram.
Face	coldness in hands with hot face	Agar., Arn., ars., asaf., chin., con., eupho., hyos., ign., ruta., sabin., Stram., sumb., thuj.
Face	coldness in leg with flushed face	Op.
Face	coldness in leg with heat on face	Arn.
Face	coldness of face	Cham., chin., hell.
Face	coldness of face during heat	Cina., nat-c.
Face	complaints of face aggravated by shaving	Carb-an.
Face	congestion of face	Acon., agar., Aml-n., ant-t., apis., arg-n., Aur., bar-c., Bell., bry., cact., calc., cann-s., caust., chin., coc-c., coloc., cop., equis., eup-per., gels., Glon., hydr-ac., hyos., ign., Ind., iod., lach., lact-ac., lil-t., meli., merc-c., mit., morph., oena., op., paeon., phos., Puls., sabin., Stram., stry., tanac., thuj., ust., ziz.
Face	congestion of face, rubbing after	Aesc.
Face	convulsion aggravated from wiping perspiration from face	Nux-v.
Face	convulsion begin in face	Absin., bufo., cina., dulc., hyos., ign., lach., sant., sec.
Face	convulsion of upper limbs in prosopalgia (a disorder of the trigeminal nerve (the fifth cranial nerve) that causes episodes of sharp, stabbing pain in the cheek, lips, gums, or chin on one side of the face)	Plat.
Face	cool air seems blowing upon face	Coloc., mez.
Face	covulsions beginning in face	Absin., bufo., cina., dulc., hyos., ign., sant., sec.
Face	covulsions in left side of face	Lach.
Face	covulsions of face before menses	Puls.
Face	covulsions of face while speaking	Plb.
Face	covulsions of right side of face	Agar.
Face	discolouration of face after anger	Con.
Face	discolouration of face black	Camph., Chin., cor-r., crot-h., hydr-ac., lach., oena., op., stry., tarent.
Face	discolouration of face blue during cough	Apis., bell., caust., coc-c., cor-r., Dros., Ip., mag-p., verat.
Face	discolouration of face blue during headache	Cact., op.
Face	discolouration of face blue in whooping cough	Ars., coc-c., cor-r., crot-h., dros., ip., nux-v.
Face	discolouration of face blue in asthma	Stram., tab.
Face	discolouration of face blue in cholera	Camph., Cupr., Verat.
Face	discolouration of face blue in croup	Brom., carb-v.

Body part/Disease	Symptom	Medicines
Face	discolouration of face blue in heart trouble	Apis., cact.
Face	discolouration of face blue spots	Ail., apis., ars., aur., bapt., crot-h., ferr., hura., kali-br., kali-p., lach., led., mur-ac.
Face	discolouration of face blue with convulsions	Cic., Cupr., hyos., ip., oena., phys., stry.
Face	discolouration of face blue with dyspnœa (difficulty in breathing, often caused by heart or lung disease)	Bry., op., stram.
Face	discolouration of face bronze	Ars-h.
Face	discolouration of face brown when angry	Staph.
Face	discolouration of face reddish	Bry., hyos., nit-ac., op., puls., samb., sep., stram., sulph.
Face	discolouration of face, blue spots following eruptions	Ant-t., ferr., Lach., thuj.
Face	discolouration of face, blue when angry	Staph.
Face	discolouration of face, blue, during maniacal rage	Acon., ars., bell., con., hyos., lach., merc., op., puls., verat.
Face	discolouration of face, changing colours	Acon., alum., ars., Bell., bor., bov., camph., caps., cham., chin., cina., croc., ferr., hyos., Ign., kali-c., laur., led., mag-c., mag-s., nux-v., olnd., op., ph-ac., Phos., Plat., puls., sec., spig., squil., sul-ac., verat., zinc.
Face	discolouration of face, copper coloured	Alum., ars-h., ars., calc-p., calc., carb-an., cupr., kreos., led., rhus-t., ruta., stram., verat.
Face	discolouration of face, copper coloured spots	Benz-ac., graph.
Face	discolouration of face, dark coloured	Ail., apis., ars., Bapt., both., carb-s., carb-v., cupr., dub., elaps., gels., hura., hydr-ac., kali-i., lach., morph., Nit-ac., op., ox-ac., plb., sulph., verat.
Face	discolouration of face, dirty looking	Apis., Arg-n., caps., card-m., chel., cupr., iod., kali-p., Lyc., mag-c., merc., phos., Psor., sanic., sec., Sulph., thuj.
Face	discolouration of face, greenish	Ars., berb., Carb-v., Chel., crot-h., cupr., dig., ferr-ar., ferr., iod., kreos., med., merc-c., merc., nux-v., puls., verat.
Face	discolouration of face, greenish spots	Ars.
Face	discolouration of face, greenish spots about the eyes	Verat.
Face	discolouration of face, mottled (patches or spots of different colors)	Ail., bapt., bell., cench., crot-h., dor., lach., rhus-t.
Face	discolouration of face, pink spots	Ars., Carb-an., merc., nat-c.
Face	discolouration, yellowish Face	Phos., vac.
Face	eczema on face like dried honey	Ant-c., Cic., mez.
Face	eczema spreading from ear to face	Ars.
Face	emaciation of face	Acet-ac., agar., anac., ars-i., ars., bar-c., calc., chin-s., cupr., guai., hura., iod., kali-bi., kali-i., lac-d., merc-c., mez., naja., nat-c., nat-p., nux-m., plb., psor., sel., sep., sil., sulph., sumb., tab.
Face	emaciation of face after neuralgia	Plb.
Face	emaciation of face and hands	Grat., sel.
Face	epistaxis from washing face	Am-c., ant-s., Arn., calc-s., dros., kali-bi., kali-c., tarent.

Body part/Disease	Symptom	Medicines
Face	epithelioma of face	Ars., cic., con., hydr., kali-ar., Kali-s., lach., lap-a., phos., sep., sil.
Face	eruption crusty black on face	Ars.
Face	eruption crusty greenish yellow on face	Merc., petr.
Face	eruption crusty offensive on face	Merc., petr., Psor.
Face	eruption crusty serpiginous on face	Sulph.
Face	eruption crusty white on face	Mez.
Face	eruption crusty yellow on face	Ant-c., calc., cic., Dulc., hyper., merc., mez., ph-ac., sulph., viol-t.
Face	eruption desquamating on face	Apis., ars., bell., canth., chin-s., hydr., kali-ar., lach., merc., ol-an., phos., psor., puls., rhus-t., rhus-v., sulph., thuj.
Face	eruption, desquamating dry on face	Ars., kali-i., led., lyc., psor., sep.
Face	eruptions on face aggravated at night	Ars., mag-m.
Face	eruptions on face aggravated at night in warm room	Mag-m.
Face	eruptions on face aggravated by cold air	Ars., dulc.
Face	eruptions on face aggravated from warmth	Euphr., mez., psor., sulph., teucr.
Face	eruptions on face aggravated from washing	Nux-v., sulph.
Face	eruptions on face ameliorated from warmth	Ars.
Face	eruptions on face before menses	Mag-m., sars.
Face	eruptions on face during menses	Calc., dulc., eug., graph., psor., sang.
Face	eruptions on face painful	Alum., apis., bell., berb., calc., cic., clem., eug., led., phos., plat., sep., staph., Sulph.
Face	eruptions on face painful at night	Viol-t.
Face	eruptions on face painful when touched	Ant-c., bell., hep., lach., led., nit-ac., par., sabad., stann., valer.
Face	eruptions on face red	Ant-c., aur., calc-p., calc., carb-s., caust., cham., cic., euphr., fago., hyper., lac-c., led., nit-ac., par., petr., phos., psor., sep., sulph.
Face	erysipela (a severe skin rash accompanied by fever and vomiting and caused by a streptococcal bacterium) extending to face	Apis.
Face	erysipela in cervical region extending to face	Rhus-t.
Face	erysipelas on face from bites of insects	Led.
Face	erysipelas on face	Ars., camph., Carb-v., chin., hippoz., Lach., mur-ac., rhus-t., Sec., sil.
Face	erysipelas on face, oedematous	Apis., ars., chin., crot-t., hell., lyc., merc., rhus-t., sulph., thuj.
Face	erysipelas on left face	Agn., bor., cham., lach.
Face	erysipelas on left to right face	Lach., Rhus-t.
Face	erysipelas on right face	Arund., bell., stram.
Face	erysipelas on right to left face	Apis., arund., Graph., lyc., sulph.
Face	excessive flow of blood in brain with redness of face	Acon., Bell., canth., coff., cop., cor-r., glon., graph., meli., merc-c., phos., sil., sol-n.

Body part/Disease	Symptom	Medicines
Face	face expression, old looking	Abrot., ambr., Arg-n., ars-h., ars-i., ars., aur-m., bar-c., Calc., chlor., con., fl-ac., Guai., hydr-ac., iod., kreos., merc-c., Nat-m., ol-j., Op., plb., sars., sep., staph., sulph.
Face	face expression, old looking, sallow, wrinkled	Sep.
Face	face expression, sleepy	Cann-i., laur., nux-m., Op., phos., phys.
Face	face expression, tired	Acon., ars., cimic., stram.
Face	fetid (having a rotten or offensive smell) eczema on face	Lyc.
Face	fever with dry burning heat extending from head and face with thirst for cold drinks	Acon.
Face	fever with intense heat on head & face but body cold	**Arn.**, bell., op., stram.
Face	fissures on face bleeding	Petr.
Face	fissures on face	Calc., Graph., merc., nicc., nit-ac., petr., psor., sil., sulph.
Face	formication in lumbar region extending to face	Arund.
Face	formication on right side of face	Alum., plat.
Face	freckles on face	Am-c., ant-c., calc., dulc., graph., kali-c., Lyc., mur-ac., nat-c., nit-ac., nux-m., Phos., puls., sep., sil., Sulph., thuj.
Face	frequent urination, with pain in face	Calc.
Face	furfuraceous in whiskers (a short stiff hair growing on somebody's face, especially on the cheeks, chin, or upper lip)	Kali-ar.
Face	gangrene of face	Merc., sul-ac.
Face	greasy face	Agar., arg-n., aur., bar-c., bry., bufo., calc., caust., chin., mag-c., med., merc., nat-m., plb., psor., rhus-t., sel., stram., thuj., tub.
Face	hair growth on child's face	Calc., nat-m., ol-j., psor., sulph.
Face	he strikes his face with motion of hands	Acon.
Face	headache extending around the face	Am-m., anac., ant-t., aran., arg-m., bry., graph., guai., indg., lyc., mag-m., nat-m., phos., puls., rhus-t., sars., seneg., sil., spig., tarent., thuj.
Face	headache on left side of head and face extending to neck	Guai.
Face	headache on left side of head and face extending to neck aggravated by lying on left side	Ars., calad., kali-bi.
Face	headache on left side of head and face, extending to neck ameliorated by lying on right side	Brom.
Face	heat in lumbar region extending to face	Arund.
Face	inflammation of bone of face	Aur., calc., fl-ac., mez., nit-ac., ph-ac., ruta., sil., staph., still., symph.
Face	itching of face ameliorated by rubbing	Rhus-v.
Face	itching of face ameliorated by scratching	Apis., grat., nat-c.
Face	itching of face, changes place on scratching	Sars.

Body part/Disease	Symptom	Medicines
Face	itching on face aggravated at night	Mez., sulph., viol-t.
Face	itching on face aggravated by warmth	Ant-c., euphr., mez., psor., sulph., teucr.
Face	leprous spots on face	Ant-t., graph., phos., Sec.
Face	lupus (tuberculosis of skin) of face	Alumn., arg-n., Ars., aur-m., carb-ac., carb-v., cist., Hydrc., kali-ar., kali-bi., kali-chl., kreos., lach., psor., sep., sil.
Face	metastasis (the spread of a cancer from the original tumor to other parts of the body by means of tiny clumps of cells transported by the blood or lymph) of face	Agar.
Face	metastasis of face	Abrot., carb-v., puls.
Face	moist eczema on face	Cic., Graph., Lyc., petr., psor., rhus-t.
Face	motion of hands toward face	Stry.
Face	motion of upper limbs toward face	Stry.
Face	nodosities like eruptions on face	Merc.
Face	oedematous swelling on face	Aeth., ant-a., ant-t., Apis., apoc., ars-h., ars-m., Ars., cact., Calc., carb-s., chel., chin., colch., crot-h., cupr-ar., dig., dulc., eupho., ferr-p., ferr, Graph., ham., hell., kali-ar., Lyc., merc-c., merc., nat-a., nat-c., nat-m., phos., plb., rhus-t., thuj., vesp., xan.
Face	oedematous swelling on one side of face	Arn., ars., aur., bell., bry., canth., cham., merc., nux-v., plb., puls., sep., staph.
Face	pain between scapula extending to shoulders and face	Valer.
Face	pain in ear extending to left face	Anac., bell., cann-s., merc., nux-v., stram., thea.
Face	pain in ear with face-ache	Bell., merc., ph-ac.
Face	pain in eye extending to over side of face	Lyc., op.
Face	pain in sacral region ameliorated from lying on face	Bapt.
Face	pain in upper limb extending from face to fingers	Coff.
Face	pain of face after eating	Agar., chin., iris., mang., nux-v., phos., zinc.
Face	pain of face after menses	Spig.
Face	pain of face after suppressed ereuption	Dulc., kalm., mez., thuj.
Face	pain of face aggravated by bathing	Am-c., coff.
Face	pain of face aggravated by blowing nose	Merc.
Face	pain of face aggravated by change of weather	Rhod.
Face	pain of face aggravated by chewing	Acon., agar., Ars., bell., carb-s., colch., dulc., kali-ar., kali-c., kali-p., mag-c., Mag-p., merc., phos., rhod., Rhus-t., ruta., sulph., verb.
Face	pain of face aggravated by cold application	Aesc., bell., con., ferr., hep., mag-c., Mag-p., phos., rhod., Rhus-t., sanic., Sil., stann.
Face	pain of face aggravated during stool	Spig.
Face	pain of face aggravated from dry cold wind	Acon., caust., Hep., lac-c., Mag-p., rhod.
Face	pain of face aggravated from motion	Acon., Bell., Bry., cact., calc-p., calc., chin-a., chin., colch., coloc., ferr-p., gels., lac-c., mez., Nux-v., phos., rhod., sep., Spig., squil., staph., verb.
Face	pain of face aggravated from odors	Sep.

Body part/Disease	Symptom	Medicines
Face	pain of face aggravated from pressure	Bell., caps., cina., coloc., cupr., dros., gels., mag-c., merc-i-f., nux-v., verb.
Face	pain of face aggravated from rising from bed	Chin., olnd., rhus-t., spig.
Face	pain of face aggravated from swallowing	Kali-n., phos., staph.
Face	pain of face aggravated from talking	Bry., chel., euphr., mez., phos., puls., rhod., spig., squil., verb.
Face	pain of face aggravated from touch	Arn., aur., Bell., bry., caps., chel., chin-s., chin., cina., cocc., Coff., coloc., cor-r., cupr., dig., dros., Hep., Lach., lyc., mag-c., mag-p., nat-m., nux-v., par., ph-ac., phos., puls., sep., spig., spong., staph., verb., zinc.
Face	pain of face aggravated from walking	Agar., mag-c., sulph.
Face	pain of face aggravated from warm drinks	Cham.
Face	pain of face aggravated from warm food	Mez., puls., sep.
Face	pain of face aggravated from warmth	Clem., glon., merc., mez., plat., puls., verat.
Face	pain of face aggravated from wine	Bell., cact.
Face	pain of face aggravated from yawning	Arn., ign., op., rhus-t., sabad., staph.
Face	pain of face aggravated in bed	Carb-v., mag-c., mag-p., puls., sil., spong., verb., viol-t.
Face	pain of face aggravated in damp weather	Calc-p., calc., chin-s., dulc., merc., nat-s., sep., sil., spig., verat.
Face	pain of face aggravated in open air	Alum., ars., bell., calc., carb-an., chin-a., chin., cocc., guai., hep., kali-ar., kali-c., kali-p., kreos., laur., mag-c., mag-p., merc-c., merc., phos., plat., puls., rhus-t., sars., sep., sil., spig., spong., Sulph., thuj., valer.
Face	pain of face aggravated while lying on affected side	Acon., arn., chin., clem., puls., spig., syph.
Face	pain of face alternating with pain in limbs	Kali-bi.
Face	pain of face alternating with pain in shoulder	Mag-p.
Face	pain of face ameliorated from hard pressure	Bell., bry., chin-s., chin., rhus-t., spig.
Face	pain of face ameliorated from pressure	Ail., bry., coloc., cupr., dig., guai., lepi., mag-c., Mag-p., mez., sang., sep., spig., stann., staph., syph.
Face	pain of face ameliorated after eating	Chin., kali-p., kalm., spig.
Face	pain of face ameliorated by chewing	Cupr.
Face	pain of face ameliorated by chewing	All-c., Kali-s., nicc., puls.
Face	pain of face ameliorated by cold application	Apis., arg-m., ars-m., asar., bism., bry., caust., chin., coff., ferr-p., fl-ac., kali-p., lac-c., nicc., puls., sabad., sep.
Face	pain of face ameliorated from excitement	Kali-p., pip-m.
Face	pain of face ameliorated from motion	Agar., bism., ferr., iris., kali-p., lyc., mag-c., mag-p., meny., plat., puls., rhod., Rhus-t., ruta., valer.
Face	pain of face ameliorated from profuse urination	Acon., ferr-p., Gels., ign., kalm., sang., sil., ter., verat.
Face	pain of face ameliorated from rubbing	Ant-c., caust., Phos., plat., plb., rhus-t., valer.
Face	pain of face ameliorated from sleep	Mag-p., Phos., sep.
Face	pain of face ameliorated from talking	Kali-p.
Face	pain of face ameliorated from touch	Am-c., am-m., asaf., chin., euphr., kali-p., olnd., thuj.
Face	pain of face ameliorated from warmth	Ars., calc-p., calc., caust., cham., chin-s., coloc., cupr., Hep., kali-p., lach., Mag-p., mez., phos., rhod., rhus-t., sanic., Sil., spig., sul-ac., sulph.

Body part/Disease	Symptom	Medicines
Face	pain of face ameliorated in open air	All-c., am-m., Asar., coloc., hep., kali-bi., kali-i., kali-s., lac-c., mag-c. nat-m., nat-s., puls., sulph.
Face	pain of face ameliorated while eating	Caj., rhod.
Face	pain of face ameliorated while lying	Cact., calc-p., chin-s., coff., nux-v., sep., spig.
Face	pain of face ameliorated while lying on affected side	Bry., cupr., ign., sul-ac.
Face	pain of face before menses	Am-c., mang., stann., zinc.
Face	pain of face below eye	Acon., arg-n., ars., aur-m-n., bell., chin., coloc., gels., hydrc., iris., mag-p., mez., nux-v., plat., sil., spig., sulph., verb., zinc.
Face	pain of face come and go with sun	Kali-bi., kalm., nat-m., spig., stann., verb.
Face	pain of face during chill	Acon., caust., chin., lach., mez., nux-v., rhus-t., spig.
Face	pain of face during cough	Kali-bi.
Face	pain of face during menses	Am-c., caust., graph., lyc., mag-c., mag-m., nat-m., sep., sil., stann., zinc.
Face	pain of face extending to arms	Kalm.
Face	pain of face extending to chest	Sil.
Face	pain of face extending to ears	Bell., calc., carb-an., caust., coloc., hep., Lach., lyc., mez., plan., Puls., sang., sep., spig., thuj.
Face	pain of face extending to fingers	Coff.
Face	pain of face extending to neck	Bell., coloc., guai., puls., sang., spig.
Face	pain of face extending to nose	Spig.
Face	pain of face extending to root nose	Phos.
Face	pain of face extending to temples	Berb., hep., mez., phos., spig.
Face	pain of face from excitement	Cact., coff., cupr., lyc., sep., staph.
Face	pain of face from exposure to heat	Merc., plan., sul-ac.
Face	pain of face from fasting	Cact.
Face	pain of face from opening the mouth	Alum., ang., cham., Cocc., dros., mag-p., merc., phos., sabad., spong., thuj., verat.
Face	pain of face from sneezing	Chin., verb.
Face	pain of face from suppressed ague	Nat-m., sep., stann.
Face	pain of face inflammatory	Acon., arn., bar-c., Bell., bry., cact., ferr-p., glon., lach., Merc., phos., plat., thuj., verat.
Face	pain of face on closing eyes	Cimic., med.
Face	pain of face one sided	Acon., am-c., caps., caust., cham., colch., euon., grat., kali-bi., kalm., kreos., mez., nux-v., ol-j., phos., puls., verat., verb.
Face	pain of face suddenly coming and going	Bell., spig., sulph.
Face	pain of face when alone	Pip-m.
Face	pain of face while chewing	Acon., alum., am-m., anac., arg-n., bell., bism., bry., calc., cham., coff., cur., euphr., graph., lach., nat-m., nit-ac., osm., phos., plat., puls., sep., sil., spig., staph., verat., verb.
Face	pain of face while eating	Bry., gels., mag-p., mez., phos., plan., spig., spong., syph.

Body part/Disease	Symptom	Medicines
Face	pain of face while laughing	Bor., mang., tab.
Face	pain of face while lying	Ail., ambr., arn., bell., carb-s., cham., chel., chin., coloc., ferr., gels., graph., hep., ign., kalm., lac-c., mag-c., phos., pip-m., plat., plb., puls., ruta., sil., spig., sulph., syph., verb.
Face	pain of face with paralysis	Caust., cur., gels., kali-chl., Nat-m.
Face	pain on left side of face	Acon., ars., arund., asar., cedr., chel., chin-s., chin., coloc., cor-r., dulc., echi., glon., guai., hell., kali-bi., Lob., mag-c., merc-c., nat-h., osm., phos., plan., polyg-h., puls., sabad., sep., Spig., stann., staph., thuj., Verb., vesp.
Face	pain on right side of face	Agar., am-c., am-m., anac., arn., aur., Bell., bry., cact., calc-p., camph., carb-v., caust., cedr., Chel., chin-s., cist., clem., coff., cur., dor., ferr., hom., indg., iris., kali-i., kali-p., kalm., lil-t., lyc., lyss., mag-p., merc., nux-v., plat., psor., Puls., rhod., sanic., sep., spig., spong., stront., sul-ac., sulph., syph., ter., urt-u., verb., zinc.
Face	pain under left scapula extending to shoulders and face	Valer.
Face	pain, stitching in kidneys ameliorated from lying on face	Chel.
Face	paralysis of face	Agar., all-c., anac., bar-c., cadm., Caust., cocc., crot-h., cupr., cur., dulc., form., graph., iod., kali-chl., kali-p., nux-v., op., petr., plb., puls., ruta., seneg., stry., syph., zinc.
Face	paralysis of face after getting wet	Caust.
Face	paralysis of face after pain	Kali-chl.
Face	paralysis of face from bathing	Graph.
Face	paralysis of face from cold	Cadm., Caust., dulc., ruta.
Face	paralysis of face from riding the wind	Cadm., caust.
Face	paralysis of face one sided	Bar-c., cadm., Caust., cocc., graph., kali-chl., kali-p., puls.
Face	paralysis of face where corners of mouth drop and saliva runs out	Agar., op., zinc.
Face	paralysis of face with profuse urination	All-c.
Face	paralysis of left side of face	All-c., cadm., cur., form., graph., nux-v., spig., sulph.
Face	paralysis of right side of face	Arn., caust., hep., kali-chl., kali-p., phos., plb., sil.
Face	paroxysmal pain of face	Acon., bell., caust., cedr., cham., chin-s., chin., cocc., coloc., dulc., plat., sabad., sep., stann., thuj., verb.
Face	periodical pain of face	Ars., cact., cedr., chin-a., chin-s., chin., glon., guai., kali-ar., mag-p., Nat-m., Spig., thuj.
Face	perspiration on face after dinner	Sulph.
Face	perspiration on face after eating	Alum., Cham., nat-s., psor., viol-t.
Face	perspiration on face after eating warm food	Sep.
Face	perspiration on face during convulsions	Bufo., cocc.
Face	perspiration on face during dinner	Carb-an.

Body part/Disease	Symptom	Medicines
Face	perspiration on face during midnight	Rhus-t.
Face	perspiration on face during motion	Valer.
Face	perspiration on face during night	Puls.
Face	perspiration on face during sleep	Med., prun-s., sep., tab.
Face	perspiration on face in afternoon	Com., ign., samb.
Face	perspiration on face in evening	Hura., psor., puls., sars., spong.
Face	perspiration on face in forenoon	Phos.
Face	perspiration on face in morning	Ars., chin., puls., sulph., verat.
Face	perspiration on face in noon	Cic.
Face	perspiration on face offensive	Puls.
Face	perspiration on face on falling asleep	Sil.
Face	perspiration on face when passing flatus	Kali-bi.
Face	perspiration on face while eating	Ign., nat-m., sulph.
Face	perspiration on one side of face	Alum., ambr., bar-c., Nux-v., Puls., sulph.
Face	perspiration on right side of face	Alum., puls.
Face	perspiration on scalp and face	Puls., valer., verat.
Face	perspiration on side of face lain on	Acon., act-sp., chin.
Face	perspiration on side of face not lain on	Sil., thuj.
Face	perspiration only on face	Ign.
Face	pimples of face aggravated at night	Mag-m.
Face	pimples of face blue	Lyss.
Face	pimples on face aggravated by cold air	Ars.
Face	pimples on face burning	Aphis., cic.
Face	pimples on face copper coloured	Kali-i.
Face	pimples on face inflamed	Bry., chel., stann., sulph.
Face	pimples on face itching	Ant-c., asc-t., caust., con., Graph., hep., mur-ac., ol-an., pall., psor., sep., til., zinc.
Face	pimples on face itching aggravated before menses	Mag-m.
Face	pimples on face itching aggravated during menses	Dulc., eug., graph.
Face	pimples on face itching when warm	Ant-c., cocc., til.
Face	pimples on face moist after scratching	Graph.
Face	plethora (an excess of blood in a part of the body, especially in the facial veins, causing a reddish complexion)	Acon., alum., am-c., ambr., arn., ars., **Aur.**, bar-c., **Bell.**, bov., **Bry.**, **Calc.**, canth., carb-an., carb-s., carb-v., caust., cham., chel., chin., clem., cocc., coloc., con., croc., cupr., dig., dulc., ferr-ar., ferr-p., ferr., graph., guai., hep., **Hyos.**, ign., iod., ip., **Kali-bi.**, kali-c., kali-n., lach., led., **Lyc.**, mag-m., merc., mosch., nat-c., **Nat-m.**, nit-ac., nux-v., op., petr., ph-ac., **Phos.**, puls., rhod., rhus-t., sabin., sars., sec., sel., seneg., **Sep.**, **Sil.**, spig., spong., stann., staph., stram., stront., **Sulph.**, thuj., valer., verat., zinc.
Face	quivering on face	Agar., chin., coloc., gels., kali-c., lyss., mag-m., phel., plb., stront., thuj.

Body part/Disease	Symptom	Medicines
Face	rash on face aggravated from warmth	Euphr., teucr.
Face	rash on face bluish	Lach., phos., sulph.
Face	rash on face burning	Teucr.
Face	rash on face itching	Teucr.
Face	risus sinodicus (expression of smiling broadly, usually showing the teeth caused by involuntary prolonged contraction of the facial muscles, especially as a result of tetanus)	Bell., caust., colch., con., hyos., ign., nux-m., oena., plb., ran-s., sec., sol-n., stram., stry., verat., zinc.
Face	rosacea (recurring inflammatory disorder of the skin of the nose, cheeks, and forehead that is characterized by swelling, dilation of capillaries, pimples, and a reddened appearance)	Ars., aur-m., aur., calc-p., Calc-sil., canth., caps., carb-ac., Carb-an., carb-s., Carb-v., Caust., chel., cic., clem., Eug., hydr-ac., iris., kali-br., kreos., Lach., led., mez., petr., plb., Psor., rad., Rhus-t., ruta., sep., sil., sul-ac., sulph., tub., verat., viol-o., viol-t.
Face	rosacea on face appearing in group	Caust.
Face	rosacea on face biting	Bry., merc., nat-m., plat., sil.
Face	rosacea on face blackish	Ars., spig.
Face	rosacea on face bluish	Lach., sulph.
Face	sensation of hair on face	Carl., chlol., graph., laur.
Face	shaking chill with heat of face	Thuj.
Face	shriveled (become shrunken or wrinkled) face	Ant-t., apis., crot-t., merc., op., plb., rob., sin-n., ter., zinc-s.
Face	sleeps on the knees with face forced into pillow	Med.
Face	small blood boils on face	Alum., iris., sil.
Face	sudden pain of face	Ign., kalm., valer.
Face	swelling in face at night	Lach.
Face	swelling in face before menses	Bar-c., graph., kali-c., merc., puls.
Face	swelling in face during menses	Aeth., sulph.
Face	swelling in face during pregnancy	Merc-c., phos.
Face	swelling in face from bee stings	Carb-ac., lach., led.
Face	swelling in face in afternoon	Ars., phos.
Face	swelling in face in evening	Rhus-t.
Face	swelling in face in morning	Crot-h., dirc.
Face	swelling in face in morning	Ars., aur., calc., crot-h., dirc., kali-c., manc., merc., nit-ac.
Face	swelling in face in scarlet fever	Apis., Arum-t., calc., hell., kali-s., lyc., zinc.
Face	swelling in face nodular	Alum.
Face	swelling in face with shining cheeks	Apis., arn., aur., spig.
Face	swelling in left side of face	Anac., arg-n., com., kali-c., Lach., lyss., phyt., zinc.
Face	swelling in right side of face	Elaps., merc., nicc.
Face	tingling in left side of face	Euon.
Face	tingling in right side of face	Aur., elaps., gymn.
Face	trembling in face	Ambr., merc., op., plb., sabad., sec.
Face	trembling in face when talking	Merc.

Body part/Disease	Symptom	Medicines
Face	twitching in right side of face	Caust., puls.
Face	twitching of left side of face	Agar.
Face	ulcer in face	Anan., ant-t., Ars., aur-m-n., con., cund., hep., iod., kali-ar., kali-bi., kali-chl., kali-i., lach., merc., nat-m., nit-ac., phos., phyt., psor., thuj., vesp.
Face	ulcer in face burning	Nux-v.
Face	ulcer in face putrid (decaying with disgusting smell)	Merc.
Face	ulcer in face wart (a small benign rough lump that grows, usually, on the hands, feet, or genitals, caused by a virus) like	Ars.
Face	veins of face distended	Bapt., Chin., ferr., glon., Lach., op., sang., sars., thuj.
Face	vesicles on ears extending to face	Graph., sep.
Face	vesicles on face burning	Agar., anac., aur., caust., cic., nat-m., ran-b.
Face	vesicles on face itching	Anac., ant-c., ars., cic., mez., sep.
Face	warts on face	Calc., Caust., Dulc., kali-c., lyc., nit-ac., sep., sulph., thuj.
Face	wrinkled face	Abrot., aeth., ant-t., apis., ars., bar-c., bell., Calc., carb-h., crot-t., hell., lyc., merc., nat-m., nit-ac., op., plb., rob., sars., sec., sin-n., stram., ter., zinc-s., zinc.
Faint	faintness after anger	Gels.
Faint	faintness after breakfast	Bufo., naja.
Faint	faintness after coition	**Agar.**, asaf., dig., nat-p., sep.
Faint	faintness after diarrhoea	Ars.
Faint	faintness after dinner when taking exercise in open air	Am-m.
Faint	faintness after eating	Bar-c., bufo., caust., mag-m., nux-v., ph-ac., plan., sang.
Faint	faintness after emission	**Asaf.**, ph-ac.
Faint	faintness after eructation	Nux-v.
Faint	faintness after every pain	Hep., nux-v.
Faint	faintness after fright	**Acon.**, gels., ign., lach., **Op.**, verat.
Faint	faintness after getting wet	Sep.
Faint	faintness after lying	Calad., mag-c.
Faint	faintness after menses	Chin., lach., lyc.
Faint	faintness after rapidly walking in open air	Petr.
Faint	faintness after reading	Asaf., cycl., tarax.
Faint	faintness after stool	Ars., calc., cocc., colch., **Con.**, cur., dios., lyc., morph., nat-s., nux-m., phos., phyt., plan., **Podo.**, sulph., ter., verat.
Faint	faintness after urinating	**Acon.**, all-c., med.
Faint	faintness after vomiting	**Ars.**, dig., elaps., gamb.
Faint	faintness after walking	Berb., paeon.
Faint	faintness after walking in open air	Nux-v.
Faint	faintness after writing	Calad., mosch., op.

Body part/Disease	Symptom	Medicines
Faint	faintness ameliorated after continuing walking	Anac.
Faint	faintness ameliorated after eructation	Mag-m.
Faint	faintness ameliorated from acidic fruit	Naja.
Faint	faintness ameliorated from deep breath	Asaf.
Faint	faintness ameliorated from taking cold water	Glon.
Faint	faintness ameliorated in morning during eating	Nux-v.
Faint	faintness ameliorated on moving	Jug-c.
Faint	faintness ameliorated while lying	Alumn., dios., merc-i-f., nux-v.
Faint	faintness at 1.00 p.m.	Lycps.
Faint	faintness at 11.00 a.m.	Ind., *lach.,* **Sulph.**
Faint	faintness at 2.00 p.m. after chill	Gels.
Faint	faintness at 3.00 a.m.	Dios.
Faint	faintness at 5.30 p.m.	Nux-m.
Faint	faintness at 6.00 p.m.	Glon.
Faint	faintness at 7.00 a.m.	Dios.
Faint	faintness at 7.00 p.m.	Lycps., seneg.
Faint	faintness at 8.00 to 9.00 a.m.	Phos.
Faint	faintness at 8.00 to 9.00 p.m.	Nux-v.
Faint	faintness at 9.00 p.m.	Mag-m., meli., rhus-t.
Faint	faintness at midnight	Sep.
Faint	faintness at night	Am-c., bar-c., mosch., nit-ac., nux-m., sil., ther.
Faint	faintness at sight of blood	Nux-m.
Faint	faintness before diarrhoea	Ars., sulph., sumb.
Faint	faintness before eating	Asaf., bufo., Ind., phos., ran-b., sulph.
Faint	faintness before menses	Cocc., lach., lyc., murx., nux-m., nux-v., sep., thuj.
Faint	faintness before stool	Ars., dig., glon., puls., sars., sumb.
Faint	faintness before thunderstorm	Petr., sil.
Faint	faintness during chill	Ars., asar., **Sep.**
Faint	faintness during cough	Ars., coff.
Faint	faintness during dinner	Asaf., lyc., mag-m., nux-v.
Faint	faintness during fever	Acon., arn., bell., nat-m., nux-v., op., phos., **Sep.**
Faint	faintness during headache	Glon., stram., verat., zing.
Faint	faintness during labor	Cimic., coff., **Nux-v.**, **Puls.**, **Sec.**, verat.
Faint	faintness during menses	Apis., berb., calc., cham., cimic., cocc., ign., **Lach.**, mag-m., mosch., nat-m., nux-m., **Nux-v.**, plb., puls., raph., sars., **Sep.**, sulph., verat.
Faint	faintness during palpitation	Cact., cimic., cocc., iod., **Lach.**, **Nux-m.**, petr., verat.
Faint	faintness during stool	Aloe., coll., dios., dulc., nux-m., ox-ac., puls., sars., sulph.
Faint	faintness from constriction of chest	Acon.
Faint	faintness from hunger	Phos., sulph.

Body part/Disease	Symptom	Medicines
Faint	faintness from looking steadily at any object directly before eye	Sumb.
Faint	faintness from loss of fluid	**Chin.**, ph-ac., tril.
Faint	faintness from many lights being in room	Nux-v.
Faint	faintness from menstrual pain	Kali-s., lap-a.
Faint	faintness from noise	Asaf., merc.
Faint	faintness from odor of stool	Dios.
Faint	faintness from odors	Ign., **Nux-v.**, phos.
Faint	faintness from odors of cooking food	**Colch.**, ip.
Faint	faintness from odors of fish	Colch.
Faint	faintness from odors of flowers	Phos., sang.
Faint	faintness from pain	Apis., asaf., cham., cocc., coloc., hep., nux-m., nux-v., phyt., valer., verat.
Faint	faintness from pain in abdomen	Cocc., plb.
Faint	faintness from pain in heart	Aur., **Lach.**
Faint	faintness from pain in stomach	Coll., puls., ran-s.
Faint	faintness from pain in teeth	Chin., puls., verat.
Faint	faintness from raising arms above head	Lac-d., lach., spong.
Faint	faintness from raising the head	Apoc., bry., ip.
Faint	faintness from rubbing of temples with both hands	Merc.
Faint	faintness from running up stairs	Sumb.
Faint	faintness from sensation of something rising from stomach	Am-br.
Faint	faintness from sitting up	**Acon.**, arn., **Bry.**, carb-v., dios., ip., nux-v., phyt., sulph., verat-v., vib.
Faint	faintness from sleeping on left side	Asaf.
Faint	faintness from slight wounds	Verat.
Faint	faintness from suddenly sitting up	Ery-a., verat-v.
Faint	faintness from summer heat	Ant-c., ip.
Faint	faintness from taking cold	Petr., sil.
Faint	faintness from urging to stool	Cocc.
Faint	faintness from walking in open air	Lycps., seneg., sep.
Faint	faintness from warm bath	Lach.
Faint	faintness in afternoon	Phos., sep., staph., stram.
Faint	faintness in afternoon	Anac., asar., bor., dios., sulph.
Faint	faintness in afternoon while standing erect	Dios.
Faint	faintness in bed	Caust., dios.
Faint	faintness in class room	Acon., asaf., ip., lach., **Puls.**, tab.
Faint	faintness in cold weather	Sep.
Faint	faintness in crowded room	Am-c., ambr., ars., bar-c., con., ign., lyc., nat-c., nat-m., nux-m., nux-v., phos., plb., **Puls.**, sulph.
Faint	faintness in crowded street	Asaf.

Body part/Disease	Symptom	Medicines
Faint	faintness in dark places	Stram.
Faint	faintness in evening	Alet., am-c., asaf., calc., glon., hep., lyc., lycps., mosch., nat-m., nux-v., phos., sep.
Faint	faintness in evening from cardiac depression	Lycps.
Faint	faintness in evening on exertion	Nat-m.
Faint	faintness in evening on undressing	Chel.
Faint	faintness in forenoon while walking in open air	Lycps.
Faint	faintness in morning	Alumn., **Ars.**, carb-v., cocc., con., dios., kreos., med., nat-m., **Nux-v.**, plb., puls., sang., stram., stry., **Sulph.**
Faint	faintness in morning before eating	Calc.
Faint	faintness in morning during eating	Lach.
Faint	faintness in morning during stool	Phys.
Faint	faintness in morning in open air	Mosch., nux-v.
Faint	faintness in morning on entering house	Petr.
Faint	faintness in morning on rising	**Bry., Carb-v.**, cocc., iod., kreos., lach., sep.
Faint	faintness in morning on rising quickly from stooping or turning head quickly	Sang.
Faint	faintness in noon	Bov.
Faint	faintness in warm room	Acon., ip., kreos., lach., lil-t., lyc., nat-m., nux-v., **Puls.**, **Sep.**, spig., tab.
Faint	faintness on ascending hill	Agar.
Faint	faintness on ascending stairs	Anac., iod., lycps., plb.
Faint	faintness on excitement	Acon., am-c., asaf., camph., caust., cham., **Coff.**, **Ign.**, **Lach.**, nat-c., nux-m., **Op.**, ph-ac., **Sumb.**, verat.
Faint	faintness on exertion	Ars., calc., carb-v., caust., cocc., hyper., nat-m., nux-v., plan., plb., senec., **Sep.**, sulph., ther., verat.
Faint	faintness on hearing music	Cann-i., sumb.
Faint	faintness on moving	**Ars.**, cocc., cupr., kali-c., nit-ac., phys., **Spong.**, verat.
Faint	faintness on moving quickly	Samb.
Faint	faintness on rising	Ambr., bry., calad., chel., crot-h., cupr., Ind., plb.
Faint	faintness on rising from bed	Acon., **Bry.**, calad., carb-v., cina., iod., op., **Phyt.**, rhus-t., rob., sep.
Faint	faintness on rising from seat	Staph., sumb., trom.
Faint	faintness on smelling freshly beaten egg	Colch.
Faint	faintness on smoking	Sil.
Faint	faintness on speaking	Ars.
Faint	faintness on stooping	Elaps., sumb.
Faint	faintness on thinking of drug	Asaf.
Faint	faintness on turning the head	Ptel.
Faint	faintness on waking	**Carb-v.**, dios., graph., lach., ptel.
Faint	faintness on waking if sleeping on left side	Asaf.
Faint	faintness when attempting to read while standing	Glon.

Body part/Disease	Symptom	Medicines
Faint	faintness when discouraged	Ars.
Faint	faintness when drowsy	Ars.
Faint	faintness while kneeling in church	**Sep.**
Faint	faintness while lying	Calad., iod., lyc., sulph.
Faint	faintness while lying on one side	Lyc., sil.
Faint	faintness while meditating	Calad.
Faint	faintness while riding	Berb., grat., sep., sil.
Faint	faintness while sitting	Iod., kali-n., nat-s.
Faint	faintness while standing	**Alum.**, apis., bry., dig., lil-t., nux-m., nux-v., phyt., rhus-r., sil., sulph., zinc.
Faint	faintness while standing in church during menses	Lyc., nux-m., puls.
Faint	faintness while walking	Arn., ars., bov., cur., dor., ferr., nat-s., verat-v.
Faint	faintness with about heart pressure	Cimic., petr., plb.
Faint	faintness with heat then coldness	**Sep.**
Faint	frequent faintness	**Ars.**, phos., **Sulph.**
Faint	headache after fainting	Mosch.
Faint	menses, copious, with faintness	Acon., apis., chin., cocc., helon., Ip., lach., sulph.
Faint	nausea faint-like	Alum., arg-n., calc., carb-s., cham., chel., Cocc., fago., glon., graph., Lach., nat-m., Nux-v., op., sul-ac., sulph., verat.
Faint	pain burning in kidney with oppressed breathing and faintness	Bufo.
Faint	pain in abdomen with fainting	Bism., nux-v., ran-s.
Faint	periodical faintness	Cact., fl-ac., lyc.
Faint	periodical faintness during pregnancy	Bell., nux-m., nux-v., puls., sec., sep.
Faint	periodical unconsciousness	Cic., fl-ac., lyc.
Faint	prolonged faintness	Hydr-ac., laur.
Faint	shaking of extremities after faintness	Arn., asaf., colch., kali-br., kreos., lyc., merc-c., sec., stry.
Fainting	burning in kidneys with oppressed breathing and faintness	Bufo.
Fainting	catalepsy after fright	Acon., bell., gels., ign., **Op.**
Fainting	catalepsy (actual or apparent unconsciousness during which muscles become rigid and remain in any position in which they are placed)	Acon., agar., aran., art-v., bell., cann-i., cham., chlol., cic., cocc., coff., con., cur., ferr., gels., **Graph.**, hyos., ign., ip., lach., nat-m., nux-m., op., petr., ph-ac., plat., staph., stram., sulph., thuj., verat.
Fainting	catalepsy after grief	Ign., ph-ac., staph.
Fainting	catalepsy during menses	Plat.
Fainting	catalepsy from jealousy	Hyos., **Lach.**
Fainting	catalepsy from joy	**Coff.**
Fainting	catalepsy from love not felt in response, or not returned in the same way or to the same degree	Hyos., ign., lach., ph-ac.
Fainting	catalepsy from religious excitement	Stram., sulph., verat.
Fainting	catalepsy from sexual excitement	Con., plat., stram.

Body part/Disease	Symptom	Medicines
Fainting	catalepsy in evening in bed	Cur.
Fainting	chill in morning during menses after faintness	**Nux-v.**
Fainting	convulsion alternating with unconsciousness	Agar., aur.
Fainting	cough with loss of consciousness	Cadm., cina., cupr.
Fainting	fever with complete stupor	**Hell., Hyos.,** lyc., **Op.,** *ph-ac.,* stram.
Fainting	fever with intense heat with stupefaction (amazement) and unconsciousness	Bell., cact., **Nat-m., Op.,** phos.
Fainting	frequent spells of unconsciousness	Ars., bapt., hyos., ign., merc-cy., nat-m., phos.
Fainting	hiccough when unconscious	Cupr.
Fainting	hysteriacal fainting	Ars., cham., cimic., Cocc., Ign., lac-d., mosch., nat-m., nux-m., nux-v., puls., samb., ter.
Fainting	hysterical faintness	Ars., cham., cimic., **Cocc., Ign.,** lac-d., mosch., nat-m., nux-m., nux-v., puls., sumb., ter.
Fainting	lies unconscious as if dead	Arn.
Fainting	pulse imperceptible with stupor (dazed state/ unconsciousness)	Hep.
Fainting	seminal discharge while unconscious	Caust., dios., ham., Ind., lach., merc-i-f., nat-p., plan., plb., sel., sep., uran.
Fainting	sighing breath during unconsciousness	Glon.
Fainting	stiffness during swoon (usually brief loss of consciousness)	Bov.
Fainting	stitching pain in chest with fainting	Arn.
Fainting	sudden faintness	Phos., rhus-t., sep.
Fainting	sudden unconsciousness	Bufo., Op., plb.
Fainting	sudden unconsciousness	Absin., cann-i., canth., carb-h., carb-o., cocc., kali-c., plb.
Fainting	suffocation during swoon	Stram.
Fainting	suppression of urine with unconsciousness	Dig., plb.
Fainting	triffles from faintness	Sep.
Fainting	unconsciousness	Agar., camph., cann-s., stram.
Fainting	unconsciousness after diarrhœa	Ars.
Fainting	unconsciousness after emotion	Acon., am-c., camph., caust., cham., Coff., Ign., Lach., nux-m., op., ph-ac., verat.
Fainting	unconsciousness after excitement	Nux-m.
Fainting	unconsciousness after exertion	Ars., calc-ar., calc., caust., cocc., hyper., senec., ther., verat.
Fainting	unconsciousness after menses	Chin., lach., lyc.
Fainting	unconsciousness after suppressed menses	Acon., cham., chin., con., lyc., Nux-m., nux-v., verat.
Fainting	unconsciousness after suppression of eruptions	Zinc.
Fainting	unconsciousness ameliorated by cold water poured over head	Tab.
Fainting	unconsciousness ameliorated from rubbing soles of feet	Chel.

Body part/Disease	Symptom	Medicines
Fainting	unconsciousness before menses	Murx., nux-m.
Fainting	unconsciousness between attacks of cough	Ant-t., cadm.
Fainting	unconsciousness cannot open eyes	Gels.
Fainting	unconsciousness does not know, where he is	Glon., merc., nux-m., petr., ran-b.
Fainting	unconsciousness during menses	Apis., cocc., ign., Lach., nux-m., nux-v., plb., puls., sars., sep., sulph., verat.
Fainting	unconsciousness during parturition	Cimic., coff., Nux-v., puls., sec.
Fainting	unconsciousness during pregnancy	Nux-m., nux-v., sec.
Fainting	unconsciousness from pain	Hep., nux-m., phyt., valer.
Fainting	unconsciousness in crowded room	Ambr., ars., bar-c., con., ign., lyc., nat-c., nat-m., nux-m., phos., Puls., sulph.
Fainting	unconsciousness on sight of blood	Nux-m.
Fainting	unconsciousness while sitting	Asaf., bell., carb-an., caust., mosch., nat-m., sil., tarax.
Fainting	unconsciousness while walking	Stram.
Fainting	unconsciousness with fixed eyes	Aeth., ars., bov., camph., canth., caust., cupr., stram.
Fainting	violent chill with unconsciousness (unable to see, hear, or otherwise sense what is going on, usually temporarily and often as a result of an accident or injury)	Ars., bell., camph., hep., lach., **Nat-m.**, nux-v., op., puls., stram., valer.
Fainting	vomiting after fainting	Ars.
Fainting	vomiting during fainting	Ars., benz-n.
Fasting	ailments from fast	Ars., ip., led., nux-v., sulph.
Fasting	constriction in chest in morning during fasting	Sulph.
Fasting	constriction in stomach when fasting	Carl.
Fasting	cramping pain in abdomen from lying on back	Phys.
Fasting	cutting pain in abdomen from fasting	Dulc.
Fasting	distension of abdomen fasting while	Dulc.
Fasting	eructations tasting bitter while fasting	Nux-v.
Fasting	eructations while fasting	Acon., bov., cina., croc., nit-ac., nux-v., plat., valer.
Fasting	feeling of tightness in abdomen during fasting	Carb-an.
Fasting	headache from fasting	Ars-i., caust., cist., elaps., Ind., iod., kali-c., kali-s., lyc., nux-v., phos., ptel., ran-b., sang., sil., spig., sulph., thuj., uran.
Fasting	nausea while fasting	Alum., aur-m., bar-c., calc., graph., Lyc., sep., sil.
Fasting	pain in abdomen on fasting	Dulc., gran., hell.
Fasting	pain in abdomen while fasting	Bar-c., calc., caust., cocc., fago., Graph., hura., ign., lach., lob., nit-ac., petr., psor., rhod., seneg., sep.
Fasting	pain in back when fasting	Kali-n.
Fasting	pain in chest from fasting	Iod.
Fasting	pain of face from fasting	Cact.
Fasting	retching while fasting	Berb., kali-c.
Fasting	weakness in morning after fasting	Con.
Felon	Felon (a pus-filled infection on the skin at the side of a fingernail or toenail) ameliorated from cold application	Apis., fl-ac., led., **Nat-s.**, **Puls.**

Body part/Disease	Symptom	Medicines
Felon	Felon at root of nail	Caust., graph.
Felon	Felon beginning in nail	Par., petr., phyt., plb., puls., rhus-t., sep., **Sil.**, sulph.
Felon	felon in palm	Lach., sil., sulph.,Hep.
Felon	felon in thumb	All-c., am-m., bor., bufo., eug., fl-ac., gran., hep., kali-c., kali-i., nux-v., op., sep., sil., sul-ac., sulph.
Felon	felon under nail	Alum., caust., coc-c., sulph.
Felon	felon with caries of bone	Asaf., aur., fl-ac., lach., lyc., merc., mez., ph-ac., **Sil.**, sulph.
Felon	felon with caries of bone and deep seated pain aggravated from warmth of bed	Sep.
Felon	felon, bone caries with offensive pus	Fl-ac.
Felon	felon, burning panaritium	**Anthr.**
Felon	felon, deep seated panaritium	Bry., hep., lyc., rhus-t.
Felon	felon, from hangnails	Lyc., nat-m., sulph.
Felon	felon, from injury	Led.
Felon	felon, gangrenous	Ars., lach.
Felon	felon, itching	**Apis.**
Felon	felon, lymphatic (a network of vessels that transport fluid, fats, proteins, and lymphocytes to the bloodstream) inflamed	All-c., bufo., hep., lach., rhus-t.
Felon	felon, malignant (likely to spread or cause death) with burning	Anthr., ars., **Tarent-c.**
Felon	felon, maltreated (treat somebody or something badly)	Hep., phos., sil., stram., sulph.
Felon	felon, panaritium	All-c., alum., **Am-c.**, am-m., anac., **Anthr.**, **Apis.**, arn., asaf., bar-c., benz-ac., berb., bov., bufo., calc., caust., chin., cist., con., cur., **Dios.**, eug., ferr., **Fl-ac.**, gins., **Hep.**, hyper., iod., iris., kali-c., kalm., lach., led., lyc., merc., nat-c., nat-h., nat-m., nat-s., **Nit-ac.**, par., petr., phyt., plb., puls., rhus-t., sang., sep., **Sil.**, sulph., **Tarent-c.**, teucr.
Felon	felon, periosteum (tissue around bone)	Am-c., asaf., calc-p., calc., canth., dios., fl-ac., mez., phos., sep., **Sil.**, sulph.
Female	chorea after coition in women	Agar., cedr.
Female	cysts (a protective covering around a parasite, produced by a host or by the parasite itself) in female	Sabin.
Female	desire diminished in female	Agn., alum., ambr., bar-c., bell., berb., bor., camph., cann-s., carb-an., Caust., ferr-p., ferr., graph., helon., hep., kali-i., lyc., mag-c., mur-ac., nat-m., ph-ac., phos., rhod., sep., sil., sulph.
Female	desire increased in female	Am-c., ant-c., apis., arg-n., ars-i., ars., asaf., aster., aur., bar-c., bar-m., bell., bov., cact., calad., Calc-p., Calc., Camph., cann-i., cann-s., Canth., carb-v., chin., coff., Con., cub., cur., dulc., Fl-ac., form., gels., Grat., Hyos., ign., iod., kali-br., kali-p., kreos., lac-c., Lach., lil-t., lyc., lyss., merc., mosch., murx., mygal., nat-a., nat-c., nat-m., nat-p., nit-ac., Nux-v., op., orig., Phos., pic-ac., Plat., plb., Puls., raph., sabin., sil., stann., staph., stram., sul-ac., tarent., thuj., Verat., zinc.

Body part/Disease	Symptom	Medicines
Female	desire increased in female during headache	Sep.
Female	desire increased in female during menses	Agar., bell., bufo., camph., canth., chin., cina., coff., dulc., hyos., kali-br., lach., Lyc., mosch., nux-v., orig., plat., Puls., sul-ac., tarent., verat.
Female	desire increased in old women	Mosch.
Female Genitalia	burning pain in inner side of thigh near female genitalia	Bor., kreos., laur., sulph.
Female Genitalia	condylomata (growth resembling a wart) on female genital	Calc., euphr., lyc., merc., Nat-s., Nit-ac., sabin., sars., staph., Thuj.
Female Genitalia	condylomata on female genital like dry cauliflower	Lyc.
Female Genitalia	condylomata on female genital dry, red and fleshy	Nat-s.
Female Genitalia	condylomata on female genital like cauliflower	Nit-ac.
Female Genitalia	crusts on eruptions on genitalia	Caust., Nit-ac., sars., thuj.
Female Genitalia	eruption on female gentialia with vesicles	Graph., lyc., nat-s., Rhus-t., sep., staph., sulph.
Female Genitalia	eruption on female gentialia with vesicles	Graph., lyc., nat-s., Rhus-t., sep., staph., sulph.
Female Genitalia	eruptions on female genitalia moist	Sep.
Female Genitalia	eruptions on female gentialia, erysipelatous	Rhus-t.
Female Genitalia	formication in female private parts	Elaps., plat.
Female Genitalia	hard black pustules in females gentialia	Bry.
Female Genitalia	herpetic eruptions in female genitalia	Bufo., carb-v., caust., cench., dulc., kali-c., kreos., merc., nat-m., nux-v., Petr., Sep., thuj.
Female Genitalia	herpetic eruptions in female genitalia from every cold	Dulc.
Female Genitalia	itching in eruptions in female genitalia during menses	Agar., aur-m., bry., calc., caust., con., dulc., graph., kali-c., merc., nux-v., petr., sep., staph.
Female Genitalia	itching in eruptions in female genitalia	Ambr., graph., lach., nit-ac., nux-v., sep., sil., sulph., urt-u.
Female Genitalia	itching in eruptions in female genitalia before menses	Aur-m., dulc., verat.
Female Genitalia	itching in eruptions in female Genitalia when warm	Aeth.
Female Genitalia	itching in female genitalia aggravated by scrartching	Am-c., onos.
Female Genitalia	itching in female genitalia aggravated on contact of urine	Merc.
Female Genitalia	itching in female genitalia ameliorasted by scrartching	Crot-t.
Female Genitalia	itching in female genitalia before menses	Bufo., carb-v., caust., colch., Graph., kali-c., lac-c., lil-t., merc., sulph., tarent., zinc.
Female Genitalia	itching in female genitalia from becoming cold	Nit-ac.
Female Genitalia	itching in female genitalia from leucorrhoea	Agar., alum., anac., ars., calc-s., Calc., carb-v., caust., chin., coll., cub., cur., fl-ac., hydr., kali-bi., kali-c., kali-p., Kreos., merc., nat-m., Nit-ac., onos., ph-ac., puls., sabin., Sep., sulph., zinc.
Female Genitalia	itching in female genitalia from leucorrhoea ameliorated on lying	Berb.
Female Genitalia	nodule in female genitalia	Calc., lac-c., merc., phos.
Female Genitalia	ovaries painful extending to genitals	Lach.

Body part/Disease	Symptom	Medicines
Female Genitalia	pain in abdomen extending to genitals	Alumn., calc., crot-t., dig., lyc., plb., Puls., rhus-t., sep., tep., teucr., verat.
Female Genitalia	pain in ilium extending to the genitals	Carl., dros., erig.
Female Genitalia	pain in kidneys extending from genitals , anus and thighs	Kreos.
Female Genitalia	pimples, burning on female genitalia	Alum., calc.
Female Genitalia	Pubic hair falling out in female	Hell., Nat-m., nit-ac., rhus-t., sel., sulph., zinc.
Female Genitalia	tumors (an uncontrolled growth or mass of body cells, which may be malignant or benign and has no physiological function) in female genitalia pediculated bluish as large as a cherry	Con., thuj.
Female Genitalia	varicose vein of female genitalia with soreness	Graph., ham., puls.
Femur	hernia (part of an internal organ projects through the wall of the cavity that contains it, especially the projection of the intestine from the abdominal cavity. It may be present at birth, especially in the region of the navel, be caused by muscular strain or injury, or result from a congenital weakness in the cavity wall) femoral (involving the thigh or femur)	Lyc., nux-v.
Femur	inflammation in femur (main bone in human thigh)	Aur., mez., phyt.
Fever	Aching in back during fever	Eug., ziz.
Fever	Aching in lumbar region in afternoon during fever	Trom.
Fever	appetite, increased before attack of fever	Eup-per., staph.
Fever	appetite, increased during fever	Chin., cina., cur., eup-pur., hell., Phos.
Fever	appetite, insatiable before attack of fever	Eup-per., staph.
Fever	asthma catching during fever	Sil.
Fever	asthmatic with intermittent fever	Mez.
Fever	bleeding from mouth in scarlet fever (Bacterial infection marked by fever, a sore throat, and a red rash, mainly affecting children	Arum-t.
Fever	burning pain in hand during fever	Hura.
Fever	catarrhal (inflammation of a mucous membrane, especially in the nose or throat, causing an increase in the production of mucus, as happens in the common cold) fever	**Acon.**, ars., bar-m., **Bry.**, carb-v., con., ferr-p., **Hep.**, kali-chl., kali-i., lach., **Merc.**, ph-ac., rhus-t., sabad., sep.
Fever	catarrhal fever during menses	Graph.
Fever	cerebral fever	Apis., arn., bapt., bry., canth., cic., gels., **Hyos.**, lach., lyc., nux-m., op., ph-ac., phos., rhus-t., **Stram.**, verat-v., verat.
Fever	cerebro spinal (involving the brain and spinal cord) fever	Acon., aeth., agar., am-c., ant-t., **Apis.**, arg-n., arn., ars., bapt., **Bell.**, bry., cact., camph., canth., cic., cimic., cocc., crot-h., cupr., dig., **Gels.**, glon., hell., hydr-ac., hyos., ign., lyc., nat-m., **Nat-s.**, nux-v., **Op.**, phos., plb., rhus-t., sol-n., tarent., **Verat-v.**, verat., zinc.
Fever	chest fever	Am-c., ant-t., **Bry.**, carb-v., chel., chin., hyos., kali-bi., lyc., nit-ac., **Phos.**, rhus-t., sulph.

Body part/Disease	Symptom	Medicines
Fever	chill after exposure to malarial influences	**Arn.**, carb-ac., **Cedr.**, chin-a., chin-s., chin., eucal., eup-per., ferr., ip., nat-m., nat-s., nux-v., **Psor.**, sulph.
Fever	chill ameliorated from wrapping up followed by severe fever and sweat	Sil.
Fever	chill at day time with fever at night	Alum.
Fever	chill in fever alternating with thirst, then sweat	Sabad.
Fever	chill in fever followed by heat with sweat of the face	Alum.
Fever	chill in fever followed by heat without sweat	Graph., nat-m.
Fever	chill in fever followed by heat, then sour sweat	Lyc.
Fever	chill in fever followed by thirst then sweat	Kali-c.
Fever	chill in fever followed by thirst then sweat then heat without thirst	Hep., kali-n., nat-m.
Fever	chill in fever followed with internal chill, then heat and sweat	Phos.
Fever	chill in fever followed with thirst	Rhus-t.
Fever	chill in fever followed without thirst	Am-m., nit-ac.
Fever	coldness during fever	Carb-an., kali-ar., sep., Stram.
Fever	coldness in foot during fever	Am-c., arn., ars., bar-c., bell., bufo., calad., calc., caps., carb-an., carb-v., chin., hell., ign., ip., iris., kali-c., kali-s., lach., meny., nux-v., petr., ptel., puls., ran-b., rhod., samb., stann., stram., sulph.
Fever	coldness in hands during fever	Arn., asaf., canth., cycl., euphr., hell., ip., nit-ac., puls., ran-b., sabad.
Fever	coldness in leg during fever	Carb-an., eup-pur., meph., sep., Stram.
Fever	coldness in upper limbs after fever	Sil.
Fever	coldness in wrist (joint at base of hand) from puerperal (blood poisoning following childbirth) fever	Puls.
Fever	coldness of skin during fever	Camph., iod.
Fever	congestive fever with threatened brain paralysis with collapse	Carb-v.
Fever	congestive fever with threatened brain paralysis with paralysis of lungs	Ant-t., ars., carb-v., lyc., mosch., phos., sulph.
Fever	congestive fever with threatened brain paralysis	Hell., lach., lyc., **Op.**, ph-ac., phos., tarent., zinc.
Fever	congestive fever with threatened brain paralysis	Hell., lach., lyc., **Op.**, ph-ac., phos., tarent., zinc.
Fever	congestive fever	Arn., bry., gels., glon., lach., sang., verat.
Fever	constant urging to urinate during fever	Acon., ant-t., Apis., bell., bry., canth., caust., dulc., graph., hell., hyos., kali-c., lyc., nux-v., ph-ac., puls., rhus-t., sabin., sars., squil., staph., sulph.
Fever	continued , typhus , typhoid fever at midnight	Ars., lyc., rhus-t., stram., sulph., verat.
Fever	continued , typhus , typhoid fever at night	Am-c., apis., **Ars.**, arum-t., **Bapt.**, **Bry.**, calad., **Carb-v.**, cham., **Chin-a.**, **Chin.**, cocc., colch., kali-bi., **Lach.**, lyc., **Merc.**, mur-ac., nux-v., op., ph-ac., phos., puls., **Rhus-t.**, stram., sul-ac., **Sulph.**

Body part/Disease	Symptom	Medicines
Fever	continued , typhus , typhoid fever at night with temperature running very high	**Bell.**, bry., hyos., rhus-t., stram.
Fever	continued , typhus , typhoid fever before midnight	Ars., bapt., **Bry.**, calad., **Carb-v.**, lach., lyc., nux-v., stram.
Fever	continued , typhus , typhoid fever in afternoon	Agar., apis., ars., bry., canth., chin., colch., dig., gels., hyos., ip., **Lach.**, lyc., nit-ac., nux-v., ph-ac., **Phos.**, puls., rhus-t., stram., sul-ac., sulph.
Fever	continued , typhus , typhoid fever in evening	Arn., ars., **Bry.**, carb-v., cham., chin., hell., ign., ip., lach., **Lyc.**, mur-ac., nit-ac., nux-v., **Ph-ac.**, **Phos.**, **Puls.**, **Rhus-t.**, sul-ac., sulph.
Fever	continued , typhus , typhoid fever in evening at 10.00 p.m.	Lach.
Fever	continued , typhus , typhoid fever in evening at 5.00 p.m.	Kali-n., rhus-t., sulph.
Fever	continued , typhus , typhoid fever in evening at 7.00 p.m.	Lyc., rhus-t.
Fever	continued , typhus , typhoid fever in evening at 8.00 p.m.	Hep., mur-ac., phos., sulph.
Fever	continued , typhus , typhoid fever in evening at 9.00 to 12.00 p.m.	Bry.
Fever	continued , typhus , typhoid fever in evening from 4.00 p.m. till midnight	Stram.
Fever	continued , typhus , typhoid fever in evening from 4.00 to 8.00 p.m.	Lyc.
Fever	continued , typhus, (an infectious disease that causes fever, severe headaches, a rash, and often delirium. It is spread by ticks and fleas carried by rodents) typhoid (a serious and sometimes fatal bacterial infection of the digestive system, caused by ingesting food or water contaminated with the bacillus Salmonella typhi. It causes fever, severe abdominal pain, and sometimes intestinal bleeding) fever after midnight	**Ars.**, bry., chin-a., chin., lyc., nux-v., **Phos.**, **Rhus-t.**, sulph.
Fever	continued typhus, typhoid fever with external coldness	**Agar.**, ail., am-c., anthr., apis., arg-n., arn., **Ars.**, **Arum-t.**, **Bapt.**, **Bry.**, calad., calc., camph., canth., caps., carb-ac., carb-an., **Carb-v.**, cham., chel., chin-a., chin-s., **Chin.**, **Chlor.**, cic., cocc., **Colch.**, **Crot-h.**, **Echi.**, **Gels.**, hell., hydr-ac., **Hyos.**, iod., ip., kali-p., **Lach.**, lyc., lycps., mang., merc., mosch., mur-ac., nit-ac., nux-m., op., petr., ph-ac., **Phos.**, psor., puls., pyrog., **Rhus-t.**, rhus-v., sang., sec., sil., **Stram.**, sul-ac., sulph., ter., verat-v., verat., zinc.
Fever	cough after scarlet fever	Ant-c., con., hyos.
Fever	cough as after intermittent fever	Nat-m.
Fever	cough as before intermittent fever in spells	Eup-per., rhus-t., samb.
Fever	cough during remittent fever	Podo.
Fever	cough from suppression of intermittent (Occurring at irregular intervals) fever	Eup-per.

Body part/Disease	Symptom	Medicines
Fever	cough remittent during intermittent fever	Podo.
Fever	cramping pain in abdomen during fever	Caps., carb-v., elat., rhus-t., rob.
Fever	diarrhoea during hectic fever	Aesc.
Fever	diarrhoea during intermittent fever	Ars., chin-a., Cina., cocc., con., gels., puls., rhus-t., thuj.
Fever	discharge from ears after scarlet fever	Apis., asar., aur., bar-m., bov., brom., calc-s., Carb-v., crot-h., graph., hep., kali-bi., Lyc., merc., nit-ac., Psor., puls., sulph., tell., verb.
Fever	discoloration of skin after intermittent fever	Am-c., ars., chin-s., con., ferr., nat-c., nat-m., nux-v., sang., **Sep.**, tub.
Fever	distension of blood vessels during fever	Agar., bell., camph., chin-s., **Chin., Hyos., Led., Puls.**
Fever	dry cough before intermittent fever	Eup-per., rhus-t., tub.
Fever	dry cough during fever	Acon., ang., ant-c., apis., arn., ars., bell., brom., Bry., calc., carb-v., caust., cham., chin-a., chin., cina., coff., Con., cupr., dros., hep., hyos., ign., Ip., Kali-c., kali-p., lach., lyc., Nat-m., nit-ac., nux-m., Nux-v., op., petr., Phos., plat., puls., rhus-t., Sabad., samb., sep., spig., spong., squil., staph., sul-ac., sulph., tarent., verat., verb.
Fever	dysuria during fever	Ant-c., cann-s., canth., cham., colch., dulc., nit-ac., nux-v., staph., sulph.
Fever	emptyness of abdomen, during fever	Zinc.
Fever	eructations during apyrexia	Am-c.
Fever	eruption, red rash like scarlet fever in upper limbs	Cocc.
Fever	eruptions herpetic in fever	Carb-v., **Nat-m.**, rhus-t.
Fever	eruption, rash fiery receding in eruptive fevers	**Bry.**
Fever	faintness during fever	Acon., arn., bell., nat-m., nux-v., op., phos., **Sep.**
Fever	fever after abuse of homœopathic potencies	**Sep.**
Fever	fever after abuse of quinine	Arn., ars., elat., eup-per., ferr., ign., ip., nux-v., **Puls.**
Fever	fever after breakfast	Bar-c., calc., croc., ign., iod., sabad., sulph.
Fever	fever after breakfast	Bar-c., *dig.*, nit-ac., phos., plan., ptel., sabin., sep., sul-ac., til.
Fever	fever after coition	Graph., nux-v.
Fever	fever after eating	Alum., ang., arg-n., asaf., bell., bor., bry., calc., caust., cham., cycl., dig., fl-ac., graph., ign., Ind., lach., lyc., mag-c., mag-m., nat-m., nit-ac., nux-v., petr., **Phos.**, psor., pyrog., raph., sep., sil., sul-ac., sulph., viol-t.
Fever	fever after exertion	Am-m., brom., fl-ac., pyrog., rhus-t., sep.
Fever	fever after getting out of bed	Acon., agn., am-c., ambr., ant-t., ars., asar., bell., calc., carb-an., carb-v., chel., chin., coloc., dros., hell., ign., iod., kali-c., mang., merc., mez., petr., plat., sel., sep., spig., stront., sul-ac., sulph., valer., verat.
Fever	fever after mental exertion	Ambr., bell., nux-v., olnd., phos., sep., sil.
Fever	fever after stool	Ars., bry., caust., nux-v., rhus-t., sel.
Fever	fever aggravated from drinking	Bar-c., calc., cham., cocc.
Fever	fever aggravated from drinking beer	Bell., ferr., rhus-t., sulph.
Fever	fever aggravated from drinking coffee	Canth., cham., rhus-t.

Body part/Disease	Symptom	Medicines
Fever	fever aggravated from drinking cold water with shivering	Bell., calen., **Caps.**, eup-per., nux-v.
Fever	fever aggravated from drinking water	*Calc., canth., ign., rhus-t., sep.*
Fever	fever aggravated from drinking wine	Ars., carb-v., fl-ac., gins., iod., nat-m., nux-v., sil.
Fever	fever aggravated from standing	Arg-m., con., mang., puls., rhus-t.
Fever	fever aggravated from warm covering	Acon., **Apis.**, calc., cham., coff., ferr., **Ign.**, led., lyc., mur-ac., nux-v., op., petr., **Puls.**, rhus-t., staph., sulph., verat.
Fever	fever aggravated from warm drinks	Sumb.
Fever	fever aggravated from warmth	**Apis.**, bry., ign., op., **Puls.**, staph.
Fever	fever aggravated from washing	Am-c., rhus-t., sep., sulph.
Fever	fever aggravated in warm room	Am-m., ang., **Apis.**, bry., ip., lyc., mag-m., nat-m., nicc., plan., **Puls.**, sul-ac., sulph., zinc.
Fever	fever aggravated on motion	Agar., alum., am-m., ant-c., ant-t., ars., bell., bry., camph., canth., chin-s., **Chin.**, con., cur., nux-v., sep., stann., stram., sul-ac.
Fever	fever aggravated while sitting	Phos., sep.
Fever	fever alternating with chill during menses	Am-c., thuj.
Fever	fever alternating with chill after eating	Sep.
Fever	fever alternating with chill at night	**Acon.**, ang., bar-c., hura., ip., mag-s., merc., phos., sabad., sep., sulph.
Fever	fever alternating with chill at night with perspiration	Ip.
Fever	fever alternating with chill in afternoon	Calc., chin-s., chin., kali-n., lob., myric., rhus-t., sep., sulph.
Fever	fever alternating with chill in evening	All-c., all-s., alum., am-c., ant-s., bar-c., cocc., kali-c., kali-n., lyc., merc., ph-ac.
Fever	fever alternating with chill in evening in bed	Am-c.
Fever	fever alternating with chill in forenoon	Chin., colch., elaps., thuj.
Fever	fever alternating with chill in open air	Chin.
Fever	fever alternating with chill on motion	Ant-t.
Fever	fever alternating with chill then heat	Verat.
Fever	fever alternating with chill then heat then finally sweat	Bry., kali-c., spig.
Fever	fever alternating with chill then sweat then cold sweat	Caps., verat.
Fever	fever alternating with chill with fright	Lyc.
Fever	fever alternating with chill, followed by sweat	Kali-c., meny., verat.
Fever	fever alternating with chilliness, dry burning heat	Bell., sang.
Fever	fever alternating with hot twitches	Nat-m.
Fever	fever alternating with perspiration	Apis., ars., bell., calad., calc., eupho., kali-bi., kali-i., led., lyc., nux-v., phos., puls., sabad., sacc., sulph., thuj., verat.
Fever	fever alternating with shivering	Agar., ars., bov., caust., chin., cycl., elaps., hep., lach., lob., merc., mosch., nicc., ph-ac., podo., sabad., sang.

Body part/Disease	Symptom	Medicines
Fever	fever alternating with shuddering	Ars., mag-s., mosch.
Fever	fever ameliorated after dinner	**Anac.**, ars., **Chin.**, cur., ferr., ign., iod., nat-c., phos., rhus-t., stront.
Fever	fever ameliorated after exertion	Ign., sep., stann.
Fever	fever ameliorated after mental exertion	Ferr., nat-m.
Fever	fever ameliorated after sleep	**Calad.**, chin., colch., hell., nux-v., phos., sep.
Fever	fever ameliorated after walking in open air	Ars., caust., petr., **Ran-s.**, rhus-t., sabin., sep.
Fever	fever ameliorated by uncovering	Acon., ars., bov., cham., chin-a., chin., coloc., ferr., ign., led., lyc., mur-ac., nux-v., plat., puls., staph., verat.
Fever	fever ameliorated during vomiting	Acon., dig., puls., sec.
Fever	fever ameliorated from drinking coffee	Ars.
Fever	fever ameliorated from drinking cold water	Bism., **Caust.**, cupr., fl-ac., lob., op., phos., sep.
Fever	fever ameliorated from standing	Bell., cann-s., iod., ip., phos., sel.
Fever	fever ameliorated from walking in open air	Alum., asar., caps., cic., lyc., mag-c., mosch., phos., puls., sabin., tarax.
Fever	fever ameliorated from washing	**Apis.**, bapt., **Fl-ac.**, **Puls.**
Fever	fever ameliorated in bed	Agar., bell., canth., caust., cic., cocc., con., hyos., lach., laur., nux-v., sil., squil., staph., stram.
Fever	fever ameliorated on motion	Agar., apis., **Caps.**, cycl., ferr., lyc., merc-c., puls., rhus-t., sabad., samb., sel., tarax., valer.
Fever	fever ameliorated while eating	**Anac.**, ign., lach., mez., zinc.
Fever	fever ameliorated while sitting	Nux-v.
Fever	fever at after midnight	Ang., **Ars.**, bor., caust., chin., cic., cimic., dros., elaps., ferr-ar., ferr., ign., kali-c., lyc., mag-c., mag-m., merc., nat-m., phos., ran-b., ran-s., sabad., sars., sulph., thuj.
Fever	fever at before midnight	Acon., agar., alum., ant-c., ars., **Bry.**, cadm., **Calad.**, carb-v., cham., chin-s., elaps., eug., graph., hydr., laur., lyc., mag-m., mag-s., nit-ac., petr., phos., puls., sabad., sep., verat.
Fever	fever at midnight	**Ars.**, coc-c., elaps., lyc., mag-m., mag-s., nux-v., petr., rhus-t., sep., stram., sulph., verat.
Fever	fever at midnight and noon	Ars., elaps., spig., stram., sulph.
Fever	fever at midnight before menses	Lyc.
Fever	fever at midnight with perspiration when lying on back	Cham.
Fever	fever at night with anxiety & sweat	Alum., calc.
Fever	fever at night with chilli during day and heat at night	Dros.
Fever	fever at night with chilliness	Acon., agar., apis., ars., bapt., carb-s., carb-v., caust., cham., coca, coff., colch., cur., elaps., graph., kali-bi., rhus-t., sil., **Sulph.**, thuj., tub.
Fever	fever at night with dry burning heat	**Acon.**, anac., arn., **Ars.**, bar-c., **Bell.**, **Bry.**, calc., carb-v., caust., cedr., chel., chin-s., cina, coc-c., coff., colch., coloc., con., dulc., graph., hep., kali-n., lach., lyc., nit-ac., nux-m., nux-v., **Phos.**, puls., ran-s., rhod., **Rhus-t.**, rhus-v., spig., thuj., tub.

Body part/Disease	Symptom	Medicines
Fever	fever at night with dry burning heat and anxiety	Acon., apis., **Ars.**, bar-c., bry., rhus-t.
Fever	fever at night with dry burning heat and sleeplessness	Bar-c., cham., graph., hyos., phos.
Fever	fever at night with dry burning heat without thirst	Apis., **Ars.**
Fever	fever at night with perspiration	Agar., alum., am-m., ant-c., **Bell.**, bor., bry., calc., caps., carb-an., cedr., cina., colch., con., ferr., glon., ign., mag-c., mag-m., **Merc.**, nat-m., nit-ac., nux-v., op., **Phos.**, psor., **Puls.**, **Rhus-t.**, sabad., sep., staph., stram., **Sulph.**, thuj., verat.
Fever	fever at night with perspiration ameliorated on waking	Calad.
Fever	fever at night with perspiration as if hot water were poured over one	Ars.
Fever	fever at night with perspiration on waking	**Bar-c.**, benz-ac., carb-v., coloc., **Sulph.**, zinc.
Fever	fever at night with perspiration with cold and damp sweat and quick pulse	Cimic.
Fever	fever before menses	Am-c., calc., carb-an., con., cupr., iod., kali-c., lyc., nit-ac., puls., sep., thuj.
Fever	fever before stool	Calc., crot-t., cupr., mag-c., merc., phos., samb., verat.
Fever	fever brought on by paroxysms of anger	Acon., **Cham.**, cocc., coloc., ign., nat-m., nux-v., petr., **Sep.**, **Staph.**
Fever	fever comes on after sleep	Agar., anac., arn., ars., bell., bor., calad., calc., caust., cic., cina., cocc., coloc., con., ferr-ar., ferr-p., ferr., hep., ip., kreos., lyc., mag-m., merc., mosch., nat-m., nit-ac., op., petr., ph-ac., phos., ptel., puls., samb., sep., sil., **Sulph.**, **Tarax.**, thuj., zinc.
Fever	fever comes on during sleep	Acon., alum., anac., ant-t., apis., ars., astac., bar-c, bell., bor., bov., bry., **Calad.**, calc., caps., cham., chin-a., chin., cic., cina., con., cycl., dulc., gels., gins., ign., lach., led., lil-t., lyc., merc., **Mez.**, nat-c., nat-m., nat-p., nit-ac., nux-m., **Op.**, petr., ph-ac., phos., puls., ran-b., rheum., rhus-t., **Samb.**, sep., sil., stram., tarax., thuj., ust., vario., viol-t.
Fever	fever comes on during sleep with cold feet and sweat on waking	**Samb.**
Fever	fever driving him out of bed at night	Graph., merc.
Fever	fever during menses	Acon., aesc., bell., bry., calc., carb-an., gels., graph., helon., kali-bi., kreos., mag-c., mag-m., merc., nat-m., nux-v., phos., rhod., **Sep.**, sulph.
Fever	fever during stool	Ars., cham., puls., rhus-t., sulph.
Fever	fever during vomiting	Ant-c., arn., ars., cham., lach., nux-v., stram., verat.
Fever	fever followed chill then cold sweat	Ars., verat.
Fever	fever followed chill then cold sweat then heat	**Bell.**
Fever	fever followed chill then cold sweat then sweat then heat	Bell.
Fever	fever followed chill then cold sweat then sweat without heat or thirst	Am-m., bry., caust., staph.
Fever	fever followed heat then chill then heat	Am-m., stram.

Body part/Disease	Symptom	Medicines
Fever	fever followed heat then chill then sweat	Rhus-t.
Fever	fever from conversation	Sep.
Fever	fever from exertion	Acon., alum., ant-c., ant-t., arg-m., ars., camph., chin., ferr., merc., nit-ac., nux-v., olnd., ox-ac., rhus-t., samb., sep., spig., spong., stann., stram., sumb., valer.
Fever	fever from gastric	Acon., **Ant-c.**, **Ant-t.**, **Ars.**, bapt., bell., **Bry.**, canth., carb-v., cham., chel., chin., colch., coloc., cupr., eup-per., gels., ign., **Ip.**, iris., mag-m., mag-s., merc., mur-ac., nat-s., nux-v., phos., podo., **Puls.**, rheum., rhus-t., sec., sulph., tarax., verat.
Fever	fever from noise	Bry.
Fever	fever from pain	Carb-v., cham.
Fever	fever from pain in stomach	Sec.
Fever	fever from smoking tobacco	Cic., ign., sep.
Fever	fever from walking in heat of sun	Ant-c.
Fever	fever from walking in open air	Am-c., am-m., arg-m., bell., bor., bry., **Camph.**, caust., chin., cur., hep., hyos., meny., nux-v., ph-ac., rhus-t., sabad., sep., spig., staph., tarax., thuj.
Fever	fever in afternoon	Acon., agar., alum., am-m., ambr., anac., ang., ant-t., **Apis.**, arg-n., ars., asaf., asar., aster., **Bell.**, berb., bov., bry., cahin., calad., calc-ar., calc-s., calc., calen., canth., caps., caust., chel., chin., cina., coff., colch., con., croc., cur., dig., dros., eup-per., eupi., ferr-ar., ferr-i., ferr., **Gels.**, hep., hyos., **Ign.**, iod., ip., iris., kali-ar., kali-c., kali-n., kali-p., lach., lact-ac., lyc., lyss., mag-c., mag-m., mag-s., nat-m., nicc., nit-ac., nux-v., ph-ac., **Phos.**, phyt., podo., psor., **Puls.**, ran-b., rhod., rhus-t., ruta., sang., sarr., senec., sep., sil., spong., squil., staph., stram., sul-ac., sulph., trom., zinc.
Fever	fever in afternoon after dinner	Alum., bar-c., dig., lach., nit-ac., phos., plan., ptel., raph., sabin., sul-ac., til.
Fever	fever in afternoon after lying down	Bry., carb-an., chel., coff., mag-m., nicc., **Puls.**, sul-ac., sulph., zinc.
Fever	fever in afternoon after sleep	Bor., calad., ferr., nat-m.
Fever	fever in afternoon after walking in the open air	Meny.
Fever	fever in afternoon alternating with chill	**Calc.**, kali-n.
Fever	fever in afternoon during dinner	Mag-m., sul-ac., thuj., valer.
Fever	fever in afternoon followed by chilliness	Kali-n.
Fever	fever in afternoon followed by chilliness in the open air	Kali-c.
Fever	fever in afternoon while walking	Bry., thuj.
Fever	fever in afternoon with chilliness	Anac., **Apis.**, ars., caust., coff., colch., cur., hyos., kali-c., podo., rhus-t., sil., sulph.
Fever	fever in afternoon with external coldness	Sulph.

Body part/Disease	Symptom	Medicines
Fever	fever in bed	Acon., agar., agn., am-c., am-m., ant-c., ant-t., apis., arg-m., arn., asar., bapt., bor., bry., calc., calen., carb-an., carb-v., cham., chel., chin-s., clem., coc-c., **Coff.**, con., eug., hell., hep., kali-c., kali-chl., kali-p., led., mag-c., **Mag-m.**, mag-s., **Merc.**, mez., mosch., nicc., nit-ac., nux-v., ph-ac., phos., **Puls.**, rhus-t., samb., sars., sil., spong., squil., **Sul-ac.**, sulph., thuj.
Fever	fever in evening after chill	Acon., apis., ars., berb., graph., guai., petr., sulph.
Fever	fever in evening after eating	Anac., ang., raph.
Fever	fever in evening in bed	Acon., agn., arg-m., bor., calen., coc-c., coff., hep., kali-c., mosch., sars., thuj.
Fever	fever in evening in bed after lying down	Acon., asar., bar-c., **Bry.**, carb-ac., chel., coff., hell., mag-m.
Fever	fever in evening in bed with sweat	Bor., bov., calc.
Fever	fever in evening lasting all night	Acon., bol., cocc., graph., hep., lach., lyc., puls., rhus-t., sarr., sil.
Fever	fever in evening lasting all night followed by shuddering	Cocc.
Fever	fever in evening on entering the room	Ang., nicc., **Puls.**, sul-ac., sulph., zinc.
Fever	fever in evening with chilliness	Acon., anac., apis., arn., ars., bapt., bor., carb-v., caust., cham., coff., elaps., ferr-i., hep., kali-c., kali-i., nat-m., sabin., sil., sulph., thuj.
Fever	fever in evening with delirium (state marked by extreme restlessness, confusion, and sometimes hallucinations, caused by fever, poisoning, or brain injury)	Psor.
Fever	fever in forenoon	Alum., am-c., am-m., arg-m., ars., bapt., berb., bry., cact., calc., caps., cedr., **Cham.**, eup-per., gels., ham., kali-c., lyc., mag-c., **Nat-m.**, nux-m., nux-v., phos., rhus-t., sars., sep., sil., sol-n., spig., sulph., thuj., verat., zinc.
Fever	fever in forenoon alternating with chill	Calc., cham., thuj.
Fever	fever in forenoon before menses	Am-c.
Fever	fever in forenoon with chilliness	Ars., bapt., **Cham.**, kali-c., sil., sulph., thuj.
Fever	fever in forenoon with heat in whole body except head	Arg-m.
Fever	fever in heat of sun	Ant-c., bell., cact., glon., lyss., nat-c., puls., sep.
Fever	fever in morning	Aeth., ail., ang., **Apis.**, arn., ars., bell., bor., bry., calc., carb-an., caust., cham., chel., chin., cimic., coff., cycl., dros., eup-per., fl-ac., glon., hep., ign., kali-bi., kali-c., kali-i., lach., mag-c., nat-m., nicc., nux-m., nux-v., ox-ac., petr., phyt., podo., rhus-t., sabad., sang., sarr., sulph., teucr., thuj., vip.
Fever	fever in morning & evening	Hep.
Fever	fever in morning after breakfast	Bar-c., calc., croc., ign., iod., sabad., staph.
Fever	fever in morning after rising	Calc., carb-an., lach., mag-c., rhus-t., sabad.
Fever	fever in morning after rising and walking about	Aeth., camph., chel., petr., sep., sulph.

Body part/Disease	Symptom	Medicines
Fever	fever in morning after walking in open air	Nux-v.
Fever	fever in morning in bed	Ars., ign., nicc., nux-v., petr., **Puls.**, sulph.
Fever	fever in morning in bed at 5.00 a.m. followed by shaking chill	Apis.
Fever	fever in morning on waking	Acon-c., aeth., camph., chel., eup-per., lac-c., petr., sep., sulph.
Fever	fever in morning with chilliness	**Apis.**, arn., **Ars.**, caust., cham., coff., kali-bi., kali-c., kali-i., sulph., thuj.
Fever	fever in noon	Ars-h., ars., ferr-i., merc., spig., stram., sulph.
Fever	fever in summer (hot season)	Ant-c., ars., bell., bry., calc., caps., carb-v., cedr., chin., cina., eup-per., gels., ip., lach., nat-m., puls., sulph., thuj., verat.
Fever	fever in winter	Calc., carb-v., chin., nux-m., puls., rhus-t., sulph., verat.
Fever	fever while dinner	Mag-m., sul-ac., thuj., valer.
Fever	fever while eating	Am-c., bar-c., cham., mag-m., nux-v., psor., sil., spig., sul-ac., thuj., valer., viol-t.
Fever	fever while scarlatina (contagious bacterial infection marked by fever, a sore throat, and a red rash, mainly affecting children)	**Ail., Am-c., Apis.**, arg-n., arn., ars., arum-t., **Bell.**, bry., calc., canth., carb-ac., carb-v., cham., chin., crot-c., crot-h., cupr., **Echi.**, gels., hep., hyos., ip., **Lach., Lyc., Merc.**, mur-ac., **Nit-ac.**, nux-m., ph-ac., phos., **Rhus-t.**, sec., stram., sulph., **Ter.**, zinc.
Fever	fever while skin rash, measles	**Acon.**, am-c., ant-c., **Apis.**, ars., **Bry.**, camph., carb-v., cham., chel., chin., chlor., coff., cop., crot-h., dros., **Euphr.**, gels., hep., hyos., ign., ip., kali-bi., phos., **Puls.**, rhus-t., squil., stram., **Sulph.**, verat., zinc.
Fever	fever with aversion to uncovering	Acon., arg-n., ars., aur., **Bell.**, calc., camph., carb-an., chin-s., clem., coff., colch., con., gels., graph., hell., hep., **Mag-c.**, mag-m., manc., merc., nat-c., nux-m., **Nux-v.**, ph-ac., phos., **Psor., Puls., Pyrog., Rhus-t., Samb.**, sil., **Squil., Stram.**, stront., tarent., **Tub.**
Fever	fever with burning heat after midnight	**Ars.**, ign., lyc., merc., nat-m., phos., sulph., thuj.
Fever	fever with burning heat alternating with chill	Laur.
Fever	fever with burning heat alternating with chilliness	**Bell.**
Fever	fever with burning heat at midnight	**Ars.**, lyc., rhus-t., stram., sulph., verat.
Fever	fever with burning heat at night	**Acon.**, agar., apis., **Ars.**, arund., bapt., **Bell.**, berb., bry., **Cact.**, cann-s., canth., carb-s., carb-v., cham., cina., con., hep., ign., lyc., merc., nat-m., nit-ac., nux-v., op., petr., **Phos., Puls.**, rhus-t., staph., stram., sulph., thuj., verat.
Fever	fever with burning heat at night in bed with intolerable burning heat	**Puls.**
Fever	fever with burning heat before midnight	Agar., ars., **Bry.**, cham., laur., puls., sep., verat.
Fever	fever with burning heat in afternoon	**Apis.**, ars., **Bell.**, berb., bry., hep., hyos., ign., lyc., nat-m., nit-ac., nux-v., **Phos.**, puls., rhus-t., stram., sulph.
Fever	fever with burning heat in afternoon with transient (short in duration) chill	Cur.

Body part/Disease	Symptom	Medicines
Fever	fever with burning heat in evening	Acon., agar., apis., ars., **Bell.**, berb., bry., carb-v., cham., cina., hell., hep., hyos., ign., ip., **Lyc.**, merc-c., mosch., nat-m., nit-ac., nux-v., **Phos.**, **Puls.**, **Rhus-t.**, staph., sulph., thuj., verat.
Fever	fever with burning heat in forenoon	Bry., lyc., **Nat-m.**, nux-v., phos., rhus-t., sulph., thuj., verat.
Fever	fever with burning heat in morning	Ars., bry., cham., ign., nat-m., nux-v., rhus-t., sulph., thuj.
Fever	fever with burning heat with distended blood vessels	Aloe., bell., chin-s., **Chin.**, cycl., dig., ferr., hyos., led., **Merl.**, puls., sars.
Fever	fever with changing symptoms	Elat., eupi., **Ign.**, meny., psor., **Puls.**, sep.
Fever	fever with chill	**Acon.**, ambr., anac., ant-c., ars-i., **Ars.**, asar., **Bell.**, benz-ac., bry., bufo., **Calc.**, caps., carb-v., **Cham.**, chel., chin-s., chin., cocc., coff., coloc., dig., dros., ferr-ar., ferr., graph., **Hell.**, **Ign.**, iod., ip., kali-ar., kreos., led., lyc., merc., mez., nat-c., nat-m., nat-s., nicc., **Nit-ac.**, **Nux-v.**, olnd., petr., phos., plb., podo., puls., pyrog., ran-b., **Rhus-t.**, sabad., sabin., samb., sang., sep., sil., spig., staph., stram., **Sulph.**, tarent., thuj., verat., zinc.
Fever	fever with chill with and shaking	Sec.
Fever	fever with chill without subsequent perspiration	Graph.
Fever	fever with chilliness	Acon., agar., anac., **Apis.**, arn., ars., bapt., bar-m., bell., bor., **Calc.**, carb-v., caust., cham., **Coff.**, colch., cur., dros., elaps., hep., kali-ar., **Kali-bi.**, kali-c., kali-i., kali-s., lach., lachn., led., merc., nat-m., phos., podo., **Puls.**, pyrog., sabin., sec., sep., sil., spig., squil., sulph., tarent., **Thuj.**, tub., **Verat.**, zinc.
Fever	fever with chilliness alternating with heat not perceptible to the touch	Merc.
Fever	fever with chilliness and pain from uncovering	Squil.
Fever	fever with chilliness from putting the hands out of bed	Arn., bar-c., bor., hep., **Nux-v.**, pyrog., stram., tarent., **Tub.**
Fever	fever with chilliness from uncovering	Acon., agar., apis., **Arn.**, bar-c., bell., calc., carb-an., cham., chin-s., **Chin.**, **Nux-v.**, psor., pyrog., **Rhus-t.**, sarr., sep., squil., tarent., **Tub.**
Fever	fever with chilliness from uncovering in any stage of symptoms	Arn., ars., aur., carb-an., chin., gels., graph., hell., hep., **Nux-v.**, pyrog., **Rhus-t.**, **Samb.**, squil., stram., tarent.
Fever	fever with complete stupor	**Hell.**, **Hyos.**, lyc., **Op.**, *ph-ac.*, stram.
Fever	fever with constant shuddering with one cheek hot and red	Coff.
Fever	fever with cough which increases the heat	Am-c., ambr., ant-t., arn., ars., bell., carb-v., hep., hyos., iod., ip., kreos., lach., led., lyc., mag-m., nat-c., nux-v., phos., puls., sabad., squil., sulph.
Fever	fever with desire for uncovering	**Acon.**, **Apis.**, arn., ars-i., ars., asar., bar-c., bor., bov., bry., calad., calc., cham., chin-a., **Chin.**, coff., **Eupho.**, ferr-i., **Ferr.**, fl-ac., hep., **Ign.**, iod., lach., led., lyc., mag-c., med., **Mosch.**, **Mur-ac.**, **Nat-m.**, nit-ac., **Op.**, **Petr.**, phos., plat., **Puls.**, rhus-t., **Sec.**, spig., **Staph.**, sulph., thuj., verat.

Body part/Disease	Symptom	Medicines
Fever	fever with dry burning heat and desire to be covered	Manc.
Fever	fever with dry burning heat during sleep	Gins., **Samb.**, thuj.
Fever	fever with dry burning heat except head and face, which are covered with sweat	Stram.
Fever	fever with dry burning heat except head and face, which are covered with sweat which he does not feel	Canth.
Fever	fever with dry burning heat extending from head and face with thirst for cold drinks	Acon.
Fever	fever with dry burning heat in parts lain on	Lyss., manc.
Fever	fever with dry burning heat increased by walking in open air	Chin.
Fever	fever with dry burning heat lasting all day	Chin., thuj.
Fever	fever with dry burning heat mostly internal, blood seems to burn in the veins	**Ars.**, bry., med., **Rhus-t.**
Fever	fever with dry burning heat outside & cold inside	Ars.
Fever	fever with dry burning heat spreading from the hands over the whole body	**Chel.**
Fever	fever with dry burning heat with and without body turning hot	**Bell.**
Fever	fever with dry burning heat with pricking over the whole body	**Chin.**, gels.
Fever	fever with dry burning heat with stinging sensation	Apis., merc-c.
Fever	fever with dry burning heat with sweat even when bathed in with red face	Op.
Fever	fever with dry burning heat with thirst for cold drinks	Acon., **Phos.**
Fever	fever with dry burning heat with unquenchable thirst	**Ars.**, bell., colch., hep., **Phos.**
Fever	fever with dry heat at day time	Bar-m.
Fever	fever with dry heat at night	**Acon.**, anac., ant-t., arn., **Ars.**, bapt., bar-c., bar-m., **Bell.**, bry., calc., carb-an., carb-s., carb-v., caust., cedr., chel., chin-a., chin-s., cina., clem., cocc., coff., colch., coloc., con., dulc., ferr., graph., hep., kali-n., lach., lyc., mur-ac., nit-ac., nux-m., nux-v., **Phos.**, puls., ran-s., raph., **Rhus-t.**, rhus-v., sumb., tarent., thea., thuj.
Fever	fever with dry heat at night after coition	Nux-v.
Fever	fever with dry heat at night as if hot vapors rise up to the brain	Ant-t., sarr., sulph.
Fever	fever with dry heat at night before menses	Con.
Fever	fever with dry heat at night driving him out of bed	Ant-t.
Fever	fever with dry heat at night during sleep	Bov., bry., gins., ph-ac., **Samb.**, thuj., viol-t.
Fever	fever with dry heat at night from noise	Bry.
Fever	fever with dry heat at night of covered parts	Thuj.
Fever	fever with dry heat at night on going to sleep	Samb.

Body part/Disease	Symptom	Medicines
Fever	fever with dry heat at night on motion	Bry.
Fever	fever with dry heat at night while walking in open air	*Arg-m., nat-m., sumb.*
Fever	fever with dry heat at night with delirium	**Ars., Bell.,** bry., chin-s., coff., lach., lyc., phos., **Rhus-t.**
Fever	fever with dry heat at night with pricking as from needles	Bol., chin., gels., nit-ac.
Fever	fever with dry heat at night with rising heat and glowing redness of cheeks, without thirst, after sleep	Cina.
Fever	fever with dry heat at night with spasmodic gagging (choking)	**Cimx.**
Fever	fever with dry heat at night without thirst with swollen veins of arms and hands	**Chin.,** sumb.
Fever	fever with dry heat in afternoon	Alum., ars., elaps., ferr., gels., nat-s.
Fever	fever with dry heat in afternoon during sleep	Alum.
Fever	fever with dry heat in afternoon with chilliness	Arg-n.
Fever	fever with dry heat in evening	Aesc., apis., ars., bapt., bell., calc-p., carb-v., **Chin.,** coff., coloc., elaps., graph., kali-c., plb., **Puls.**
Fever	fever with dry heat in evening between 7.00 to 9.00 p.m. followed by chill until 10 p.m.	Elaps.
Fever	fever with dry heat in evening in bed with chilliness in back	Coff.
Fever	fever with dry heat in evening with distended veins and burning hands that seek out cool places	**Puls.**
Fever	fever with dry heat in morning	Ail., ars., bry., calc., cocc., nit-ac., sulph.
Fever	fever with dry heat in morning on waking	Arn.
Fever	fever with dry heat with sweaty hands at night when put out of bed	Hep.
Fever	fever with external coldness	Arn., ars., bell., bry., calc., chin., eupho., hell., iod., merc., mez., mosch., ph-ac., phos., puls., rhus-t., sabad., spong., stann., verat.
Fever	fever with external heat	**Acon.,** aeth., ail., alum., am-c., anac., ant-t., apis., arn., ars-i., **Ars.,** asaf., bapt., **Bell.,** bism., **Bry.,** calc., **Canth.,** caps., carb-s., carb-v., cedr., **Cham.,** chel., chin-s., chin., chlor., cic., cimic., coc-c., cocc., coff., colch., coloc., con., cor-r., crot-h., cupr., dig., dulc., hell., hep., hyos., **Ign.,** iod., ip., jatr., kali-ar., kali-bi., kali-c., kali-chl., kali-i., kali-n., lach., lyc., mag-c., merc-c., merc., nux-v., op., phos., phyt., plb., **Puls., Rhus-t.,** ruta., sec., sel., sep., **Sil.,** spig., **Stram.,** sul-ac., sulph., tarent., verat., zinc.
Fever	fever with external heat after dinner	Ptel.
Fever	fever with external heat at night	Bry., colch., kali-bi., phos., rhus-t.
Fever	fever with external heat at night on waking at 2.00 a.m.	Hep.
Fever	fever with external heat at night without internal heat	**Cham.,** ign.

Body part/Disease	Symptom	Medicines
Fever	fever with external heat desire to fanned in place of thirst during the heat	**Carb-v.**
Fever	fever with external heat in afternoon and redness without internal heat	**Ign.**
Fever	fever with external heat in afternoon with chilliness	Ars.
Fever	fever with external heat in evening	Anac., iod., plb., rhus-t., sulph.
Fever	fever with external heat in evening after lying down	Coff.
Fever	fever with external heat in morning	Bell.
Fever	fever with external heat with chilliness	Acon., agn., alum., anac., arn., **Ars.**, asar., atro., bell., berb., bry., calc-ar., **Calc.**, cann-i., cocc., coff., coloc., dig., dros., gamb., hell., hep., **Ign.**, kali-n., lac-c., lach., laur., lyc., meny., merc., mur-ac., nat-m., **Nux-v.**, par., phos., plb., **Pyrog.**, ran-b., raph., rat., rheum., **Sep.**, sil., squil., sulph., tab., **Thuj.**, verat.
Fever	fever with external heat with sensation of coldness of the whole body	Bar-c.
Fever	fever with external heat with yellow skin	Merc-c.
Fever	fever with febrile heat only during the day	Ail., ant-t., bell., berb., carb-v., eup-per., ox-ac., sep., sulph., thuj.
Fever	fever with febrile heat periodically during the day	Sil.
Fever	fever with feeling of heat in bed yet aversion to uncovering	Coff., merc.
Fever	fever with fever with inflammed body part	Acon., arn., **Ars.**, bapt., bell., bry., camph., canth., carb-v., cham., chin., cocc., crot-t., cupr., dig., gels., hell., hyos., **Lach.**, lyc., merc., mur-ac., nat-m., nux-v., op., ph-ac., podo., puls., rhus-t., sec., sulph., verat.
Fever	fever with heat absent	Agar., am-m., **Aran.**, benz., bov., camph., canth., caps., caust., cimx., cocc., gamb., graph., hep., kali-c., kali-n., led., lyc., mag-c., mez., mur-ac., nat-c., ph-ac., ran-b., rhus-t., sabad., **Staph.**, sul-ac., **Sulph.**, thuj., verat.
Fever	fever with heat on rising from bed	Thuj.
Fever	fever with heat on rising from bed and walking about	Nicc.
Fever	fever with intense heat	Abrot., **Acon.**, ant-t., apis., **Arn.**, **Ars.**, arum-t., aur., **Bell.**, bry., cact., canth., caps., chel., chin-s., chin., cina., coff., colch., **Con.**, croc., crot-h., cupr., dig., dulc., ferr-ar., **Gels.**, hep., hyos., kali-ar., kali-i., lach., lyc., mag-c., meny., merc-c., **Mez.**, **Nat-m.**, nat-s., nit-ac., nux-m., nux-v., op., ph-ac., phos., **Puls.**, **Pyrog.**, **Rhus-t.**, samb., sang., **Sec.**, sil., staph., stram., thuj., tub.
Fever	fever with intense heat after sleep	Cina., op.
Fever	fever with intense heat during sleep	Ant-t., apis., caps., chin., gels., lach., lyc., **Mez.**, nat-m., nux-m., **Op.**, rhus-t., stram.
Fever	fever with intense heat on head & face but body cold	**Arn.**, bell., op., stram.
Fever	fever with intense heat with convulsions	**Bell.**, cic., hyos., op., **Stram.**

Body part/Disease	Symptom	Medicines
Fever	fever with intense heat with delirium	Ant-t., apis., **Ars.**, **Bell.**, bry., carb-v., chin-s., chin., chlor., coff., hep., hyos., iod., **Nat-m.**, nux-v., **Op.**, **Puls.**, sarr., sec., **Stram.**
Fever	fever with intense heat with stupefaction (amazement) and unconsciousness	Bell., cact., **Nat-m.**, **Op.**, phos.
Fever	fever with internal burning heat	Ars., bell., brom., caps., hyos., mez., mosch., **Sec.**
Fever	fever with internal burning heat at 9.00 a.m.	Brom.
Fever	fever with internal heat at night must uncover, which causes chilliness	**Mag-c.**
Fever	fever with internal heat in evening	Anac., puls.
Fever	fever with internal heat in morning	Alum.
Fever	fever with internal heat in morning at 8.00 a.m.	Caust.
Fever	fever with internal heat while the body feels cold to the touch	Carb-v., ferr., sars.
Fever	fever with internal heat with cold perspiration	Anac.
Fever	fever with internal heat with external chill	**Acon.**, arn., ars-i., **Ars.**, bell., bry., calc., **Camph.**, caps., cham., chel., ferr-ar., ferr-i., ferr., ign., iod., ip., kali-ar., kali-c., mez., **Mosch.**, nit-ac., ph-ac., phos., puls., rhus-t., sabad., sang., sec., sil., squil., sul-ac., sulph., **Verat.**, zinc.
Fever	fever with internal heat with external chill with coldness of single parts	Chin., ign., nux-v., rhus-t.
Fever	fever with long lasting heat	Acon., ant-t., apis., arn., ars., aster., bar-m., bell., bol., cact., calc-f., caps., **Cham.**, chin., colch., elaps., eup-per., ferr., **Gels.**, graph., hep., hyos., lach., laur., lyc., nat-m., nux-v., sec., sil., sulph., tarent.
Fever	fever with long lasting heat followed by chill	Apis.
Fever	fever with long lasting heat with sleep	Chin.
Fever	fever with no two symptoms alike	**Puls.**
Fever	fever with shivering	Acon., anac., ant-t., apis., **Arn.**, bell., bov., bry., calc., carb-s., carb-v., **Caust.**, cham., chin-s., chin., cina., cocc., coff., cur., cycl., dros., elaps., eup-per., **Gels.**, graph., **Hell.**, hep., ign., lach., mag-m., mag-p., meny., merc., **Nux-v.**, petr., ph-ac., podo., psor., puls., rhus-t., sabad., sep., **Sulph.**, tarent., verat., zinc.
Fever	fever with shivering alternating with heat	Acon., ars., bell., bov., bry., calc., caust., chin., cocc., cycl., dros., elaps., hep., ip., kali-bi., lach., lob., merc., mosch., nux-v., ph-ac., plat., sabad.
Fever	fever with shivering and perspiration with heat	**Nux-v.**, podo., rhus-t., sulph.
Fever	fever with shivering from drinking	Bell., **Caps.**, eup-per., **Nux-v.**
Fever	fever with shivering from motion	Apis., arn., **Nux-v.**, podo., stram.
Fever	fever with shivering from uncovering	Apis., **Arn.**, bar-c., calc., chin-s., chin., lach., **Nux-v.**, psor., rhus-t., stram., tarent., **Tub.**
Fever	fever with shuddering (shiver violently) alternating with heat	Bov.
Fever	fever with shuddering (shiver violently) with the heat	Acon., bell., caps., **Cham.**, hell., ign., kali-i., nat-m., nux-v., rheum., rhus-t., zinc.

Body part/Disease	Symptom	Medicines
Fever	fever with skin rash	Ail., **Apis.**, arn., ars., arum-t., **Bell.**, bry., calc., carb-v., chlor., euphr., lach., merc., mur-ac., nux-m., ph-ac., phos., **Rhus-t.**, sec., stann., sulph.
Fever	fever with skin rash with cold, viscous (thick and sticky) sweat	Chlor.
Fever	fever with symptoms frequently changing	Elat., ign., psor., puls.
Fever	fever without chill	Acet-ac., acon., aesc., alum., ambr., anac., ang., ant-c., **Apis.**, arn., **Ars.**, bapt., **Bell.**, benz-ac., bov., **Bry.**, cact., calc., carb-s., carb-v., caust., **Cham.**, chin-a., chin., cina., clem., coff., con., cur., elaps., eup-per., ferr-ar., ferr-p., ferr., **Gels.**, graph., hep., ip., kali-ar., kali-bi., kali-c., lach., lyc., lyss., mang., merl., nat-m., nicc., nux-m., nux-v., petr., podo., puls., **Rhus-t.**, spig., stann., stram., sulph., thuj.
Fever	fever without chill after midnight	**Ars.**, bor., ferr., kali-c., lyc., nat-m., sulph., tax., thuj.
Fever	fever without chill at 5.30 p.m. with pricking in tongue	Cedr.
Fever	fever without chill at midnight	**Ars.**, nux-v., stram., sulph.
Fever	fever without chill at night	Acon., ang., ant-t., apis., **Ars.**, **Bapt.**, **Bell.**, **Bry.**, calc., carb-v., caust., cham., cina., coff., ferr-ar., ferr., gels., hep., ip., kali-bi., lachn., lyc., nat-m., nicc., nux-v., petr., phos., podo., puls., **Rhus-t.**, stram., sulph., thuj.
Fever	fever without chill before midnight	Acon., ant-c., ars., **Bry.**, carb-v., cham., elaps., lyc., mag-m., mag-s., nat-m., petr., puls., sabad.
Fever	fever without chill in afternoon	Aesc., anac., ang., apis., **Ars.**, **Bell.**, bry., calc., caust., chin-a., chin., clem., coff., con., cur., eup-per., ferr-ar., ferr., gels., graph., ip., kali-ar., kali-bi., kali-c., lyc., nat-m., nux-v., puls., rhus-t., sang., sil., sulph.
Fever	fever without chill in afternoon lasting all night	Ars., hep., puls., stann.
Fever	fever without chill in evening	Acon., aesc., alum., ambr., anac., ang., ant-t., apis., arn., ars., bapt., **Bell.**, bor., **Bry.**, calc., carb-v., caust., cham., chin-a., chin., cina., coff., coloc., eup-per., ferr-ar., ferr-p., ferr., hep., ip., kali-ar., kali-bi., kali-c., lach., lyc., nat-m., nicc., nux-m., nux-v., petr., plat., podo., **Puls.**, **Rhus-t.**, stann., sulph., thuj.
Fever	fever without chill in evening at same hour, daily fever, with short breath	Cina.
Fever	fever without chill in evening lasting all night	Cham., lyc., nux-v., rhus-t.
Fever	fever without chill in forenoon	Ars., bapt., cact., calc., cham., Gels., lyc., nat-m., nux-m., nux-v., rhus-t., spig., sulph., thuj.
Fever	fever without chill in morning	Arn., ars., bry., calc., caust., eup-per., hep., kali-bi., kali-c., nat-m., petr., podo., rhus-t., sulph., thuj.
Fever	fever without chill in noon	Ars., spig., stram., sulph.
Fever	fever without chill with very ill humored	Con.
Fever	frequent urination, during fever	Arg-m., bell., kreos., lyc., merc., ph-ac., rhus-t., staph., stram.

Body part/Disease	Symptom	Medicines
Fever	haemorrhagic fever including Ebola (a virus transmitted by blood and body fluids that causes the linings of bodily organs and vessels to leak blood and fluids, usually resulting in death) & Dengue (a tropical disease caused by a virus that is transmitted by mosquitoes and marked by high fever and severe muscle and joint pains)	Carb-v., **Crot-h.**, lach., mill., **Phos.**, sul-ac.
Fever	haemorrhagic fever with oozing of dark thin blood from capillaries	Crot-h., sul-ac.
Fever	headache after Scarlatina	Am-c., bell., bry., carb-v., cham., dulc., hell., hep., lach., merc., rhus-t.
Fever	hearing impaired after scarlet fever	Carb-v., crot-h., graph., hep., lach., Lyc., nit-ac., puls., sil., Sulph.
Fever	hearing impaired after suppressed intermittent fever	Calc., chin-s.
Fever	hearing impaired after typhoid fever(a serious and sometimes fatal bacterial infection of the digestive system, caused by ingesting food or water contaminated with the bacillus Salmonella typhi. It causes fever, severe abdominal pain, and sometimes intestinal bleeding)	Apis., arg-n., ars., nit-ac., ph-ac.
Fever	heaviness in extremities during fever	**Calc., Gels., Nux-v., Rhus-t.**, sulph.
Fever	hectic (recurrent afternoon fever, especially one accompanying tuberculosis) fever	Abrot., acet-ac., am-c., arg-m., arn., **Ars-i., Ars.,** aur-m., bol., bry., calc-p., calc-s., calc., **Caps.**, carb-an., carb-v., chin-a., chin., chlor., cocc., crot-h., cupr., ferr-p., hep., **Iod.**, ip., **Kali-ar.**, kali-c., kali-p., kali-s., lach., **Lyc.**, med., merc., mez., mill., nit-ac., nux-v., ph-ac., **Phos.**, puls., pyrog., **Sang.**, senec., **Sep., Sil.**, stann., sul-ac., sulph., tarent., thuj., **Tub.**
Fever	hectic fever daily forenoon	Arg-m.
Fever	hectic fever with haemoptysis (coughing up of blood)	Mill.
Fever	hiccough during fever	Crot-h., mag-p.
Fever	hiccough in typhoid	Phos.
Fever	hot breath during fever	Zinc.
Fever	impossible to swallow in typhus (fever, severe headaches, a rash, and often delirium)	Bapt., camph.
Fever	inflammation during scarlet fever (a contagious bacterial infection marked by fever, a sore throat, and a red rash, mainly affecting children) in which eruptions do not develop	Dulc.
Fever	inflammation of lungs with typhoid	Ant-t., bad., benz-ac., Bry., hyos., laur., Lyc., nit-ac., Phos., rhus-t., sang., Sulph., ter.
Fever	inflammatory (caused by inflammation) fever	Acet-ac., acon., apis., arn., ars., **Bell., Bry.**, cact., canth., cham., chin., colch., con., dig., dulc., gels., hep., hyos., ip., kali-c., lach., lyc., **Merc.**, nit-ac., nux-v., phos., **Puls., Rhus-t.**, sep., sil., sul-ac., sulph., verat.
Fever	insidious (gradual and harmful) fever	Acet-ac., ars., chin., cocc., colch., con., sec., sulph., tub.

Body part/Disease	Symptom	Medicines
Fever	intermittent chronic fever	Agar., alum., apis., ars-i., **Ars.**, calc-p., calc-s., **Calc.**, carb-ac., carb-v., chin-a., ferr-ar., ferr-i., **Ferr.**, graph., hep., iod., kali-ar., kali-c., **Kali-s.**, lach., **Lyc.**, **Nat-m.**, **Nat-s.**, **Nit-ac.**, nux-v., phos., **Psor.**, **Pyrog.**, sep., sil., **Sulph.**, **Tarent.**, **Tub.**
Fever	intermittent chronic fever occuring in old people with coma	Alum., nux-m., op.
Fever	intermittent chronic fever with enlarged liver	Ferr-ar., ferr-i., lyc., nat-m., **Nit-ac.**
Fever	intermittent chronic fever with enlarged spleen	Carb-ac., ferr-ar., ferr-i.
Fever	intermittent chronic fever with gout	Ferr., led.
Fever	intermittent chronic fever with long lasting heat	**Ant-t.**, cact., canth., colch., ferr., hep., ip., sec., sil., tarent.
Fever	intermittent chronic fever with pulmonary (lung) haemorrhage	Arg-n.
Fever	intermittent chronic fever with rheumatism	Led.
Fever	intolerance of both cold and warm air from warm covering in fever	Cocc.
Fever	involuntary urination in typhoid fever	Arg-n., arn., ars., colch., hell., Hyos., lach., lyc., mosch., mur-ac., op., ph-ac., phos., psor., rhus-t., stram., sulph., verat-v., verat.
Fever	involuntary urination in typhoid fever	Arg-n., arn., ars., colch., hell., Hyos., lach., lyc., mosch., mur-ac., op., ph-ac., phos., psor., rhus-t., stram., sulph., verat-v., verat.
Fever	itching in mouth in scarlatina	Arum-t.
Fever	lameness in lower limbs during fever	Rhus-t., tub.
Fever	loose cough during fever	Alum., anac., apis., arg-m., Ars., bell., bism., brom., bry., Calc., carb-v., chin., cic., cub., dig., dros., dulc., ferr., iod., Kali-c., kreos., lyc., ph-ac., phos., puls., ruta., seneg., sep., sil., spong., squil., stann., staph., sulph., thuj.
Fever	masked (not detectable) intermittent chronic fever	Ars., ip., nux-v., sep., spig., tarent., tub.
Fever	motion between convulsions in fever	Arg-n.
Fever	motion between convulsions in fever	Arg-n.
Fever	motion brings on chilliness during fever	Ant-t., apis., arn., chin-s., merc., **Nux-v.**, podo., **Rhus-t.**, stram.
Fever	nausea after fever	Ars., dros., fl-ac.
Fever	nausea during fever	Arg-n., ars., bry., carb-v., cham., cimx., cocc., eup-per., eup-pur., guare., ip., kali-c., lyc., Nat-m., nit-ac., nux-v., op., phos., ptel., sang., sel., sep., thuj., vinc., zinc.
Fever	numbness in fingers before an attack of intermittent fever	Puls.
Fever	numbness in fingers during fever	Thuj.
Fever	numbness in upper arm in intermittent fever	Agar., am-m., ars-s-r., cocc., merc-sul., zinc.
Fever	pain in back during fever	Alst., arn., ars., bell., calc., caps., carb-v., caust., chin-s., chin., cocc., eug., eup-per., hyos., ign., kali-ar., kali-c., lach., laur., lyc., nat-m., nat-s., Nux-v., puls., rhus-t., sulph., ziz.

Body part/Disease	Symptom	Medicines
Fever	pain in back without fever	Arn., ars., calc., caps., cham., cina., ign., nat-m., nit-ac., nux-v., petr., samb., sep., sil., spig., stram., thuj., verat.
Fever	pain in ear after suppression of ague (a feverish condition involving alternating hot, cold, and sweating stages, especially as a symptom of malaria)	Puls.
Fever	pain in extremities during fever	Arn., ars., bell., **Bry.**, calc., chin., **Eup-per.**, ferr., merc., nat-m., **Nux-v.**, phos., ptel., puls., pyrog., rhod., rhus-t., sec., sep., sulph., tub., valer.
Fever	pain in hand from uncovering hands during fever	Nux-v., stram.
Fever	pain in leg with fever	Puls., ran-a., **Rhus-t.**, spong.
Fever	pain of face from suppressed ague	Nat-m., sep., stann.
Fever	pain under nails of toes in intermittent fever	Eup-per.
Fever	palpitation of heart during fever	Acon., aesc., Ars., bar-c., Calc., cocc., crot-h., merc., Nit-ac., phos., Puls., sars., sep., sulph.
Fever	paralysis agitans after intermittent fever	**Nat-m.**
Fever	paralysis in typhoid	Agar., lach., rhus-t.
Fever	perspiration absent in fever	Acon., alum., am-c., apis., aran., arg-n., arn., ars-i., **Ars.**, **Bell.**, bism., bov., **Bry.**, **Cact.**, calc., caps., carb-s., cham., chin., coff., colch., cor-r., corn., crot-h., dulc., eup-per., **Gels.**, graph., hyos., ign., iod., ip., kali-ar., kali-bi., kali-c., kali-p., kali-s., lach., led., lyc., mag-c., merl., nat-a., nat-c., nat-m., nit-ac., **Nux-m.**, nux-v., olnd., op., ph-ac., phel., phos., plat., plb., psor., puls., ran-b., rhus-t., sabad., sang., sec., sil., spong., squil., staph., sulph., tub., verb.
Fever	perspiration after fever	Ant-t., **Ars.**, bell., bov., bry., calad., calc., carb-v., chin-a., chin-s., chin., coloc., cupr., ferr., gels., glon., graph., hell., hep., kali-n., lach., lyc., nat-a., nat-c., nat-m., nat-s., nux-v., phos., puls., rhus-t., spig., tab., thuj., zinc.
Fever	perspiration at night without fever	Cimx.
Fever	perspiration in knees after fever	Plb.
Fever	petechial (tiny purplish red spot on the skin caused by the release into the skin of a very small quantity of blood from a capillary) fever with fetid stool intestinal hæmorrhage, sopor so weak that he settles down in bed into a heap	**Mur-ac.**
Fever	petechial fever with foul smell	**Arn.**
Fever	petechial fever with foul smell, putrid, foul, cadaverous smell to stool, brown, dry, leathery-looking tongue, extreme prostration	**Ars.**
Fever	petechial fever	Anthr., arn., ars., bapt., camph., caps., carb-v., chin., **Chlor.**, lach., **Mur-ac.**, nit-ac., phos., rhus-t., sec., sulph.
Fever	profuse perspiration in evening with high fever	Con.
Fever	puerperal (relating to child birth) fever	Apis., arg-n., arn., ars., bapt., bell., bry., **Carb-s.**, cham., cimic., coff., coloc., **Echi.**, ferr., gels., hyos., ign., ip., kali-c., **Lach.**, **Lyc.**, mill., mur-ac., nux-v., op., phos., plat., **Puls.**, **Pyrog.**, **Rhus-r.**, **Rhus-t.**, sec., sil., **Sulph.**, verat-v., verat.

Body part/Disease	Symptom	Medicines
Fever	puerperal fever from suppressed lochia (vaginal discharge after childbirth)	Lyc., mill., puls., **Sulph.**
Fever	pulsation in head during fever	Bell., eup-per.
Fever	pulsation in lumbar region from fever	Hura.
Fever	pulse febrile (relating to fever)	Acon., alum., ars., bell., bov., lact-ac., merc-c., mez., plb., sars., sec., stram., thuj.
Fever	relapsing fever (infectious disease, characterized by chills and recurring fever, caused by a bacterium transmitted to people by ticks and lice)	Ars., **Calc.**, **Ferr.**, **Psor.**, **Sulph.**, tub.
Fever	remitent (getting better and the worse) fever after riding in a carriage in the wind	Nit-ac.
Fever	remitent fever ameliorated while riding in a carriage	Kali-n., nit-ac.
Fever	remitent fever at night	Acon., ant-t., **Ars.**, bapt., cham., coff., lyc., mag-c., mag-s., **Merc.**, nux-v., ph-ac., phos., puls., **Rhus-t.**, sulph.
Fever	remitent fever in afternoon	**Ars.**, **Bell.**, bry., chin., **Gels.**, ign., **Lach.**, lyc., nux-v.
Fever	remitent fever in evning	Acon., arn., **Bell.**, bry., chin., lach., **Lyc.**, mag-c., merc., mur-ac., nux-v., ph-ac., phos., puls., **Rhus-t.**, sulph.
Fever	remitent fever in infants	**Acon.**, ars., **Bell.**, bry., **Cham.**, **Gels.**, ip., nux-v., sulph.
Fever	remitent fever in morning	Arn., bry., mag-c., podo., rhus-t., sulph.
Fever	remitent fever occuring every autumn	Carb-ac.
Fever	remitent fever prone to become typhoid from the use of quinine	Arn., **Ars.**, ip., puls., **Rhus-t.**
Fever	remitent fever prone to become typhoid	Ant-t., **Ars.**, bapt., **Bry.**, carb-ac., colch., gels., mur-ac., ph-ac., phos., **Psor.**, **Rhus-t.**, sec., ter., tub.
Fever	remitent fever while riding in a carriage	Graph., psor.
Fever	remitent fever with redness of one cheek, paleness of the other	Acon., **Cham.**
Fever	respiration arreasted during fever	Ruta.
Fever	septic (full of or generating pus) fever	Acet-ac., **Anthr.**, apis., **Arn.**, **Ars.**, **Bapt.**, bell., berb., **Bry.**, cadm., carb-v., **Crot-c.**, **Crot-h.**, cur., **Echi.**, **Kali-p.**, **Lach.**, **Lyc.**, merc., **Mur-ac.**, op., ph-ac., **Phos.**, puls., **Pyrog.**, rhus-t., rhus-v., **Sulph.**, **Tarent-c.**
Fever	sighing breath in typhoid	Calad.
Fever	skin, crawling during fever	Kali-br.
Fever	skin, heat without fever	Aloe., arn., ars., bell., bor., bry., chin., cocc., coloc., dulc., graph., hep., hyos., iod., kali-bi., lach., mag-c., mur-ac., nux-v., phos., puls., rhus-t., sang., sep., sil., sulph.
Fever	sleeplessness from low fevers	Stram.
Fever	sole hot during fever	Aesc., canth., cupr., ferr., graph., lach., Sulph.
Fever	spoiled intermittent chronic fever	Ars., calc., ferr., ip., nat-m., nux-v., **Sep.**, sulph., tarent.

Body part/Disease	Symptom	Medicines
Fever	spoiled intermittent chronic fever that tends towards typhoid	Ars., gels.
Fever	stitching sensation in chest during fever	Acon., Bry., kali-c., nux-v.
Fever	stretching during fever	Thuj.
Fever	suppression of urine with fever	Arn., ars., bell., cact., canth., colch., crot-h., hyos., op., plb., sel., stram.
Fever	sweating on forehead during fever	Ant-t., ip., mag-s., sars., staph., Verat.
Fever	swelling in face in scarlet fever	Apis., Arum-t., calc., hell., kali-s., lyc., zinc.
Fever	swelling in glands after scarlet fever	**Bar-c.**
Fever	swelling in left parotid gland after exanthemata (a disease characterized by the appearance of a skin rash, e.g. measles or scarlet fever)	Anthr., arn., bar-c., Brom., carb-v., dulc., iod., kali-bi., mag-c., sulph.
Fever	swelling in lower limbs after scarlet fever	**Apis.**, bar-m., crot-h., hell.
Fever	trembling during fever	Ars., calc., camph., cist., eup-per., kali-c., lach., mag-c., mygal., sep., Zinc.
Fever	trembling in hand in typhoid	Arg-n., zinc.
Fever	trembling in hand on moving them in typhoid	Gels.
Fever	typhus fever with swelled parotid, and sensitive bones	Mang.
Fever	urine albuminous after scarlet fever	Apis., ars., asc-t., aur-m., bell., bry., canth., carb-ac., coch., colch., con., cop., crot-h., dig., dulc., glon., hell., helon., hep., kali-c., kali-chl., kali-s., lach., Lyc., merc-c., Nat-s., phos., phyt., rhus-t., sec., senec., stram., ter., uran.
Fever	urine copious with amenorrhoea during fever	Ant-c., arg-m., ars., aur-m-n., cedr., cham., colch., dulc., eup-pur., lyc., med., mur-ac., ph-ac., phos., squil., Stram.
Fever	urine inadequate during fever	Apis., ars., cann-s., canth., cocc., colch., eup-pur., lyc., nat-m., nit-ac., nux-v., op., puls., staph.
Fever	urine offensive during fever	Arg-m., kreos., lyc., merc., ph-ac., rhus-t., squil., staph., sulph.
Fever	urine offensive, disgusting smell during fever	Ph-ac.
Fever	urticaria during fever	**Apis.**, chlor., cop., cub., **Ign.**, **Rhus-t.**, rhus-v., sulph.
Fever	vomiting bile during fever	Ars., bry., cham., chin., cina., crot-h., cupr., dros., Eup-per., ign., ip., iris., merc., nat-m., nux-v., op., phos., psor., puls., sec., sep., sulph., thuj., verat.
Fever	wants to be quiet in any stage of fever	**Bry.**, gels.
Fever	weakness after fever	Aran.
Fever	weakness during fever	Acon., ant-t., aran., **Ars.**, bapt., bry., carb-v., eup-pur., ferr., ign., lyc., mur-ac., nat-c., nat-m., nit-ac., ph-ac., **Phos.**, puls., rhus-t., rob., sarr., sulph.
Fever	weakness following prolonged fever	**Sel.**
Fever	weakness in back after typhoid fever	Sel.
Fever	weakness in foot after fever	Nat-s.
Fever	weakness in hand at night after fever	Nat-s.

Body part/Disease	Symptom	Medicines
Fever	weakness in lower limbs during getting catarrhal (inflammation of a mucous membrane) fever	Sep.
Fever	weakness in lumbar region during fever	Hura.
Fever	yellow fever	Acon., arg-n., ars-h., **Ars.**, bell., bry., cadm., calc., camph., **Canth.**, **Carb-v.**, chin., coff., **Crot-h.**, daph., hep., ip., lach., lob., nat-s., **Nux-v.**, phos., psor., rhus-t., ter., verat.
Fever	yellow fever (often fatal viral disease of warm climates, transmitted by mosquitoes and marked by high fever, hemorrhaging, vomiting of blood, liver damage, and jaundice) third stage with hæmorrhages, with great paleness of face, violent headache, great heaviness of limbs and trembling of the body	**Carb-v.**
Fever	yellow fever when sweat is checked from exposure to a draft of air	Cadm.
Fibre	fibroids in ovaries	Apis., calc., coloc., fl-ac., hep., iod., lach., merc., plat., podo., staph., thuj.
Fibre	fibroids in uterus	Apis., aur-m-n., brom., bufo., Calc-f., calc-p., calc-s., Calc., con., kali-br., kali-c., kali-i., lach., led., lil-t., lyc., merc-c., merc-i-r., merc., nit-ac., nux-v., Phos., plat., sec., sil., sul-ac., ter., thuj., tub., ust., vinc.
Fibre	Fibrous (The coarse fibrous substances, largely composed of cellulose, that are found in grains, fruits, and vegetables, and aid digestion) Deposits	Acetic Acid
Fibre	metrorrhagia from fibroids (fibrous tissue growth)	Calc-p., calc., hydr., lyc., merc., nit-ac., Phos., sabin., sil., sul-ac., sulph.
Fibre	recurrent fibroid (benign growth composed of fibrous and muscle tissue, especially one that develops in the wall of the womb and is associated with painful and excessive menstrual flow) tumours in external throat	Sil.
Fibre	tumours fibroid (a benign growth composed of fibrous and muscle tissue, especially one that develops in the wall of the womb)	**Calc-f.**, calc-s., calc., con., **Phos.**, **Sil.**
Fibre	vomiting fibrous	Iod., ox-ac., phos., sul-ac.
Finger	abscess in fingers	Fl-ac., hep., lach., mang.
Finger	ankylosis (stiffness of a joint bones) of first joint of fingers	Crot-h.
Finger	ankylosis of last joint of fingers	Fl-ac.
Finger	arthritic nodosities on condyles on finger joints	Aesc., agn., ant-c., Apis., Benz-ac., calc-f., calc-p., Calc., Caust., clem., colch., dig., Graph., hep., Led., Lith., Lyc., ox-ac., ran-s., rhod., sil., staph., sulph., urt-u.
Finger	arthritic nodositieson condyles on finger joints with stiffness	Carb-an., graph., Lyc.
Finger	automatic motion of fingers	Zinc.
Finger	Biting fingers	Arum-t., op., plb.
Finger	boring fingers in ears	Agar., chel., mez., mill., phys., ruta., sal-ac., sil., thuj.

Body part/Disease	Symptom	Medicines
Finger	boring in nose with fingers	Arum-t., aur., bufo., Cina., con., ph-ac., phos., psor., sel., stict., verat., zinc.
Finger	brittle (hard and breakable) finger nails	Alum., ambr., ant-c., ars., calc., cast-eq., dios., fl-ac., Graph., merc., nit-ac., Psor., sep., sil., squil., sulph., thuj.
Finger	burning pain & crawling in first finger	Agar.
Finger	burning pain between fingers	Alum., rhus-v.
Finger	burning pain between index finger and thumb	Alum., berb., iod., rhus-t., sulph.
Finger	burning pain in back of finger	Brom., cocc., ran-s., sil.
Finger	burning pain in ball of finger	Sulph., Zinc.
Finger	burning pain in finger in evening	Alum.
Finger	burning pain in finger in forenoon	Fago.
Finger	burning pain in first finger	Acon., agar., alum., arund., berb., card-m., chel., ferr-ma., hura., kali-c., olnd., sil.
Finger	burning pain in fourth finger	Spig., stann., tarax.
Finger	burning pain in joints of finger	Apis., bufo., cann-i., carb-v., caust., vinc.
Finger	burning pain in joints of fingers	Nat-c.
Finger	burning pain in nail of second finger	Kali-c.
Finger	burning pain in second finger	Apis., coloc., kali-c., mez., sul-ac.
Finger	burning pain in third finger	Osm., tarax.
Finger	burning pain in tip of fourth finger	Apis., aur-m-n., fl-ac., kali-c., sul-ac.
Finger	burning pain in tips of finger	Am-m., anthr., apis., bell., caust., con., croc., crot-c., gins., mag-m., mur-ac., nat-s., sabad., sars., sil., sulph., tab.
Finger	burning pain in upper limbs extending to fingers	Mag-m.
Finger	burning pain in wrist extending to index finger	Arund.
Finger	burning pain in wrist extending to index finger & thumb	Agar., asar.
Finger	burning pain in wrist extending to little finger	**Sulph.**
Finger	caries of fingers	Sil.
Finger	caries of hands metacarpal bone (any bone in the human hand between the wrist and digits)	Sil.
Finger	chapped (to become sore and cracked by exposure to wind or cold) fingers	Nat-m.
Finger	chapped tips of fingers	Bar-c.
Finger	chilblains on fingers	Berb., carb-an., lyc., nit-ac., nux-v., petr., puls., sul-ac., sulph.
Finger	chilblains on fingers with itching	Sulph.
Finger	chilblains on fingers, painful	Sul-ac.
Finger	children put finger in mouth	Calc., cham., Ip.
Finger	chill beginning in and extending from fingers	Bry., coff., dig., **Nat-m.**, nux-v., sep., sulph.
Finger	chill beginning in and extending from tips of fingers	**Bry.**, nat-m., puls.
Finger	chill beginning in and extending from tips of fingers and toes	**Bry.**, cycl., dig., meny., nat-m., **Sep.**, stann., sulph.

Body part/Disease	Symptom	Medicines
Finger	chill in and extending from abdomen to fingers and toes	Calad.
Finger	closed (little space between) fingers	Lyc., stry.
Finger	closed fingers during sleep	Hyos., sul-ac.
Finger	coldness in finger joints	Chel.
Finger	coldness in fingers alternating with headache	Cupr.
Finger	coldness in fingers at night	Mur-ac.
Finger	coldness in fingers extending to middle of upper arms	Graph.
Finger	coldness in fingers extending to nape	Coff.
Finger	coldness in fingers extending to palms and soles	Dig.
Finger	coldness in fingers in afternoon	Plan.
Finger	coldness in fingers in evening	Sulph., thuj.
Finger	coldness in fingers in morning	Chin-s., rat.
Finger	coldness in fingers while sitting	Cham.
Finger	coldness in first finger	Rhod.
Finger	coldness in fourth finger	Lyc.
Finger	coldness in joints of second finger	Agar.
Finger	coldness in second finger	Mur-ac., phos., rhod.
Finger	coldness in third finger	Rhod., sulph.
Finger	coldness in third finger in evening	Sulph.
Finger	coldness in tips of finger	Abrot., ant-t., arn., brom., caps., carb-v., carl., Chel., cist., coloc., hell., jatr., lac-d., lob., meny., merc., mur-ac., ph-ac., ran-b., sal-ac., sars., spig., sulph., sumb., tarax., thuj., zinc.
Finger	coldness in tips of finger after writing	Carl.
Finger	coldness in tips of finger during chill	Ran-b.
Finger	coldness in tips of finger during heat	Caps.
Finger	coldness in tips of finger in morning after rising	Coloc.
Finger	coldness in tips of finger in open air	Ph-ac.
Finger	coldness in tips of finger sensitive to cold	Sec.
Finger	coldness in tips of finger with rest of body hot	Thuj.
Finger	coldness in upper limbs from cold air as if passing down to fingers	Fl-ac.
Finger	constant motion of fingers	Kali-br., stram., sulph.
Finger	constrictions in fingers	Aeth., carb-an., croc., dros., elaps., lach., nux-v., phos., sep., spong.
Finger	constrictions in fingers periodical	Phos.
Finger	contraction of muscles & tendons of fingers after vomiting blood	Ars.
Finger	contraction of muscles & tendons of fingers before chill	Cimx.
Finger	contraction of muscles & tendons of fingers from abductors (a muscle that pulls the body or a limb away from a midpoint or midline)	Arg-n.
Finger	contraction of muscles & tendons of fingers from flexors muscle	Ars., caust., cimx., sil.

Body part/Disease	Symptom	Medicines
Finger	contraction of muscles & tendons of fingers in afternoon	Morph.
Finger	contraction of muscles & tendons of fingers in cholera	Cupr.
Finger	contraction of muscles & tendons of fingers in epilepsy	Lach., mag-p., merc.
Finger	contraction of muscles & tendons of fingers in morning	Phos.
Finger	contraction of muscles & tendons of fingers periodical	Phos.
Finger	contraction of muscles & tendons of fingers when yawning	Crot-t., nux-v.
Finger	contraction of muscles & tendons of fingers while grasping	Arg-n., dros., stry.
Finger	contraction of muscles & tendons of fingers while lying on that side	Crot-t.
Finger	contraction of muscles & tendons of first finger	Alum., cycl., graph.
Finger	contraction of muscles & tendons of fourth finger	Sabad., sulph.
Finger	contraction of muscles & tendons of second finger	Cina., sil.
Finger	contraction of muscles & tendons of third finger	Sabad.
Finger	convulsion begin in finger & toes	Cupr.
Finger	convulsion of first finger	Cycl.
Finger	convulsion of upper limbs extending to fingers	Acon.
Finger	convulsion with wounds in the soles, finger and palm	Bell., **Hyper.**, led.
Finger	convulsive trembling of first finger	Calc.
Finger	cracking in finger from closing the hand	Ars-m.
Finger	cracking in finger joints	Ars-m., caps., carb-an., kali-n., merc., sulph.
Finger	cracking in third joint of finger	Hydr., phos.
Finger	cracks between fingers	Ars., aur-m., graph., sulph., zinc.
Finger	cracks in fingers	Am-m., bar-c., Calc., cist., hep., kali-c., mag-c., merc., Petr., phos., Sars., sil., zinc.
Finger	cracks in first finger	Sil.
Finger	cracks in joints of fingers	Graph., mang., merc., phos., sanic.,sulph.
Finger	cracks in joints of fingers that ulcerate	Merc.
Finger	cramp in fingers at midnight in bed	Nux-v.
Finger	cramp in fingers at night in bed	Ars.
Finger	cramp in fingers during parturition (act of giving birth)	Cupr., Dios.
Finger	cramp in fingers from playing piano or violin	Mag-p.
Finger	cramp in fingers in evening	Ars.
Finger	cramp in fingers in morning	Tab.
Finger	cramp in fingers on moving	Merc.
Finger	cramp in fingers when stretching them	Ars.
Finger	cramp in fingers while sewing	Kali-c.

Body part/Disease	Symptom	Medicines
Finger	cramp in fingers while shoe making	Stann.
Finger	cramp in fingers while writing	Brach., cycl., mag-p., Stann., tril.
Finger	cramp in fingers with cholera (an acute and often fatal intestinal disease that produces severe gastrointestinal symptoms and is usually caused by the bacterium Vibrio cholerae)	Colch., Cupr., sec., Verat.
Finger	cramp in fingers, on attempting to pick a small object	Stann.
Finger	cramp in fingers, periodical	Phos.
Finger	cramp in first finger	Cycl., kali-chl., nat-p.
Finger	cramp in first finger while writing	Cycl.
Finger	cramp in fourth finger	Cocc., com., sulph.
Finger	cramp in fourth finger while writing	Cocc.
Finger	cramp in second finger	Am-m., hura., lil-t., plb., sulph.
Finger	cramp in third finger	Hura., sep., sulph.
Finger	cramp in third finger from extending to elbow	Sep., sulph.
Finger	cramp in third finger in evening	Sep., sulph.
Finger	crushed and ulcerated finger ends	**Hyper.**, led.
Finger	curved finger nails	Nit-ac.
Finger	curved finger nails in consumption (any condition that causes progressive wasting of the tissues, especially tuberculosis of the lungs)	Med., tub.
Finger	dificult motion of fingers	Plb., rob., tarent., vip.
Finger	dificult motion of fingers in afternoon	Mag-s.
Finger	discoloration of fingers	Act-sp.
Finger	discoloration of fingers black	Sep., vip.
Finger	discoloration of fingers blue	Benz-n., caust., cocc., corn., crot-h., cupr., nat-m., nux-m., nux-v., op., petr., sil., vip.
Finger	discoloration of fingers blue in morning	Petr.
Finger	discoloration of fingers with brown spots	Ant-t.
Finger	discoloration of first finger with black spots	Apis., rhus-t.
Finger	discoloration of first finger with red blotches	Arg-n.
Finger	discoloration of nail tip of first finger	Phos.
Finger	discoloration of second joint of second finger	Ars-h.
Finger	discoloration red of back of first finger	Arg-n.
Finger	discoloration, blotches on fingers	Arg-n.
Finger	discoloration, ecchymoses of fingers	Coca.
Finger	discoloration, in joints of fingers	Cann-s., cham., chel., cinnb., lyc., pall., spong., sulph.
Finger	discoloration, red points on fingers	Lach.
Finger	discoloration, red spots on fingers	Benz-ac., cor-r., plb., zinc.
Finger	discoloration, red stripes on fingers	Apis.
Finger	discoloration, redness of fingers	Agar., apis., apoc., arg-n., arum-i., benz-ac., berb., bor., cann-i., cit-v., fl-ac., graph., kali-bi., lach., lyc., nux-v., plb., sil., sulph., ther., zinc.

Body part/Disease	Symptom	Medicines
Finger	discoloration, redness of fingers in evening	Sulph.
Finger	discoloration, redness of fourth finger	Lyc.
Finger	discoloration, spots on fingers	Con., corn., lyc., mang., nat-m., ph-ac., plb.
Finger	discoloration, violet of fingers	Stry.
Finger	discoloration, white of fingers	Gins., lach., vip.
Finger	discoloration, white of fingers during coldness	Gins.
Finger	discoloration, yellow of fingers	Ant-t., chel., con., elaps., ph-ac., sabad.
Finger	discoloration, yellow of fingers in spots	Ant-t., bism., con., elaps., sabad.
Finger	disecting wounds of fingers	Apis., **Ars., Lach.**
Finger	dislocated feeling in finger joints	Phos.
Finger	emaciation of fingers	Lach., sil., thuj.
Finger	emaciation of index finger	Lach., thuj.
Finger	emaciation of tips of fingers	Ars.
Finger	eruption in fingers	Arn., ars., bor., canth., caust., cist., cupr., cycl., fl-ac., graph., hep., kali-s., lach., mez., mur-ac., ph-ac., ran-b., rhus-t., rhus-v., sars., sep., sil., spig., sulph., tab., tarax., thuj.
Finger	eruption, vesicles between second and third fingers	Sulph.
Finger	eruption, between first and second fingers	Cic.
Finger	eruption, between second and third fingers	Sulph.
Finger	eruption, between third and fourth fingers	Mag-c.
Finger	eruption, blotches in fingers	Ant-c., arg-n., ars., berb., caust., cocc., con., lach., led., nat-c., rhus-t., verat.
Finger	eruption, burning vesicles between the fingers	Canth.
Finger	eruption, desquamation between index finger and thumb	Am-m.
Finger	eruption, desquamation between the fingers	Am-m.
Finger	eruption, herpes between index finger and thumb	Ambr.
Finger	eruption, herpes between the fingers	Ambr., graph., merc., nit-ac.
Finger	eruption, itching between the fingers	Canth., lyc., **Psor., Sulph.**
Finger	eruption, itching pimples between index finger and thumb	Ars., sulph.
Finger	eruption, itching vesicles between the fingers	Canth., psor., **Sulph.**
Finger	eruption, moist between the fingers	Graph.
Finger	eruption, pimples between index finger and thumb	Agar., bry., canth., ham., sulph., thuj.
Finger	eruption, pimples between index finger and thumb burning on touch	Canth.
Finger	eruption, pimples between the fingers	Ars., lyc., ph-ac., puls.
Finger	eruption, pimples between the fingers	Canth.
Finger	eruption, pustules between the fingers	Caps., rhus-t.
Finger	eruption, scaly between the fingers	Laur.
Finger	eruption, urticaria between the fingers	Hyper., merc.

Body part/Disease	Symptom	Medicines
Finger	eruption, vesicles between index finger and thumb	Grat., nat-s., **Sulph.**
Finger	eruption, vesicles between the fingers	Anag., apis., calc., canth., hell., iod., laur., nat-m., olnd., phos., **Psor.**, puls., rhus-t., rhus-v., ruta., sel., **Sulph.**
Finger	eruption, vesicles between third and fourth fingers	Mag-c.
Finger	eruptions in nails of fingers	Eug., merc., sel.
Finger	eruptions, blisters in tips of fingers	Alum., cupr.
Finger	eruptions, bluish vesicles in fingers	Ran-b.
Finger	eruptions, boils in fingers	Calc., lach., sil.
Finger	eruptions, burning in fingers	Ran-b.
Finger	eruptions, burning vesicles in fingers	Ran-b.
Finger	eruptions, copper coloured spots in fingers	Cor-r.
Finger	eruptions, crusts in nails of fingers	Ars.
Finger	eruptions, desquamation in fingers	Agar., bar-c., elaps., graph., merc., mez., rhus-v., sabad., sep., still., sulph.
Finger	eruptions, desquamation in nails of fingers	Chlol.
Finger	eruptions, desquamation in tips of fingers	Bar-c., elaps., ph-ac., phos.
Finger	eruptions, dry in fingers	Anag., psor.
Finger	eruptions, dry in joints of fingers	**Psor.**
Finger	eruptions, eczema in fingers	Lyc., sil., staph.
Finger	eruptions, elevated spots in fingers	Syph.
Finger	eruptions, excrescences in fingers	Ars., thuj.
Finger	eruptions, greenish excrescences in fingers	Ars.
Finger	eruptions, herpes in fingers	Ambr., caust., cist., **Graph.**, kreos., merc., nit-ac., psor., ran-b., thuj., zinc.
Finger	eruptions, in first finger	Agar., calc., kali-c., mag-c., nat-c., sil.
Finger	eruptions, in fourth finger	Cycl.
Finger	eruptions, in joints of fingers	Cycl., hydr., mez., **Psor.**
Finger	eruptions, in sides of fingers	Mez., sabad., tax.
Finger	eruptions, in third finger	Cycl.
Finger	eruptions, in tips of fingers	Ars., bar-c., cist., cupr., elaps., nat-c., psor.
Finger	eruptions, itching in fingers	Ran-b.
Finger	eruptions, itching ulcer in joints of fingers	Mez.
Finger	eruptions, itching vesicles in fingers	Ran-b.
Finger	eruptions, painful eczema in fingers	Arn.
Finger	eruptions, painful nodules in fingers	Calc.
Finger	eruptions, pemohigus (large blisters on the skin and mucous membranes, often accompanied by itching or burning sensations) in fingers	Lyc.
Finger	eruptions, phagedenic blisters in fingers	Calc., graph., hep., kali-c., mag-c., nit-ac., ran-b., sil., sulph.
Finger	eruptions, phagedenic in first finger after washing with cold water	Nat-c.
Finger	eruptions, phagedenic in first finger discharging water	Calc.

Body part/Disease	Symptom	Medicines
Finger	eruptions, pimples in fingers	Anac., ant-c., arn., ars., bar-c., berb., canth., carb-ac., cycl., elaps., graph., kali-c., lyc., mez., mur-ac., ph-ac., sars., spig., tab., tarax., ther., zinc.
Finger	eruptions, pimples in first finger	Sulph.
Finger	eruptions, pimples in tips of fingers	Elaps.
Finger	eruptions, psoriasis in fingers	Lyc., teucr.
Finger	eruptions, psoriasis in first finger	Anag., teucr.
Finger	eruptions, psoriasis in second finger	Anag.
Finger	eruptions, pustules in fingers	Anac., bar-c., bor., cinnb., cocc., cupr., kali-bi., rhus-t., sang., sars., spig., zinc.
Finger	eruptions, pustules in nails of fingers spreading over hand to wrist	Kali-bi.
Finger	eruptions, pustules in tips of fingers	Psor.
Finger	eruptions, rash in fingers	Hydr., sil.
Finger	eruptions, scabs in fingers	Anag., cit-v., kali-bi., lyc., mur-ac., rhus-v., thuj.
Finger	eruptions, scales in fingers	white : Lyc., sep.
Finger	eruptions, tubercles in between thumb & index finger	Ars.
Finger	eruptions, tubercles in fingers	Berb., caust., con., hydrc., lach., led., lyc., nat-c., rhus-t., verat., zinc.
Finger	eruptions, ulcer in nails of fingers	Ars.
Finger	eruptions, urticaria in fingers	Hep., thuj., urt-u.
Finger	eruptions, urticaria in fingers on becoming cold	Thuj.
Finger	eruptions, vesicles becoming ulcer in fingers	Calc., graph., kali-c., mag-c., nit-ac., ran-b., sil.
Finger	eruptions, vesicles in fingers on becoming cold	Bell., bor., calc., cit-v., clem., cupr-ar., cupr., cycl., fl-ac., graph., hep., kali-c., kali-s., lach., mag-c., mang., mez., nat-c., nat-m., nat-s., nit-ac., ph-ac., phos., plb., puls., ran-b., rhus-t., rhus-v., sars., sel., sep., sil., sulph.
Finger	eruptions, vesicles in first finger	Calc., kali-c., mag-c., nat-c., sil., sulph.
Finger	eruptions, vesicles in first finger discharging water	Kali-c.
Finger	eruptions, vesicles in fourth finger	Graph.
Finger	eruptions, vesicles in nails of fingers	Ail., nat-c.
Finger	eruptions, vesicles in tips of fingers	Ail., ars., cupr., nat-c.
Finger	eruptions, vesicles in tips of fingers filled with blood	**Ars.**
Finger	eruptions, wart-like excrescences in fingers	Thuj.
Finger	erysipelatous inflammation in fingers	Rhod., rhus-t., sulph., thuj.
Finger	exostoses on fingers	Calc-f.
Finger	extension of fingers difficult	Arn., ars., camph., carb-s., coloc., cupr-ar., cupr., hyos., merc., mosch., plat., plb., stram., syph., tab.
Finger	feels impelled to crack the fingers	Meph.
Finger	Finger nails thick	Alum., **Graph.**, sabad.
Finger	fingers abducted spasmodically (Involuntary muscle contraction)	Glon., lac-c., Sec.
Finger	fingers hot	Apis., bor., fago., lact., mag-c., par., rhus-t., thuj.

Body part/Disease	Symptom	Medicines
Finger	fingers nails hot	Hura.
Finger	fingers sensitive to cold	Agar., sec.
Finger	fingers tips hot	Daph., fago., hura., nat-c., rhod.
Finger	flexed finger	Ambr., ars., caust., colch., **Cupr.**, hyos., **Merc.**, nux-m., nux-v., phos., plat., **Plb.**, sec., stram.
Finger	formication in back extending to fingers and toes	Sec.
Finger	formication in back of fingers	Bar-ac., ran-b.
Finger	formication in fingers	**Acon.**, aeth., agar., alum., ars., brom., calc., caust., colch., gins., graph., hep., kali-c., kreos., lach., **Lyc.**, mag-c., mag-s., mez., mur-ac., nat-c., nat-m., nit-ac., op., paeon., phos., plat., plb., psor., ran-b., rhod., rhus-t., samb., sep., sil., staph., sul-ac., thuj., verat.
Finger	formication in fingers as from anxiety	Verat.
Finger	formication in fingers in evening	Alum., ars., colch.
Finger	formication in fingers in morning in bed	Psor.
Finger	formication in fingers while writing	Acon.
Finger	formication in first finger	Croc., mag-s., phos., tab.
Finger	formication in fourth finger	Agar., aran., mag-s., phos., rhod.
Finger	formication in second finger	Acon., mag-s., mez., tab.
Finger	formication in third finger	Aran., caust., mag-s., sulph., tab.
Finger	formication in tip of first finger	Graph., nat-m.
Finger	formication in tip of second finger	Kali-c.
Finger	formication in tips of fingers	**Am-m.**, cann-s., cupr., glon., graph., hep., mag-s., morph., **Nat-m.**, nat-s., plat., **Sec.**, sep., spig., stry., sulph., tep., thuj.
Finger	formication in tips of fingers in afternoon	Am-m.
Finger	formication in tips of fingers in evening	Nat-c.
Finger	gangrene in fingers	Sec.
Finger	gouty stiffness of fingers	**Agar.**, carb-an., lyc., sulph.
Finger	gouty swelling of joints of fingers	Anag., kali-i., **Lyc.**, sulph.
Finger	hardness of skin of finger nails	Ars.
Finger	headache extending around the finger tips	
Finger	heaviness in hand in fingers	Berb., par., phos., plb., rhus-v.
Finger	horny warts on first finger	Caust.
Finger	hypertrophy of heart with numbness in left arm and fingers	Acon., Rhus-t.
Finger	induration (hardening) of fingers	Caust., crot-h., graph., med., phyt.
Finger	induration (hardness in body tissue) of tendons (tough band connecting muscle to bone) of fingers	Carb-an., Caust.
Finger	inflammation in bone of fingers	Staph.
Finger	inflammation in fingers	**Am-c.**, apis., calc-s., con., cupr., hep., kali-c., lyc., mag-c., mang., nat-m., nit-ac., puls., ran-b., sil., tarent.
Finger	inflammation in joints of fingers	Lyc.

Body part/Disease	Symptom	Medicines
Finger	inflammation in periosteum (tissue around bones) of fingers	**Led.**
Finger	irregular motion of fingers	Cupr.
Finger	itching between fingers	Alum., anac., aur., brom., carb-s., carb-v., caust., cycl., grat., nat-s., ph-ac., psor., puls., rhod., rhus-v., sel., **Sulph.**
Finger	itching between fingers in evening	Ran-s.
Finger	itching between fingers in morning on walking	Rhus-v., sulph.
Finger	itching between fingers in morning	**Sulph.**
Finger	itching between thumb and index finger	Agar., ambr., aur., grat., hura., iod., jatr., kreos., plb., sumb.
Finger	itching in back of fingers	Ars., berb., carb-an., **Con.**, merc-i-r., nat-m., sars., sulph.
Finger	itching in back of joints of fingers	Bor.
Finger	itching in ball of fingers	Con., graph., sep.
Finger	itching in ball of fingers in spots	Sep.
Finger	itching in fingers	Agar., alum., am-c., **Anac.**, apis., ars-h., ars., arum-d., asc-t., aur., berb., calad., calc., cann-s., carb-v., caust., cit-v., coc-c., con., eupho., hep., jatr., jug-r., lach., lact., lyc., mag-c., mang., merc., mez., nat-c., nat-m., nux-v., ox-ac., petr., phos., plan., plat., prun-s., puls., ran-b., rhod., rhus-v., sel., sil., stry., sul-ac., **Sulph.**, tarent., thuj., **Urt-u.**, zinc.
Finger	itching in fingers aggravated from scratching	Ars., arum-t.
Finger	itching in fingers aggravated in warm room	Nux-v.
Finger	itching in fingers as if they were frozen	Agar.
Finger	itching in fingers from smoking	Calad.
Finger	itching in fingers in afternoon	Coc-c., jug-r.
Finger	itching in fingers in evening	Calad., sulph.
Finger	itching in fingers in evening in bed	Nat-m.
Finger	itching in fingers on going to bed	Nux-v.
Finger	itching in fingers when cool	Thuj.
Finger	itching in fingers while lying	Calad.
Finger	itching in first finger	Agar., anac., calc., carb-an., caust., crot-h., fl-ac., hell., hura., lach., nat-m., sil., teucr.
Finger	itching in first finger in evening	Fl-ac.
Finger	itching in fourth finger	Asc-t., con., lach., lyc., ol-an.
Finger	itching in fourth finger at night	Sulph.
Finger	itching in joints of fingers	Alum., apis., bor., bry., camph., hydr., nux-v., petr.
Finger	itching in joints of last finger	Petr.
Finger	itching in joints of middle finger	Manc.
Finger	itching in metacarpal joints of first finger	Berb., fl-ac., verat.
Finger	itching in palm near root of fingers	Kali-c., lyc.
Finger	itching in second finger	Ars-h., ars., chel., crot-h., crot-t., gran., kali-n., lith., nat-m., olnd., ph-ac., rhod., teucr., verat., verb.

Body part/Disease	Symptom	Medicines
Finger	itching in third finger	Asc-t., crot-h., crot-t., lith., rhod., teucr., ther.
Finger	itching in tip of finger	Am-m., nat-m.
Finger	itching in tip of finger and scratching does not ameliorate	Am-m.
Finger	itching in tip of finger in morning	Am-m.
Finger	itching in tips of fingers	Ambr., plat., prun-s., spig., sul-ac.
Finger	jerking and fingers painful while writing	Cocc.
Finger	jerking in fourth fingers	Com., meny.
Finger	jerking into joints of fingers	Carb-s.
Finger	jerking of fingers	Cadm., calc., **Cic., Cina.**, cocc., merc-c., merc., nat-c., op., stram.
Finger	jerking of fingers in epilepsy	**Cic.**
Finger	knobby finger ends	Laur.
Finger	lacerations of nails of fingers	**Hyper.**
Finger	lameness in fingers	Bor., calc., carb-v., hyper., kali-c., sep.
Finger	lameness in second finger	Cimic., rhus-t.
Finger	lameness in third finger	Bry.
Finger	lameness in third finger after writing	Bry.
Finger	motion as if he were counting with fingers	Mosch.
Finger	motion of fingers	Agar., fl-ac., lach., ox-ac., stram., tarent.
Finger	nodular (small mass of cells or tissue, which may be a normal part of the body or a growth such as a tumor) swelling of fingers	Anac., lyc., mag-c.
Finger	numbness in elbow extending to tips of fingers	Jatr.
Finger	numbness in fingers after eating	Con.
Finger	numbness in fingers after writing	Carl.
Finger	numbness in fingers at night	Am-c., mur-ac., puls.
Finger	numbness in fingers before an attack of intermittent fever	Puls.
Finger	numbness in fingers between convulsiions	Sec.
Finger	numbness in fingers during chill	Cedr., cimx., ferr., **Sep.**, stann., thuj.
Finger	numbness in fingers during epileptic	Cupr.
Finger	numbness in fingers during fever	Thuj.
Finger	numbness in fingers during perspiration	Nux-v.
Finger	numbness in fingers extending upwards	Ars.
Finger	numbness in fingers from carrying load on arm	Carl.
Finger	numbness in fingers from chest affection	Carb-an.
Finger	numbness in fingers grasping anything	Acon., am-c., calc.
Finger	numbness in fingers in afternoon	Fl-ac., sulph.
Finger	numbness in fingers in cold air	Nit-ac.
Finger	numbness in fingers in evening	Sep., ter.
Finger	numbness in fingers in evening on lying down	Mag-m.

Body part/Disease	Symptom	Medicines
Finger	numbness in fingers in morning in bed	Puls.
Finger	numbness in fingers in morning in bed on rising	Stram.
Finger	numbness in fingers while playing piano	Sulph.
Finger	numbness in fingers while sitting	Cham.
Finger	numbness in first finger	Agar., apis., caust., euphr., hura., kreos., lyc., nat-m., par., phos., rhod., rhus-t.
Finger	numbness in first finger in morning	Lyc., nat-m., rhus-t.
Finger	numbness in first finger of left hand	Anac., nat-m., rhus-t.
Finger	numbness in first finger up radial (radius bone of the forearm) side of arm	Anac., carb-an., phos.
Finger	numbness in forearm extending to end of little finger	Cinnb.
Finger	numbness in forearm extending to finger	Pall.
Finger	numbness in fourth finger	Alum., anac., aran., arg-n., calad., calc-s., coca., com., dios., eupi., inul., lyc., med., nat-c., nat-m., op., plat., sars., sulph., sumb., thuj.
Finger	numbness in fourth finger after sitting	Alum.
Finger	numbness in fourth finger ameliorated from rubbing	Nat-c.
Finger	numbness in fourth finger in afternoon	Calc-s., nicc.
Finger	numbness in fourth finger in evening	Sulph.
Finger	numbness in fourth finger in evening in bed	Sulph.
Finger	numbness in fourth finger in morning	Calc-s., lyc.
Finger	numbness in fourth finger in morning on walking	Lyc.
Finger	numbness in fourth finger on walking	Coca., lyc.
Finger	numbness in fourth finger while writing	Com.
Finger	numbness in left fourth finger	Dios., sumb., thuj.
Finger	numbness in left third finger	Sumb., thuj.
Finger	numbness in right fingers	Hydrc., nat-p., sep.
Finger	numbness in right fingers in morning	Am-c., caust., cham., dios., ferr., kreos., merc., phos., puls., rhus-t., sulph.
Finger	numbness in right fourth finger	Inul.
Finger	numbness in right third finger	Rat.
Finger	numbness in third finger	Anac., aran., arg-n., calc., carb-o., com., eupi., lyc., nat-m., nicc., op., phys., rat., sabad., sars., sulph., sumb., thuj.
Finger	numbness in third finger in morning	Lyc.
Finger	numbness in third finger in afternoon	Nicc.
Finger	numbness in third finger in evening	Phys.
Finger	numbness in third finger in evening in bed	Sulph.
Finger	numbness in third finger on waking in morning	Lyc.
Finger	numbness in third finger while writing	Com.
Finger	numbness in tip of first finger	Graph., spong.

Body part/Disease	Symptom	Medicines
Finger	numbness in tip of fourth finger	Plb.
Finger	numbness in tip of second finger	Calc., carb-o., dig., euphr., gamb., lyc., mur-ac., nat-m., phos., rat., rhus-t.
Finger	numbness in tip of second finger at night	Mur-ac.
Finger	numbness in tip of second finger in cold air	Phos.
Finger	numbness in tip of second finger in morning	Lyc., nat-m., rhus-t.
Finger	numbness in tips of finger after a wetting	Rhus-t.
Finger	numbness in tips of finger during whooping cough	Spong.
Finger	numbness in tips of finger on stretching hands	Tell.
Finger	numbness in tips of fingers	Ant-t., apis., arg-n., ars., cann-s., carb-an., carb-s., caust., chel., graph., kali-c., kali-p., lach., mag-m., mez., mur-ac., ph-ac., **Phos.**, sec., spong., stann., staph., sumb., tab., tell., thuj.
Finger	numbness in tips of fingers during chill	Stann.
Finger	numbness in tips of fingers in morning	Kali-c., lach.
Finger	one sided numbness in fingers	Cact., ph-ac.
Finger	pain between fingers in evening	Rhus-t.
Finger	pain in arm extending to finger	Chel.
Finger	pain in axilla extending down to little finger	Nat-a.
Finger	pain in ball of fifth finger as from chillblains	Nit-ac.
Finger	pain in bones of fingers	Alum., apis., ars., crot-h., dios., mez., **Sil.**, verat.
Finger	pain in bones of fingers when grasping	Verat.
Finger	pain in cervical region extending arm and fingers	Kalm., nux-v., par.
Finger	pain in elbow extending to little finger	Aesc., arund., jatr., lyc., phyt., puls., seneg.
Finger	pain in fingers after rising	Coloc.
Finger	pain in fingers after walking	Croc.
Finger	pain in fingers aggravated from cold	Stram.
Finger	pain in fingers ameliorated from cold	Caust., lac-c.
Finger	pain in fingers ameliorated from grasping	Lith.
Finger	pain in fingers ameliorated from pressure	Lith.
Finger	pain in fingers ameliorated from warmth	Agar., ars., bry., calc., **Hep.**, lyc., rhus-t., stram.
Finger	pain in fingers ameliorated when moving	Lith.
Finger	pain in fingers at night	Bor., kali-n., mag-s., merc., puls., sulph.
Finger	pain in fingers during chill	Nux-v.
Finger	pain in fingers extending to elbow	Nat-m., plat., plb.
Finger	pain in fingers extending to shoulder	Nux-m., plb.
Finger	pain in fingers from putting warm water in hands	Caust., phos.
Finger	pain in fingers from stretching them apart	Am-c.
Finger	pain in fingers from writing	Acon., bry., calc-p., cist., iris., mur-ac.
Finger	pain in fingers in cold air	Agar.
Finger	pain in fingers in evening	Lyc., sulph.
Finger	pain in fingers in forenoon	Thuj.

Body part/Disease	Symptom	Medicines
Finger	pain in fingers in morning	Coloc., crot-h., kali-c., merc-i-r.
Finger	pain in fingers in variola	Thuj.
Finger	pain in fingers of amputed (cut off part of body) stump (leg)	Phos., staph.
Finger	pain in fingers on exertion	Bry.
Finger	pain in fingers when closed	Nat-s., verat.
Finger	pain in fingers when moving	Guai., hep., kali-c., nit-ac., rhus-t.
Finger	pain in fingers while writing	Calc-p.
Finger	pain in first finger	Arund., iris., upa.
Finger	pain in first finger as of dislocation	Alum., ruta.
Finger	pain in first phalanx (finger bone) of first finger	Osm., plat.
Finger	pain in forearm extending to finger	Asc-t., cocc., con., cycl., puls.
Finger	pain in forearm extending to little finger	Agar., kreos.
Finger	pain in forearm from moving finger	Asaf.
Finger	pain in joints of fingers	**Ant-c.**, ars., arund., aur., benz-ac., bry., calc-p., calc., carb-v., **Caul.**, **Caust.**, cist., colch., coloc., fl-ac., guai., hydr-ac., iris., kali-bi., kali-n., lact-ac., led., lith., manc., mez., nat-s., onos., ox-ac., phos., polyg-h., pyrus., rhod., sep., sil., staph., still., sulph., tarent., upa.
Finger	pain in joints of fingers extending upward	Brom.
Finger	pain in joints of fingers in evening	Calc., staph.
Finger	pain in joints of fingers when moved	Ang., ars., sep.
Finger	pain in joints of first finger	Acon., **Act-sp.**, arg-n., berb., caul., coloc., nat-m., nat-p., nat-s., phys., rhus-t., spong., verat-v., viol-o., zinc.
Finger	pain in joints of fourth finger	All-c., aloe., canth., chel., cinnb., coca., coloc., con., dios., gels., hyos., kalm., lith., naja., nat-p., phyt., rhod., rhus-t., stry., tarent.
Finger	pain in joints of second finger	Carb-ac., iris., nat-a., nat-m., puls-n., stann., verat-v.
Finger	pain in joints of third finger	All-c., arn., colch., crot-h., gymn., led., lil-t., naja., pip-m., thuj.
Finger	pain in nail of fifth finger	Aloe., anag., asar., asc-t., blatta., chel., con., fl-ac., hura., lith., merc-i-f., rumx., staph., ther.
Finger	pain in nail of fifth finger as from chillblains	Aloe.
Finger	pain in nail of fifth finger in morning	Anag.
Finger	pain in nail of fifth finger while walking	Nit-ac.
Finger	pain in nail of fourth finger	Asc-t., brom., calc-s., chel., dios., fl-ac., form., merc-i-f., mur-ac.
Finger	pain in nail of second finger	Berb., bry., coloc., fl-ac., mur-ac., nat-s.
Finger	pain in nail of third finger	Aloe., berb., chel., fl-ac., form., mag-m., mur-ac., thuj.
Finger	pain in nail of third finger in morning	Mag-m.
Finger	pain in palm extending to fingers	Sabin.
Finger	pain in second finger	Jac., lil-t.
Finger	pain in second phalanx of first finger	Staph.

Body part/Disease	Symptom	Medicines
Finger	pain in shoulder extending to fingers	Apis., calc-p., cocc., elat., ferr., fl-ac., naja., nux-v., rhus-t., thuj.
Finger	pain in third finger	Ang., sep.
Finger	pain in third finger on motion	Ang., sep.
Finger	pain in third phalanx of first finger	Mosch.
Finger	pain in upper limb extending from axilla to little finger	Nat-a.
Finger	pain in upper limb extending from face to fingers	Coff.
Finger	pain in upper limb extending from heart to fingers	Aur., cocc., cycl., guai., lat-m.
Finger	pain in upper limb extending to little finger	Hura., nat-a.
Finger	pain of face extending to fingers	Coff.
Finger	pain stitching outward to tips of fingers	Lob.
Finger	pain under nipples extending to fingers	Aster.
Finger	pain, drawing extending to fingers	Apis.
Finger	painful stiffness of fingers while lying	Manc.
Finger	paralysis of fingers	Calc-p., calc., caust., cocc., Mag-c. mez., phos., plb.
Finger	paralysis of first finger with cramps	Carb-s.
Finger	paralysis of fourth finger	Plb.
Finger	paralysis of third finger	Plb.
Finger	paralytic weakness in fingers	**Ars.**, carb-v.
Finger	perspiration between the fingers	Sulph.
Finger	perspiration in fingers	Agn., ant-c., bar-c., carb-v., ign., rhod., sulph.
Finger	perspiration in tips of fingers	Carb-an., carb-v.
Finger	roughness in fingers	Ph-ac., zinc.
Finger	roughness in tips of fingers	**Petr.**
Finger	sensation as if air passing down from shoulder to finger	Fl-ac.
Finger	sensation as if cold wind were bpassing over the shoulder and extending to fingers	Fl-ac.
Finger	sensation of electrical current in fingers on touching things	Alum.
Finger	sensation of enlargement of fingers	Benz-ac., calad.
Finger	sensation of enlargement of fingers when touching something	Caust.
Finger	sensation of paralysis in fingers	Acon., ars., asar., aur., bry., carb-v., chin., cycl., dig., euon., gran., kreos., lact., lil-t., meny., mez., phos., plb., staph.
Finger	sensation of paralysis in fingers when grasping	Carb-v., mez.
Finger	sensation of paralysis in fourth finger	Hell., lact., nat-m.
Finger	sensation of paralysis in fourth finger ameliorated on rest	Hell.
Finger	sensation of paralysis in joints of fingers	Aur., calc-p., par., ptel., verb.
Finger	sensation of paralysis of third fingers	Nat-m.

Body part/Disease	Symptom	Medicines
Finger	sensitive finger nails	Berb., nat-m., nux-v., petr., sil., squil., sulph.
Finger	sensitive fingers	Lac-c., lach., led., sec.
Finger	sensitive fingers must keep fingers separated	Lac-c., lach.
Finger	shocks in fingers if he touch anything	Alum.
Finger	slow growth of finger nails	Ant-c.
Finger	splinters in nails of fingers	Sil.
Finger	stiffness in fingers after exertion	**Rhus-t.**, stann.
Finger	stiffness in fingers after grasping any thing	Graph.
Finger	stiffness in fingers during chill	Eup-per., ferr., rhus-t.
Finger	stiffness in fingers in evening	Petr.
Finger	stiffness in fingers in forenoon	Fl-ac.
Finger	stiffness in fingers in morning	Am-c., ars., calc-s., calc., ferr., lach., led., rhus-t., thuj.
Finger	stiffness in fingers when grasping any thing	Am-c., carb-an., dros.
Finger	stiffness in fingers when stretching out arm	Dulc.
Finger	stiffness in fingers while holding a book	Lyc.
Finger	stiffness in fingers while lying	Hep.
Finger	stiffness in fingers while writing	Aesc., cocc., stann.
Finger	stiffness in fingers with spinal affections	Apis.
Finger	stiffness in first finger	Acon., arg-n., calc., kali-c., sabad.
Finger	stiffness in first finger while writing	Kali-c.
Finger	stiffness in fourth finger	Aloe., calc-s., con., hell., mur-ac., sil.
Finger	stiffness in fourth finger ameliorated at rest	Hell.
Finger	stiffness in fourth finger at night	Sil.
Finger	stiffness in fourth finger in morning	Calc-s.
Finger	stiffness in second finger	Bor., calc-s., carb-an., dros., phos., **Sil.**
Finger	stiffness in third finger	Mur-ac., sulph., til.
Finger	stiffness in third finger at night	Mur-ac.
Finger	stiffness in third finger in evening	Sulph.
Finger	suppuration from fingers	Bor., mang.
Finger	suppuration under nails of first finger	Calc., nat-s.
Finger	swelling in bones of fingers	Carb-an.
Finger	swelling in fingers after walking	Act-sp.
Finger	swelling in fingers at midnight	Carb-an.
Finger	swelling in fingers at night	Dig.
Finger	swelling in fingers from dissecting wound	**Ars.**, lach.
Finger	swelling in fingers in afternoon	Calc-s.
Finger	swelling in fingers in evening	Stront., sulph.
Finger	swelling in fingers in forenoon	Calc-s.
Finger	swelling in fingers in morning	Ars., calc-s., nat-c., nit-ac., ran-s., sec., sulph.
Finger	swelling in fingers with burning	Olnd.
Finger	swelling in fingers with eruptions	Psor.

Body part/Disease	Symptom	Medicines
Finger	swelling in first joint of fingers	Merc., vinc.
Finger	swelling in joints of fingers	Am-c., anag., ang., apis., ars., berb., bry., bufo., calc., caul., caust., cham., chin., colch., euphr., hep., hyos., iod., lact-ac., lyc., med., merc., nit-ac., phyt., rhod., rhus-t., spong.
Finger	swelling in joints of fingers with burning	Bufo.
Finger	swelling in tips of fingers	Fl-ac., kreos., mur-ac., rhus-t., tab., thuj.
Finger	swelling in tips of first finger	Chin-s., fl-ac., lach., lact-ac., lyc., mag-c., merc., phos., staph., sulph., thuj.
Finger	swelling in tips of fourth finger	Bry., hyos., mang., rhus-t.
Finger	swelling in tips of second finger	Apis., bor., calc-s., iris., phos., sulph., syph., thuj.
Finger	swelling in tips of third finger	Bry., calc., olnd., sulph., thuj.
Finger	tetanic convulsion of fingers	Am-c., arn., ars., bell., calc., cann-s., cham., Chel., cic., clem., cocc., coff., cupr., dros., ferr., hell., ign., iod., ip., kali-n., lach., lyc., merc-c., mosch., nat-m., nux-v., phos., plb., sant., sec., stann., staph., sulph., tab., verat.
Finger	Thrilling sensation of finger tips	Ail.
Finger	tingling in fingers at night on waking	Bar-c.
Finger	tingling in fingers in morning	Dios.
Finger	tingling in fingers in morning on waking	Ail.
Finger	tingling in fingers while sitting	Alum.
Finger	tingling in first finger	Plat.
Finger	tingling in forearm extending to fingers	Carb-ac., phys., pip-m.
Finger	tingling in fourth finger	Alum., carb-an.
Finger	tingling in fourth finger while sitting	Alum.
Finger	tingling in second finger	Apis.
Finger	tingling in third finger	Alum., sil.
Finger	tingling in tips of fingers	Acon-c., acon-f., acon., **Am-m.**, cact., cann-s., colch., croc., fl-ac., hep., **Kali-c.**, lach., nat-m., nat-s., rhod., rhus-t., sec., sep., sulph., thuj.
Finger	tingling in tips of fingers in morning	Kali-c.
Finger	tingling in tips of fingers when grasping	Rhus-t.
Finger	tingling in tips of fingers when hanging down the arms	Sulph.
Finger	tingling under nail of fingers	Cann-s., colch., nat-s.
Finger	tips of fingers sensitive to cold	Cist.
Finger	tonic in convulsion of fingers	Ars.
Finger	tough finger nails	Chin-s.
Finger	trembling in fingers	Ars., bry., cic., cupr-ar., glon., hyper., iod., merc., morph., nat-m., nit-ac., olnd., phos., plat., plb., rhus-t., sep., stront.
Finger	trembling in fingers at night	Olnd.
Finger	trembling in fingers on motion	Plb.
Finger	trembling in fingers while writing	Cimic.
Finger	trembling in first finger	Calc.
Finger	twitching between index finger & thumb	Mag-s., stann.

Body part/Disease	Symptom	Medicines
Finger	twitching in fingers in evening after lying down	Puls.
Finger	twitching in fingers with toothache	Mag-c.
Finger	twitching in fingers at day time	Phos.
Finger	twitching in fingers at night	Mag-c., nat-c.
Finger	twitching in fingers during motion	Bry.
Finger	twitching in fingers during sleep	Anac., cupr., lyc., nat-c., sulph.
Finger	twitching in fingers in evening	Lyc., puls., sulph.
Finger	twitching in fingers in morning	Pall.
Finger	twitching in fingers in morning after rising	Mag-c.
Finger	twitching in fingers when sewing	Kali-c.
Finger	twitching in fingers while writing	Caust.
Finger	twitching in first finger	Am-m., dig., lyc., mang., nat-a., pall., rhod., sil.
Finger	twitching in first finger in evening	Am-m., mang.
Finger	twitching in first finger while sitting	Pall.
Finger	twitching in fourth finger	Chin., com., kali-bi., meny., phos.
Finger	twitching in second finger	Arn., chin., fl-ac., kali-n., nat-a., sil., stann., thuj.
Finger	twitching in third finger	Chin., kali-n., mang., nat-c.
Finger	twitching in tips of fingers	**Ars.**, merc., phos., staph., sul-ac., thuj.
Finger	ulcerative pain in nail of third finger	Berb.
Finger	ulcer around fingers nails	**Carb-s.**, chlol., con., hell., nat-s., phos., rhus-t., sang., **Sil.**, sulph.
Finger	ulcer in fingers	Alum., ars., bor., bov., bry., calc., carb-an., carb-v., caust., cupr-ac., kali-bi., kreos., lyc., mang., mez., nat-m., petr., plat., ran-b., sep., sil., sulph.
Finger	ulcer in first finger	Calc., kali-bi.
Finger	ulcer in joints of fingers	Bor., mez., sep.
Finger	ulcer in nail of first finger	Iod., nat-s.
Finger	ulcer in nails of fingers	Alum., bar-c., bor., caust., con., hep., iod., kali-c., lach., lyc., merc., nat-m., plat., puls., sang., sep., **Sil.**, sul-ac., **Sulph.**, thuj.
Finger	ulcer in second finger	Aloe.
Finger	ulcer in tips of fingers	Alum., ant-t., **Ars.**, carb-v., fl-ac., nat-c., petr., plat., sars., sec., sep.
Finger	ulcer under fingers nails	**Ars.**
Finger	ulcer with burning in tips of fingers	**Ars.**, sep.
Finger	wandering pain in first finger	Polyg-h.
Finger	wandering pain in joints of fingers	Coloc., polyg-h., psor., sulph.
Finger	warts on finger close to nails	**Caust.**, dulc., fl-ac.
Finger	warts on fingers	Ambr., bar-c., berb., calc., carb-an., caust., dulc., ferr., fl-ac., **Lac-c.**, lach., lyc., nat-m., nit-ac., petr., psor., ran-b., rhus-t., sang., sars., sep., sulph., thuj.
Finger	warts on first finger	Caust., thuj.
Finger	warts on joints of fingers	Sars.

Body part/Disease	Symptom	Medicines
Finger	warts on knuckles (finger joints)	Pall.
Finger	warts on second finger	Berb., lach.
Finger	warts on third finger	Nat-s.
Finger	warts on tips of fingers	**Caust.**, dulc., thuj.
Finger	weakness in fingers	Ambr., **Ars.**, bov., carb-an., carb-v., cic., crot-h., cur., fago., hipp., hura., kali-n., lact., led., lyc., nat-m., par., phos., **Rhus-t.**, sil., zinc.
Finger	weakness in fingers at day time	Phos.
Finger	weakness in fingers at night	Ambr.
Finger	weakness in fingers drops things	Ars., carb-an., nat-m., sil., stann.
Finger	weakness in fingers when grasping	**Ars.**, carb-an., carb-v., kali-br., sil.
Finger	weakness in fingers while writing	Fago., kali-c.
Finger	weakness in first finger while writing	Kali-c.
Finger	weakness in first fingers	Kali-c., nat-m.
Finger	weakness in second finger	Nat-m.
Finger	weakness in third finger	Plb.
Finger	wrinkled fingers	Ambr., cupr., ph-ac., sol-n.
Fissure	fissure (a break in the skin lining the anal canal, usually causing pain during bowel movements and sometimes bleeding. Anal fissures occur as a consequence of constipation or sometimes of diarrhoea) in Anus	Aesc., agn., all-c., alum., ant-c., arg-m., ars., arum-t., berb., calc-f., calc-p., calc., carb-an., caust., Cham., cund., cur., fl-ac., Graph., grat., hydr., ign., kali-c., lach., med., merc-i-r., merc., mez., mur-ac., nat-m., Nit-ac., nux-v., paeon., petr., phos., phyt., plat., plb., Rat., rhus-t., Sep., sil., sulph., syph., Thuj.
Fissure	fissured throat	Bar-c., elaps., ph-ac., phos.
Fissure	fissures in larynx	Bufo.
Fissure	fissures on face bleeding	Petr.
Fissure	fissures on face	Calc., Graph., merc., nicc., nit-ac., petr., psor., sil., sulph.
Fissure	pain in fissure of anus	Graph.
Fistula	fistula (an anal fistula may develop after an abscess in the rectum has burst , creating an opening between the anal canal and the surface of the skin) in eye	Sil.
Fistula	fistula (an anal fistula may develop after an abscess in the rectum has burst , creating an opening between the anal canal and the surface of the skin) in inguinal (Groin) glands	Hep., lach., phos., sil., sulph.
Fistula	fistula (an opening or passage between two organs or between an organ and the skin, caused by disease, injury, or congenital malformation) on back	Calc-p., hep., ph-ac., Phos., Sil., Sulph.
Fistula	fistula in external throat	Phos., sil.
Fistula	fistula in gums	Aur-m., aur., bar-c., calc., canth., Caust., coch., Fl-ac., kali-chl., lyc., mag-c., nat-m., nit-ac., petr., phos., Sil., staph., sulph.
Fistula	fistula in gums near upper incisors/flat sharp front tooth and the first bicuspids/one of the eight teeth with two points	Canth.

Body part/Disease	Symptom	Medicines
Fistula	fistula in vagina	Asar., Calc., carb-v., caust., lach., lyc., nit-ac., puls., Sil.
Fistula	fistula lacrymalis	Agar., apis., arg-n., aur-m., brom., Calc., chel., Fl-ac., hep., lach., lyc., mill., nat-c., nat-m., nit-ac., Petr., phyt., Puls., Sil., stann., sulph.
Fistula	fistula lacrymalis discharging pus on pressure	Puls., sil., stann.
Fistula	fistula of glands	Phos., sil., sulph.
Fistula	fistulous openings in ankle	Calc-p.
Fistula	fistulous openings in axilla	Calc., sulph.
Fistula	fistulous openings in hip	Calc., carb-v., caust., **Lach.**, ph-ac., **Phos.**, sil.
Fistula	fistulous openings in joints	Calc., hep., ol-j., **Phos., Sil.**, sulph.
Fistula	fistulous openings in knee	Iod.
Fistula	fistulous openings in leg	Ruta.
Fistula	fistulous openings in mammæ	Caust., hep., merc., phos., phyt., Sil.
Fistula	fistulous openings in palm	Ars.
Fistula	fistulous openings in thigh	Calc.
Fistula	fistulous openings on scrotum	Iod., phyt., spong.
Fistula	fistulous ulcer in lower limbs	Calc., ruta.
Fistula	fistulous ulcer on ankle	Calc-p., sil.
Fistula	ulcer in skin, fistulous	Agar., ant-c., ars., asaf., aur., bar-c., bell., **Bry.**, calc-p., calc-s., **Calc.**, carb-ac., carb-s., carb-v., **Caust.**, chel., cinnb., clem., con., fl-ac., hep., hippoz., kreos., led., **Lyc.**, merc., nat-c., nat-m., nat-p., nit-ac., petr., **Phos., Puls.**, rhus-t., ruta., sabin., sel., sep., **Sil.**, staph., stram., sulph., thuj.
Flatulance	asthmatic from flatulance	Carb-v., cham., chin., lyc., mag-p., nux-v., op., phos., sulph., zinc.
Flatulance	breathing difficult from flatulence	Carb-v., cast., cham., lyc., nat-s., ol-an., sang., zinc.
Flatulance	constriction in chest from flatulance	Nux-v., rheum., sil.
Flatulance	flatulence (causing gas in digestive system) after acids	Ph-ac.
Flatulance	flatulence after breakfast	Caust., nat-p., Nat-s.
Flatulance	flatulence after eating	Arg-n., aster., aur., bor., bufo., calc., carb-an., carb-v., caust., coc-c., dios., ferr-m., kali-n., Lyc., mag-m., nat-p., Nux-v., puls., rumx., thuj., zinc.
Flatulance	flatulence after milk	Carb-v., merc., nat-c., nat-s., sul-ac.
Flatulance	flatulence before breakfast	Agar.
Flatulance	flatulence before menses	Zinc.
Flatulance	flatulence during menses	Kali-c., vesp.
Flatulance	flatulence during urination	Merc.
Flatulance	flatulence from fruit	Chin.
Flatulance	flatulence in afternoon after eating	Fago.
Flatulance	flatulence in afternoon during stool	Fago.
Flatulance	flatulence obstructed with hard stool	Caust.

Body part/Disease	Symptom	Medicines
Flatulance	flatulence of aged people	Carb-ac., phos.
Flatulance	flatulence on rising from bed	Zinc.
Flatulance	flatulence with constipation	Aur., iod., lyc., rhod., sulph.
Flatulance	flatus after dinner	Ant-c., arg-n., cycl., grat., nat-m., sulph.
Flatulance	impeded, obstructed breath from flatulancy	Carb-v., ol-an., zinc.
Flatulance	pain in abdomen after flatulent food	Carb-v.
Flatus	Aching in lumbar region ameliorated after flatus	Coc-c.
Flatus	anxiety ameliorated from flatus	Calc.
Flatus	anxiety from flatus	Coff., nux-v.
Flatus	cough ameliorated from passing flatus	Sang.
Flatus	cramping pain in abdomen ameliorated from passing flatus	Acon., am-c., cimx., coloc., con., echi., graph., hydr., lyc., mag-c., merc-c., nat-a., nat-m., nux-m., ol-an., psor., rumx., sil., spong., squil., sulph.
Flatus	cutting pain in abdomen ameliorated from passing flatus	Anac., ars-i., bapt., bov., bry., calc-p., Con., eupi., gamb., hydr., laur., plb., psor., sel., sulph., viol-t.
Flatus	distension of abdomen ameliorated by passing flatus	All-c., am-m., ant-t., bov., bry., carb-v., kali-i., Lyc., mag-c., mang., nat-c., nat-m., ph-ac., sulph.
Flatus	distesion of abdomen, ameliorated after passing flatus	Rat.
Flatus	dry cough ameliorated by discharge of flatus up and down and must sit up	Sang.
Flatus	emission of prostatic fluid while passing flatus	Con., mag-c.
Flatus	emmission of prostatic fluid while passing flatus	Con., mag-c.
Flatus	even an emission of flatus causes easy discharge of prostatic fluid	Mag-c.
Flatus	feeling of tightness in abdomen ameliorated by passing flatus	Sil.
Flatus	flatus difficult	All-c., calc-p., cocc., coff., hyos., lyss., nat-s., op., ox-ac., phos., plat., sul-ac.
Flatus	flatus during stool	Gels.,Ph-ac.
Flatus	flatus from vagina	Apis., bell., Brom., calc., chin., hyos., lac-c., Lyc., mag-c., nat-c., nux-m., nux-v., orig., Ph-ac., sang., sep., sulph., tarent.
Flatus	flatus from vagina during menses	Brom., kreos., nicc.
Flatus	flatus hot	Acon., agar., Aloe., ant-t., bapt., carb-v., cham., cocc., dios., phos., plb., psor., puls., staph., sulph., sumb., teucr., zinc.
Flatus	flatus loud during stool	Aloe., Nat-s., ph-ac., thuj.
Flatus	flatus loud, after sugar	Arg-n.
Flatus	flatus moist	All-c., ant-c., carb-v., zinc.
Flatus	flatus odorless	Agar., arg-n., bell., carb-v., lyc., nicc., phos., plat., Sulph., thuj.
Flatus	haemorrhage during emission of flatus	Phos.
Flatus	headache ameliorated from emmission of flatus	Aeth., cic.

Body part/Disease	Symptom	Medicines
Flatus	involuntary stool while passing flatus	Acon., Aloe., apoc., bell., carb-v., caust., cench., ferr-ma., ign., jatr., kali-c., mur-ac., nat-c., nat-m., Nat-p., nat-s., nux-v., Olnd., Ph-ac., Podo., pyrog., sanic., staph., sulph., tub., Verat.
Flatus	involuntary urination when expelling flatus	Puls., sulph.
Flatus	involuntary urination while fully conscious supposing it to be flatus	Ars.
Flatus	pain in abdomen aggravated on passing flatus	Aur., canth., fl-ac., nat-a., squil.
Flatus	pain in abdomen ameliorated by passing flatus	Agar., chel., dig., hep., lact., tarent.
Flatus	pain in abdomen before passing flatus	Calc-p., Chin., nit-ac.
Flatus	pain in anus on passing flatus	Camph., carb-v.
Flatus	pain in back ameliorated from flatus	Berb., coc-c., ruta.
Flatus	pain in lumbar region ameliorated from flatus passing	Am-m., bar-c., coc-c., kali-c., Lyc., pic-ac., ruta.
Flatus	pain in sacral region ameliorated from passing flatus	Pic-ac.
Flatus	perspiration on face when passing flatus	Kali-bi.
Flatus	perspiration when passing flatus	Kali-bi.
Flatus	prolapsus of anus when passing flatus	Valer.
Flatus	restlessness in lumbar region ameliorated from passing flatus	Bar-c., calc-f., cedr., chin-s.
Flatus	stitching pain in urethra on passing flatus	Mang.
Flatus	urging for stool but only flatus is passed	Aloe., ant-c., cahin., carb-an., carb-v., colch., lac-c., laur., mag-c., mag-m., myric., Nat-s., osm., ruta., sang., sep.
Flatus	urging for stool when passing flatus	Aloe., ruta., spig.
Flatus	urging to urinate in bladder when passing flatus	Puls.
Flushes of Heat	flushes of heat after eating	Alum., arg-n., carb-v., par., sumb.
Flushes of Heat	flushes of heat after mental exertion	Olnd.
Flushes of Heat	flushes of heat alternating with chill	Acon., ars., asar., calc., chin-s., corn., iod., kali-bi., med., sep., spig.
Flushes of Heat	flushes of heat as if warm water were dashed over	Calc., cann-s., nat-m., phos., puls., rhus-t., sep.
Flushes of Heat	flushes of heat as if warm water were poured over	**Ars.**, bry., ph-ac., phos., **Psor.**, puls., rhus-t., **Sep.**
Flushes of Heat	flushes of heat at after anger	Phos.
Flushes of Heat	flushes of heat at night	Bar-c., spig.
Flushes of Heat	flushes of heat at night at 3.00 a.m. feeling as if sweat would break out	Bapt.
Flushes of Heat	flushes of heat before menses	Alum., iod.
Flushes of Heat	flushes of heat downward	Glon., sang.
Flushes of Heat	flushes of heat downward from head to stomach	Sang.
Flushes of Heat	flushes of heat during menses	Nat-p.
Flushes of Heat	flushes of heat during sleep	Cham., nat-m., phos., sil., zinc.
Flushes of Heat	flushes of heat followd by chill	**Caust.**, sang.
Flushes of Heat	flushes of heat from emotions	Lach., phos.
Flushes of Heat	flushes of heat from least exertion	Alum., sep., sumb.

Body part/Disease	Symptom	Medicines
Flushes of Heat	flushes of heat from motion	Helon.
Flushes of Heat	flushes of heat from walking in open air	Caust.
Flushes of Heat	flushes of heat in afternoon	Ambr., bell., colch., con., laur., meny., nat-p., plb., samb., **Sep.**
Flushes of Heat	flushes of heat in afternoon during dinner	Calc-s., nux-v.
Flushes of Heat	flushes of heat in back	Acon., bapt., brom., clem., dig., mang., merl., Sumb.
Flushes of Heat	flushes of heat in back after stool	Podo.
Flushes of Heat	flushes of heat in back extending to body	Sumb.
Flushes of Heat	flushes of heat in back in during stool	Podo.
Flushes of Heat	flushes of heat in back in evening	Ph-ac., sol-n.
Flushes of Heat	flushes of heat in back in evening after stool	Podo.
Flushes of Heat	flushes of heat in back in evening after supper	Spig.
Flushes of Heat	flushes of heat in back in evening on continued walking	Glon.
Flushes of Heat	flushes of heat in back in morning	Lil-t.
Flushes of Heat	flushes of heat in cervical region	Aesc., fl-ac., hydr., lach., med., Phos., podo., sarr.
Flushes of Heat	flushes of heat in evening	Acon., all-c., arum-t., bor., carb-an., carb-v., elaps., lyc., merc-c., nat-p., nat-s., nit-ac., phos., psor., **Sep.**, sulph.
Flushes of Heat	flushes of heat in evening after eating	Carb-v.
Flushes of Heat	flushes of heat in evening at 8.00 p.m. with nausea	Ferr.
Flushes of Heat	flushes of heat in evening at 8.30 p.m.	Arum-t., cina., sep.
Flushes of Heat	flushes of heat in evening before falling asleep	Carb-v.
Flushes of Heat	flushes of heat in foot	Colch., stann., **Sulph.**
Flushes of Heat	flushes of heat in hand	Colch., hydr., pip-m., **Sulph.**
Flushes of Heat	flushes of heat in leg	Cob.
Flushes of Heat	flushes of heat in morning	Bism., bor.
Flushes of Heat	flushes of heat in morning after eating	Thuj.
Flushes of Heat	flushes of heat in palm	Cub.
Flushes of Heat	flushes of heat in spine	Bol.
Flushes of Heat	flushes of heat in spine as if warm air streaming up spine into head	Ars., sumb.
Flushes of Heat	flushes of heat in spine up in waves	Lyc.
Flushes of Heat	flushes of heat upwards	Alum., alumn., ars., asaf., calc., carb-an., carb-v., chin., cinnb., ferr-ar., ferr., **Glon.**, graph., indg., iris., kali-bi., kali-c., laur., lyc., mag-m., mang., nat-s., nit-ac., phos., plb., psor., **Sep.**, spong., sulph., sumb., tarent., valer.
Flushes of Heat	flushes of heat upwards from the hips	Alumn.
Flushes of Heat	flushes of heat while eating	Calc-s., nux-v., psor.
Flushes of Heat	flushes of heat with chilliness	Agar., apis., ars., carb-v., colch., corn., eup-per., kali-bi., lach., lob., merc., plat., puls., sep., sulph., ter., thuj.
Flushes of Heat	flushes of heat with palpitation	**Kali-c.**
Flushes of Heat	flushes of heat with perspiration	Acet-ac., am-m., ant-c., aur., bell., carb-v., hep., kali-bi., lach., op., sep., sul-ac., sulph., **Tub.**, xan.

Body part/Disease	Symptom	Medicines
Flushes of Heat	flushes of heat with perspiration and anxiety	Ang., kali-bi.
Fontanelles	open fontanelles (a soft, membrane-covered space between the bones at the front and the back of a young baby's skull)	Apis., Calc-p., Calc., ip., merc., sep., Sil., sulph., syph.
Foot	abscess in foot (part of the leg below the ankle joint that supports the rest of the body and maintains balance when standing and walking)	Merc., sil., tarent.
Foot	arthritic nodosities on condyles on foot	Bufo., kali-i., Led., nat-s.
Foot	back of foot hot	Calc., coloc., cupr-s., plb., puls., rhus-t.
Foot	bleeding from ulcer of foot	Ars.
Foot	bubbling sensation in foot	Bell., berb., chel., lach.
Foot	bunions (an inflammation of the sac bursa around the first joint of the big toe, accompanied by swelling and sideways displacement of the joint) of foot	Am-c., hyper., kali-chl., ph-ac., phos., plb., Sil., zinc.
Foot	burning pain in foot after walking	Kali-c.
Foot	burning pain in foot aggravated from touch	Bor.
Foot	burning pain in foot at night	Ars-m., coloc., lac-c., nat-c., sep., sil., **Sulph.**
Foot	burning pain in foot at night in bed	Nat-p., **Sulph.**
Foot	burning pain in foot at night in bed during menses	Nat-p.
Foot	burning pain in foot at night in bed during sleep	Ars-m.
Foot	burning pain in foot from climacteric	Sang.
Foot	burning pain in foot from warmth of bed	Agar., calc., merc., stront., **Sulph.**
Foot	burning pain in foot in bed in evening	Agar.
Foot	burning pain in foot in bed in morning	Hep.
Foot	burning pain in foot in evening	Calc., nat-s., sang., sulph.
Foot	burning pain in foot in evening in bed	Calc., hep., merc., stront., **Sulph.**
Foot	burning pain in foot in morning in bed	Hep., nat-s.
Foot	burning pain in foot in noon	Am-c., hura.
Foot	burning pain in foot while walking	Carb-an., nat-c., nat-m., phyt.
Foot	burning pain in foot with perspiration	Sil.
Foot	burning pain in toes with cold feet	Apis.
Foot	burning swelling of foot	Canth.
Foot	caries of foot	Asaf., calc., hecla., merc., Sil.
Foot	chilblains on feet cracked	Merc., nux-v., petr.
Foot	chilblains on feet suppurating	Lach., sil., sulph.
Foot	chilblains on feet swollen	Merc.
Foot	chilblains on feet with inflammation	Lach., merc., nit-ac., Petr.
Foot	chilblains on feet with purple	Lach., merc., puls., sulph.
Foot	chill beginning in and extending from feet	Apis., arn., bar-c., bor., calc-s., calc., chel., cimx., dig., **Gels.**, hyos., kali-bi., lyc., mag-c., **Nat-m.**, nux-m., nux-v., puls., rhus-t., sabad., sarr., sep., sulph.
Foot	chill beginning in and extending from hands and feet	Apis., bry., carb-v., chel., dig., ferr., gels., **Nat-m.**, nux-m., op., sabin., samb., sulph.

Body part/Disease	Symptom	Medicines
Foot	chill beginning in and extending from right foot	Chel., lyc., sabin.
Foot	chilliness in feet	Agar., ant-c., bry., cedr., dros., nit-ac., petr., phos., rhus-t., sulph., thuj.
Foot	chilliness in feet after motion	Calc.
Foot	chilliness in feet in summer	Ant-c.
Foot	coldness in back extending down to feet	Croc.
Foot	coldness in back extending down to feet	Croc.
Foot	coldness in foot after dinner	Cann-i., carb-v., sulph.
Foot	coldness in foot after eating	Aloe., calc., camph., caps.
Foot	coldness in foot after emission	Aloe., nux-v.
Foot	coldness in foot after menses	Ferr.
Foot	coldness in foot after motion	Cocc.
Foot	coldness in foot after stool	Sulph.
Foot	coldness in foot after supper	Lyc.
Foot	coldness in foot after vomiting	Sin-a.
Foot	coldness in foot after walking	Nit-ac.
Foot	coldness in foot after wine	Lyc.
Foot	coldness in foot ameliorated while lying	Phos.
Foot	coldness in foot ameliorated after menses	Carb-v., chin-s.
Foot	coldness in foot ameliorated before menses	Calc., hyper., lyc., nux-m.
Foot	coldness in foot ameliorated during menses	Arg-n., calc., cop., crot-h., graph., nat-p., nux-m., phos., sabin., Sil.
Foot	coldness in foot ameliorated in cold air	Camph., led.
Foot	coldness in foot ameliorated in house	Mang.
Foot	coldness in foot ameliorated while sitting	Mang.
Foot	coldness in foot at day time	Hep., mag-s., nit-ac., phos., sep., sil., sulph.
Foot	coldness in foot at day time during menses	Nat-p.
Foot	coldness in foot at midnight	Calad.
Foot	coldness in foot at midnight alternating with cold hands	Aloe., sep., zing.
Foot	coldness in foot at midnight alternating with heat	Alum.
Foot	coldness in foot at midnight alternating with heat with pain in limbs	Rhus-t.
Foot	coldness in foot at night	Aloe., am-c., am-m., ant-c., aur., bov., bry., calad., Calc., carb-s., carb-v., chel., com., cop., ferr-i., ferr., iod., kali-ar., nit-ac., par., petr., phos., psor., raph., rhod., sars., sep., sil., sulph., thuj., verat., zinc.
Foot	coldness in foot at night in bed	Am-m., aur., Calc., carb-v., chel., ferr., nit-ac., petr., phos., raph., rhod., sil., sulph., thuj., zinc.
Foot	coldness in foot at night on waking	Nit-ac., zinc.
Foot	coldness in foot during anxiety	Cupr., graph., puls., sulph.
Foot	coldness in foot during dinner	Sulph.
Foot	coldness in foot during excitement	during : Mag-c.

Body part/Disease	Symptom	Medicines
Foot	coldness in foot during fever	Am-c., arn., ars., bar-c., bell., bufo., calad., calc., caps., carb-an., carb-v., chin., hell., ign., ip., iris., kali-c., kali-s., lach., meny., nux-v., petr., ptel., puls., ran-b., rhod., samb., stann., stram., sulph.
Foot	coldness in foot during headache	Arg-n., ars., aur., bell., bufo., cact., calc., camph., carb-s., carb-v., chin., chr-ac., coca., dirc., ferr-p., ferr., Gels., lac-d., lach., laur., Meli., meny., naja., nat-m., phos., plat., psor., sars., Sep., stram., sulph., verat-v.
Foot	coldness in foot during pregnancy	Lyc., Verat.
Foot	coldness in foot during sleep	Samb., zinc.
Foot	coldness in foot during sleep with heat of body	Samb.
Foot	coldness in foot during supper	Ign.
Foot	coldness in foot during urination	Dig.
Foot	coldness in foot extending to calves	Aloe., crot-t.
Foot	coldness in foot extending to knees	Aeth., chel., ign., meny., nat-m.
Foot	coldness in foot from fast walking	Phos.
Foot	coldness in foot from mental exertion	Agar., am-c., ambr., anac., Aur., bell., calc-p., Calc., carb-v., caust., chin., cocc., cupr., gels., kali-c., lach., lyc., Nat-c., nat-m., nit-ac., Nux-v., petr., ph-ac., Phos., psor., Puls., Sep., Sil.
Foot	coldness in foot from walking in open air	Anac., bar-c., plan., plb.
Foot	coldness in foot from walking in sun	Lach.
Foot	coldness in foot in a warm room	Kali-br.
Foot	coldness in foot in afternoon	Bar-c., chel., chin-s., coca., colch., gels., mez., nux-v., sang., sep., squil., sulph.
Foot	coldness in foot in afternoon with hot face	Hura.
Foot	coldness in foot in bed	Alum., ferr., kali-c., lach., naja., raph., rhod., thuj.
Foot	coldness in foot in evening	Acon., aloe., am-br., am-c., ars., Calc., carb-an., carb-s., carb-v., cham., chel., chin., con., graph., hell., kali-s., lyc., mag-c., mang., nat-n., nux-v., ox-ac., petr., ph-ac., plan., puls., rhod., Sep., Sil., stront., sulph., til., verat., zinc.
Foot	coldness in foot in evening ameliorated in bed	Sulph.
Foot	coldness in foot in evening in bed	Aloe., Am-c., am-m., aur., Calc., carb-an., carb-s., carb-v., carl., chel., ferr-p., ferr., Graph., kali-ar., kali-c., kali-s., lyc., merc., nat-c., nit-ac., nux-v., par., petr., ph-ac., phos., raph., rhod., Sep., Sil., staph., sulph., thuj., zinc.
Foot	coldness in foot in evening in the open air	Mang.
Foot	coldness in foot in forenoon	Carb-an., chin-s., cop., fago., hura., mez., petr., sep.
Foot	coldness in foot in hottest weather	Asar.
Foot	coldness in foot in morning	Anac., caps., chel., coc-c., graph., hura., lyc., mag-m., merc., nux-v., Sep., spig., stram., sumb.
Foot	coldness in foot in morning after breakfast	Verat.
Foot	coldness in foot in morning during headache	Sep.
Foot	coldness in foot in noon	Chin-s., nit-ac., zing.

Body part/Disease	Symptom	Medicines
Foot	coldness in foot in noon during heat and redness of the face	Sep.
Foot	coldness in foot in noon while the other one burns	Hura.
Foot	coldness in foot on walking	Chel., samb., verat., zinc.
Foot	coldness in foot while ameliorated walking	Aloe.
Foot	coldness in foot while eating	Ign.
Foot	coldness in foot while lying	Tell.
Foot	coldness in foot while sitting	Ars., sep.
Foot	coldness in foot while talking	Am-c.
Foot	coldness in foot while walking	Anac., aran., asaf., chin., mang., mez., sil.
Foot	coldness in foot while writing	Chin-s., sep.
Foot	coldness in foot with burning soles	Cupr.
Foot	coldness in foot with burning soles during chill	Ant-c., aur., ferr., Meny., phos., sep., Verat., zinc.
Foot	coldness in foot with diarrhoea	Dig., lyc., nit-ac.
Foot	coldness in foot with heat of face	Acon., asaf., cocc., gels., ign., ruta., samb., sep., Stram.
Foot	coldness in foot with heat of feet ameliorated from bath	Glon.
Foot	coldness in foot with heat of hands	Acon., calad., com., nux-m., sep.
Foot	coldness in foot with heat of head	Alum., am-c., anac., arn., ars., aur., bar-c., bell., cact., calc., com., ferr., gels., laur., nat-c., ph-ac., sep., squil., thuj.
Foot	coldness in foot with heat of one side of body	Ran-b.
Foot	coldness in foot with heat of one side of body during sleep	Samb.
Foot	coldness in foot with heat of thighs	Cocc., thuj.
Foot	coldness in foot with one cold, the other hot	Chel., dig., ip., Lyc., puls.
Foot	coldness in hands alternating with cold feet	Aloe., sep., zing.
Foot	coldness in hands with hot feet	Aloe., calc., coloc., ph-ac., sep.
Foot	coldness in left foot	Aeth., hydrc., pip-m., sumb., tub.
Foot	coldness in right foot while walking	Bar-c.
Foot	coldness in right foot	Ambr., bar-c., chel., lyc., sulph.
Foot	coldness of feet during heat	Acon., calad., com., nux-m., sep.
Foot	compression of foot	Ang., cimic.
Foot	constant motion of foot	Lach.
Foot	constant perspiration in foot	**Sil.**, thuj.
Foot	constriction in chest after suppressed foot sweat	Sil.
Foot	constrictions in foot	Anac., graph., nat-m., nit-ac., petr., stront.
Foot	contraction of muscles & tendons of foot	Acon., cann-s., carb-an., caust., ferr-s., guare., Ind., merc-c., nat-c., nat-m., plat., sec., sep.
Foot	contraction of muscles & tendons of hand alternating with feet	Stram.
Foot	contraction of muscles & tendons of left foot	Cycl.

Body part/Disease	Symptom	Medicines
Foot	contraction of muscles & tendons of left foot with cramp like pain	Nat-m., phos.
Foot	convulsion after suppressed foot sweat	**Sil.**
Foot	convulsion of foot	Bar-m., calc., camph., cupr., iod., merc-c., nat-m., nux-v., op., phos., sec., stram., zinc.
Foot	convulsion of foot at night	Iod.
Foot	convulsion of foot during menses	Hyos.
Foot	convulsion of foot extending to knees	Stram.
Foot	convulsion of foot from touch	Nux-v.
Foot	convulsive motion of foot	zinc.
Foot	convulsive trembling of foot	Hyos., kali-cy.
Foot	cough aggravated from uncovering feet or head	Sil.
Foot	cough from becoming feet cold	Bar-c., bufo., sil., sulph.
Foot	cracking in foot	Caust., petr., ph-ac., sars., sulph., thuj.
Foot	cracks on feet	Aur-m., com., hep., Sars., sulph.
Foot	cramp in calf at night from bending foot	Chin.
Foot	cramp in calf from lifting the foot	Agar.
Foot	cramp in calf on crossing feet	Alum.
Foot	cramp in calf when stretching foot after waking	Aspar.,Chin., nit-ac., thuj.
Foot	cramp in calf when stretching foot in bed after waking	**Calc.**, carl., cham., lyss., nat-c., pin-s., sulph.
Foot	cramp in calf when turning foot while sitting	Nat-m.
Foot	cramp in first toe on stretching out foot	Psor.
Foot	cramp in foot at day time	Ox-ac., petr., sep.
Foot	cramp in foot at night	Form., lachn., lyc., nat-c., sanic.
Foot	cramp in foot at night alternating with dim vision	Bell.
Foot	cramp in foot during chill	Cupr., elat., nux-v.
Foot	cramp in foot during menses	Lachn., sulph.
Foot	cramp in foot in attempting to coition	Cupr.
Foot	cramp in foot in bed	Bry., graph., sanic.
Foot	cramp in foot in cholera	**Cupr.**, sec., **Verat.**
Foot	cramp in foot in evening on drawing up limbs	Ferr.
Foot	cramp in foot in morning	Lachn.
Foot	cramp in foot on going to sleep	Hyper.
Foot	cramp in foot on motion	Calc., ph-ac.
Foot	cramp in foot on motion after resting	Plb.
Foot	cramp in foot on sitting	Eupho.
Foot	cramp in foot on stretching	Caust., verat.
Foot	cramp in foot when standing	Eupho.
Foot	cramp in foot while walking	Verat.
Foot	cramp in foot while walking	Sil.,Ran-b.

Body part/Disease	Symptom	Medicines
Foot	cramp in hand alternating with cramps in feet	Stram.
Foot	cramp in leg when stretching out the feet	Sulph.
Foot	cramp in lower limbs from bending foot forward	Coff.
Foot	cramp in sole from hanging foot down	Berb.
Foot	cramp in sole in bed aggravated from putting foot out of bed	Chel.
Foot	cramp in toes from stretching out foot	Psor., sulph.
Foot	dark red inflammation in foot	Rhus-v., sil.
Foot	desquamating inflammation in foot	Dulc.
Foot	difficult motion of foot	Nat-m.
Foot	difficult to raise foot	Tab., zinc.
Foot	difficult to raise foot in forenoon	Mang.
Foot	dislocated feeling in foot	Arum-t., bell.
Foot	downward motion of foot as if stamping	Cina.
Foot	emaciation of foot	Ars., **Caust.**, chin., nat-m., plb.
Foot	eruption in back of foot	Aster., bov., carb-o., caust., lach., led., med., merc., petr., psor., puls., sars., tarax., thuj., zinc.
Foot	eruption in foot	Anan., ars., aster., bar-c., bov., calc., carb-o., caust., chin-s., con., croc., crot-c., elaps., genist., lach., med., mez., phos., rhus-t., rhus-v., sec., sep., stram., sulph.
Foot	eruption, black in foot	Ars., sec.
Foot	eruption, black vesicles in foot	**Ars.**, nat-m.
Foot	eruption, bleeding in foot	Calc.
Foot	eruption, blotches in foot	Ant-c., jug-r., kreos., lyc., sep., sulph.
Foot	eruption, boils in foot	Anan., calc., led., sars., sil., **Stram.**
Foot	eruption, burning in foot	Bov., mez.
Foot	eruption, confluent in foot	Cop., rhus-v.
Foot	eruption, coppery spots in foot	Graph.
Foot	eruption, desquamating in sole of foot	Ars., chin-s., elaps., manc., sulph.
Foot	eruption, desquamation in foot	Chin-s., dulc., **Mez.**
Foot	eruption, dry in foot	Mez.
Foot	eruption, eczema in back of foot	Merc., psor.
Foot	eruption, elevations in back of foot	Petr., puls., thuj.
Foot	eruption, elevations in foot	Cop.
Foot	eruption, herpes in foot	**Alum.**, mez., nat-m., petr., **Sulph.**
Foot	eruption, impetigo (contagious infection of the skin characterized by blisters that form yellow-brown scabs) in back of foot	Carb-s.
Foot	eruption, itching biting in foot	Calc.
Foot	eruption, itching burning in foot	Bov., mez.
Foot	eruption, itching in back of foot	Aster., calc., lach., psor., tarax.
Foot	eruption, itching in foot	Aster., bov., calc., con., mez., sep., sil.

Body part/Disease	Symptom	Medicines
Foot	eruption, itching vesicles in back of foot	Aster.
Foot	eruption, like flee bite in foot	Sec.
Foot	eruption, miliary in foot	Ars.
Foot	eruption, nodes in foot	Ang.
Foot	eruption, nodules (Cell or tissue mass) in back of foot	Petr.
Foot	eruption, painful in back of foot	Bov., psor.
Foot	eruption, painful in foot	Lyc., phos., spig., sulph.
Foot	eruption, phagedenic (rapidly spreading ulcer) vesicles in foot	Con., sel., sulph., zinc.
Foot	eruption, pimples in back of foot	Caust., led., mosch.
Foot	eruption, pimples in foot	Ars., bar-c., bov., bry., carb-s., con., crot-c., cupr., led., mosch., sel., sep., sulph., zinc.
Foot	eruption, psoriasis in sole of foot	Phos.
Foot	eruption, pustules in back of foot	Calc., con., sars., sep.
Foot	eruption, pustules in foot	Calc., con., merc., rhus-t., sep.
Foot	eruption, rash in foot	Bov., bry.
Foot	eruption, red in foot	Bov., crot-c.
Foot	eruption, scabs in foot	Calc., rhus-v., sil.
Foot	eruption, scaly in back of foot	Psor.
Foot	eruption, scaly in foot	Rhus-v.
Foot	eruption, scurfy in foot	Sil.
Foot	eruption, suppurating vesicles in foot	Con., graph., nat-c., sel.
Foot	eruption, tubercles in foot	Carb-an., rhus-t.
Foot	eruption, ulcerative vesicles in back of foot	Zinc.
Foot	eruption, urticaria in foot	Calc., sulph.
Foot	eruption, vesicles in back of foot	Aster., bov., carb-o., lach., zinc.
Foot	eruption, vesicles in foot	Ars., aster., carb-o., caust., con., elaps., graph., lach., manc., nit-ac., phos., rhus-v., sec., sel., sep., sulph., tarax., vinc., vip.
Foot	eruption, vesicles in foot from rubbing	Caust.
Foot	eruption, watery vesicles in foot	Rhus-v.
Foot	eruption, white vesicles in foot	Cycl., graph., lach., sulph.
Foot	erysipelatous inflammation in foot	Apis., arn., bry., dulc., nux-v., puls., rhus-t., sil., sulph.
Foot	erysipelatous inflammation in foot after dancing	Berb.
Foot	erysipelatous spots in foot	Apis.
Foot	excoriating with perspiration in foot	Bar-c., calc., carb-v., coff., **Fl-ac.**, graph., hell., iod., lyc., nit-ac., ran-b., sanic., sec., sep., sil., squil., zinc.
Foot	feet becoming cold	Bar-c., cham., con., cupr., puls., **Sil.**
Foot	Feet knocked together	Cann-s.
Foot	Felon (a pus-filled infection on the skin at the side of a fingernail or toenail) ameliorated from cold application	Apis., fl-ac., led., **Nat-s., Puls.**

Body part/Disease	Symptom	Medicines
Foot	fever comes on during sleep with cold feet and sweat on waking	**Samb.**
Foot	flaky (thin dry flaking scales of skin) suppuration of foot	Sil.
Foot	flushes of heat in foot	Colch., stann., **Sulph.**
Foot	foot alternatly hot & cold	Gels., graph., sec.
Foot	foot burning	Agar., ars., aster., calc., cham., cocc., fl-ac., graph., kali-ar., kali-c., lyc., **Med.**, nat-s., **Ph-ac.**, phyt., plan., **Puls.**, sang., sanic., **Sec.**, sep., stann., **Sulph.**, zinc.
Foot	foot burning uncovers them	Agar., cham., mag-c., **Med.**, **Puls.**, sang., sanic., **Sulph.**
Foot	foot hot	Acon., agar., ang., apis., arn., ars-h., ars., arund., aster., brom., bufo., calad., calc., camph., carb-an., carb-s., carb-v., caust., **Cham.**, cimic., cocc., coff., coloc., crot-h., cub., glon., hyos., ign., kali-ar., kali-bi., kali-chl., kali-i., lach., laur., led., lyc., merc., mez., mill., morph., nat-c., nat-m., nat-p., nat-s., nit-ac., nux-v., par., petr., ph-ac., phos., phyt., psor., ptel., **Puls.**, rheum., rhus-t., rhus-v., ruta., sec., sep., sil., spig., spong., stann., staph., **Sulph.**, sumb., til., vip., zinc.
Foot	foot hot after cold perspiration	Hura.
Foot	foot hot after dinner	Calen., phos.
Foot	foot hot after eating	Calen.
Foot	foot hot after midnight	Calad.
Foot	foot hot after walking	Carl., puls.
Foot	foot hot as if fire were forcing to head	Zinc.
Foot	foot hot at night	Calc., ign., nat-s., ph-ac., sep., sil., staph., **Sulph.**
Foot	foot hot at night in bed	Sil.
Foot	foot hot at night in bed after walking in open air	Alum.
Foot	foot hot at night while lying on back	Ign.
Foot	foot hot before midnight	Mag-m.
Foot	foot hot during chill	Cann-s., rat., spong.
Foot	foot hot in afternoon	Gels., hura.
Foot	foot hot in bed	Calc., fago., hep., hura., merc., mez., sang., sil., stront., **Sulph.**
Foot	foot hot in evening	Alum., bell., bry., carb-s., caust., led., mag-m., nat-s., nit-ac., nux-m., sil.
Foot	foot hot in evening after lying down	Stront.
Foot	foot hot in evening with cold hands	Aloe.
Foot	foot hot in morning	Apis., nat-s., nux-v., ptel.
Foot	foot hot when going to sleep	Alum.
Foot	foot hot while lying on back	Ign.
Foot	foot hot with body cold	Calad.
Foot	foot hot with cold sweat in hands	Hura.
Foot	foot hot with hands cold	Aloe., calc., coloc., ph-ac., sep.

Body part/Disease	Symptom	Medicines
Foot	foot hot with tingling	Berb., merc., sumb.
Foot	foot pricking (hurt in stinging way) hot	Rhus-v.
Foot	foot sensitive to cold	Alum., am-c., zinc.
Foot	formication beginning at feet and extending upwards	Nat-m.
Foot	formication in foot	Acon., aeth., **Agar.**, alum., am-c., ang., ant-c., apis., arn., ars-h., ars-i., ars., arund., bell., bor., canth., caps., carb-an., carb-s., carl., caust., chel., cic., clem., coloc., con., croc., crot-c., dulc., eupho., graph., guai., hep., hyper., ign., jatr., kali-c., kali-n., kreos., lyc., mag-c., manc., mang., mez., nat-c., nat-m., nat-p., nux-v., op., par., phos., plb., rhod., rhus-t., rhus-v., sars., **Sec.**, sep., spong., stann., stram., stront., sulph., tarax., tax., zinc.
Foot	formication in foot after heat	Sulph.
Foot	formication in foot ameliorated from open air	Bor., zinc.
Foot	formication in foot at night	Phos.
Foot	formication in foot during chill	Canth.
Foot	formication in foot extending over body	Caps., nat-m.
Foot	formication in foot in morning	Hyper., nat-c.
Foot	formication in foot in morning in bed	Rhus-t.
Foot	formication in foot in morning on stepping	Puls.
Foot	formication in foot while sitting	Carl.
Foot	formication in foot while standing	Mang., sep.
Foot	ganglion on instep (upper middle area of foot)	Bufo-s.
Foot	gangrene in foot	Ant-c., ant-t., ars., calen., lach., merc., **Sec.**, vip.
Foot	gangrene in foot with burning tearing pains	**Sec.**
Foot	hand hot at night with cold feet	Sulph.
Foot	hand hot at night with cold feet and legs	Com.
Foot	hands hot & feet cold alternating with cold hands & hot feet vice versa	Cocc., sec.
Foot	hands hot with cold feet	**Sep.**
Foot	heaviness in foot after dinner	Carb-v.
Foot	heaviness in foot after eating	Bry., cann-s., op.
Foot	heaviness in foot after walking	Alum., arn., cann-s., caust., con., murx., rhus-t., ruta.
Foot	heaviness in foot ameliorated during menses	**Cycl.**
Foot	heaviness in foot ameliorated from motion	Nicc., zinc.
Foot	heaviness in foot ameliorated while walking	Ars-i., **Mag-c.**, nat-m., sulph.
Foot	heaviness in foot at night	Apis., caust.
Foot	heaviness in foot at night in bed	Caust.
Foot	heaviness in foot before menses	Bar-c., cycl., lyc., zinc.
Foot	heaviness in foot during chilliness	Hell.
Foot	heaviness in foot during menses	Colch., nat-m., sulph., zinc.
Foot	heaviness in foot in afternoon	Lyc., nux-v.

Body part/Disease	Symptom	Medicines
Foot	heaviness in foot in afternoon while sitting	Lyc.
Foot	heaviness in foot in afternoon while waking	Lyc.
Foot	heaviness in foot in evening	Am-c., apis., bor., mang., nat-m., thuj.
Foot	heaviness in foot in evening when undressing	Apis.
Foot	heaviness in foot in evening while walking	Lyc.
Foot	heaviness in foot in forenoon	Bry., coloc.
Foot	heaviness in foot in morning	Apis., carl.
Foot	heaviness in foot in morning in bed	Mag-m., nat-m., sep., sulph.
Foot	heaviness in foot in morning on waking	Nat-s.
Foot	heaviness in foot while ascending stairs	Cann-s., lyc., mag-c.
Foot	heaviness in foot while sitting	Alum., anac., **Mag-c.**, plat., **Rhus-t.**
Foot	heaviness in foot while standing	Nat-m., phos.
Foot	heaviness in foot while walking	Cann-i., kreos., manc., phos., plb., sep., sulph., verat.
Foot	heaviness in right foot	Agn.
Foot	icy coldness in foot	Agar., apis., aur., cact., calad., Camph., Carb-v., cedr., Crot-c., cupr., dor., Elaps., eup-per., gels., graph., hep., Lach., lyc., manc., meny., merc-c., merc., nat-p., nux-m., par., Phos., psor., samb., sars., Sep., Sil., squil., sulph., Verat., zinc.
Foot	impossible to raise foot	Ars., nux-v.
Foot	inclination to uncover feet	Agar., **Cham.**, cur., fl-ac., mag-c., **Med.**, petr., **Puls.**, sang., sanic., sep., **Sulph.**
Foot	inclination to uncover feet toward morning	Cur.
Foot	inflammation in back of foot	Calc., mag-c., puls., thuj.
Foot	inflammation in foot	Acon., arn., ars., bor., **Bry.**, calc., calen., carb-an., com., dulc., kali-bi., merc., mygal., phos., puls., rhus-v., sil., **Sulph.**, zinc.
Foot	inflammation in foot bone	Acon., arn., ars., bor., **Bry.**, calc., calen., carb-an., com., dulc., kali-bi., merc., mygal., phos., puls., rhus-v., sil., **Sulph.**, zinc.
Foot	inflammation in periosteum of foot	Aur-m., guai.
Foot	Inflammation of eye with swelling of feet	Ars.
Foot	inflammed swelling of foot	Calc., carb-an., zinc.
Foot	inversion (a typical positioning of an organ, especially the turning inward or inside out of an organ) of foot	Nux-v., sec.
Foot	itching in back of foot	Agar., alum., anac., apis., asaf., bell., berb., bism., calc., **Caust.**, chel., dig., hep., lach., **Led.**, mag-m., nat-m., nat-s., nit-ac., puls., ran-s., rhus-t., sars., spig., stann., tarax., thuj.
Foot	itching in back of foot aggravated from scratching	Berb., bism., led.
Foot	itching in back of foot ameliorated from scratching	Mag-m., nat-s., tarax.
Foot	itching in back of foot at night	Dig.
Foot	itching in back of foot from warmth of bed	Apis., **Led.**, merc-i-f., sulph., zinc.
Foot	itching in back of foot in evening	Nat-s.

Body part/Disease	Symptom	Medicines
Foot	itching in back of foot in evening while undressing	Apis., nat-s.
Foot	itching in back of foot in morning in bed	Puls.
Foot	itching in back of foot with biting	Berb.
Foot	itching in back of foot with burning	Berb.
Foot	itching in foot	Agar., alum., am-c., anac., apis., ars., arum-t., aur., bell., berb., bism., bov., bry., calc., cann-s., canth., caust., cham., chel., cocc., coloc., con., corn., crot-c., dios., dulc., fago., hura., ign., jug-r., kali-ar., kali-c., lach., **Led.**, lyc., mag-c., merc-i-f., mur-ac., nat-m., nat-p., nit-ac., nux-v., ol-an., phyt., psor., puls., ran-s., rhus-t., rhus-v., sabad., sars., sel., **Sep.**, spong., stram., sul-i., **Sulph.**, tarent., tell., thuj., verat-v., verat., zinc.
Foot	itching in foot after walking	Alum.
Foot	itching in foot aggravated from rubbing	Corn.
Foot	itching in foot aggravated from scratching	Bism., corn., led.
Foot	itching in foot aggravated from warming up	Rhus-v.
Foot	itching in foot ameliorated from motion	Psor., rhus-v., spig.
Foot	itching in foot ameliorated from scratching	Cann-i.
Foot	itching in foot as if frozen	**Agar.**, kali-c.
Foot	itching in foot at night	Apis., canth., **Led.**, lith., rhus-t., sabad.
Foot	itching in foot before midnight	Puls.
Foot	itching in foot from cold	Tarent.
Foot	itching in foot in afternoon	Fago.
Foot	itching in foot in bed	Apis., **Led.**, merc-i-f., sulph., zinc.
Foot	itching in foot in evening	Kali-c., nux-v., sel., zinc.
Foot	itching in foot with biting	Bell., berb., spong.
Foot	itching in foot with burning	Berb., stram.
Foot	itching in foot with tickling (make somebody laugh and twitch)	Bry.
Foot	itching in innerside of foot	Ambr., bov., bufo., laur.
Foot	itching in joints of foot	Aur., calc., dig., kali-c., mez., mur-ac., ph-ac., stann.
Foot	itching in leg on touching foot	**Kali-c.**
Foot	itching in outerside of foot	Grat., merc-i-f., sars.
Foot	itching in outerside of foot with stinging	Merc-i-f.
Foot	jerking in foot	Anac., ars., bar-c., bar-m., cic., cina., graph., hyos., ip., kali-br., lyc., nat-c., nat-s., nux-v., puls., sep., **Stram.**, sul-ac.
Foot	jerking in foot in sleep	Nat-c., phos., sep.
Foot	jerking in foot in spasm	Cina.
Foot	jerking in foot on going to sleep	Bell., kali-c., zinc.
Foot	lameness in foot	Abrot., am-br., aur., bell., colch., com., fl-ac., hyper., merc-i-f., nat-m., rhus-t., sil., thuj., tub.
Foot	lameness in foot during pregnancy	Sil.
Foot	lameness in foot in afternoon	Thuj.

Body part/Disease	Symptom	Medicines
Foot	lameness of left arm and foot after fright	Stann.
Foot	numbness in foot after dinner	Kali-c., mill.
Foot	numbness in foot after eating	**Kali-c.**
Foot	numbness in foot alternating with hands	**Cocc.**
Foot	numbness in foot at day time	Carb-an.
Foot	numbness in foot at night	Am-m., bry., ferr., lyc., mag-m., zinc.
Foot	numbness in foot at night in bed	Alumn., calc.
Foot	numbness in foot before menses	Hyper.
Foot	numbness in foot during dinner	Kali-c.
Foot	numbness in foot during excitement	Sulph.
Foot	numbness in foot from crossing limbs	Laur., phos.
Foot	numbness in foot in afternoon	Fago., mang., mez., phos.
Foot	numbness in foot in evening	Calc., phos., puls., zinc.
Foot	numbness in foot in evening in bed	Carb-an.
Foot	numbness in foot in forenoon	Am-m., nat-c.
Foot	numbness in foot in morning	Alum., dios., nux-v., sil.
Foot	numbness in foot in morning in bed	Alum., calc-p., mag-s.
Foot	numbness in foot on ascending steps	Nat-m.
Foot	numbness in foot on motion	Bapt.
Foot	numbness in foot painful	Puls.
Foot	numbness in foot when pressing on spine	Phos.
Foot	numbness in foot while lying	Caust., sulph.
Foot	numbness in foot while riding	Calc-p.
Foot	numbness in foot while riding in cold wind	Ham.
Foot	numbness in foot while sitting	Am-c., ant-t., calc-p., calc., cann-s., caust., cham., coloc., eupho., graph., grat., helon., jug-c., laur., lyc., mill., nat-c., phos., plat., puls., rhod., sep., sul-ac.
Foot	numbness in foot while standing	Mang., merc., sec.
Foot	numbness in foot while stooping	Coloc.
Foot	numbness in foot while stooping	Coloc.
Foot	numbness in foot while stretching	Cham.
Foot	numbness in foot while walking	Ant-c., graph., ph-ac., sec.
Foot	numbness in foot while walking in open air	Graph.
Foot	numbness in foot with chill	Cedr., cimx., ferr., lyc., nux-m., **Puls.**, sep., stann., stram.
Foot	numbness in hollow of foot	Bry., merc-sul.
Foot	numbness in joints of foot	Cann-i.
Foot	numbness in left foot	Glon., nat-m., ph-ac., thuj.
Foot	numbness in left foot only while walking	Ph-ac.
Foot	numbness in left foot then right	Mill.
Foot	numbness in right foot	Alum., ant-c., ars., mang., sep., zinc.
Foot	numbness in right foot then left	Coloc., mill.

Body part/Disease	Symptom	Medicines
Foot	odors of feet offensive without perspiration	Graph., sep., sil.
Foot	oedematous swelling of one foot only	Kali-c.
Foot	offensive perspiration in foot	Am-c., am-m., anan., arg-n., ars-i., ars., arund., **Bar-c.**, bufo., calc-s., calc., carb-ac., carb-s., cob., coloc., cycl., fl-ac., **Graph., Kali-c.**, kalm., **Lyc.**, nat-m., **Nit-ac.**, petr., phos., plb., psor., **Puls.**, rhus-t., sanic., sec., sep., **Sil.**, staph., sulph., **Tell., Thuj.**, zinc.
Foot	offensive perspiration in foot after menses	Sep., sil.
Foot	offensive perspiration in foot like rotten eggs	Staph.
Foot	offensive perspiration in foot like sole leather	Cob.
Foot	one foot hot the other cold	Chel., dig., ip., **Lyc.**, puls.
Foot	pain alternately in each foot	Lac-c., nat-p.
Foot	pain in back extending to feet	Bor., sep.
Foot	pain in back of foot	Aesc., agar., alum., asaf., aur., card-m., chel., coloc., cop., eup-per., ferr-i., ferr., guai., hell., lach., lil-t., merc-i-f., mez., nat-s., nux-m., phyt., plan., plb., puls., sang., sil., syph., tarax., xan.
Foot	pain in back of foot aggravated from stepping	Nux-m.
Foot	pain in back of foot ameliorated from warnth of bed	**Caust.**
Foot	pain in back of foot during menses	Lyss.
Foot	pain in back of foot extending to pelvis	Ferr-i.
Foot	pain in back of foot extending to toes	Syph.
Foot	pain in back of foot in evening	Agar., ferr., led.
Foot	pain in back of foot in evening while walking	Agar.
Foot	pain in back of foot on motion	Cop.
Foot	pain in back of foot on stretching out	Bry.
Foot	pain in back of foot on touch	Puls.
Foot	pain in back of foot while sitting	Asaf., tarax.
Foot	pain in back of foot while walking	Agar., bry., calc., coloc.
Foot	pain in bones of foot	Acon., agar., alum., ars., asaf., aur., bell., bism., carb-v., chin., cocc., cupr., lach., led., merc., mez., nit-ac., plat., ruta., sabin., spig., stann., staph., teucr., verat., zinc.
Foot	pain in calf ameliorated from drawing feet	Cham.
Foot	pain in calf on bending foot	Calc.
Foot	pain in calf on motion of feet	Cham.
Foot	pain in ear when feet become cold	Stann.
Foot	pain in foot after dinner	Carb-s.
Foot	pain in foot after walking in open air	Rhus-t.
Foot	pain in foot aggravated from touch	Acon., bor., bry., chin., ferr-ma.
Foot	pain in foot aggravated from warmth	Guai.
Foot	pain in foot ameliorated after coffee	Calo.
Foot	pain in foot ameliorated in warm bed	**Caust.**

Body part/Disease	Symptom	Medicines
Foot	pain in foot ameliorated on motion	Abrot., calo., cur., dios., psor., rhod., **Rhus-t.**, verat.
Foot	pain in foot ameliorated on motion	Abrot., calo., cur., dios., psor., rhod., **Rhus-t.**, verat.
Foot	pain in foot ameliorated while walking	Dig., puls., **Rhus-t.**, verat.
Foot	pain in foot as from chillblains	Berb., bor., caust., cham., nux-v.
Foot	pain in foot at night	Caul., cham., kali-c., lyc., mez., phos., sil., spong., stront., syph., verat.
Foot	pain in foot during chill	Cupr.
Foot	pain in foot during menses	Am-m., ars., mag-c.
Foot	pain in foot evening	Acon., all-c., ars-h., ferr-m., fl-ac., led., lyc., mag-c., phos., puls., sil., sulph.
Foot	pain in foot extending to body	Plb.
Foot	pain in foot extending to calves	Dros.
Foot	pain in foot extending to hips	Nux-v.
Foot	pain in foot extending to knees	Dirc.
Foot	pain in foot extending to tibia	Nat-m.
Foot	pain in foot extending to toes	Chel.
Foot	pain in foot from ascending	**Led.**, mag-c.
Foot	pain in foot from exertion	Bar-c., caust., phos., **Rhus-t.**
Foot	pain in foot from heat	Ran-a.
Foot	pain in foot from lifting	Berb.
Foot	pain in foot in afternoon	Lith., mez., phos., rhus-v.
Foot	pain in foot in morning	Dios., **Rhus-t.**, sulph.
Foot	pain in foot in noon	Arund.
Foot	pain in foot in warm bed	Mag-c., verat.
Foot	pain in foot in wet weather	Dulc., rhod., rhus-t.
Foot	pain in foot on motion	Acon., bry., bufo., caust., coff., guai., led., puls., sel., thuj.
Foot	pain in foot when bending	Coff., sel.
Foot	pain in foot when stepping	Bry., caust., **Ruta.**, thuj.
Foot	pain in foot when uncovering	Stront.
Foot	pain in foot while sitting	Alum., aur-m-n., dig., nat-c., **Rhus-t.**, tarax., valer.
Foot	pain in foot while standing	Chin., eup-per., puls., rhus-v., tarax.
Foot	pain in foot while walking	Agn., ambr., ang., ant-t., ars-h., bar-c., carb-s., caust., clem., coloc., crot-h., ferr., guai., lith., mag-c., nat-c., nit-ac., petr., phyt., plb., puls., rhus-v., sabad., stry., sulph., tax.
Foot	pain in heel ameliorated from elevating the feet	Phyt.
Foot	pain in hip extending to feet	Berb., cact., fago., lach., lyc., mag-p.
Foot	pain in ilium extending to feet	Bor., lyc., lyss., sep., still.
Foot	pain in ilium extending to right upper arm and left lower feet	Alum.
Foot	pain in joints of foot	Ambr., aster., bell., bry., calc., cedr., clem., coloc., con., graph., guai., hell., kali-c., mez., nat-m., nat-s., osm., ph-ac., phos., staph., stront., tarent., verat.

Body part/Disease	Symptom	Medicines
Foot	pain in kidney extending to thighs and feet	Pareir.
Foot	pain in knee extending to feet	Phos., tarent.
Foot	pain in knee extending to instep (upper middle area of foot)	Elat.
Foot	pain in left foot	Ail., crot-h., hyper., mur-ac., murx., sang.
Foot	pain in leg alternating with cold feet	Rhus-t.
Foot	pain in leg ameliorated from elevating feet	Bar-c., dios.
Foot	pain in leg extending to feet	Kalm., pic-ac., ptel., rhod., still.
Foot	pain in leg on flexing foot	Bad.
Foot	pain in lower limb extending to foot	Apis., colch., lach., merc-i-f., phyt., sang., zinc.
Foot	pain in right foot	Kalm., lith.
Foot	pain in sacral region extending to feet	Lyc.
Foot	pain in sacral region when stepping with left foot	Spong.
Foot	pain in ureters extending to thighs & feet	Pareir.
Foot	painful swelling of foot	Apis., ars., aur., chin., led., merc., ph-ac., phos., rhus-t., sabad., sulph.
Foot	painful tingling in foot	Mag-m.
Foot	paralysis of foot	Ang., apis., arn., ars., bar-m., bell., carb-o., chin., cocc., colch., con., crot-h., hydr-ac., laur., lyc., nux-v., olnd., phos., plb., rhus-t., stram., sulph., vip., zinc.
Foot	paralysis of foot from right	Stann.
Foot	paralytic weakness in foot	Cham., nat-m., olnd., tab.
Foot	perspiration in foot after menses	Calc., lil-t., sep., sil.
Foot	perspiration in foot after stool	Sulph.
Foot	perspiration in foot at 11.00 p.m.	Hura.
Foot	perspiration in foot at 2.00 a.m.	Ars.
Foot	perspiration in foot at day time	Pic-ac.
Foot	perspiration in foot at night	Coloc., nit-ac., sulph., thuj.
Foot	perspiration in foot during & before menses	Calc.
Foot	perspiration in foot during chill	Cann-s.
Foot	perspiration in foot in afternoon	Graph., lact-ac.
Foot	perspiration in foot in cold & damp	Acon., cann-i., pic-ac., sep., sulph.
Foot	perspiration in foot in evening	**Calc.**, cocc., graph., mur-ac., pic-ac., podo.
Foot	perspiration in foot in evening in bed	Calc., clem., mur-ac.
Foot	perspiration in foot in forenoon	Fago.
Foot	perspiration in foot in injuries of spine	**Nit-ac.**
Foot	perspiration in foot in morning	Am-m., bry., coc-c., lyc., merc., sulph.
Foot	perspiration in foot in morning after rising	Am-m.
Foot	perspiration in foot in morning in bed	Bry., lach., merc., phos., puls., sabin.
Foot	perspiration in foot in warm	Led.
Foot	perspiration in foot like urine	Canth., coloc.
Foot	perspiration in foot while walking	Carb-v., graph., nat-c.

Body part/Disease	Symptom	Medicines
Foot	perspiration in foot with burning	Calc., lyc., mur-ac., petr., sep., sulph., thuj.
Foot	perspiration in foot with swelling of feet	Graph., iod., kali-c., kreos., lyc., petr., ph-ac., plb., sabad.
Foot	perspiration in foot worse during winter	Arg-n., med.
Foot	perspiration in left foot	Cham., nit-ac.
Foot	profuse perspiration in foot	Ars., arund., carb-an., carb-s., carb-v., cham., coloc., fl-ac., graph., Ind., ip., kali-c., kreos., lach., lact-ac., **Lyc.**, merc., **Nit-ac.**, petr., phyt., psor., puls., sabad., sal-ac., sanic., sec., sep., **Sil.**, staph., sulph., thuj., zinc.
Foot	raises his foot unnecessarily high in stepping over small objects when walking	Eupho., Onos.
Foot	reddish blue swelling of foot	Ars.
Foot	retarded urination, can only pass urine while standing with feet wide apart and body inclined forward	Chim.
Foot	retention of urine after getting feet wet	All-c., rhus-t.
Foot	retention of urine painful after getting feet wet	All-c., rhus-t.
Foot	rheumatic swelling of foot	Chel.
Foot	sensation as if cold feet had been put in hot water	Raph.
Foot	sensation as if cold water were poured on foot	Verat.
Foot	sensation as if foot bandaged with iron	Ferr.
Foot	sensation as if foot dipped into cold water	Carb-v.
Foot	Sensation as if foot frozen	Pic-ac., puls.
Foot	sensation of electrical current in foot	
Foot	sensation of enlargement of foot	**Apis.**, coloc., daph., mang.
Foot	sensation of enlargement of foot after walking in open air	Mang.
Foot	sensation of glow (a redness of the face or complexion, especially one caused by embarrassment) from foot to head	Visc.
Foot	sensation of paralysis in foot	Asaf., asar., cham., chel., eug., kali-bi., led., mur-ac., nat-m., phos., sil., tab., zinc.
Foot	sensation of paralysis in foot after rising in morning	Phos.
Foot	sensation of paralysis in foot in morning in bed	Nat-m.
Foot	sensation of paralysis in foot on stepping	Asaf.
Foot	Sensation of paralysis in left arm & right foot	Hyper., stann.
Foot	sensitive foot	Agar., aloe., anac., ant-c., apis., calc-s., kali-c., lac-f., lach., led., **Lyc.**, med., merc-i-r., mez., petr., rumx., sil., stann., staph., sulph.
Foot	sensitive foot while walking	Alum.
Foot	shaking of feet	Tab.
Foot	shocks in foot	Agar., all-s., cadm., phos., spig., stann.
Foot	shocks in foot before falling asleep	Phos.
Foot	shocks in foot during sleep	All-s., cadm.
Foot	sleeplessness from coldness of feet	Aloe., am-m., carb-v., chel., nit-ac., petr., phos., raph., rhod., sil., zinc.

Body part/Disease	Symptom	Medicines
Foot	sour perspiration in foot	Calc., cob., nat-m., nit-ac., sil.
Foot	sour perspiration in foot in evening	Sil.
Foot	stiffness in foot after eating	Graph.
Foot	stiffness in foot after rising from sitting	Bry., caps., laur.
Foot	stiffness in foot ameliorated after rising from sitting	Alum.
Foot	stiffness in foot ameliorated while walking	Alum., laur.
Foot	stiffness in foot at night	**Apis.**
Foot	stiffness in foot in evening	Calc-s., kali-s.
Foot	stiffness in foot in evening when undressing	Apis.
Foot	stiffness in foot in morning	Apis., ign., led.
Foot	stiffness in foot in open air	Nux-v.
Foot	stiffness in foot on waking in morning	Alum.
Foot	stiffness in foot on walking	Alum.
Foot	stiffness in foot while walking	Ign.
Foot	stinging swelling of foot	Carb-v., lyc., merc., phos., **Puls.**
Foot	sudden swelling of foot	Arn., cham., verat.
Foot	suppuration of foot	Rhus-v., sec., vip.
Foot	swelling of back of foot	Ars., **Bry.**, calc., lyc., merc., puls., rhus-t., staph., thuj.
Foot	swelling of foot after walking	Aesc., lach., phos., sep.
Foot	swelling of foot after walking in open air	Nit-ac., sulph.
Foot	swelling of foot after washing	Aesc.
Foot	swelling of foot extending to calf	Am-c., puls.
Foot	swelling of foot from warmth of bed	Sulph.
Foot	swelling of foot while walking	Sil.
Foot	swelling in foot after dancing	Bov.
Foot	swelling in foot after unusual exertion	Rhod.
Foot	swelling in foot ameliorated in evening	Dig., sil.
Foot	swelling in foot ameliorated when out of bed	Sulph.
Foot	swelling in foot at day time	Dig.
Foot	swelling in foot at night	**Apis.**, carb-v.
Foot	swelling in foot before menses	Bar-c., lyc.
Foot	swelling in foot during menses	Calc., graph., lyc., merc., sulph.
Foot	swelling in foot in bed in evening	Am-c.
Foot	swelling in foot in evening	Apis., bell., **Bry.**, carb-s., caust., chin-s., crot-h., phos., puls., rhus-t., sang., sars., stann., thuj.
Foot	swelling in foot in hydrothorax (result of failing circulation caused by heart disease)	Apis., merc-sul.
Foot	swelling in foot in morning	Apis., aur., manc., phyt., sabad., sil.
Foot	swelling in foot in phthisis (wasting disease/Lung disease)	Acet-ac., stann.
Foot	swelling in foot in pregnancy	Merc-c., zinc.

Body part/Disease	Symptom	Medicines
Foot	swelling in foot left to right	Kali-c.
Foot	swelling in foot while ascending steps	Nat-m.
Foot	swelling in foot while sitting	Carb-an., lach.
Foot	swelling in foot while walking in evening	Mang.
Foot	swelling in foot with iron deficiency	Ferr.
Foot	swelling in foot with itching	Ars., sol-n.
Foot	swelling in foot with shining	Alum., **Ars.**, sabin., sulph.
Foot	swelling in left foot	Apis., com., elaps., lach., lyc., sang., sil.
Foot	swelling in right foot	Sec., spig., sulph.
Foot	swelling in toes after wetting feet	Nit-ac.
Foot	swelling of foot with red spots	Elaps., lach.
Foot	takes cold through coldness in foot	Con., sil.
Foot	tetanic convulsion of foot	Camph., nux-v.
Foot	thigh hot with hands & feet cold	**Thuj.**
Foot	Thrilling sensation of foot	Bapt.
Foot	tingling in back of foot	Am-c., ran-s.
Foot	tingling in foot after eating	Kali-c.
Foot	tingling in foot aggravated from heat	Lachn.
Foot	tingling in foot alternating with hands	**Cocc.**
Foot	tingling in foot ameliorated while walking	Am-c., puls.
Foot	tingling in foot at night	Am-m., mag-m.
Foot	tingling in foot extending upwards	**Acon.**
Foot	tingling in foot in evening in bed	Carb-an.
Foot	tingling in foot in morning	Calc-p.
Foot	tingling in foot when rising from sitting	Puls.
Foot	tingling in foot while lying in bed	Carb-an., hyper.
Foot	tingling in foot while sitting	Grat.
Foot	tingling in foot while sitting	Grat.
Foot	tingling in foot while standing	Naja., puls., sec.
Foot	tingling in foot while walking	Ant-c., berb., sec.
Foot	tingling in hand alternating with feet	Carb-an., cocc.
Foot	tingling in left foot	Crot-h., grat.
Foot	tingling in right foot	Alum., carb-an.
Foot	toes hot with cold feet	Apis.
Foot	tonic in convulsion of foot	Phos.
Foot	trembling in foot after dinner	Mag-m.
Foot	trembling in foot ameliorated during motion	Mag-m.
Foot	trembling in foot ameliorated while sitting	Ol-an.
Foot	trembling in foot ameliorated while walking in open air	Bor.
Foot	trembling in foot as from fright	Coloc.
Foot	trembling in foot as from menses	Coloc.

Body part/Disease	Symptom	Medicines
Foot	trembling in foot at 11.00 a.m. on rising from bed	Nat-m.
Foot	trembling in foot during chill	Canth.
Foot	trembling in foot during menses	Hyos., zinc.
Foot	trembling in foot during motion	Camph.
Foot	trembling in foot from music	Thuj.
Foot	trembling in foot in evening in bed	Canth., nat-m.
Foot	trembling in foot on standing	Bar-c., ol-an.
Foot	trembling in foot while descending stairs	Thuj.
Foot	trembling in foot while sitting	Mag-m., zinc.
Foot	trembling in foot while walking	Merc., par., puls.
Foot	trembling in foot with suppression of menses	Puls.
Foot	twitching in foot after midnight during sleep	Nat-s.
Foot	twitching in foot ameliorated when ltying on painless side	Nux-v.
Foot	twitching in foot at daytime	Sulph.
Foot	twitching in foot at midnight	Nat-c.
Foot	twitching in foot at night	Canth., mag-c., nat-s.
Foot	twitching in foot during sleep	Hyos., nat-s., sulph.
Foot	twitching in foot in afternoon during sleep	Ruta.
Foot	twitching in foot in bed	Arg-m., cimic., nat-c.
Foot	twitching in foot in evening	Alum., arg-m.
Foot	twitching in foot in evening on going to sleep	Carb-an.
Foot	twitching in foot in morning after rising	Mag-c.
Foot	twitching in foot on going to sleep	Carb-an.
Foot	twitching in foot while bending them	Led.
Foot	twitching in foot while crawling	Thuj.
Foot	twitching in foot while lying on back	Nux-v.
Foot	twitching in foot while sitting	Crot-t.
Foot	twitching in foot while standing	Verat.
Foot	ulcerative pain in foot	Bry., caust., hep., lyc., mag-c., **Nat-m.**, nat-s.
Foot	ulcer in back of foot	Psor., sep., sulph.
Foot	unsteadiness of foot	Agar., camph., merc., sumb.
Foot	varices of foot	Ant-t., ferr., lac-c., lach., **Puls.**, sul-ac., sulph., thuj.
Foot	vertigo ameliorated when feet become warm	Lach.
Foot	vision, dimness from suppresed foot sweat	Sil.
Foot	walks on wider side of foot	Cic.
Foot	wandering pain in foot	Ars-h., coloc., iris., puls.
Foot	wandering pain in joints of foot	Coloc.
Foot	wants hands & feet fanned	**Med.**
Foot	weakness in foot after coition	Calc-p.
Foot	weakness in foot after dinner	Cahin., ferr. Mag-m.

Body part/Disease	Symptom	Medicines
Foot	weakness in foot after fever	Nat-s.
Foot	weakness in foot ameliorated from lying	Mag-c., nat-m.
Foot	weakness in foot ameliorated when riding	Nat-m.
Foot	weakness in foot ameliorated while sitting	Nat-m.
Foot	weakness in foot ameliorated while walking	Laur., nat-m., zinc.
Foot	weakness in foot at night	Carb-an., mag-s., nit-ac.
Foot	weakness in foot at night before menses	Mang.
Foot	weakness in foot during chillinss	Hell.
Foot	weakness in foot during headache	Ol-an.
Foot	weakness in foot during menses	Ant-t., cast., graph., mang., ol-an., zinc.
Foot	weakness in foot in afternoon	Alum., bov., hydr-ac., lith., lyc., nux-v.
Foot	weakness in foot in afternoon at 4.00 p.m.	Lyc.
Foot	weakness in foot in afternoon at 5.00 p.m.	Cham.
Foot	weakness in foot in afternoon while walking	Lyc.
Foot	weakness in foot in evening	Agar., ign., merc-c., pic-ac., puls.
Foot	weakness in foot in evening after walking	Coc-c.
Foot	weakness in foot in evening at 7.00 p.m.	
Foot	weakness in foot in forenoon	Seneg.
Foot	weakness in foot in morning	Caust., lyc., mag-m.
Foot	weakness in foot in morning at 4.00 a.m.	Plb.
Foot	weakness in foot in morning in bed	Zinc.
Foot	weakness in foot in morning on rising	Nat-m.
Foot	weakness in foot in morning while walking	Lyc., mag-c., mag-m.
Foot	weakness in foot in noon	Kali-bi.
Foot	weakness in foot on bending	Led.
Foot	weakness in foot on waking	Nat-m.
Foot	weakness in foot when trying to raise them	Merc.
Foot	weakness in foot while ascending stairs	Acon., bor., bry., led., lyc., mag-c., nux-v.
Foot	weakness in foot while sitting	Anac., coc-c., led., plat., rhus-t., thuj.
Foot	weakness in foot while standing	Kali-n., nat-m., sars.
Foot	weakness in foot while walking	Camph., chin., clem., croc., graph., ham., kali-n., par.
Foot	weakness in foot while walking in open air	Agar., arn., olnd., thuj.
Foot	weakness in foot with trembling	Caps.
Foot	weakness in lower limbs after getting foot wet	Phos., rhus-t.
Foot	weakness while washing the feet	Merc.
Foot	wooden sensation of foot	Carl.
Foot	wrinkled feet	Ars.
Forearm	abscess in forearm (the part of the human arm between the elbow and the wrist, or the corresponding part of an animal's foreleg)	Plb.
Forearm	arthritic nodosities on condyles on forearm	Am-c.

Body part/Disease	Symptom	Medicines
Forearm	bubbling sensation in forearm	Spong., zinc.
Forearm	bubbling sensation in posterior part of forearm (human arm between the elbow and the wrist)	Colch.
Forearm	burning pain in forearm ameliorated from rubbing	Ol-an.
Forearm	burning pain in forearm after scratching	Bor., caust., clem., laur., sulph.
Forearm	burning pain in forearm aggravated from pressure	Bell.
Forearm	burning pain in forearm at night on lying on it	Graph.
Forearm	burning pain in forearm at night	Graph., zinc.
Forearm	burning pain in forearm during motion	Thuj.
Forearm	burning pain in forearm near the wrist	Agar., bov., caust., kali-bi., rhus-v., zinc.
Forearm	burning pain in forearm with stinging in spots	Ran-s.
Forearm	carbuncles on forearm	Hep.
Forearm	coldness in forearm (the part of the arm between the elbow and the wrist)	Arg-n., ars., brom., bry., calc., caust., cedr., con., crot-c., Graph., hydrc., kali-chl., nux-v., Phos., plb., rhus-t., verat-v.
Forearm	coldness in forearm during menses	Arg-n.
Forearm	coldness in forearm icy cold	Brom., rhus-t., thuj.
Forearm	coldness in forearm in morning after rising	Nux-v.
Forearm	coldness in forearm in morning	Nux-v.
Forearm	coldness in right forearm	Med.
Forearm	compression of forearm	Led., nat-s.
Forearm	compression of left forearm	Led., nat-s.
Forearm	constrictions in forearm	Cupr., gins.
Forearm	constrictions in forearm from walking in open air	Mez.
Forearm	constrictions in right forearm (between the elbow and the wrist)	Cupr.
Forearm	contraction of muscles & tendons of forearm	Calc-ar., calc., caust., cina., coloc., con., hydrc., meny., mez., nat-c., plb., rheum., rhod., sep., stann., verat.
Forearm	contraction of muscles & tendons of forearm while walking	Viol-t.
Forearm	contraction of muscles & tendons of hand extending over forearm	Coloc.
Forearm	convulsion of forearm	Chen., sec., zinc.
Forearm	convulsion of radial (muscles of radius bone of the forearm) muscles	Merc.
Forearm	cramp in anterior part of forearm (part of the human arm between the elbow and the wrist)	Berb., plat., plb.
Forearm	cramp in extensor muscle of forearm	Merc.
Forearm	cramp in flexor muscle of forearm	Chin-s.
Forearm	cramp in forearm	Am-c., anac., arn., berb., calc-p., calc., cina., coloc., corn., ferr-ma., kali-i., lyc., mur-ac., ph-ac., plat., plb., ruta., sep.
Forearm	cramp in forearm aggravated from motion	Kali-i., plb.
Forearm	cramp in forearm at night in bed	Anac.
Forearm	cramp in forearm from flexing arm	Arn., mur-ac.

Body part/Disease	Symptom	Medicines
Forearm	cramp in forearm in afternoon	Lyc.
Forearm	cramp in forearm in morning	Calc.
Forearm	cramp in forearm while walking	Sep.
Forearm	cramp like stiffness of forearm	Plat., stann.
Forearm	cramp like twitching of forearm	Asaf.
Forearm	difficult motion of forearm	Chel., con., merc.
Forearm	discoloration, blue on forearm with blotches	Apis., arg-n., bism., plat., sep.
Forearm	discoloration, bluish spots on forearm	**Sul-ac.**
Forearm	discoloration, dark on forearm	Acon., ant-c., ars., caust., com., sep.
Forearm	discoloration, purple spots on forearm	Kali-c., kali-p.
Forearm	discoloration, red on forearm with blotches	Hura., kreos.
Forearm	discoloration, redness in spots on forearm	Ars., berb., bor., chel., eupho., merc., olnd., rhus-v., sulph., tarent., tax., thuj., vesp.
Forearm	discoloration, redness on forearm	Anac., apis., arn., bell., colch., kreos., mang., rhus-t.
Forearm	discoloration, spots on forearm with blotches	Cimx., hura.
Forearm	discoloration, with red streaks on forearm	Anthr.
Forearm	discoloration, with spots on forearm	Carb-o., mang., mill., nat-m.
Forearm	discoloration, with white spots on forearm	Berb.
Forearm	emaciation of forearm	Phos., **Plb.**
Forearm	eruption in forearm aggravated from scratching	Mang., mez.
Forearm	eruption, boils in forearm	Calc., carb-v., cob., iod., lach., lyc., mag-m., nat-s., petr., sil.
Forearm	eruption, burning vesicles in forearm	Sil.
Forearm	eruption, crusts in forearm	Mez.
Forearm	eruption, eczema in forearm	Graph., merc., mez., sil., thuj.
Forearm	eruption, forearm moist	Alum., merc., mez., rhus-t.
Forearm	eruption, herpes in forearm	Alum., con., mag-s., mang., **Merc.**, nat-m., sulph.
Forearm	eruption, in forearm	Alum., ant-t., ars., bry., calad., carb-an., caust., cinnb., con., cupr., graph., mag-s., mang., merc., mez., phos., rhus-t., sel., spong., tarax., zinc.
Forearm	eruption, itching in forearm	Mez.
Forearm	eruption, nodules in forearm	Hippoz.
Forearm	eruption, painful pustules in forearm	Tarent.
Forearm	eruption, pimples after scratching in forearm	Am-m.
Forearm	eruption, pimples burning in forearm	Am-c., calad., mang., nat-s.
Forearm	eruption, pimples from washing in forearm	Mag-c.
Forearm	eruption, pimples in forearm	Am-c., am-m., ant-t., ars., asc-t., bell., bor., bry., calad., calc-p., carb-s., caust., cit-v., fago., gamb., iod., kali-bi., kali-n., lach., laur., lyc., mag-c., mag-s., mang., merc., nat-m., nat-s., ol-an., osm., ph-ac., rat., rhod., sabad., sars., sulph., tax., thuj., valer., zinc.
Forearm	eruption, pimples in forearm alternating with asthma	Calad.
Forearm	eruption, pimples in forearm during menses	Sulph.

Body part/Disease	Symptom	Medicines
Forearm	eruption, pimples itching in forearm	Am-m., calad., carb-s., caust., gamb., lyc., nat-s., sabad., sulph., zinc.
Forearm	eruption, pimples oozing after scratching in forearm	Kali-n.
Forearm	eruption, psoriasis in forearm	Rhus-t.
Forearm	eruption, pustules in forearm	Anac., ant-t., calc., cop., rhod., rhus-t., staph., tarent.
Forearm	eruption, rash in forearm	Am-c., ant-t., bry., calad., merc., mez., rheum., sel.
Forearm	eruption, rash in forearm alternating with asthma	Calad.
Forearm	eruption, raw in forearm	Petr., rhus-t.
Forearm	eruption, red in forearm	Petr.
Forearm	eruption, scaly in forearm	Alum., merc., petr.
Forearm	eruption, skin teared off in forearm	Rhus-t.
Forearm	eruption, stinging vesicles in forearm	Rhus-t.
Forearm	eruption, transparent vesicles in forearm	Rhus-t.
Forearm	eruption, tubercles in forearm	Agar., am-c., jug-r., kali-n., lach., mur-ac., ph-ac.
Forearm	eruption, urticaria in forearm	Am-c., calad., chin., clem., lyc., nat-m., sil.
Forearm	eruption, urticaria in forearm after scratching	Calad., calc., chin.
Forearm	eruption, urticaria in forearm during heat	Calad.
Forearm	eruption, urticaria in forearm in evening	Lyc.
Forearm	eruption, urticaria in forearm in morning	Chin.
Forearm	eruption, vesicles after scratching in forearm	Sars.
Forearm	eruption, vesicles in forearm	Anac., ant-t., arn., ars., calad., carb-o., caust., chin., cit-v., hura., merc., petr., phos., rhus-r., rhus-t., rhus-v., sars., sil., spong., staph., sulph.
Forearm	eruption, white vesicles in forearm	Calad.
Forearm	eruption, with purulent discharge in forearm	Rhus-t.
Forearm	eruption, with white scales in forearm	Merc.
Forearm	eruption, with white scales in forearm smelling like cheese	Calc.
Forearm	eruption, with yellow scales in forearm	Rhus-t.
Forearm	erysipelatous inflammation in forearm	Anan., ant-c., apis., bufo., kali-c., **Lach.**, merc., petr.
Forearm	exostoses on forearm	Dulc.
Forearm	forearm hot	Anac., apis., aur-m-n., bry., nit-ac., rhus-t., tarent.
Forearm	formication in forearm	Acon., alum., arn., carb-an., carb-s., caust., chin., chlor., con., lach., merc., plb., sec.
Forearm	gangrenous swelling of forearm	**Lach.**
Forearm	goose flesh (pimply skin) in fore arm	Ign., ran-b.
Forearm	heaviness in forearm	Acon., aeth., alum., am-m., anac., aran., **Arg-n.**, aur., berb., cann-i., croc., laur., lyc., mur-ac., nux-v., ph-ac., sabad., spig., spong., sulph., tell., teucr., thuj.
Forearm	heaviness in forearm after coition	Sabin.
Forearm	heaviness in forearm at night	Tell.
Forearm	heaviness in forearm during rest	Aur.

Body part/Disease	Symptom	Medicines
Forearm	heaviness in forearm in forenoon	Lyc.
Forearm	heaviness in forearm on waking	Aran.
Forearm	induration of forearm	Sil.
Forearm	inflammation in forearm	Ars., lyc., rhus-t.
Forearm	inflammation in periosteum of forearm	Aur.
Forearm	insensibility (without feeling or consciousness) in forarm to heat of stove	Plb., thuj.
Forearm	insensibility in forarm to pain	Kreos., plb.
Forearm	itching in anterior part of forearm in spots	Am-c., am-m., berb., bor., carb-an., mag-c., ol-an., sars.
Forearm	itching in forearm	Agar., am-c., am-m., anac., berb., bol., bor., bov., carb-an., carb-s., caust., chin-s., cit-v., clem., colch., cop., dulc., eupho., gels., hura., kali-bi., kali-n., laur., mag-c., mag-m., mag-s., mang., merc-i-f., mez., mur-ac., myric., ol-an., psor., puls., rat., rhus-t., rhus-v., rumx., sars., spig., stront., sulph., tax., til., verb.
Forearm	itching in forearm after lying down	Kali-bi.
Forearm	itching in forearm ameliorated after scratching	Mag-c., mill., ol-an.
Forearm	itching in forearm at night	Am-m., anac., asc-t., mez.
Forearm	itching in forearm in evening	Am-m.
Forearm	itching in forearm in evening aggravated in bed	Sars.
Forearm	itching in forearm in morning	Am-m., mag-c., tax.
Forearm	itching in forearm with burning	Agar., calad., kali-bi.
Forearm	itching in spots of forearm	Kali-n.
Forearm	jerking of forearm	Caps., **Cic.**, cupr., hyper., ign., jal., staph.
Forearm	jerking of forearm in evening	Ign.
Forearm	lameness in forearm	Agar., bell., berb., caust., colch., dulc., fl-ac., merc-i-f., myric., nat-m., sil., stront., sulph., thuj.
Forearm	lameness in forearm near the wrist	Myric.
Forearm	nodular swelling of forearm	Eupi., mez., mur-ac., nat-m., zinc.
Forearm	nodules on forearm	Calc., mur-ac.
Forearm	numbness in anterior part of forearm	Aloe., cham., fl-ac.
Forearm	numbness in forearm aggravated from raising arm	Puls., sep.
Forearm	numbness in forearm ameliorated from motion	Cinnb., puls.
Forearm	numbness in forearm at night	Rhus-t.
Forearm	numbness in forearm extending to end of little finger	Cinnb.
Forearm	numbness in forearm extending to finger	Pall.
Forearm	numbness in forearm in afternoon at 5 p.m.	Phys.
Forearm	numbness in forearm in evening at 10 p.m.	Tell.
Forearm	numbness in forearm in forenoon at	Fl-ac., zinc.
Forearm	numbness in forearm in morning	Mag-m., nux-v.
Forearm	numbness in forearm in morning after rising	Mag-m., nux-v.
Forearm	numbness in forearm in morning from lying on right side	Fl-ac.

Body part/Disease	Symptom	Medicines
Forearm	numbness in forearm in morning on waking	Kali-c.
Forearm	numbness in forearm oedematous	Chel.
Forearm	numbness in forearm painful	Com.
Forearm	numbness in forearm when bending	Chin.
Forearm	numbness in forearm when grasping anything	**Cham.**
Forearm	numbness in forearm when hangs down	Berb.
Forearm	numbness in forearm when writing on table	Lyc.
Forearm	numbness in forearm while lying	Puls.
Forearm	numbness in forearm while sitting	Fl-ac., merc.
Forearm	numbness in left forearm	**Acon.**, alum., cinnb., fl-ac., kali-c., med., onos.
Forearm	numbness in posterior part of forearm	Berb., caj., plb.
Forearm	numbness in radial side of forearm	Fl-ac.
Forearm	numbness in right forearm	Am-m., chin., coloc., euphr., hep., nit-ac., sulph.
Forearm	pain in forearm aggravated from touch	Cupr., sabin., staph.
Forearm	pain in forearm ameliorated from touch	Bism., meny.
Forearm	pain in forearm ameliorated from warm application	Chel., chin., dulc., ferr., gran., kali-c., kalm., lyc., nit-ac., **Nux-v.**, **Rhus-t.**, sil., zinc.
Forearm	pain in forearm ameliorated on motion	Alum., aur-m-n., bar-c., bism., camph., cocc., **Rhus-t.**, spig., stront.
Forearm	pain in forearm at day time	Plb., sulph.
Forearm	pain in forearm at night	Agar., aloe., arg-n., lyc., mez., plan.
Forearm	pain in forearm extending to elbow	Spig.
Forearm	pain in forearm extending to extensor (muscle capable of extending) muscles	Coloc., hep., mur-ac., sil.
Forearm	pain in forearm extending to finger	Asc-t., cocc., con., cycl., puls.
Forearm	pain in forearm extending to Flexor muscles	Arn., calc., gels., nux-v.
Forearm	pain in forearm extending to little finger	Agar., kreos.
Forearm	pain in forearm extending to thumb	Agar., croc.
Forearm	pain in forearm from moving finger	Asaf.
Forearm	pain in forearm in afternoon	Agar., nat-s., sulph., thuj.
Forearm	pain in forearm in bed	Aloe., am-c., am-m., mez., sulph.
Forearm	pain in forearm in evening	All-c., alum., am-c., calc-s., cast-eq., fl-ac., stront., sulph.
Forearm	pain in forearm in forenoon	Sil., trom., verat-v.
Forearm	pain in forearm in morning	Ars., bar-c., bry., chin-s., coloc., dios., kali-bi., lyc., nat-a., thuj.
Forearm	pain in forearm in noon	Cedr., trom.
Forearm	pain in forearm on grasping	Chel., lach.
Forearm	pain in forearm on jerking	Led., sil.
Forearm	pain in forearm on motion	Anac., calc., chel., croc., led., rhus-t., sabin., staph.
Forearm	pain in forearm while lying	Aur-m-n.
Forearm	pain in forearm while sitting	Aur-m-n., led.
Forearm	pain in forearm while writing	Acon., anac., cycl., fago., fl-ac., **Mag-p.**, merc-i-f.

Body part/Disease	Symptom	Medicines
Forearm	pain in left forearm	Agar., med.
Forearm	pain in right forearm	Cycl., merc-i-f.
Forearm	pain in wrist extending to forearm while writing	Ferr-p.
Forearm	painful stiffness of forearm	**Rhus-t.**, thuj.
Forearm	paralysis of forearm	Bar-c., calc-p., caust., colch., phos., plat., plb., **Sil.**
Forearm	paralysis of forearm as from pressure	Cham.
Forearm	paralysis of forearm when palm turned upward	Plb.
Forearm	paralysis of left forearm	Bar-c., calc-p.
Forearm	paralysis of right forearm	Plb., rhus-t.
Forearm	perspiration in forearm	Petr.
Forearm	red swelling of forearm	Lac-d., sep., **Sil.**
Forearm	roughness in forearm	Rhus-t.
Forearm	roughness in forearm in evening	Peti.
Forearm	sensation of heat in anterior part of forearm	Lyc.
Forearm	sensation of heat in posterior part of forearm	Bell.
Forearm	sensation of paralysis in forearm	Acon., all-s., ambr., apis., bism., bov., chel., cocc., fl-ac., kreos., par., prun-s., **Rhus-t.**, seneg., staph., stront., sulph.
Forearm	sensation of paralysis in forearm while writing	Cocc., ferr-i.
Forearm	stiffness in forearm	Aur-m., bry., calc-s., caust., cham., coloc., hydr-ac., plat., prun-s., rhus-t., stann., thuj.
Forearm	stiffness in forearm on grasping anything	Cham.
Forearm	stiffness in forearm while writing	Caust., prun-s.
Forearm	swelling in forearm dark blue	Samb.
Forearm	swelling in forearm near elbow	Lyc.
Forearm	swelling in forearm on posterior (behind) part	Plb.
Forearm	tetanic convulsion of forearm	Zinc.
Forearm	tingling in forearm extending to fingers	Carb-ac., phys., pip-m.
Forearm	trembling in forearm	Agar., bar-c., calc-p., carb-s., caust., cimic., colch., fl-ac., merc., nit-ac., onos., plb., spong., zing.
Forearm	trembling in forearm extending to thumb	Agar.
Forearm	trembling in forearm when anything is grasped	Verat.
Forearm	trembling in forearm while writing	Caust., com., **Merc.**
Forearm	trembling in right forearm	Dulc., nit-ac.
Forearm	twitching in forearm during chill	Nux-m.
Forearm	twitching in forearm during rest	Asaf., spig., staph.
Forearm	twitching in forearm in evening at 4.00 a.m.	Zing.
Forearm	twitching in forearm in morning after walking	Puls.
Forearm	twitching in forearm when grasping anything	Nat-c.
Forearm	twitching in forearm when sneezing	Cast.
Forearm	twitching in forearm while writing	Caust., ox-ac.
Forearm	ulcer in forearm	Kali-bi.

Body part/Disease	Symptom	Medicines
Forearm	voluptuous (sensual pleasure) itching in forearm in spots	Merc.
Forearm	wandering pain in forearm	Nat-a.
Forearm	warts on bend of forearm	Sil.
Forearm	weakness in forearm at night	Kali-n.
Forearm	weakness in forearm in evening	Dig.
Forearm	weakness in forearm in morning on waking	Arg-m.
Forearm	weakness in forearm while knitting	Aeth.
Forearm	weakness in forearm while writing	Agar., arg-m., coloc.
Forehead	blotches on forehead	Nat-c.
Forehead	boils above the eyes	Calc-s., nat-m.
Forehead	boils on forehead	Am-c., led., mag-c., phos., sep.
Forehead	coldness in hands with hot forehead	Ars., asaf., asar.
Forehead	coldness of forehead ameliorated from walking	Gins.
Forehead	coldness of forehead ameliorated on lying	Calc.
Forehead	coldness of forehead ameliorated when covered	Aur., grat., kali-i., nat-m., sanic.
Forehead	coldness of forehead as from cold water	Cann-s., croc., cupr., glon., sabad., tarent.
Forehead	coldness of forehead as from ice	Agar., glon., laur.
Forehead	coldness of forehead as if a cold spot	Sulph.
Forehead	coldness of forehead during headache	Ars., sulph.
Forehead	coldness of forehead during menses	Ant-t., calc., mag-s., sep., sulph., verat.
Forehead	coldness of forehead during menses	Sulph.
Forehead	coldness of forehead even when covered	Mang.
Forehead	coldness of forehead from being heated	Carb-v.
Forehead	coldness of forehead which penetrates painfully	Zinc.
Forehead	coldness of forehead with heat	Chin., puls.
Forehead	coldness of forehead with pain	Gels., phos.
Forehead	coldness of forehead with perspiration	Merc-c.
Forehead	comedones on forehead	Sulph.
Forehead	crawling of worm in forehead	Alum.
Forehead	erysipela extending to forehead	Apis., kali-i., ruta., sulph.
Forehead	external coldness of forehead	Cinnb., cist., gels., laur., sulph.
Forehead	feeling of insects crawling on forehead	Apis., arn., arund., benz-ac., chel., cic., colch., glon., kali-c., laur., manc., nux-v., ph-ac., rhus-t., rhus-v., tarax., zinc.
Forehead	gouty pain in joints alternates with pain in forehead	Sulph.
Forehead	greasy forehead	Hydr., psor.
Forehead	greasy sweating on forehead	Coloc., psor.
Forehead	heaviness of forehead after mental exertion	Calc.
Forehead	heaviness of forehead at 4 p.m.	Mang.
Forehead	heaviness of forehead during menses	Zinc.
Forehead	heaviness of forehead from heat of sun	Brom., nat-c.

Body part/Disease	Symptom	Medicines
Forehead	heaviness of forehead in afternoon	Am-c., chel., chin-s., kali-i., mang., nicc., pall., sil.
Forehead	heaviness of forehead in evening	Coloc., lith., mag-m., nat-m., sulph.
Forehead	heaviness of forehead in forenoon	Carb-an., gamb., mang., nicc., sarr.
Forehead	heaviness of forehead in noon	Sulph.
Forehead	heaviness of forehead on motion	Bism., fl-ac.
Forehead	heaviness of forehead on waking	Calc., nat-m.
Forehead	heaviness of forehead on waking	Bell., sulph.
Forehead	heaviness of forehead while standing	Mag-c.
Forehead	heaviness of forehead while walking	Camph., con., sulph.
Forehead	heaviness of forehead while writing	Calc.
Forehead	heaviness of forehead with frontal sinuses	Puls.
Forehead	icy coldness of forehead	Agar., ars., bar-c., calc-p., Calc., Ind., laur., nux-v., phos., sep., valer.
Forehead	impetigo on forehead	Ant-c., kreos., led., merc., rhus-t., sep., sulph., viol-t.
Forehead	inclination to rub forehead	Glon.
Forehead	internal coldness of forehead	Arn., bell., Calc.
Forehead	itching of forehead	Sars.
Forehead	itching of Forehead ameliorated by rubbing	Ol-an., samb., tab.
Forehead	itching of Forehead ameliorated by scratching	Bov., mag-c., squil.
Forehead	itching of Forehead ameliorated in open air	Gamb.
Forehead	itching of Forehead in evening	Sulph., zinc.
Forehead	itching of Forehead with burning	Kali-bi.
Forehead	offensive sweating on forehead	Led., sil.
Forehead	oily forehead	Hydr., psor.
Forehead	pain in cervical region extending to forehead while walking	Rat.
Forehead	pain in cervical region extending to forehead	Daph., mez., rat., sars.
Forehead	pain in ear extending to left forehead	Dig., nux-v., ptel.
Forehead	pain in eye extending to forehead	Agar., croc., hura., kalm., ran-b.
Forehead	pain in joints alternating with pain in forehead	Sulph.
Forehead	pain in nose extending to forehead	Bufo., calc., kali-i., nat-s., sil.
Forehead	Prickling sensation on forehead	Apis., aur., chin-s., ferr., lil-t., mur-ac., sabad., sep., thuj., verat., viol-o.
Forehead	pulsation by beating from pressure upon forehead	Mag-m.
Forehead	pulsation in cervical region extending to forehead and occiput	Chel.
Forehead	pulsation in cervical region extending to forehead on moving or stooping	Ter.
Forehead	rash on forehead	Ail., arn., indg., lil-t., rheum., teucr.
Forehead	rosacea on forehead	Ant-c., ars., aur., bar-c., bell., calc., caps., Carb-an., Carb-s., Carb-v., Caust., cic., clem., Hep., kreos., led., nat-m., nit-ac., Nux-v., ph-ac., Psor., Rhus-t., Sep., Sil., Sulph., viol-t.

Body part/Disease	Symptom	Medicines
Forehead	sensation as of lump in forehead	Cham., pip-m., staph.
Forehead	sticky sweating on forehead	Cocc.
Forehead	sweating on forehead during cough	Ant-t., chlor., ip., verat.
Forehead	sweating on forehead during diarrhœa	Sulph.
Forehead	sweating on forehead during fever	Ant-t., ip., mag-s., sars., staph., Verat.
Forehead	sweating on forehead while eating	Carb-v., nit-ac., nux-v., sul-ac., sulph.
Forehead	tingling in forehead	Ambr., stram.
Fracture	fracture of hand with laceration (cutting or gashing the skin in a way that leaves a deep jagged wound)	Hyper.
Freckle	discoloration, freckles	Ferr.
Freckle	freckles (a harmless small brownish patch on skin) in chest	Nit-ac.
Freckle	freckles on face	Am-c., ant-c., calc., dulc., graph., kali-c., Lyc., mur-ac., nat-c., nit-ac., nux-m., Phos., puls., sep., sil., Sulph., thuj.
Freckle	freckles on nose	Phos., Sulph.
Fullness	fullness after breakfast	Carb-s., carb-v., sulph.
Fullness	fullness after drinking	Carb-v., caust., nux-v., sars.
Fullness	fullness ameliorated after drinking	Rhus-t.
Fullness	fullness ameliorated on passing flatus	Grat., hell., rhod., sulph.
Fullness	fullness ameliorated on walking	Mag-c.
Fullness	fullness during constipation (a condition in which a person has difficulty in eliminating solid waste from the body and the feces are hard and dry)	Bry., dios., ery-a., graph., hyos., iod., lach., nit-ac., nux-v., phos., ter.
Fullness	fullness during diarrhoea (frequent and excessive discharging of the bowels producing thin watery feces, usually as a symptom of gastrointestinal upset or infection)	Nat-s.
Fullness	fullness during hunger	Asar.
Fullness	fullness in chest after coffee	Canth.
Fullness	fullness in chest after eating	Ant-c., caps., lyc.
Fullness	fullness in chest after eating in evening	Alumn.
Fullness	fullness in chest ameliorated after expectoration	Ail.
Fullness	fullness in chest before menses	Brom., Sulph.
Fullness	fullness in chest during exertion	Nat-a.
Fullness	fullness in chest if desire to urinate is delayed	Lil-t.
Fullness	fullness in chest in afternoon	Alumn., coca.
Fullness	fullness in chest in bed in evening	Nat-s., sulph.
Fullness	fullness in chest in evening	Carb-v., eupi., lact., Puls., sulph.
Fullness	fullness in chest in morning	Con., lyc., sulph.
Fullness	fullness in chest in morning after smoking	Cycl.
Fullness	fullness in chest in open air	Lyc.
Fullness	fullness in chest on deep inspiration	Kali-n., nat-a., sulph.
Fullness	fullness in chest on waking	Con., ph-ac.

Body part/Disease	Symptom	Medicines
Fullness	fullness in chest on walking	Ferr.
Fullness	fullness in chest when ascending	Bar-c.
Fullness	fullness in chest while sitting	Caps.
Fullness	fullness in chest while walking in forenoon	Acon.
Fullness	fullness in chest while writing in forenoon	Fl-ac.
Fullness	fullness in hypogastrium region	Aesc., bar-c., bell., carb-v., sulph.
Fullness	fullness in inguinal region	Cocc., nat-s., sep.
Fullness	fullness in larynx	Cob., naja.
Fullness	fullness in larynx in morning	Cob.
Fullness	fullness in liver region	Ferr., kreos., lach., nat-m., nux-v., podo., sep., sulph., thuj.
Fullness	fullness in region of heart at night	Colch.
Fullness	fullness in region of heart during menses	Puls.
Fullness	fullness in region of heart in evening	Puls.
Fullness	fullness in region of heart while ascending stairs	Aur-m., Aur.
Fullness	fullness in region of heart while lying on left side	Colch.
Fullness	fullness in sides	Am-c.
Fullness	fullness in spleen region	Kali-i., lec.
Fullness	fullness of stomach after stool	Aesc., alum., lyc., sep.
Fullness	fullness of stomach, after bread and milk in noon	Arg-n.
Fullness	fullness of stomach, after dinner at night	Agar., ant-c., cast., clem., dig., grat., kalm., nat-m., petr., zinc.
Fullness	fullness of stomach, after eating in evening	
Fullness	fullness of stomach, after eating in noon	Ox-ac.
Fullness	fullness of stomach, after soup	Prun-s.
Fullness	fullness of stomach, after supper	Carb-v., chin-s.
Fullness	fullness of stomach, after wine	Rhus-t.
Fullness	fullness of stomach, ameliorated by eructation	Carb-v., euphr., iris., mag-c., nux-v., phos., sil.
Fullness	fullness of stomach, ameliorated by sleeping	Phos.
Fullness	fullness of stomach, during menses	Am-c., kali-c., kali-p.
Fullness	fullness of stomach, in bed in evening	Nat-s.
Fullness	fullness of stomach, on going to bed at night	Rumx.
Fullness	fullness of stomach, with opression in breathing	Nat-s., nux-m., nux-v., prun-s.
Fullness	fulness in ear from swallowing	Arum-d., mang.
Fullness	fulness in ear when blowing nose	Mang., puls.
Fullness	fulness in ear while eating	Nat-c.
Fullness	fulness in ear, after stitching pains in ear	Iod.
Fullness	fulness in ear, ameliorated by boring in ear	Mez.
Fungus	excrescences on skin, fungus medullary (describes nerve fibers that are surrounded by a sheath of myelin)	Bell., carb-an., phos., sil., sulph., thuj.

Body part/Disease	Symptom	Medicines
Fungus	excrescences on skin, fungus syphilitic	**Ars-i.**, ars., aur-m-n., aur-m., aur., iod., **Lach.**, manc., **Merc-c.**, **Merc.**, **Nit-ac.**, **Sil.**, staph., thuj.
Fungus	fungal growth on lower jaw	Hep., phos., thuj.
Fungus	fungoid growth in urethra	Calc., con., graph., lyc., thuj.
Fungus	fungoid growths in bladder	Calc.
Fungus	fungoid growths in urethra	Calc., con., graph., lyc., thuj.
Fungus	fungus excrescence (a growth that sticks out from the body) in ear	Merc.
Fungus	fungus growth in eye	Bell., Calc., lyc., Phos., sep., sil., thuj.
Fungus	fungus growth on skin of coccyx	Thuj.
Fungus	ulcer in skin fungus	Alum., alumn., ant-c., arg-n., **Ars.**, bell., calc., carb-an., carb-s., carb-v., caust., cham., cinnb., clem., crot-c., graph., hydr., kreos., lach., merc., nit-ac., petr., phos., sabin., **Sep.**, **Sil.**, staph., sulph., thuj.

INDEX

9 781642 499452